RUSH
UNIVERSITY

REVIEW
OF
SURGERY

STEVEN G. ECONOMOU, M.D.
Helen Shedd Keith Professor
General Surgery
Rush Medical College
Senior Attending Surgeon and
Chairman
Department of General Surgery
Presbyterian–St. Luke's Hospital

STEVEN D. BINES, M.D.
Assistant Professor
General Surgery
Rush Medical College
Assistant Attending Surgeon and
Associate Director, Surgical Research Laboratories
Department of General Surgery
Presbyterian–St. Luke's Hospital

DANIEL J. DEZIEL, M.D.
Assistant Professor
General Surgery
Rush Medical College
Assistant Attending Surgeon and
Associate Coordinator, Resident Clinical Activities
Department of General Surgery
Presbyterian–St. Luke's Hospital

THOMAS R. WITT, M.D.
Assistant Professor
General Surgery
Rush Medical College
Associate Attending Surgeon and
Coordinator of Clinical Conferences
Department of General Surgery
Presbyterian–St. Luke's Hospital

W. B. SAUNDERS COMPANY
Harcourt Brace Jovanovich, Inc.
Philadelphia • London • Toronto
Montreal • Sydney • Tokyo

W. B. SAUNDERS COMPANY
Harcourt Brace Jovanovich, Inc.

The Curtis Center
Independence Square West
Philadelphia, PA 19106

Rush University review of surgery / Steven G. Economou . . . [et al.].
        p.   cm.
    ISBN 0-7216-2070-1
    1. Surgery.   I. Economou, Steven G., 1922-   . II. Rush
University. III. Title: Review of Surgery.
    [DNLM: 1. Surgery. WO 10-0 R953]
RD31.R85 1988
617 —dc19
DNLM/DLC   87-35626
for Library of Congress   CIP

Editor: W. B. Saunders Staff
Designer: Karen O'Keefe
Production Manager: Bill Preston
Manuscript Editor: Mark Coyle
Illustration Coordinator: Lisa Lambert

RUSH UNIVERSITY REVIEW OF SURGERY   ISBN   0–7216–2070–1

© 1988 by W. B. Saunders Company.   Copyright under the Uniform Copyright Convention.   Simultaneously published in Canada.   All rights reserved.   This book is protected by copyright.   No part of it may be reproduced, stored in a retrieval system, or transmitted in any form or by any means, electronic, mechanical, photocopying, recording, or otherwise, without written permission from the publisher. Made in the United States of America. Library of Congress catalog card number 87-35626.

Last digit is the print number: 9   8   7   6   5   4   3   2

Contents

Preface

A written work is best when it fills a clearly defined need; it is more on target when those who have that need suggest a way by which this can be accomplished. Such was the case with the RUSH UNIVERSITY REVIEW OF SURGERY. While a resident, one of the authors (S.B.) perceived a need for a systematic way to review the totality of surgery that would benefit general surgeons and then to continue refreshing their storehouse of knowledge. This would offer a solution to the commonplace but ill-advised practice of chief residents cramming through a textbook of surgery just before completion of their residency, in preparation for the taking of Boards. Also it would meet the need of the far-sighted younger residents trying on their own to establish a habit of regular programmed reading. Our initial effort consisted of a weekly assignment of twenty pages of reading in a textbook, with each general surgery resident, in rotation, constructing an examination of twenty questions—one per page of text—highlighting the key points of the text. The twenty-question examination was taken and then on to another twenty pages. Very early, we saw the need to discuss the reasons an answer was correct or not, rather than to just cite its source. As the residents became more skilled at constructing the questions—an interesting and instructive exercise in itself— it became necessary to read both text and questions with greater care; likewise, the discussion that followed became more analytic and then more erudite.

We began recording our discussions, and when they were transcribed, we were pleasantly surprised to realize we were raising many questions, the answers to which were not in our reference textbooks or were outside the purview of standard texts. We solved this problem and, as well, enriched the content of these exercises by having appropriately experienced consultants join us each week.

The current format enables us to read, examine, and discuss the content of a major textbook of surgery twice in the course of a 5-year residency. It further offers residents the repeated experience of constructing and answering questions similar to those which they will encounter in their In-Service and Board examinations.

Originally, we had planned to simply assemble and organize into book form the several years' worth of examinations constructed by the residents. We soon realized, however, that in too many questions the intent was only to test for recall of information, or the structure of the questions was such that a resident moderately skilled in the art of test-taking could deduce the correct answers without the requisite knowledge of content.

The editors, therefore, attempted to construct questions that in themselves were instructive, with a scope of inquiry that was inclusive and a balance of content that was in keeping with the perceived needs of our audience. More importantly, perhaps, there was a need to extract more information from the individual questions than the correct answer alone would provide. This need was met by the writing of a comment following each question, the purpose of which is to amplify the correct answer, to explain away the incorrect answers, or to make conceptual sense of the factual details brought out in the question. We expect, of course, to refine all these goals with subsequent editions.

In choosing our source references, we felt that there was no one textbook that met all our needs; furthermore, readers have preferences in the order, style, and breadth and depth of presentation. These wants were met by the two most widely read works of surgery: TEXTBOOK OF SURGERY (Thirteenth edition, 1986) by David C. Sabiston, Jr., M.D., and PRINCIPLES OF SURGERY (Fourth Edition, 1984) by Seymour I. Schwartz, M.D., as the Editor-in-Chief. As these textbooks have about 90% commonality of content, we felt secure that not much of importance would be missed if we did not include additional resource texts.

From early on, however, and even more so when consultants joined our review sessions, we found that we occasionally disagreed with the writings in our source textbooks in one of several ways: the information in the textbook was correct when written, but more current information superseded it; the facts as stated in the textbook were correct but could profit by further expansion or even clarification; and rarely, we simply did not agree with a statement or concept as presented. For validity of the latter, we relied on our pooled clinical experience and that of our consultants. So, the reader should be aware that while the questions and answers are gated either to Sabiston's or Schwartz's textbook, the Comments do not necessarily have that proscription.

We purposely chose a conversational and informal writing style that mimics what takes place in our Review Sessions. Hopefully, it is informative; we trust it is not ponderous.

S.E.
S.B.
D.D.
T.W.

Contributing Editors

GILBERT C. CARROLL, M.D.
Assistant Professor
Anesthesiology
Rush Medical College

Assistant Attending
Department of Anesthesiology
Presbyterian–St. Luke's Hospital

MICHAEL J. DaVALLE, M.D.
Assistant Professor
Cardiovascular-Thoracic Surgery
Rush Medical College

Assistant Attending
Department of Cardiovascular-Thoracic
 Surgery
Presbyterian–St. Luke's Hospital

FREDERIC A. dePEYSTER, M.D.
Professor Emeritus
General Surgery
Rush Medical College

Attending Surgeon Emeritus
Department of General Surgery
Presbyterian–St. Luke's Hospital

ALEXANDER DOOLAS, M.D.
Professor
General Surgery
Rush Medical College

Senior Attending
Director, Undergraduate Surgical
 Education
Department of General Surgery
Presbyterian–St. Luke's Hospital

HOWARD M. GEBEL, Ph.D.
Associate Professor
Immunology/Microbiology
Rush Medical College

Associate Scientist
Department of General Surgery
Department of
 Immunology/Microbiology
Presbyterian–St. Luke's Hospital

STEPHEN C. JENSIK, M.D., Ph.D.
Assistant Professor
General Surgery
Rush Medical College

Assistant Attending
Department of General Surgery
Presbyterian–St. Luke's Hospital

C. FREDERICK KITTLE, M.D.
Professor
Cardiovascular-Thoracic Surgery
Rush Medical College

Director, Section of Thoracic Surgery
Presbyterian–St. Luke's Hospital

GARY J. MERLOTTI, M.D.
Assistant Professor
General Surgery
Rush Medical College

Assistant Professor
Department of Surgery
University of Illinois
School of Medicine

Provisional Associate Staff
Director of Trauma Service
Department of Surgery
Christ Hospital and Medical Center

GEORGE F. MESLEH, M.D.
Assistant Professor
General Surgery
Rush Medical College

Active Attending Staff
Department of General Surgery
Christ Hospital and Medical Center

JACK C. ROBERTS, M.D.
Assistant Professor
Cardiovascular-Thoracic Surgery
Rush Medical College

Associate Director
Rush Affiliated Program
Department of General Surgery

Active Attending
Department of Surgery
Christ Hospital and Medical Center

THEODORE J. SACLARIDES, M.D.
Instructor
Rush Medical College (LOA)

Adjunct Attending
Department of General Surgery
Presbyterian–St. Luke's Hospital
    (LOA)

Fellow
Colon and Rectal Surgery
Mayo Clinic

RAJENDRA R. SHAH, M.D.
Assistant Professor
Plastic & Reconstructive Surgery
Rush Medical College

Associate Attending
Research Fellow
Department of Plastic & Reconstructive
    Surgery
Christ Hospital and Medical Center

EDGAR D. STAREN, M.D.
Instructor
Rush Medical College

Adjunct Attending
Department of General Surgery
Presbyterian–St. Luke's Hospital

KENNETH J. TUMAN, M.D.
Assistant Professor
Anesthesiology
Rush Medical College

Assistant Attending
Department of Anesthesiology
Presbyterian–St. Luke's Hospital

JAMES W. WILLIAMS, M.D.
Jack Fraser Smith Professor
General Surgery
Rush Medical College

Senior Attending
Director, Section of Transplantation
Presbyterian–St. Luke's Hospital

Consulting Editors

HERAND ABCARIAN, M.D.
Lecturer
General Surgery
Rush Medical College

Professor of Surgery
University of Illinois

Senior Attending Surgeon
Head, Surgical Endoscopy
Department of General Surgery
Presbyterian–St. Luke's Hospital

Attending Surgeon
Department of General Surgery
Chairman, Section of Colon and Rectal
  Surgery
Cook County Hospital

ROBERT AKI, M.D.
Instructor
General Surgery
Rush Medical College

Provisional Associate Staff
Department of Surgery
Christ Hospital and Medical Center

GUNNAR ANDERSSON, M.D., Ph.D.
Professor
Orthopedic Surgery
Rush Medical College

Associate Chairman
Senior Attending
Department of Orthopedic Surgery
Presbyterian–St. Luke's Hospital

JOHN A. BARRETT, M.D.
Lecturer
General Surgery
Rush Medical College

Assistant Professor of Surgery
University of Illinois

Director, Trauma Unit
Cook County Hospital
Attending Surgeon
Division of General Surgery
Cook County Hospital

ANGEL B. BASSUK, M.D.
Assistant Professor
General Surgery
Assistant Professor
Pediatrics
Rush Medical College

Associate Attending
Department of General Surgery
Section of Pediatric Surgery
Assistant Attending Surgeon
Department of Pediatrics
Presbyterian–St. Luke's Hospital

Provisional Associate Staff
Director, Pediatric Trauma
Christ Hospital and Medical Center

MARC L. CULLEN, M.D.
Attending Surgeon
Department of Pediatric/General
  Surgery
Children's Hospital of Michigan

GIACOMO A. DeLARIA, M.D.
Assistant Professor
Cardiovascular-Thoracic Surgery
Rush Medical College

Senior Attending
Department of Cardiovascular-Thoracic
Surgery
Director, Peripheral Vascular
Laboratory
Presbyterian–St. Luke's Hospital

GORDON H. DERMAN, M.D.
Assistant Professor
Plastic & Reconstructive Surgery
Rush Medical College

Assistant Attending
Department of Plastic & Reconstructive
Surgery
Presbyterian–St. Luke's Hospital

L. PENFIELD FABER, M.D.
Professor of Cardiovascular-Thoracic
Surgery
Rush Medical College

Associate Dean, Surgical Sciences &
Services
Senior Attending
Department of Cardiovascular-Thoracic
Surgery
Presbyterian–St. Luke's Hospital

STEVEN GITELIS, M.D.
Associate Professor
Orthopedic Surgery
Rush Medical College

Associate Attending
Department of Orthopedic Surgery
Presbyterian–St. Luke's Hospital

MARSHALL D. GOLDIN, M.D.
Associate Professor
Cardiovascular-Thoracic Surgery
Rush Medical College

Senior Attending
Department of Cardiovascular-Thoracic
Surgery
Director, Surgical Intensive Care Unit
Presbyterian–St. Luke's Hospital

JAMES E. GRAHAM, Jr., M.D.
Assistant Professor
Obstetrics & Gynecology
Rush Medical College

Associate Attending
Department of Obstetrics &
Gynecology
Presbyterian–St. Luke's Hospital

ALAN A. HARRIS, M.D.
Associate Professor
Internal Medicine
Associate Professor
Preventive Medicine
Rush Medical College

Senior Attending
Department of Internal Medicine
Associate Attending
Section of Preventive Medicine
Presbyterian–St. Luke's Hospital

JEROME HOEKSEMA, M.D.
Assistant Professor
Urology
Rush Medical College

Associate Attending
Department of Urology
Presbyterian–St. Luke's Hospital

WILLIAM M. HOPKINS, Jr., M.D.
Assistant Professor
General Surgery
Rush Medical College

Active Attending
Department of General Surgery
Christ Hospital and Medical Center

JAMES A. HUNTER, M.D.
Professor
Cardiovascular-Thoracic Surgery
Rush Medical College

Senior Attending
Department of Cardiovascular-Thoracic
Surgery
Presbyterian–St. Luke's Hospital

GERALD KLOMPIEN, M.D.
Assistant Professor
General Surgery
Rush Medical College

Active Attending Staff
Department of General Surgery
Christ Hospital and Medical Center

STEPHEN M. KORBET, M.D.
Assistant Professor
Internal Medicine
Rush Medical College

Assistant Attending
Section of Nephrology
Department of Internal Medicine
Presbyterian–St. Luke's Hospital

KEN N. KUO, M.D.
Associate Professor
Orthopedic Surgery
Rush Medical College

Associate Attending
Department of Orthopedic Surgery
Presbyterian–St. Luke's Hospital

DAVID O. MONSON, M.D.
Assistant Professor
Cardiovascular-Thoracic Surgery
Rush Medical College

Associate Attending
Department of Cardiovascular-Thoracic
  Surgery
Presbyterian–St. Luke's Hospital

HASSAN NAJAFI, M.D.
Professor
Cardiovascular-Thoracic Surgery
Rush Medical College

Senior Attending & Chairman
Department of Cardiovascular-Thoracic
  Surgery
Presbyterian–St. Luke's Hospital

AARON G. ROSENBERG, M.D.
Assistant Professor
Orthopedic Surgery
Rush Medical College

Assistant Attending
Department of Orthopedic Surgery
Presbyterian–St. Luke's Hospital

HOWARD SANKARY, M.D.
Assistant Professor
General Surgery
Rush Medical College

Assistant Attending
Department of General Surgery
Section of Transplantation
Presbyterian–St. Luke's Hospital

RICHARD J. SASSETTI, M.D.
Associate Professor
Internal Medicine
Rush Medical College

Senior Attending
Department of Internal Medicine
Director, Blood Center
Presbyterian–St. Luke's Hospital

ROBERT R. SCHENCK, M.D.
Associate Professor
Plastic & Reconstructive Surgery and
  Orthopedic Surgery
Rush Medical College

Senior Attending
Department of Plastic & Reconstructive
  Surgery and Department of
  Orthopedic Surgery
Presbyterian–St. Luke's Hospital

MITCHELL BEN SHEINKOP, M.D.
Associate Professor
Orthopedic Surgery
Rush Medical College

Associate Attending
Department of Orthopedic Surgery
Presbyterian–St. Luke's Hospital

JOHN L. SHOWEL, M.D.
Associate Professor
Internal Medicine
Rush Medical College

Senior Attending
Department of Internal Medicine
Presbyterian–St. Luke's Hospital

PETER SHROCK, M.D.
Assistant Professor
Surgery
Assistant Professor
Pediatrics
Rush Medical College

Associate Attending Surgeon
Department of General Surgery
Director
Section of Pediatric Surgery
Presbyterian–St. Luke's Hospital

BRUCE D. SPIESS, M.D.
Assistant Professor
Department of Anesthesiology
Rush Medical College

Associate Attending
Department of Anesthesiology
Presbyterian–St. Luke's Hospital

KELVIN A. VON ROENN, M.D.
Assistant Professor
Neurological Surgery
Rush Medical College

Assistant Attending
Department of Neurological Surgery
Presbyterian–St. Luke's Hospital

WILLIAM H. WARREN, M.D.
Assistant Professor
Cardiovascular-Thoracic Surgery
Assistant Professor
Pathology
Rush Medical College

Assistant Attending
Department of Cardiovascular-Thoracic
  Surgery
Assistant Attending
Department of Pathology
Presbyterian–St. Luke's Hospital

NORMAN L. WOOL, M.D.
Assistant Professor
General Surgery
Rush Medical College

Associate Attending
Coordinator, Resident Clinical
  Activities
Department of General Surgery
Presbyterian–St. Luke's Hospital
Director of Surgery
Sheridan Road Hospital

Acknowledgments

A book such as this, whose origin was oblique to a pragmatic need, has been sustained by recurring infusions of assistance by faculty, residents, and medical students, all of whom deserve genuine acknowledgment. Foremost are the residents who, by desire and expectations, kept the examinations in a constant motion of readiness and use; that it all was mostly for their benefit, is irrelevant to their cardinal contribution.

Then there were the wizards of the word processor: Jan Nunnally, Joan Stone, Irma Parker, and ever-faithful Julie Bjorklund, who were cajoled and pleaded with by tardy residents wanting their creations typed and ready for the very next morning's session. For the actual writing of the book, they accepted cassettes pressed on them from several directions; briskly they produced rough copies. As these rough copies underwent editorial and consultant review and were returned to them, they reliably produced the increasingly satisfactory revisions leading to the ultimate version. That the book could be conceived and then evolve so smoothly and swiftly through all these important stages, is a tribute to their prompt and accurate contribution.

How to Use This Text

A reader's approach to any textbook may vary from rapid scanning for basic concepts to meticulous outlining, note-taking, and underlining for detail. In an effort to provide something for everyone, this book hopefully includes an appropriate mixture of detail (found primarily in the questions) and conceptual information (found primarily in the comments).

The questions are organized principally in an organ-system fashion as are the major textbooks that served as the reference sources. None of the questions are intentionally "tricky"; many however, require the careful attention to detail that should characterize all students of surgery. To allow readers the opportunity to answer the question on their own and yet to allow them to check their response without the ponderous flipping back and forth of pages, the correct answer is spatially separated from the question by the interposed comment. However, for readers who wish to go to the basic source material prior to answering the question, the appropriately referenced pages in the Sabiston and Schwartz textbooks are given immediately following the question.

The comment itself is offered to provide amplification and elucidation of the facts brought out in the question as well as to provide a conceptual framework in which to view the factual data. Of necessity, several comments enjoy the latitude of editorial license and reflect individual and pooled clinical experiences or more current literature which may or may not be found in the referenced texts. As there are many areas of controversy in surgery, the reader may disagree with some of the more judgmental or conceptual statements made in the comments. We trust, however, that our editorial and consultant review of the comments has successfully resulted in the avoidance of factual errors.

We hope that readers will find the format of this book an enjoyable means by which not only to test, but also to expand, their knowledge of the art and science of surgery.

CHAPTER 1

History of Surgery

1. Which of the following is the earliest known document about surgery?

A. *De medicina* by Aurelius Cornelius Celsus
B. *On the Surgery* by Hippocrates
C. The Edwin Smith Papyrus
D. Various treatises by Galen of Pergamum
E. The Hindu treatise *Susruta-Samhita*

Sabiston: 1

Comments: **Celsus,** the "Hippocrates of the Romans," wrote extensively on a variety of subjects that present the cumulative knowledge of medicine from Hippocrates to the beginning of the Christian era. These were in the form of an encyclopedia, but only his *De medicina* survived. Discovered by Pope Nicholas I, it was among the first to be printed (1478) after the invention of movable type. He established the four cardinal signs of inflammation: pain, redness, heat, and swelling. ● **Hippocrates,** a Greek physician (ca. 500 to 400 B.C.) from the island of Cos in the Aegean, dissociated medicine and his writings from theology and philosophy. About 70 medical works on fractures, dislocations, and other medical diseases are ascribed to him, but certainly not all were written by him. Likely, they constitute the library of the medical school of Cos. Of these, *On the Surgery* relates mostly to bandaging injuries and to the knowledge, steps in therapy, and general qualifications of the surgeon. He probably is most widely known for the Hippocratic Oath, a pledge to ethics and practices of medicine by physicans widely used during medical school commencement ceremonies. ● The **Edwin Smith Papyrus,** probably written around 1500 B.C. but based on work dating from about 3000 B.C., contains a description of clinical medicine in use at the time among the Egyptians, as well as many surprisingly accurate observations on anatomy, physiology, and pathology. It is characterized by an absence of magic and mysticism at a time when these were prevalent. It is named for the Egyptologist who found it in Luxor, Egypt in 1862. ● **Galen** (129 to 199 A.D.) was one of the most distinguished teachers of the Greco-Roman period. Chief physician of gladiators at Pergamum, and a member of the Court of Marcus Aure-

lius, he wrote 400 separate treatises concerned with all aspects of medicine and surgery. He began animal experimentation and may be thought of as the founder of experimental physiology. Nonetheless, his holding to the belief that disease was caused by the dyssynchrony of humors—yellow bile, black bile, blood, and phlegm—limited the development of surgery; after all, one could hardly operate on the humors! ● *Susruta-Samhita* is a surgical treatise attributed to **Susruta,** traditionally thought of as a surgeon. It probably had its origin within several centuries of the pre-Christian era and fixed in its present form at about the 7th century A.D. It states the existence of over 1,000 diseases. The Indian materia medica consisted largely of vegetable drugs; Susruta knew over 700 of them. According to Susruta, the surgeon should be equipped with 20 sharp and 101 blunt instruments; their number and enumeration reminds one of today's scrub nurse checking her surgical instruments prior to an operation.

Answer: C

2. Match the Nobel laureates listed below with one of their listed characteristics.

Noble Laureate	Characteristic
A. Charles Huggins	a. His research includes work on elasticity and capillary action of fluids
B. Theodor Kocher	
C. Wilhelm Roentgen	b. Urologist
D. Alexis Carrel	c. Discovered lysozyme
E. Alexander Fleming	d. A student of Billroth and teacher of Harvey Cushing
	e. Recognized as a pioneer in transplantation

Sabiston: 13

Comments: **Charles Huggins** (1901–   ): Endocrine manipulation of metastatic cancer has become very sophisticated in its complexity, almost universal in practice, and certainly one of the mainstays of cancer therapy. While the role of the endocrine glands in the control of neoplastic disease was of intense interest for a considerable period, it remained for Charles Huggins, a urologist at the University of Chicago, to show in 1940 that antiandrogenic treatment either by orchiectomy or by the giving of estrogen could produce regression in disseminated cancer of the prostate. ● **Theodor Kocher** (1841–1917): A Swiss, and considered by some the greatest surgeon of his time, who was widely trained, yet considered himself to be a student of Billroth. In turn, he was a teacher of distinction to many, among his students being the American Harvey Cushing. He was the first surgeon to be awarded the Nobel Prize, this for his work on goiters. A meticulous, inventive surgeon, he was an advocate of the Listerian school of total asepsis. In contrast to the prevalent practice of surgeons of that era who attempted to justify their mistakes, often in fractious public forums, he instead built on experience and past error; by 1912 he had brought his operative mortality from a previous 18% to less than 0.5% ● **Wilhelm Roentgen** (1845–1923): Roentgen received the first Nobel Prize in Physics in 1901 for his epochal discovery of x-rays in 1895, while Professor of Physics at the University of Wurzburg in Prussia. Clearly, x-rays revolutionized medicine; within just a few months of their discovery, x-rays were used to visualize bones; and several years later intestinal motion was studied by this means. Indeed, in the very year of their discovery, x-rays of a diseased tibia were presented for observation to Dr. Nicholas Senn, a distinguished surgeon at Rush Medical College. ● **Alexis Carrel** (1873–1944): Carrel was born and trained in France, but intermittently carried on with his research studies in the United States. A colorful individual, he earned the Nobel Prize in 1912 for his important work with blood vessel anastomoses—the technique of "triangulation" of vessels and of including all layers of the vessel wall when coapting them, which is still used throughout surgery. His unflagging interest in transplantation was the backdrop for many of his other accomplishments, a notable one being his contributions to techniques of tissue culture. ● **Alexander Fleming** (1881–1955): Fleming's essentially serendipitous discovery of penicillin in 1928 heralded the beginning of antibiotic therapy for infectious diseases. In the often written story, Fleming noticed a bacteria-free circle around a mold growth (*Penicillium notatum*) that was contaminating a culture of staphylococci. This inhibitory substance, which he named penicillin, retained its potency even when diluted 800 times. He shared the Nobel prize with Ernest Chain and Howard Florey, who carried Fleming's discovery further in isolating penicillin, purifying and testing it, and finally developing methods of producing it in quantity. Fleming also discovered lysozyme, an antibacterial agent in tears and saliva.

Answer: A–b; B–d; C–a; D–e; E–c

3. The surgeon who best related anatomy and disease to function, who developed "experimental surgery," and who established the scientific basis of surgery and medicine was:

A. John Hunter
B. Ferdinand Sauerbruch
C. Rudolph Matas
D. Ephraim McDowell

Sabiston: 5

Comments: **John Hunter** was the brother of the obstetrician William Hunter. Both brothers left Scotland to train

and practice in London. John was a tireless anatomist and his interests extended to comparative anatomy and to collecting animals and pathology specimens, many of which remain in the Hunterian Museum. His numerous experiments included injecting himself with gonorrheal pus to differentiate between the manifestations of syphilis and gonorrhea (unfortunately the source of this pus had both gonorrhea and syphilis!). Experiments in transplantation, gunshot wounds, dissection of innumerable animals from insects to whales, geology, and dentistry reflect his boundless energy and insatiable curiosity, and are described in his many books. He once wrote: "I think your solution is just; but why think? Why not try the experiment?" More than any other individual, John Hunter through his efforts placed medicine on a scientific foundation. ● Because of the problem of pneumothorax, the chest cavity and its organs were not operated on until recently. **Ferdinand Sauerbruch's** low-pressure chamber accommodated both the patient and the surgical team, the patient's head projecting into the normal atmosphere through a snugly fitting collar. This technique was soon superseded by the endotracheal tube and positive-pressure anesthesia. The many patients with tuberculosis and their variety of pulmonary problems provided Sauerbruch and his daring the opportunity of innovating many thoracic procedures. ● **Rudolph Matas** (1860–1957) was Professor of Surgery at Tulane University and a pioneer vascular surgeon in the prime of his career at the turn of the century. He was an avid follower, as well as innovator, of the current theories and practices of antisepsis. On reflection, the swift pace of progress in antisepsis can be appreciated when one realizes that many surgeons today remember Matas, yet he was one who shared 52 years in common with Lister, someone often thought of as a figure of too long ago. As prosthetic vascular material was unknown at the time, Matas introduced the technique of endoaneurysmorrhaphy in the treatment of arterial aneurysm. ● In 1809, the backwoods physician and surgeon **Ephraim McDowell** of Danville, Kentucky, operated electively on Jane Todd Crawford, who had ridden 60 miles to Danville on horseback. With the patient on a kitchen table, he removed a massive ovarian cyst without benefit of anesthesia, asepsis, or antibiotics; his patient recovered uneventfully. In modesty, and not wishing to report just a single case, McDowell waited until he had two further patients before doing so. His surgical training was with John Bell at the University of Edinburgh.

Answer: A

4. The development of asepsis, one of the most important advances in surgery, was primarily due to the work of:

A. Joseph Lister
B. Charles Bell
C. Louis Pasteur
D. Ambroise Paré

Sabiston: 4, 8, 244

Comments: As Chief Surgeon to the Royal Infirmary in Glasgow, **Joseph Lister** was faced with treating patients who were in great danger from even the simplest surgical wound. Postoperative infection rates of 75% and even higher were reported in hospitalized patients during

Lister's time (1827–1912). Recognizing the work of Pasteur that demonstrated that organisms in the air caused infection, Lister decided to sterilize the air and the wound dressings using carbolic acid. Further, he was convinced that permanent suture material aided infection, and he accordingly experimented with catgut sutures treated with carbolic acid. Thus, the use of sterile absorbable sutures was established. ● **Sir Charles Bell** (1774–1842) was an anatomist who graduated from the University of Edinburgh and who, following a number of distinguished accomplishments in London, returned to take the chair of surgery at his alma mater. Among his numerous accomplishments, he distinguished between motor and sensory nerves. His *New Idea of Anatomy of the Brain* has been called by some the "Magna Carta of neurology." ● **Louis Pasteur** (1822–1895), the originator of the germ theory of disease, made many and varied scientific contributions as a chemist and microbiologist. While he is recollected almost daily when one hears of pasteurization, his longest continued involvement was with the treatment of rabies; he carried out this research at the Pasteur Institute which he headed until his death. His initial fame came with his work on fermentation of wine and beer at a time when that industry was in grave danger from contamination by unwanted fungi. At about the same time, he was of considerable assistance to the silk industry by identifying the bacillus of two silkworm diseases. Pasteur made the cardinal contribution of being the first to utilize vaccination against anthrax, cholera, and rabies. ● **Ambroise Paré** (1510–1590) is best known for introducing the use of ligatures in amputations; podalic version in difficult obstetric deliveries; the rejection of boiling oil to treat gunshot wounds; and his statement: "I dressed him, and God healed him." He worked widely in battlefields treating various war wounds, wrote extensively, devised many new surgical instruments and artificial limbs and eyes, and used a truss to control inguinal hernia. He clearly recognized syphilis as a cause of aneurysm and described carbon monoxide poisoning.

Answer: A

5. Which of the following made important contributions to the understanding of gastric function based upon observations in the human subject?

A. William Beaumont
B. Claude Bernard
C. Rudolf Heidenhain
D. Ivan Pavlov

Sabiston: 11

Comments: Current understanding of gastric physiology is founded in the work of a number of 19th century investigators. Working at a remote Army post, **William Beaumont** performed studies on Alexis St. Martin, a patient who had suffered a close-range musket wound in the lower chest and abdomen and subsequently healed but with a resultant gastrocutaneous fistula. Beaumont's landmark observations on the secretion of hydrochloric acid by the fed stomach, and on additional digestive properties of gastric secretion, were published in 1833. ● Just 20 years later, **Claude Bernard** in France left a clinical career in surgery to devote himself entirely to the study of physiology and he performed important studies on pancreatic function, gluconeogenesis, and va-somotor function. ● The development of a denervated gastric pouch by **Rudolph Heidenhain** (1878) in Germany permitted studies leading to our current understanding of the control of gastric secretion. ● **Ivan Petrovich Pavlov,** noted for his development of the concept of a conditioned reflex, studied chemistry and physiology at the University of St. Petersburg for 10 years, following this with investigations on cardiac physiology and blood pressure at the Imperial Medical Academy. His most noted research was on intestinal secretions in an innervated gastric pouch, all this leading to his being awarded the Nobel Prize in 1903.

Answer: A

6. Match the statement or term in the left-hand column with the appropriate individual in the right-hand column.

A. Performed first successful renal transplant
B. Pediatrician
C. Did important work on physiology and treatment of shock
D. Successful operation for tetralogy of Fallot
E. Developed nerve block anesthesia

a. Alfred Blalock
b. Helen Taussig
c. Joseph Murray
d. George Crile

Sabiston: 15

Comments: **Alfred Blalock** (1889–1964) was one of the pioneers in the development of an atmosphere within the surgical sciences that promoted scientific laboratory research hand in hand with clinical medicine and surgery in a cooperative venture. While at Vanderbilt University in the 1920's and 1930's he published several papers on the pathophysiology and management of shock, and thereby helped lay the groundwork for much of our present understanding of what occurs during periods of hemorrhagic shock. Much of the later work in his career was conducted at Johns Hopkins University, where he had a particular interest in the surgery of congenital heart defects. ● Blalock teamed with **Helen Taussig,** a pediatrician, to develop the Blalock-Taussig shunt, a systemic-pulmonary shunt from the subclavian to the pulmonary artery used in the management of infants with tetralogy of Fallot. ● **Joseph Murray,** a plastic surgeon at the Peter Bent Brigham Hospital, Boston, performed the first clinically successful kidney transplant between identical twins. This was possible not merely as a demonstration of surgical virtuosity. Rather, he and his associate John Merrill, in collaboration with many distinguished investigators, were able to build on a strong scientific foundation whose groundwork was laid by Hume, Longmeier, Landsteiner, Hufnagel, Terasaki, and a host of others. ● **George Crile** was a surgeon who spanned this and the last century equally and founded the Cleveland Clinic Foundation. Crile's training after graduation was typical, his having studied in London, Vienna, and Paris. He wrote on surgical shock, may have been the first in the United States to perform a radical neck dissection, and developed nerve block anesthesia.

Answer: A–c; B–b; C–a, d; D–a; E–d

7. Of the surgeons listed below, which one was the first to successfully use the cardiopulmonary bypass machine for open heart surgery on a human?

A. C. Walton Lillehei
B. John Gibbon
C. Owen Wangensteen
D. Michael DeBakey

Sabiston: 14

Comments: **C. Walton Lillehei,** a bold and resourceful surgeon at the University of Minnesota, was the first, in 1948, to perform open heart surgery using human-to-human (parent-to-child) cardiopulmonary assist. This was the beginning of a productive career in which he then went on to play a leading role in demonstrating the feasibility of open heart surgery as a routine procedure. ● It was, however, **John Gibbon** of the Jefferson Medical College, a pioneer cardiothoracic surgeon, who, along with his wife, developed extracorporeal circulation and was the first to use a cardiopulmonary assist machine while performing open heart surgery on a human. His cardinal achievement set the stage for a surgical era of innovation and progress that is still in evolution. ● **Owen Wangensteen,** enjoying an illustrious and long career as Chairman of the Department of Surgery at the University of Minnesota, had as his main research interest the workings of the gastrointestinal tract and made many important contributions in this area. Probably of greater importance, however, was his role as a leading teacher of surgeons, typified by his words: "My principal role has been essentially that of trying to create an atmosphere friendly to learning." ● **Michael DeBakey,** an internationally renowned cardiovascular surgeon, has been in the forefront of direct surgery on greater vessels and of developing plastic prosthetic arterial substitutes. He and his colleagues have pioneered a number of "firsts," including the occlusive roller pump (1934), carotid endarterectomy (1953), and the successful use of a saphenous vein bypass graft for coronary artery occlusion (1964).

Answer: B

8. Match the individual on the left with the characteristic on the right.

A. Harvey Cushing
B. Bernhard von Langenbeck
C. Theodor Billroth
D. Benjamin Rush

a. Close friend of Johannes Brahms
b. Father of the modern residency system in surgery
c. Founded Rush Medical College
d. Devised a chart for continuous recording of respirations and blood pressure by the anesthetist
e. A psychiatrist

Sabiston: 12

Comments: Harvey Williams Cushing (1869–1939) became, for many, a legend within his lifetime. A true pioneer in a specialty of which he was a founder, he distinguished himself at Johns Hopkins (where he was Halsted's resident), at Harvard, and at Yale, as well as abroad. His demeanor, his teachings, and his practice set the high standards still the guideposts for this specialty.

He first described hyperfunctioning of the pituitary gland, thus the eponym of Cushing's disease. He devised the first anesthesia record while still a medical student at Harvard. ● **Christian Albert Theodor Billroth** (1829–1894) is generally considered to be the founder of modern abdominal surgery. His preliminary experience was at the University of Zurich, but his prolonged and rich career took place at the University of Vienna, where he eventually became Professor of Surgery. Initially he wished to become a musician, and he entered medicine only at the insistence of his mother. He developed a background in pathology and experimental surgery, and became one of the most prominent teachers of surgery of his time. He performed the first successful partial gastrectomy for cancer with primary anastomosis, and likewise for an esophageal tumor. These, and associated accomplishments, opened the door for subsequent elective gastrointestinal surgery. He was a pupil of the master German surgeon von Langenbeck, whom he helped to evolve the concept of the modern surgical residency training program. As a crowning accolade, Billroth was invited to become Professor at the prestigious University of Berlin; he declined, however, giving as his reason that he could not persuade his lifelong friend Brahms to leave Vienna. ● **Bernhard Rudolf Konrad von Langenbeck** (1810–1887) studied in Göttingen, became Professor of Surgery at Kiel, and finally at the University of Berlin, there succeeding the illustrious Johann Dieffenbach. As one of the most distinguished surgeons of the 19th century, and teacher to Billroth, Kocher, and many others, his everlasting contribution was in stressing the systematic training of young surgeons. While William Halsted was studying with Billroth, it was this "German method" that he observed and admired and that he brought to the United States as the progenitor of many American programs training surgical residents. ● Rush Medical College was named in honor of **Benjamin Rush,** physician, patriot and humanitarian. Rush was the only formally trained physician and second youngest of the signers of the Declaration of Independence. He served as Physician General of the Continental Army. He supported the adoption of the U.S. Constitution and served as Treasurer of the U.S. Mint. Rush was the first Professor of Chemistry, later becoming Professor of Medicine at the University of Pennsylvania. He was a founder of The College of Physicians of Philadelphia and founded the first medical clinic for the poor. Because of his extensive work with the mentally ill, Rush became known as "The Father of American Psychiatry." As a humanitarian, he championed the cause of the black American, the poor, the alcoholic, and the criminal. He founded the first organization for the abolition of slavery; also, he founded Dickinson College as well as Franklin and Marshall College. He even proposed a Secretary of Peace as a permanent Cabinet office. ● **Daniel Brainard** (1812–1866) founded Rush Medical College 150 years ago, indeed two days before Chicago was incorporated, the city in which it is located. Bold and forthright, he was a man of vision and drive, probably best known for investigation and treatment of nonunited fractures. He organized the county and state medical societies, and was the principal surgeon of Chicago's first general and first county hospitals. At the age of 54, only a few hours after having given a lecture on cholera, he himself died of this disease.

Answer: A–d; B–b; C–a; D– e

CHAPTER 2

Endocrine and Metabolic Response to Injury

1. Which of the following is the most important stimulus to endocrine response following injury?

A. Afferent nerve stimuli from the injured area
B. Hypovolemia
C. Tissue acidosis
D. Local wound factors
E. Temperature changes

Sabiston: 30
Schwartz: 1

Comments: The response to injury involves an integrated series of endocrine and metabolic changes designed to maintain homeostasis; a variety of stimuli are involved in triggering these responses. Of these, one of the earliest and most important stimuli is the signal carried by the afferent sensory nerves from the injured area. This directly stimulates release of ACTH and the subsequent adrenocortical response to injury as well as the elaboration of ADH. This hormonal response can be ablated experimentally by division of the peripheral nerves to the injured area and may be diminished clinically in patients with spinal anesthesia. It is for this reason that paraplegic patients show a diminished corticosteroid response to injury in the denervated areas.

Answer: A

2. Which of the following is/are elevated during the acute response to injury?

A. Glucagon
B. Glucocorticoids
C. Catecholamines
D. Insulin
E. Thyroid stimulating hormone

Sabiston: 32
Schwartz: 6, 15

Comments: Following injury, pain and hypovolemia are the primary stimuli that produce the subsequent neuro-hormonal events aimed at restoring hemodynamic stability and providing readily available energy substrates. Direct stimulation of the hypothalamic-pituitary axis results in prompt increases in circulating ACTH, cortisol, ADH, and growth hormone. Hypothalamic signals also result in sympathetic autonomic nerve stimulation that leads to the release of epinephrine and norepinephrine from the adrenal medulla and the release of glucagon from the alpha cells of the pancreas. Glucocorticoids, catecholamines, and glucagon act synergistically in producing a homeostatic physiologic response. Despite the hyperglycemia that may be observed in acute injury, insulin response is inhibited by alpha-adrenergic stimulation and by the effects of circulating catecholamines, cortisol, and glucagon. Elevated TSH levels are not thought to play an important role in the acute response to injury.

Answer: A, B, C

3. Hypothalamically mediated responses to hemorrhagic shock include production of which one or more of the following?

A. ACTH
B. Vasopressin (ADH)
C. Somatostatin
D. Growth hormone
E. Aldosterone

Sabiston: 27, 32
Schwartz: 6, 14

Comments: When acute blood loss occurs, the decrease in the effective circulating volume activates baroreceptors in the aortic arch and carotid artery and volume receptors in the left atrium, which set into motion a compensatory series of responses. Direct hypothalamic stimulation results in increases in ACTH, ADH, and growth hormone. One of the most important responses to hypovolemia, however, is the release of aldosterone for the purpose of reabsorbing sodium from the renal tubule and thereby conserving volume. Among the several mechanisms that produce aldosterone release, activation of the renin-angiotensin system as a result of stimulation of the juxtaglomerular cells due to decreased renal arterial perfusion is perhaps the most important. Aldosterone release also occurs in response to ACTH, which is elevated as a result of hypothalamic stimulation in hypovolemic shock.

Answer: A, B, D, E

4. Metabolic effects of the neuroendocrine response to injury include which one or more of the following?

A. Gluconeogenesis
B. Glycogen synthesis
C. Lipolysis
D. Proteolysis
E. Hypoglycemia

Sabiston: 27, 34
Schwartz: 26

Comments: Glucose is the primary fuel for vital organs, such as the heart, peripheral nerves, renal medulla, red blood cells, and leukocytes. In order for the human organism to survive serious injury, a ready supply of glucose must be made available, and this constitutes a critical effect of the many neurohormonal changes that are observed following injury. The supply of hepatic glucose stored as glycogen is rapidly depleted, so glucose must be obtained from other sources. Gluconeogenesis occurs from alanine and other amino acids provided by breakdown of skeletal muscle, from glycerol due to the breakdown of triglycerides in body fat, and from lactate and pyruvate formed as a result of anaerobic glycolysis of the glucose (Cori cycle). Additionally, glucose entry into cells is impaired by the action of catecholamines and cortisol and by the decrease in serum insulin; this produces hyperglycemia rather than hypoglycemia.

Answer: A, C, D

5. In which one or more of the following situations is ACTH release not inhibited by high plasma cortisol levels?

A. Somatic pain
B. Severe hypovolemia
C. Cushing's disease
D. Prolonged starvation
E. Endotoxic shock

Schwartz: 8, 19

Comments: The pituitary-adrenal axis is normally under control of a negative feedback mechanism, such that increased cortisol levels inhibit further release of ACTH. This mechanism is operable in most situations of trauma, when various stimuli lead to ACTH release. An important exception is severe hypovolemia; in such a setting, ACTH release is not cortisol-suppressable. Stimulation of ACTH persists until intravascular volume has been replenished. Lack of ACTH suppression by cortisol is also seen in the nontraumatic condition of Cushing's disease as the result of ACTH production by a pituitary adenoma.

Answer: B, C

6. Chronic adrenal insufficiency is characterized by which one or more of the following?

A. Hypothermia
B. Hypertension
C. Hyperkalemia
D. Hyponatremia
E. Hyperglycemia

Sabiston: 677
Schwartz: 11, 15, 16

Comments: Adrenocortical response is a critical mechanism of survival in situations of shock, trauma, or sepsis. When endogenous corticosteroid production is impaired and exogenous replacement insufficient, profound cardiovascular collapse will occur. Acute adrenal insufficiency may result from bilateral adrenal hemorrhage (severe sepsis, anticoagulation, or spontaneously) from adrenalectomy or, particularly, from withdrawal of exogenous steroids that have been administered for a long period of time. Chronic adrenal insufficiency may result from autoimmune destruction of the adrenal glands or, less commonly, tuberculous or fungal disease. The clinical manifestations of chronic adrenal insufficiency are those of combined mineralocorticoid and glucocorticoid deficiency. Characteristically, patients have hyperpigmentation, weakness, weight loss, gastrointestinal symptoms, and electrolyte derangement marked by hyperkalemia, hyponatremia, and hypoglycemia. Fever is a hallmark of acute addisonian crisis. Patients with adrenal insufficiency must have the condition recognized and promptly treated with exogenous supplementation; otherwise they may succumb following any stressful situation, such as an operation, injury, or infection.

Answer: C, D

7. Death following severe injury often is the result of which one or more of the following?

A. Adrenal failure
B. Respiratory failure
C. Renal failure
D. All of the above

Schwartz: 13

Comments: Death after injury does not result from adrenal exhaustion, except in patients with underlying insufficiency or those who develop acute adrenal failure during the course of their illness. Severe illness is characterized by marked adrenocortical stimulation; plasma levels of corticosteroids and their metabolites are, in fact, elevated in these patients. With recovery, plasma corticosteroid levels decline; a persistent elevation suggests ongoing injury or sepsis and is a bad prognostic factor. Death following critical illness often involves multi-system organ failure, particularly pulmonary and renal decompensation.

Answer: B, C

8. Which of the following is/are important in the restoration of blood volume after hypovolemia?

A. Hepatic albumin synthesis
B. Increased interstitial osmolality

C. Decreased interstitial osmolality
D. Transcapillary refill

Sabiston: 27
Schwartz: 28

Comments: Reduction of blood volume by 15 to 20% decreases capillary pressure and results in an initial shift of protein-free fluid from the interstitium back into the vascular compartments. This mechanism only partially compensates the volume loss, however, and is limited by the equilibrium established between intravascular oncotic pressure and interstitial fluid pressure. Further restoration of intravascular volume depends upon increases in plasma proteins, primarily albumin. This albumin comes from the interstitium itself, but can only be moved across capillary membranes into the vascular system if the interstitial pressure is adequate. Critical to increasing interstitial pressure in order to accomplish this is an increase in the extracellular interstitial osmolality that occurs following injury. This metabolic effect is the result of numerous hormonal influences, especially cortisol.

Answer: B, D

9. Which of the following is/are true regarding the renin-angiotensin system?

A. Renin is an enzyme originating from the juxtaglomerular apparatus of the kidney
B. Angiotensinogen is a potent vasoconstrictor synthesized in the liver
C. Angiotensin I is converted to angiotensin II primarily in the kidney
D. Angiotensin II stimulates aldosterone release from the adrenal cortex
E. Aldosterone increases sodium resorption in the distal renal tubule

Schwartz: 14

Comments: See Question 10.

10. For each relationship described in the left-hand column, choose the appropriate physiologic effect from the right-hand column.

Relationship	Physiologic Effect
A. Effect of decreased renal artery perfusion on renin release	a. Stimulates
B. Effect of vasopressin on renin release	b. Inhibits
C. Effect of angiotensin II on renin release	c. Neither
D. Effect of angiotensin II on ADH release	

Schwartz: 14

Comments: The renin-angiotensin pathway is a critical physiologic mechanism for maintaining perfusion following hypovolemia or injury. Renin is elaborated in the juxtaglomerular cells along the afferent renal arterioles in response to decreased perfusion pressure as well as to sympathetic stimulation and decreased delivery of sodium chloride to the distal renal tubules. Renin acts upon angiotensinogen, produced in the liver, to convert it to angiotensin I, which is an inactive intermediary peptide. In the lung, angiotensin converting enzyme converts angiotensin I to the active angiotensin II. Angiotensin II is a potent vasoconstrictor and stimulates the release of aldosterone, which in turn increases sodium and water resorption from the renal tubules. Angiotensin II has other physiologic effects, including the release of vasopressin and ACTH from the pituitary. By a negative feedback mechanism, angiotensin II also inhibits the release of renin. Renin release is inhibited by vasopressin and potassium as well.

Answer: Question 9: A, D, E
Question 10: A–a, B–b, C–b, D–a

11. Acute phase reactant proteins are:

A. Synthesized in the liver and kidney
B. Synthesized exclusively in the liver
C. Incorporated into structural proteins following resolution of acute illness
D. A primary source of gluconeogenesis in acute illness
E. Critical cofactors in anaerobic glycolysis

Schwartz: 28

Comments: Certain plasma proteins may be found exclusively or in high concentrations following injury, and these are known as acute phase reactants. These substances are synthesized only in the liver and include haptoglobin, fibrinogen, ceruloplasmin, and C-reactive protein, among others. Although the entire role of acute phase reactants is unknown, they presumably benefit the organism during the acute phase of injury by mechanisms that may include facilitation of coagulation and inactivation of various toxins. They do not serve as energy substrates, nor are they useful anabolic proteins.

Answer: B

12. Which one or more of the following statements is true about protein loss after injury?

A. It results from impaired protein synthesis
B. It occurs primarily from skeletal muscle
C. It occurs primarily from the site of injury
D. It can be prevented by total parenteral nutrition

Sabiston: 34
Schwartz: 27

Comment: Acute injury is associated with an obligatory nitrogen loss occurring primarily in the form of urinary nitrogen. Generalized catabolism of skeletal muscle is the primary source of protein loss; there is also impaired entry of amino acids into muscle cells as an effect of cortisol and other hormones. Protein may also be lost when there are large open wounds, extensive areas of necrotic tissue, peritonitis, or ascites. Protein synthesis is not impaired following injury; in fact, it may be accelerated, but because of the marked increase in catabolism, the net protein balance is negative.

Answer: B

13. Match the metabolic response in the left-hand column with the appropriate clinical situation in the right-hand column.

A. Hepatic glycogenolysis
B. Hyperglycemia
C. Protein catabolism in excess of energy needs
D. Gluconeogenesis from glycerol
E. Fat main energy source

a. Trauma
b. Fasting
c. Both
d. Neither

Sabiston: 28, 35
Schwartz: 22, 26

Comments: See Question 16.

14. Metabolic adaptation occurs with prolonged fasting. Match the metabolic characteristic in the left-hand column with the appropriate phase of starvation in the right-hand column.

Metabolic Characteristic

A. Hepatic gluconeogenesis from free fatty acids
B. Hepatic gluconeogenesis from glycerol
C. Hepatic gluconeogenesis from lactate and pyruvate
D. Hepatic gluconeogenesis from amino acids
E. Renal gluconeogenesis from amino acids
F. Brain utilization of ketone bodies

Phase of Starvation

a. Early starvation
b. Late starvation
c. Both
d. Neither

Sabiston: 28
Schwartz: 22

Comments: See Question 16.

15. The entry of acetyl CoA into which of the following metabolic pathways is the rate-limiting step during fasting?

A. Pentose phosphate shunt
B. Cori cycle
C. Tricarboxylic acid cycle
D. Glucose-alanine-glucose cycle
E. Urea cycle

Sabiston: 28
Schwartz: 22, 26

Comments: See Question 16.

16. Which of the following sources of energy provide(s) substrate utilized for gluconeogenesis in the Cori cycle?

A. Circulating triglycerides
B. Liver glycogen
C. Renal alanine
D. Wound lactate
E. Lactate from cardiac muscle

Sabiston: 35
Schwartz: 21

Comments: Response to injury or fasting requires energy substrates. Normal circulating fuel sources in the form of glucose and plasma fats and triglycerides make up a very small part of a person's total fuel composition and are not capable of providing the required calories. Stored sources of fuel include hepatic and muscle glycogen, protein, and fat. Hepatic glycogen stores are readily available, but are extremely limited and are depleted within 24 hours. The largest potential calorie source is body fat, and following starvation or injury, it is this source that becomes a main provider of energy through oxidation of fatty acids and generation of glycerol to be used in gluconeogenesis. A number of vital areas of the body, including the brain, renal medulla, red cells, leukocytes, and peripheral nerves, are glycolytic tissues, meaning that they require a glucose source of energy for metabolism and are unable to utilize fatty acids. For this reason, a continuous supply of glucose must be made available; when the limited glycogen stores are depleted, this is accomplished by gluconeogenesis and by recycling of incompletely metabolized glucose. Primary sources of gluconeogenesis are: (1) amino acids, derived from breakdown of muscle proteins, and (2) glycerol, derived from breakdown of triglycerides in adipose stores. These processes are fueled by the oxidation of fatty acids. In trauma, the hormonal milieu present results in catabolism of protein stores beyond that necessary for energy needs alone. In starvation, the body attempts to conserve proteins by adaptations that permit the use of fatty acids and ketones for fuel by nonglycolytic tissues and that promote gluconeogenesis. With prolonged fasting, ketone bodies such as acetoacetate and beta-hydroxybutyrate can be used for brain metabolism in place of glucose. Lactate and pyruvate that are derived from incomplete utilization of glucose by glycolytic tissues can be regenerated into glucose using energy provided by fatty acid oxidation; this process is known as the Cori cycle. The cycled glucose, in fact, becomes the main source of available glucose in late starvation. Another change observed in late starvation is a shift from the liver to the kidney as the primary source of gluconeogenesis; this occurs as alanine—the main source of gluconeogenesis from amino acids—is depleted in the liver. The human organism does not have the enzymes necessary to utilize free fatty acids directly for gluconeogenesis. The protein-conserving adaptations that are seen in late starvation do not occur with injury, because of the hypermetabolic effects of cortisol, catecholamines, and other circulating hormones.

Answer: Question 13: A–c; B–a; C–a; D–c; E–c
Question 14: A–d; B–c; C–c; D–a; E–b; F–b
Question 15: C
Question 16: D

17. Match the statement in the left-hand column with the appropriate response in the right-hand column:

A. High urine output
B. High urine osmolarity
C. Hypernatremia
D. Associated with head trauma

a. Inappropriate ADH secretion
b. Diabetes insipidus
c. Both
d. Neither

Schwartz: 16

Comments: Afferent neural stimulation of the hypothalamus in response to injury or hypovolemia leads to release of antidiuretic hormone (ADH or vasopressin) from the posterior pituitary. The physiologic action of ADH is to increase water resorption from the distal renal tubule. A disturbance in the release of ADH may produce a syndrome of inappropriate ADH (SIADH) or diabetes insipidus. Either of these may be associated with head injury. With SIADH there is secretion of ADH in excess of that required for normal homeostasis. Consequently, there is oliguria and urinary hyperosmolarity with dilutional hyponatremia. Hyponatremia may occur in patients with normal ADH response if they are given excess hypotonic fluids. Diabetes insipidus, in contradistinction to SIADH, is a situation in which there is a failure of ADH secretion. If not recognized and treated appropriately, it results in dehydration and hypernatremia.

Answer: A–b; B–a; C–b; D–c

CHAPTER 3

Fluids and Electrolytes

1. Correct statements regarding total body water include:

A. 50 to 70% of total body weight is water
B. On the average, the percentage of total body weight as water is higher in males than in females
C. Lean individuals have a greater proportion of water to body weight than do obese individuals
D. The percentage of total body water weight increases with age
E. Body water is divided into extracellular (intravascular and interstitial) and intracellular functional compartments

Sabiston: 64
Schwartz: 45

Comments: Management of fluid and electrolyte balance depends on an understanding of the size and composition of various body fluid compartments, usually expressed as a percentage of body weight. As an example, 60% of body weight in males and 50% of body weight in females is water (±15%). This difference relates in part to the fact that fat contains little water, and therefore, lean individuals have a greater proportion of body water than fat individuals of the same weight. Generally, females have a larger amount of subcutaneous fat relative to lean mass than do males. Total body water decreases with age as a result of decreasing lean muscle mass. In infants the high total body water to body weight ratio may be as high as 75 to 80%. By 1 year of age, the percentage of body water approaches that of the adult. • Body water is divided into three functional compartments. These are: the intracellular fluid compartment (40%), the interstitial fluid compartment (15%), and the intravascular (plasma) fluid compartment (5%). Together, the interstitial and intravascular compartments constitute the extracellular fluid compartment.

Answer: A, B, C, E

2. Which of the following statements is/are correct regarding the composition of the body fluid compartments?

A. The majority of the intracellular water is in the skeletal muscle
B. The major intracellular cation is sodium
C. The major intracellular anions are the proteins and phosphates
D. The major extracellular cation is sodium
E. The major extracellular anions are chloride and bicarbonate

Sabiston: 65
Schwartz: 46

Comments: The intracellular fluid compartment (comprising 40% of total body weight) is contained mostly in the skeletal muscle mass. The principal intracellular cations are potassium and magnesium, while the principal anions are the proteins and phosphates. The extracellular fluid compartment (20% of total body weight), subdivided into the interstitial compartment (extravascular) and plasma (intravascular) compartment, has sodium as its principal cation and chloride and bicarbonate as its principal anions. The interstitial compartment has a rapidly equilibrating functional component and a slowly equilibrating, relatively nonfunctional component (i.e., fluid within connective tissue and that contained in cerebrospinal and joint fluids). Because plasma has a higher concentration of nondiffusible organic proteins that act as anions, its total concentration of cations is higher and the concentration of inorganic anions is lower than that in the interstitial fluid. This relationship is explained by the Gibbs/Donnan equilibrium equation, but for practical purposes the differences are small and the concentrations generally are considered equal.

Answer: A, C, D, E

3. Which of the following statements is/are true regarding the chemical composition and osmolality of the body fluids?

A. From a physiologic standpoint, the numbers of millimoles, milliequivalents, and milliosmoles are interchangeable

B. The numbers of millimoles and milliosmoles within a single fluid compartment are interchangeable
C. The osmolality of body fluids is between 290 and 310 milliosmoles
D. The effective oncotic pressure of a body compartment is determined by the presence of nondiffusible proteins
E. Since water diffuses freely between compartments, the effective oncotic pressures within the various fluid compartments are considered to be equal.

Sabiston: 65
Schwartz: 47

Comments: From a physiologic as well as chemical standpoint, the terms milliosmoles, milliequivalents, and millimoles are not interchangeable. Equivalents refer to the chemical combining activity of electrolytes. In the solution, the number of milliequivalents of cations present is balanced by the same number of milliequivalents of anions (a balance the body maintains in a steady state). Osmoles refer to the number of osmotic reactive particles in solution. In each body compartment, the number of osmotically reactive particles is 290 to 310 milliosmoles. While total osmotic pressure represents the sum of osmotically active particles in a fluid compartment, the effective oncotic pressure (EOP) depends on osmotically active particles that do not freely pass between the semipermeable membranes of the body. Nonpermeable proteins in plasma are responsible for the effective oncotic pressure between the plasma and interstitial fluid compartment (the colloid osmotic pressure). The effective oncotic pressure between extracellular and intracellular compartments is contributed to mainly by sodium, the major extracellular cation that does not freely cross the cell membrane. Since water moves freely between compartments, the effective oncotic pressures are considered to be equal. An increase in the effective oncotic pressure of the extracellular fluid compartment due to an increase in sodium concentration, for example, would cause movement of water from the intracellular space to the extracellular space until the pressures equalize. Conversely, loss of sodium (hyponatremia) from the extracellular space would result in a movement of water into the intracellular space. Isotonic extracellular volume losses (volume loss without change in concentration) generally will not cause transfer of water from the intracellular space as long as osmolality remains unchanged. As a rule, most fluid shifts involve the extracellular rather than the intracellular space.

Answer: C, D, E

4. Which of the following statements is/are true regarding volume status changes of the extracellular fluid compartment?

A. Hyponatremia is the most reliable finding associated with extracellular fluid volume excess
B. Hypernatremia is the most reliable finding associated with extracellular fluid volume depletion
C. Decreased tissue turgor usually does not appear in the first 24 hours following acute volume loss
D. Extracellular volume excess is usually iatrogenic

Sabiston: 66
Schwartz: 48

Comments: The concentration of serum sodium is not necessarily related to the volume status of the extracellular fluid. Severe volume deficits can exist with high, low, or normal serum sodium concentrations. Volume deficit is the most common volume disorder encountered in surgery, with loss of fluid with a composition of water and electrolytes in the same proportion as the extracellular fluid (such as loss of gastrointestinal fluids from emesis, diarrhea, fistulas and sequestration secondary to inflammation, obstruction, or burns) being the common cause. With acute water loss, central nervous system and cardiovascular signs appear first (sleepiness and apathy progressing to stupor and coma, orthostasis, tachycardia, decreased pulses, cold extremities). Tissue signs such as decreased turgor, a soft tongue with longitudinal wrinkling, and atonic muscles usually do not appear in the first 24 hours. In response to hypovolemia, the body temperature may be decreased slightly, varying with the environmental temperature. It is important therefore to monitor the body temperature of hypovolemic patients. Extracellular excess generally is iatrogenic or the result of renal insufficiency. Both plasma and interstitial fluid spaces are involved. The signs are those of circulatory overload and include distended veins, bounding pulse, functional murmurs, edema, and basilar rales. In young, healthy patients these signs may be present, but the patient can compensate for moderate to severe volume excess without developing overt failure or pulmonary edema. In the elderly patient, however, congestive heart failure with pulmonary edema may develop quite rapidly.

Answer: C, D

5. Which statement(s) is/are true regarding derangement of the serum sodium concentration?

A. Changes in serum sodium concentration usually produce changes in the status of the extracellular fluid volume
B. The chloride ion is the main determinant of the osmolarity of the extracellular fluid space
C. Extracellular hyponatremia leads to depletion of intracellular water
D. Dry, sticky mucous membranes are characteristic of hypernatremia

Sabiston: 67
Schwartz: 49

Comments: While extracellular volume may change without a change in serum sodium concentration, changes in serum sodium concentration usually produce changes in the extracellular fluid volume. This is because serum sodium concentration is the main determinant of the osmolarity of the extracellular fluid space and alterations in this concentration produce concomitant shifts in water volume. Signs and symptoms of hyper- and hyponatremia generally are not present until the changes are severe or the change in sodium concentration occurs very rapidly. In the case of **hyponatremia**, decreased extracellular osmolality causes a shift of water into the intracellular compartment. When this occurs, central nervous system symptoms due to increased intracranial pressure develop and tissue signs of excess water are noted. The CNS symptoms include muscle twitching, hyperactive tendon reflexes, and, when severe, convulsions and hypertension due to increased intracranial pressure. Tissue signs include salivation, lacrimation, watery diarrhea, and "finger-printing" of the skin. When hyponatremia develops rapidly, signs and symptoms may appear at sodium concentrations less than 130 mEq/l. If the disorder develops gradually, however, symptoms may not develop until the level falls below 120 mEq/l. Severe hyponatremia may be associated with the onset of irreversible oliguric renal failure. The administration of hypertonic solutions of sodium salt corrects the acute problem, and free water restriction may be necessary if the underlying cause is dilution due to hypotonic fluid infusion. The signs and symptoms associated with **hypernatremia** include restlessness, weakness, delirium, and maniacal behavior. The tissue signs are characteristic and include dry, sticky mucous membranes, decreased salivation and tear production, and a red, swollen tongue. The body temperature is usually elevated, occasionally to a lethal level.

Answer: A, D

6. Which statement(s) is/are true regarding mixed volume and concentration abnormalities?

A. Extracellular fluid deficit combined with hyponatremia is one of the most common mixed volume and concentration abnormalities
B. Excessive sweating in the absence of fluid intake can lead to volume deficit combined with hypernatremia
C. Excessive water loss due to sweat or insensitive evaporative loss should be replaced by saline-containing solutions to prevent renal tubular damage.
D. In mixed volume and concentration abnormalities, the signs and symptoms produced by both tend to be additive

Sabiston: 68
Schwartz: 50

Comments: Extracellular fluid deficit combined with hyponatremia is one of the most common mixed volume and concentration abnormalities seen. It occurs in patients who drink large volumes of water to replace GI losses or in postoperative patients who receive hypotonic saline infusions to replace GI loss. Extracellular volume deficit combined with hypernatremia can occur when hypotonic fluid is lost, as during excessive sweating, in the absence of fluid intake. When pure water losses (such as secondary to sweating or excessive insensible evaporative loss) are replaced by saline-containing solutions only, extracellular fluid volume excess combined with hypernatremia may result. Extracellular volume excess combined with hyponatremia can result from the excessive infusion of water or hypotonic saline solutions into a patient with oliguric renal failure. Normal kidneys can minimize these mixed abnormalities, but the patient in oliguric or anuric renal failure is particularly prone to develop them. The signs and symptoms of mixed volume and concentration abnormalities tend to be additive, and often, opposing signs will nullify one another.

Answer: A, B, D

7. Which statement(s) is/are true regarding the acid-base buffering system of the extracellular fluid?

A. The bicarbonate–carbonic acid system is the primary extracellular buffering system
B. The functions of the extracellular buffering system are expressed in the Henderson-Hasselbalch equation
C. The ratio of the base bicarbonate to carbonic acid determines the extracellular fluid pH
D. A bicarbonate–carbonic acid ratio of 20:1 is associated with a normal pH (7.4)

Sabiston: 68
Schwartz: 51

Comments: See Question 8.

8. The Henderson-Hasselbalch equation is properly expressed by which equation?

A. $pK = pH + log\dfrac{BHCO_3}{H_2CO_3}$

B. $pK = pH + log\dfrac{H_2CO_3}{BHCO_3}$

C. $pH = pK + log\dfrac{H_2CO_3}{BHCO_3}$

D. $pH = pK + log\dfrac{BHCO_3}{H_2CO_3}$

Sabiston: 68
Schwartz: 51

Comments: Assessment of complex acid-base disorders requires an understanding of the clinical situation and of acid-base physiology. Important intracellular buffers include proteins and phosphates, while the bicarbonate–carbonic acid system is the primary extracellular buffering system. In extracellular fluids, acids (inorganic acids such as hydrochloric, sulfuric, or phosphoric acids, and organic acids such as lactic, pyruvic, and keto acids) combine with sodium bicarbonate to form the sodium salt of the acid and carbonic acid. Carbonic acid then dissociates into water and carbon dioxide. In equation form this interaction is as follows: $HCl + NaHCO_3 \rightarrow NaCl + H_2CO_3$; $H_2CO_3 \rightarrow H_2O + CO_2$. The CO_2 is excreted by the lungs; the acid anion (chloride in the case of hydrochloric acid) is excreted by the kidney with hydrogen or ammonium ions. Extracellular fluid pH is determined mainly by the ratio of the base bicarbonate to the amount of carbonic acid in the blood. This relationship is expressed in the Henderson-Hasselbalch equation, where bicarbonate is the numerator and carbonic acid is in the denominator. At a body pH of 7.4, this ratio is 20:1. As long as this ratio is kept at 20:1, the pH remains 7.4, regardless of the absolute values. The relationships between the buffering reactions of bicarbonate and carbonic acid and their respective positions in the Henderson-Hasselbalch equation are important in understanding acid-base physiology; this cannot be overemphasized. As an example, addition of an acid such as the lactic acid that accumulates during periods of hypoperfusion shifts the bicarbonate/carbonic acid equation to the right, consuming bicarbonate (thus lowering the numerator in the Henderson-Hasselbalch equation) and increasing the concentration of carbonic acid (raising the denominator). As a result, the 20:1 ratio decreases, and pH falls until increased ventilation eliminates the excess CO_2. Loss of CO_2 lowers concentration of carbonic acid, restores the 20:1 ratio, and brings the pH back to 7.4.

This is an example of the changes in pH associated with metabolic acidosis. In this setting, the ability of the lungs to rapidly eliminate excess CO_2 provides rapid compensation for the pH disturbance. Slower compensation is provided by the kidney, where excretion of excess acid occurs in exchange for bicarbonate.

Answer: Question 7: A, B, C, D
Question 8: D

9. Which of the following statements is/are true regarding respiratory acid-base abnormalities?

A. Respiratory acidosis is caused by decreased alveolar ventilation
B. Respiratory alkalosis is caused by increased alveolar ventilation
C. Hyperkalemia is a frequent complication of respiratory alkalosis
D. Potassium restriction is an important adjunct in the treatment of respiratory alkalosis

Sabiston: 71
Schwartz: 53

Comments: There are four types of acid-base disturbances: respiratory acidosis, respiratory alkalosis, metabolic acidosis, and metabolic alkalosis. **Respiratory acidosis** is due to the retention of CO_2 leading to increased carbonic acid production, which increases the denominator of the Henderson-Hasselbalch equation. This lowers the 20:1 ratio, and the pH falls. The underlying problem usually is decreased alveolar ventilation. Acute forms of this in previously healthy individuals can be corrected by restoring alveolar ventilation to normal values, such as by reversing CNS depression, removing mechanical airway obstruction, or increasing the rate of mechanical ventilation. Compensation for chronic forms of decreased alveolar ventilation occurs in the renal system. In this situation acid salts (generated by the acid anion combining with the sodium from sodium bicarbonate) are secreted in exchange for renal bicarbonate. This resorbed bicarbonate raises the numerator, thus restoring the 20:1 ratio and raising the pH to a normal value. Note that in this compensated form the plasma bicarbonate level is higher than in the normal noncompensated state. **Respiratory alkalosis** is due to excessive loss of CO_2 secondary to increased alveolar ventilation. It is characterized by a fall in arterial pCO_2 and a rise in pH. Carbonic acid production falls, lowering the denominator, and thus the 20:1 ratio increases; this leads to an increased pH. Where acid is resorbed in exchange for increased bicarbonate excretion, the compensation is renal. Increased bicarbonate excretion lowers the numerator, restores the 20:1 ratio, and brings the pH back down to 7.4. Note that in the acute phase of respiratory alkalosis, the pH is elevated, the pCO_2 falls, and the bicarbonate level may be normal. In the compensated phase, pH normalizes and the bicarbonate concentration falls. Of central importance in dealing with alkalosis is the avoidance of hypokalemia. Potassium is in competition with hydrogen ions for resorption of sodium at the level of the renal tubule. In alkalosis, preferential excretion of potassium in exchange for sodium allows conservation of hydrogen ion. It should also be noted that hypokalemia itself may contribute to alkalosis, since in hypokalemic states hydrogen ion is, by necessity, excreted for sodium resorption. An additional factor in the development of hypokalemia in alkalotic states is the exchange of extracellular potassium for intracellular hydrogen ions. It becomes clear that part of the treatment for alkalosis, whether it be respiratory, metabolic, or a combination of the two, is adequate potassium replacement.

Answer: A, B

10. Which of the following statements is/are true regarding metabolic acidosis?

A. Metabolic acidosis results from the loss of bicarbonate or a gain of fixed acids
B. The most common cause of acid excess is prolonged nasogastric suction
C. The acute compensation for metabolic acidosis is primarily renal
D. Restoration of blood pressure with vasopressors corrects the metabolic acidosis associated with circulatory failure

Sabiston: 71
Schwartz: 54

Comments: Metabolic acidosis has several causes. It results from retention or gain of fixed acids (diabetic acidosis, lactic acidosis), or the loss of bicarbonate (diarrhea, small bowel fistula, renal tubular dysfunction). Increased acid consumes bicarbonate, thus lowering the numerator of the Henderson-Hasselbalch ratio. Bicarbonate loss causes the same change. Initial compensation is pulmonary (hyperventilation), which lowers carbonic acid concentration, decreasing the denominator and restoring the 20:1 ratio. Renal compensation is slower and is the same as the renal compensation for respiratory acidosis, namely, excretion of acid salts and retention of bicarbonate. This compensation depends on normal renal function. When kidney damage interferes with the ability to excrete acid and resorb bicarbonate, metabolic acidosis may rapidly progress to profound levels. The most common cause of metabolic acidosis in surgical patients is circulatory failure with accumulation of lactic acid. It is due to tissue hypoxia and anaerobic metabolism. Resuscitation with vasopressors or infusion of bicarbonate does not correct the underlying problem. Volume replacement with lactated Ringer's or blood is slightly alkalinizing, but when circulation is restored, lactic acid is cleared, the bicarbonate is consumed, and the excess carbonic acid that is formed is cleared by the lungs. The excessive use of bicarbonate in resuscitation of these patients has the potential to lead to severe metabolic alkalosis. It appears that acidosis due to circulatory arrest is well compensated for a significant period of time if the patient is well ventilated and not previously acidotic, as when resuscitation is begun immediately after a witnessed cardiac arrest. The use of excessive bicarbonate in such situations may induce a hypernatremic, hyperosmotic state. It is recommended, therefore, that the initial dose of bicarbonate not exceed 50 ml of a 7.5% solution and that additional doses be based on results of the blood gas analysis.

Answer: A

11. Which of the following statements is/are true regarding metabolic alkalosis?

A. Metabolic alkalosis is due to a loss of fixed acid or gain of bicarbonate
B. Compensation is mainly renal
C. A common cause is prolonged nasogastric suctioning
D. Hydrochloric acid infusion to correct this disturbance has been discontinued owing to the high incidence of arrhythmias

Sabiston: 72
Schwartz: 55

Comments: Metabolic alkalosis results from the loss of fixed acids, as with prolonged nasogastric suction of an obstructed stomach, or from the gain of bicarbonate, as occurs when renal tubular damage prevents its normal excretion. Loss of acid or gain of bicarbonate lead to a relative increase in the numerator, an increase in the 20:1 ratio, and a rise in pH. Compensation is mainly renal and by the same mechanisms discussed for respiratory alkalosis. Again, in alkalosis, avoidance of hypokalemia is very important. Occasionally, there will be a component of respiratory compensation leading to hypercapnia. A common problem seen in patients with persistent emesis in the face of an obstructive pylorus is hypochloremic, hypokalemic metabolic alkalosis. To compensate for the high loss of chloride from the stomach, there is a compensatory loss of bicarbonate in the urine The bicarbonate usually is excreted as the sodium salt, but in an attempt to conserve sodium to maintain intravascular volume, potassium and hydrogen are excreted, further compounding the alkalosis and leading to a paradoxic aciduria. The principles of management of this derangement include resuscitation with isotonic saline solutions as well as aggressive replacement of potassium losses. Severe metabolic alkalosis may respond to infusions of dilute HCl formulated by the addition of 150 ml of a 0.1 normal HCl solution in 1 liter of normal saline or 5% dextrose. Such a solution yields 300 mEq of hydrogen and chloride ions. This is infused over a 6- to 24-hour period with measurement of the pH, pCO_2, and electrolytes every 4 to 6 hours. To determine what volume of the solution should be infused, the chloride deficit can be calculated using the plasma chloride concentration and the presumed volume in which the chloride is dispersed (a volume equal to 20% of body weight). For a 70-kg man with a serum chloride of 80 (normal being 103), the deficit would be: (20% of body weight) × (normal chloride minus observed plasma chloride) which equals (0.2 × 70) (103 − 80) = 322 mEq.

Answer: A, B, C

12. Which of the following statements regarding respiratory acidosis and alkalosis is/are true?

A. Respiratory acidosis is associated with an increased denominator of the Henderson-Hasselbalch equation due to CO_2 retention, resulting in a ratio less than 20:1
B. Respiratory alkalosis is associated with a decreased denominator due to a loss of CO_2, resulting in a ratio greater than 20:1
C. Compensation for respiratory acidosis is primarily renal
D. Compensation for respiratory alkalosis is primarily pulmonary

Sabiston: 69
Schwartz: 52

Comments: As previously discussed, respiratory causes of acid-base imbalance relate to changes in CO_2, which correspond to changes in carbonic acid. The carbonic acid concentration is represented in the denominator of the Henderson-Hasselbalch equation. Increases in the denominator caused by CO_2 retention result in a ratio of less than 20:1 with an associated fall in pH. Excessive loss of CO_2 causes a fall in the denominator with an increase in the 20:1 ratio and a resultant rise in pH. In both settings, compensation is primarily renal.

Answer: A, B, C

13. Which of the following statements regarding metabolic acidosis and alkalosis is/are true?

A. Metabolic acidosis results from retention of fixed acid or loss of bicarbonate, causing a rise in the denominator or a fall in the numerator of the Henderson-Hasselbalch equation and leading to a ratio less than 20:1
B. Metabolic alkalosis results from a loss of fixed acid or a gain of bicarbonate, causing an increase in the numerator or a decrease in the denominator of the Henderson-Hasselbalch equation leading to a ratio greater than 20:1
C. In metabolic acidosis and alkalosis, rapid compensation is brought about by pulmonary mechanisms
D. In metabolic acidosis and alkalosis slow compensation occurs via renal mechanisms

Sabiston: 69
Schwartz: 55

Comments: The major effects of metabolic acid-base derangements are on the numerator of the Henderson-Hasselbalch equation. Metabolic acidosis due to retention of fixed acid or loss of bicarbonate causes a fall in the numerator relative to the denominator, with a ratio of less than 20:1 and fall in pH. Conversely, metabolic alkalosis due to loss of fixed acid or gain of bicarbonate causes a relative increase in the numerator to a ratio greater than 20:1 with an associated rise in pH. As opposed to pulmonary acid-base derangements, rapid compensation for metabolic acid-base disturbances is via pulmonary mechanisms. Increased ventilation compensates for metabolic acidosis; decreased ventilation compensates for metabolic alkalosis. In both instances, slow compensation is via renal mechanisms as in respiratory acidosis and respiratory alkalosis.

Answer: A, B, C, D

14. Which of the following statements regarding the metabolism and imbalance of potassium is/are true?

A. Normal dietary intake of potassium is 50 to 100 mEq daily
B. In patients with normal renal function, the majority of ingested potassium is excreted in the urine
C. Over 90% of potassium in the body is located in the extracellular compartment
D. Dangerous hyperkalemia (greater than 6 mEq/l) rarely is encountered if the renal function is normal

For intraabdominal infections*

MEZLIN® IV/IM

mezlocillin sodium

4g q6h

*Due to susceptible strains of indicated pathogens. See indicated organisms in the Brief Summary of Prescribing Information on the back page.

MILES

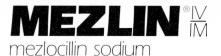

MEZLIN® IV/IM
mezlocillin sodium

MEZLIN®
Sterile mezlocillin sodium
for intravenous or intramuscular use.

BAYPEN®

BRIEF SUMMARY
CONSULT PACKAGE INSERT FOR FULL PRESCRIBING INFORMATION

INDICATIONS AND USAGE
MEZLIN® is indicated for the treatment of serious infections caused by susceptible strains of the designated microorganisms in the conditions listed below:

LOWER RESPIRATORY TRACT INFECTIONS including pneumonia and lung abscess caused by *Haemophilus influenzae*, *Klebsiella* species including *K. pneumoniae*, *Proteus mirabilis*, *Pseudomonas* species including *P. aeruginosa*, *E. coli*, and *Bacteroides* species including *B. fragilis*.

INTRA-ABDOMINAL INFECTIONS including acute cholecystitis, cholangitis, peritonitis, hepatic abscess and intra-abdominal abscess caused by susceptible *E. coli*, *Proteus mirabilis*, *Klebsiella* species, *Pseudomonas* species, *S. faecalis* (enterococcus), *Bacteroides* species, *Peptococcus* species, and *Peptostreptococcus* species.

URINARY TRACT INFECTIONS caused by susceptible *E. coli*, *Proteus mirabilis*, the indole positive *Proteus* species, *Morganella morganii*; *Klebsiella* species, *Enterobacter* species, *Serratia* species, *Pseudomonas* species, *S. faecalis* (enterococcus).

Uncomplicated gonorrhea due to susceptible *Neisseria gonorrhoeae*.

GYNECOLOGICAL INFECTIONS including endometritis, pelvic cellulitis, and pelvic inflammatory disease associated with susceptible *Neisseria gonorrhoeae*, *Peptococcus* species, *Peptostreptococcus* species, *Bacteroides* species, *E. coli*, *Proteus mirabilis*, *Klebsiella* species, and *Enterobacter* species.

SKIN AND SKIN STRUCTURE INFECTIONS caused by susceptible *S. faecalis* (enterococcus), *E. coli*, *Proteus mirabilis*, the indole positive *Proteus* species, *Proteus vulgaris*, and *Providencia rettgeri*; *Klebsiella* species, *Enterobacter* species, *Pseudomonas* species, *Peptococcus* species, and *Bacteroides* species.

SEPTICEMIA including bacteremia caused by susceptible *E. coli*, *Klebsiella* species, *Enterobacter* species, *Pseudomonas* species, *Bacteroides* species, and *Peptococcus* species.

CONTRAINDICATIONS
MEZLIN is contraindicated in patients with a history of hypersensitivity reactions to any of the penicillins.

WARNINGS
Serious and occasionally fatal hypersensitivity (anaphylactic) reactions have occurred in patients receiving a penicillin. These reactions are more apt to occur in individuals with a history of sensitivity to multiple allergens. There have been reports of individuals with a history of penicillin hypersensitivity reactions who have experienced severe hypersensitivity reactions when treated with a cephalosporin. Before therapy with mezlocillin is instituted, careful inquiry should be made to determine whether the patient has had previous hypersensitivity reactions to penicillins, cephalosporins or other drugs. Antibiotics should be used with caution in any patient who has demonstrated some form of allergy, particularly to drugs.

If an allergic reaction occurs during therapy with mezlocillin, the drug should be discontinued. SERIOUS ANAPHYLACTOID REACTIONS REQUIRE IMMEDIATE EMERGENCY TREATMENT. EPINEPHRINE, OXYGEN, INTRAVENOUS STEROIDS, AND AIRWAY MANAGEMENT, INCLUDING INTUBATION, SHOULD BE PROVIDED AS INDICATED.

PRECAUTIONS
Although MEZLIN shares with other penicillins the low potential for toxicity, as with any potent drug, periodic assessment of organ system functions, including renal, hepatic and hematopoietic, is advisable during prolonged therapy. MEZLIN has been reported rarely to cause acute interstitial nephritis.

Bleeding manifestations have occurred in some patients receiving betalactam antibiotics. These reactions have been associated with abnormalities of coagulation tests, such as clotting time, platelet aggregation and prothrombin time and are more likely to occur in patients with renal impairment. Although MEZLIN has rarely been associated with clinical bleeding, the possibility of this occurring should be kept in mind, particularly in patients with severe renal impairment receiving maximum doses of the drug.

MEZLIN has only rarely been reported to cause hypokalemia; however, the possibility of this occurring should also be kept in mind, particularly when treating patients with fluid and electrolyte imbalance. Periodic monitoring of serum potassium may be advisable in patients receiving prolonged therapy.

MEZLIN is a monosodium salt containing only 42.6 mg (1.85 mEq) of sodium per gram of mezlocillin. This should be considered when treating patients requiring restricted salt intake.

As with any penicillin, an allergic reaction, including anaphylaxis, may occur during MEZLIN administration, particularly in a hypersensitive individual.

As with other antibiotics, prolonged use of MEZLIN may result in overgrowth of non-susceptible organisms. If this occurs, appropriate measures should be taken.

Antimicrobials used in high doses for short periods to treat gonorrhea may mask or delay the symptoms of incubating syphilis. Therefore, prior to treatment, patients with gonorrhea should also be evaluated for syphilis. Specimens for dark field examination should be obtained from any suspected primary lesion and serologic tests should be performed. Patients treated with MEZLIN® should undergo follow-up serologic tests three months after therapy.

Interactions with Drugs and Laboratory Tests
As with other penicillins, the mixing of mezlocillin with an aminoglycoside in solutions for parenteral administration can result in substantial inactivation of the aminoglycoside.

Probenecid interferes with the renal tubular secretion of mezlocillin, thereby increasing serum concentrations and prolonging serum half-life of the antibiotic.

High urine concentrations of mezlocillin may produce false positive protein reactions (pseudoproteinurial) with the following methods: sulfosalicylic acid and boiling test, acetic acid test, biuret reaction, and nitric acid test. The bromphenol blue (Multi-stix®) reagent strip test has been reported to be reliable.

Pregnancy Category B
Reproduction studies have been performed in rats and mice at doses up to 2 times the human dose, and have revealed no evidence of impaired fertility or harm to the fetus, due to MEZLIN. There are however no adequate and well controlled studies in pregnant women. Because animal reproductive studies are not always predictive of human response, this drug should be used during pregnancy only if clearly needed. Mezlocillin crosses the placenta and is found in low concentrations in cord blood and amniotic fluid.

Nursing Mothers
Mezlocillin is detected in low concentrations in the milk of nursing mothers, therefore caution should be exercised when MEZLIN is administered to a nursing woman.

ADVERSE REACTIONS
As with other penicillins, the following adverse reactions may occur:

Hypersensitivity reactions: skin rash, pruritus, urticaria, drug fever, acute interstitial nephritis and anaphylactic reactions.

Gastrointestinal disturbances: abnormal taste sensation, nausea, vomiting and diarrhea. If diarrhea persists, pseudomembranous colitis should be considered.

Hematologic and Lymphatic Systems: thrombocytopenia, leukopenia, neutropenia, eosinophilia, reduction of hemoglobin or hematocrit, positive Coombs' test, and hypokalemia.

Abnormalities of hepatic and renal function tests: elevation of serum aspartate aminotransferase (SGOT), serum alanine aminotransferase (SGPT), serum alkaline phosphatase, serum bilirubin. Elevation of serum creatinine and/or BUN.

Central nervous system: convulsive seizures or neuromuscular hyperirritability.

Local reactions: thrombophlebitis with intravenous administration, pain with intramuscular injection.

COMMITTED TO THERAPEUTIC EFFICIENCY

MILES

Miles Inc.
Pharmaceutical Division
400 Morgan Lane
West Haven, CT 06516

Made in Germany

© February 1989, Miles Inc.   Printed in U.S.A.   M09019   MZR-634

Sabiston: 73
Schwartz: 56

Comments: See Question 15.

15. Which of the following statements regarding hyperkalemia is/are true?

A. The signs and symptoms of hyperkalemia are primarily neuromuscular
B. The intravenous administration of sodium lactate, calcium gluconate, and 50% dextrose can produce a rapid fall in serum potassium levels
C. Cation exchange resins administered by rectum are the treatment of choice for a rapid rise in the level of serum potassium
D. Gastrointestinal symptoms in the presence of hyperkalemia should make one suspect concomitant hypercalcemia

Sabiston: 73
Schwartz: 56

Comments: The average daily dietary intake of potassium is 50 to 100 mEq. In patients with normal renal function and normal serum potassium levels, the majority of ingested potassium is excreted in the urine. Over 90% of the body's potassium is within the intracellular compartment at a concentration of 150 mEq/l. Although the total extracellular potassium concentration is only 60 to 70 mEq (4.5 mEq/l), this concentration is critical to cardiac and neuromuscular function. While significant quantities of intracellular potassium are released in response to severe injury, surgical stress, acidosis, and a catabolic state, dangerous hyperkalemia is rarely encountered if renal function is normal. The signs of hyperkalemia are generally limited to the cardiovascular and gastrointestinal symptoms. The gastrointestinal symptoms include nausea, vomiting, intermittent intestinal colic, and diarrhea. Those of the cardiovascular system are electrocardiographic and include high-peaked T waves, a widened QRS complex, and depressed ST segments. These may be seen with potassium concentrations greater than 6 mEq/l. At higher levels of potassium concentration, the T wave may disappear, heart block follows, and diastolic cardiac arrest may ultimately develop. The treatment of hyperkalemia consists of withholding exogenous potassium, correcting the underlying cause, and instituting measures to reduce levels of serum potassium. Sudden rapid rises can be treated with the infusion of sodium lactate, calcium gluconate, and 50% dextrose in water. The dextrose stimulates synthesis of glycogen, resulting in uptake of potassium; the sodium lactate raises pH and shifts potassium intracellularly; the calcium gluconate counteracts the myocardial effects of hyperkalemia. Treatment of slow chronic increases in serum potassium levels can be controlled by the use of cation exchange resins, such as Kayexalate.

Answer: Question 14: A, B, D
Question 15: B

16. Which of the following statements regarding hypokalemia is/are true?

A. Hypokalemia occurs more commonly than does hyperkalemia in the surgical patient

B. Potassium is in competition with hydrogen ion for renal tubular excretion in exchange for sodium
C. Tubular excretion of potassium may be increased when large quantities of sodium are available for resorption
D. The signs of potassium deficit are related to abnormal contractility of skeletal, smooth, and cardiac muscle
E. Intravenous administration of potassium should not exceed 40 mEq/hr without EKG monitoring of the patient

Sabiston: 74
Schwartz: 56

Comments: Surgical patients more frequently encounter hypokalemia than hyperkalemia. This is the result of excessive renal excretion, prolonged administration of potassium-free parenteral fluids, parenteral hyperalimentation with inadequate potassium replacement, and loss of gastrointestinal secretions. Acid-base disturbances that influence potassium metabolism can result in excess excretion. These situations include both respiratory and metabolic alkalosis. In this setting, potassium is in competition with hydrogen ion for renal tubular excretion in exchange for sodium. In alkalosis, the potassium ion is preferentially excreted in an attempt to preserve hydrogen ion. Another setting leading to increased potassium excretion exists when large quantities of sodium are available for resorption from the renal tubule; potassium is exchanged for sodium and the serum levels fall. The loss of gastrointestinal fluids can present a significant cause of potassium depletion. This problem is compounded if potassium-free fluids are used for replacement. Signs of potassium deficit are related to failure of contractility of skeletal, smooth, and cardiac muscle. These include diminished or absent tendon reflexes or weakness that may progress to flaccid paralysis; and there may be paralytic ileus. Sensitivity to digitalis and EKG signs of low voltage, such as flattening of the T waves and suppression of ST segments, are characteristic. The best treatment for hypokalemia is prevention. Gastrointestinal losses should be replaced with fluids containing potassium in quantities sufficient to replace the daily obligatory loss (20 mEq/day) as well as the additional loss related to the volume of gastrointestinal drainage. As general guidelines, no more than 40 mEq of potassium should be added to each liter of intravenous fluid, the rate of administration should not exceed 40 mEq/hour without EKG monitoring, and it is wise to withhold potassium administration to the oliguric patient during the first 24 hours following severe surgical stress or trauma.

Answer: A, B, C, D, E

17. Which of the following statements regarding calcium metabolism is/are true?

A. The normal daily intake of calcium is 1 to 3 gm
B. The majority of dietary calcium is excreted via the urine
C. Nonionized calcium is the portion of serum calcium responsible for neuromuscular stability
D. Unless there is prolonged immobilization, the routine administration of calcium to the surgical patient is not needed in the absence of specific indications

Sabiston: 74
Schwartz: 57

Comments: The body contains approximately 1,000 to 1,200 gm of calcium. Normal daily intake of calcium is between 1 and 3 gm, most of which is excreted by the gastrointestinal tract. Twenty mg or less is excreted in the urine. Approximately half of the normal serum calcium level (9 to 11 mg/ml) is nonionized and bound to plasma protein. An additional 5% of nonionized calcium is bound to other substances in the plasma. The remaining 45% is ionized and is that portion responsible for neuromuscular stability. It is important, therefore, to determine the plasma protein level when assessing serum calcium levels. The ratio of ionized to nonionized calcium is affected by the pH. Acidosis increases the ionized fraction, whereas alkalosis decreases this fraction. The routine administration of calcium to the surgical patient is not needed unless there is a specific indication. An exception is the skeletal loss of calcium resulting in hypocalcemia in those subjected to prolonged immobilization.

Answer: A, D

18. Which of the following statements regarding hypocalcemia is/are true?

A. The symptoms are numbness and tingling of the circumoral region and tips of the fingers and toes
B. The signs are primarily neuromuscular without associated change in the electrocardiogram
C. Symptoms will not occur in a patient with a normal serum calcium level
D. For patients receiving rapid transfusions of blood, calcium should be administered at a dose of 0.2 gm of calcium for each 500 ml of blood transfused.

Sabiston: 75
Schwartz: 57

Comments: The signs and symptoms of hypocalcemia generally are seen at serum levels less than 8 mg per 100 ml. The symptoms include numbness and tingling of the circumoral area and of the tips of the fingers and toes. The signs include hyperactive deep tendon reflexes, positive Chvostek's sign, muscle and abdominal cramps, tetany with carpal pedal spasm, convulsions, and prolongation of the QT interval of the EKG. Symptoms may appear with a normal serum calcium level in patients with severe alkalosis due to a decrease in the physiologically active ionized fraction of the total serum calcium. Conversely, hypocalcemia may be asymptomatic in patients with hypoproteinemia but a normal ionized fraction. Common causes of hypocalcemia include acute pancreatitis, necrotizing fasciitis, renal failure, gastrointestinal fistula, and hypoparathyroidism. Acute symptoms can be relieved by the intravenous administration of calcium gluconate or calcium chloride. Patients requiring prolonged replacement can be treated with oral calcium lactate given with or without vitamin D. Presently, it is felt that the majority of patients receiving blood transfusions do not require calcium supplementation. Citrate binding of ionized calcium is compensated for by mobilization of body stores of calcium. An exception is the patient receiving blood very rapidly (500 ml over 10 minutes). In this setting, calcium should be replaced at a dose of 0.2 grams of calcium per 500 ml of blood trans-

fused. The total dose should not exceed 3 gm unless obvious signs and symptoms of hypocalcemia are present. Under ideal circumstances, calcium replacement should be monitored by measuring the concentration of calcium ion.

Answer: A, D

19. Which of the following statements regarding hypercalcemia is/are true?

A. The symptoms are of gastrointestinal, renal, musculoskeletal, and central nervous system origin
B. The critical level for serum calcium is between 16 and 20 mg per ml
C. The major causes of hypercalcemia are hyperparathyroidism and cancer with bony metastases
D. Metastatic prostate cancer is the most common cause of hypercalcemia related to metastases
E. Intravenous mithramycin is the treatment of choice for rapid reduction of acute hypercalcemia

Sabiston: 75
Schwartz: 58

Comments: The symptoms of hypercalcemia arise from the gastrointestinal, renal, musculoskeletal, and central nervous systems. Early symptoms include fatigability, lassitude, weakness, anorexia, nausea, and vomiting; at higher levels, stupor and coma may develop. Other symptoms may include headaches, back and extremity pain, thirst, polydipsia, and polyuria. The critical serum calcium level for hypercalcemia is between 16 and 20 mg/ml. At this level, prompt treatment must be instituted or the symptoms may progress to death. The two major causes of hypercalcemia are hyperparathyroidism and cancer with bony metastases. Metastatic breast cancer in patients receiving estrogen therapy is the most common cause of hypercalcemia associated with metastases. The goals of treatment in patients experiencing vomiting and polyuria are vigorous volume replacement and intravenous saline lavage combined with furosemide to increase urinary calcium excretion. Oral or intravenous phosphates are useful in reducing hypercalcemia by inhibiting bone resorption and by forming calcium phosphate complexes that are deposited in the soft tissues. Intravenous phosphorus, however, has been associated with the acute development of hypocalcemia, hypotension, and renal failure. Intravenous sodium sulfate is effective, but no more so than is saline diuresis. Corticosteroids decrease resorption of calcium from bone and reduce intestinal absorption and so are useful in treating patients with sarcoidosis, myeloma, lymphoma, or leukemia who have hypercalcemia. Its effects, however, may not be apparent for 1 to 2 weeks. Mithramycin lowers serum calcium in 24 to 48 hours by a direct action on the bones. A single dose may maintain a normal serum calcium level for up to several weeks. Calcitonin can produce a moderate decrease in serum sodium, but the effect is lost with repeated administration. Acute hypercalcemic crisis in hyperparathyroidism is treated by immediate corrective operation.

Answer: A, B, C

20. Which of the following statements is/are true regarding magnesium?

A. The distribution of magnesium is similar to that of potassium
B. The normal dietary intake of magnesium is 240 mg a day, most of which is excreted in the feces
C. Magnesium depletion is characterized by depression of the neuromuscular and central nervous systems
D. Treatment of magnesium deficiency is by the oral administration of magnesium phosphate

Sabiston: 76
Schwartz: 58

Comments: The majority of magnesium in the body is located in the intracellular space, similar in distribution to that of potassium. Plasma levels range between 1.5 and 2.5 mEq/l. Normal dietary intake is 240 mg, most of which is excreted in the feces. The kidneys excrete some magnesium and demonstrate a remarkable ability to conserve magnesium in the face of deficiency. Deficiency is characterized by neuromuscular and central nervous system hyperactivity. Deficiency is known to occur with starvation, malabsorption, protracted losses of gastrointestinal fluid, and prolonged parenteral therapy without proper magnesium supplementation. The signs and symptoms of neuromuscular and central nervous hyperactivity are similar to those of calcium deficiency. Magnesium deficiency is treated by parenteral administration of magnesium sulfate or magnesium chloride. In a patient with normal renal function, up to 2 mEq magnesium/kg of body weight can be given on a daily basis to restore severe depletion. When large doses of magnesium are given, the heart rate, blood pressure, respiration, and EKG should be monitored for signs of magnesium toxicity. The adverse effects of a rapidly rising plasma magnesium level can be countered by infusion of calcium chloride or calcium gluconate. In depleted states, the extracellular concentration can be rapidly restored, but therapy must be continued for 1 to 2 weeks in order to replenish the intracellular component. In order to avoid the development of magnesium deficiency, patients on hyperalimentation should receive 12 to 24 mEq of magnesium daily. Finally, magnesium should not be given to the oliguric patient unless magnesium depletion has actually been demonstrated.

Answer: A, B

21. Which statement(s) is/are true regarding hypermagnesemia?

A. It is most commonly seen in patients with severe renal insufficiency
B. It can occasionally occur in patients with severe alkalosis
C. The acute symptoms can be controlled by intravenous administration of calcium chloride or calcium gluconate
D. Persistent symptoms may be an indication for dialysis

Sabiston: 76
Schwartz: 59

Comments: Symptomatic hypermagnesemia is most commonly seen in patients with severe renal insufficiency. The serum magnesium levels tend to parallel changes in potassium concentration in these cases. The use of magnesium-containing antacids and laxatives can produce symptomatic hypermagnesemia in patients with impaired renal function; therefore they should be avoided. Other causes of symptomatic hypermagnesemia include burns, massive trauma, surgical stress, severe extracellular volume deficit, and severe acidosis. The signs and symptoms include lethargy, weakness, and progressive loss of deep tendon reflexes. The electrocardiographic changes resemble those seen with hyperkalemia. In extreme cases, somnambulance leading to coma and muscular paralysis may occur. Treatment is aimed at correcting any existing acidosis, restoring depleted extracellular volume deficit, and withholding exogenous magnesium. Acute symptoms can be temporarily controlled by the infusion of 5 to 10 mEq of calcium chloride or calcium gluconate. If elevated levels of magnesium or the symptoms persist, peritoneal dialysis or hemodialysis may be required.

Answer: A, C, D

22. Which of the following statements regarding water exchange is/are true?

A. The normal daily consumption of water is 2,000 to 2,500 ml
B. Normal daily losses include 600 ml of insensible loss
C. Excretion of the normal daily products of catabolism requires 500 to 800 ml of urine
D. Insensible loss is mainly from the lungs
E. In the febrile patient, loss by sweating may reach 250 ml per day for each degree of fever

Sabiston: 77
Schwartz: 59

Comments: The average individual has an intake of 2,000 to 2,500 ml of water per day—1,500 ml as fluid and the remainder as that contained in solid food. Daily losses include 250 ml in the stool, 800 to 1,500 ml in urine, and approximately 600 ml as insensible loss. To excrete the products of normal daily catabolism, an individual must produce at least 500 to 800 ml of urine. In the normal individual, 75% of insensible loss is through the skin and 25% is through the lungs. Insensible loss from the skin is by loss of water vapor formed within the body and lost through the skin and not by evaporation of water from sweat glands. In the febrile patient, losses due to sweating may increase to 250 ml per day for each degree of fever. In a patient with a tracheostomy who is ventilated with unhumidified air, insensible loss from the lung may increase to 1,500 ml per day.

Answer: A, B, C, E

23. Which of the following statements regarding gain and loss of salt is/are true?

A. The intake of salt is normally 50 to 90 mEq/day
B. Normal kidneys can reduce sodium loss to less than 1 mEq/day
C. Sweat represents a hypertonic loss of fluids and sodium
D. Gastrointestinal losses are usually isotonic or slightly hypotonic

Sabiston: 77
Schwartz: 60

Comments: Normal daily salt intake varies between 50 and 90 mEq of sodium chloride, with normal kidneys maintaining balance and excreting excess salt as it is encountered. Under conditions of reduced intake or increased extrarenal loss, the kidney can reduce sodium excretion to less than 1 mEq/day. In patients with nonfunctioning kidneys, sodium loss may be as high as 200 mEq/l of urine. ● Sweat represents a hypotonic loss of fluids. The average sodium concentration is between 15 and 60 mEq/l. ● Insensible loss from skin and lungs is pure water. ● Although the different types of gastrointestinal secretions vary in composition, gastrointestinal losses are usually isotonic or slightly hypotonic. Pancreatic fluids are high in bicarbonate concentration; stomach, small intestine, and biliary fluids are relatively high in chloride concentration. Duodenal, ileal, pancreatic, and biliary fluids contain levels of sodium that approximate those seen in the plasma. ● Saliva is relatively high in potassium, a fact important to remember in managing a patient with a salivary fistula.

Answer: A, B, D

24. Match the listed solution with its appropriate composition.

Solution	Composition
A. 0.9% saline	a. 130 mEq sodium, 109 mEq chloride, 28 mEq lactate
B. Lactated Ringer's	b. 154 mEq sodium, 154 mEq chloride
C. M/6 sodium lactate	c. 167 mEq sodium, 167 mEq lactate
D. 5% sodium chloride	d. 1,000 mEq sodium, 1000 mEq lactate
E. M (molar) sodium lactate	e. 513 mEq sodium, 513 mEq chloride
F. 3% sodium chloride	f. 855 mEq sodium, 855 mEq chloride

Sabiston: 78
Schwartz: 61

Comments: See Question 25.

25. A 30-year-old woman weighing 70 kg has symptomatic hyponatremia. Her serum sodium is 120 mEq/l. Her sodium deficit is calculated to be:

A. 500 mEq/l
B. 600 mEq/l
C. 700 mEq/l
D. 800 mEq/l

Sabiston: 80
Schwartz: 62

Comments: In utilizing fluid and electrolyte therapy, the choice of fluids depends on the volume, status, and type of fluid and electrolyte abnormality present. Lactated Ringer's is an excellent isotonic salt solution for replacing gastrointestinal losses and pre-existing volume deficits, if there are no abnormalities in gross composition and concentration, of the lost fluid. Isotonic sodium (0.9% saline) is ideal for the initial correction of depletion of extracellular fluid volume associated with hyponatremia, hypochloremia, and metabolic alkalosis. The high chloride concentration may exceed the capacity of the kidney to excrete it and has the potential to cause a dilutional aci-

dosis. M/6 sodium lactate is an alternative fluid for hyponatremic, hypochloremic states associated with moderate metabolic acidosis. Molar sodium lactate or 3% or 5% sodium chloride may be useful in correcting symptomatic hyponatremic states. The choice of lactate or chloride is dependent on the accompanying acid-base disorder. ● The sodium deficiency is estimated by multiplying the sodium deficit (normal sodium concentration minus observed sodium concentration) by the liters of total body water (60% of body weight in males, 50% of body weight in females). For the patient in question, the calculation is as follows: Total body water = 70 kg × 0.5 = 35 liters. Sodium deficit = (140 − 120 mEq/l) × 35 liters = 700 mEq sodium chloride. Initially, one-half the calculated amount of sodium is infused; the patient should then be reassessed before additional infusion of sodium salt is begun. Care must be take when treating hyponatremia associated with volume excess; in this setting, water restriction is the treatment of choice. If severe symptoms exist, a small amount of hypertonic saline can be given to alleviate symptoms. This, however, has the potential to further expand extracellular intravascular volume and is contraindicated in patients with compromised cardiac reserve. In such a case, peritoneal dialysis or hemodialysis is the preferred treatment to remove excess water.

Answer: Question 24: A–b; B–a; C–c; D–f; E–d; F–e
Question 25: C

26. True or False: Using 5% dextrose in water for rapid correction of severe symptomatic hypernatremia associated with volume deficit may result in convulsions and coma.

Sabiston: 80
Schwartz: 62

Comments: The rapid correction of symptomatic hypernatremia associated with volume deficit by using 5% dextrose in water may lead to rapid reduction in extracellular osmolarity. This has the potential to cause convulsions and coma. It may be safer, therefore, to correct this deficit with half-strength sodium chloride or lactated Ringer's solution. In the absence of significant volume deficit, hypervolemia may result with the injudicious infusion of water. In treating symptomatic hypernatremia, frequent clinical observation and determination of serum sodium concentrations are mandatory.

Answer: True

27. Which of the following statements regarding intraoperative management of fluids is/are true?

A. In a healthy person up to 500 ml of blood loss may be well tolerated without the need for replacement
B. During an operation, the functional extracellular fluid volume is reduced without actual loss of fluid from the body
C. Functional extracellular fluid losses should be replaced with plasma
D. Administration of albumin plays an important role in the replacement of functional extracellular fluid volume loss.

Sabiston: 81
Schwartz: 63

Comments: Functional extracellular fluid volume decreases during major abdominal operations. This is largely the result of sequestered loss into the operative site as a consequence of extensive dissection, collection within the lumen and wall of the small bowel, and accumulations of fluid in the peritoneal cavity. It is generally agreed that this volume loss should be replaced during the course of an operation using isotonic saline solution as a "mimic" for sequestered extracellular fluid. Useful guidelines for replacement include: (1) Blood is replaced as lost regardless of additional fluid therapy. (2) Extracellular fluid losses should be replaced during the operative procedure; delay of replacement until after the operation is complicated by adrenal compensatory mechanisms that respond to operative trauma in the immediate postoperative period. (3) Approximately 0.5 to 1 liter of fluid per hour is needed during the course of an operation, but only to a **maximum** of 2 to 3 liters during a 4-hour procedure, unless there are measurable losses. ● It is now felt that the addition of albumin to blood and extracellular fluid replacement intraoperatively is not indicated and may be potentially harmful. The maintenance of cardiac and pulmonary function by replacement of blood with blood products, and extracellular fluid with "mimic" solutions can be obtained without the addition of albumin. Generally it is felt that blood should be replaced as it is lost. It is usually unnecessary to replace blood loss of less than 500 ml. Operative blood loss is usually underestimated by the operative surgeon by a factor of 15 to 40% less than when isotopically measured, a factor that may contribute to the detection of anemia in the immediate postoperative period.

Answer: A, B

28. Which of the following statements regarding postoperative fluid management is/are true?

A. Insensible loss is approximately 600 ml/day
B. Insensible loss may increase to 1,500 ml/day
C. 800 to 1,000 ml of fluid is needed to secrete the catabolic end-products of metabolism
D. Urine losses should be replaced ml for ml
E. GI losses should be replaced ml for ml
F. In a healthy individual, potassium administration should be approximately 40 mEq/day to replace renal losses and 20 mEq/liter to replace GI losses

Schwartz: 65
Sabiston: 81

Comments: Administration of fluids daily to the postoperative patient begin with an assessment of the patient's volume status and a check for concentration or compositional disorders. All measured and insensible losses should be replaced with appropriate fluids. The amount of potassium given is 40 mEq daily for replacement of renal excretion in addition to 20 mEq/liter for replacement of gastrointestinal losses. Insensible losses usually are constant in the range of 600 ml/day; this can be increased to 1,500 ml/day by hypermetabolism, hyperventilation, or fever. Insensible loss is replaced with 5% dextrose in water. Insensible loss may be offset by an insensible gain of water from excessive tissue catabolism in the postoperative patient requiring prolonged intravenous fluid therapy. Approximately 800 to 1,000 ml/day of fluid is needed to excrete the catabolic end-products of metabo-

lism. Since kidneys are able to conserve sodium in a healthy individual, this can be replaced with 5% dextrose in water. A small amount of salt is usually added, however, to relieve the kidneys of the stress of sodium resorption. If there is a question regarding urinary sodium loss, measurement of urinary sodium will help determine the type of fluid that can best be used. Urine volume should not be replaced milliliter for milliliter, since a high output may represent diuresis of fluids given during operation or the diuresis taking place to eliminate excessive fluid administration. Sensible or measurable losses such as those from the gastrointestinal tract are usually isotonic and therefore should be replaced in equal volumes with isotonic salt solutions. The type of salt solution selected depends upon determinations of serum sodium, potassium, and chloride levels. Generally, replacement fluids are administered at a steady rate over 18 to 24 hours as losses are incurred.

Answer: A, B, C, E, F

29. Which of the following statements regarding volume excess in the postoperative patient is/are true?

A. This situation can be produced by the overadministration of isotonic salt in excess of volume loss
B. Acute overexpansion of the extracellular fluid space is usually well tolerated in healthy individuals
C. Avoidance of volume excess requires daily monitoring of intake and output and determinations of serum sodium concentrations so as to guide accurate fluid administration
D. The earliest sign of volume excess is weight gain
E. Peripheral edema is a reliable sign of volume excess

Schwartz: 66
Sabiston: 83

Comments: The earliest sign of volume excess is weight gain during the catabolic period, when the patient should be losing weight on a daily basis. Circulatory and pulmonary signs of overload appear late and usually represent a massive overload. Peripheral edema does not necessarily indicate volume excess. In a patient with edema but without additional evidence of volume overload, other causes of peripheral edema should be considered. The commonest cause of volume excess in a surgical patient is administration of isotonic salt solutions in excess of volume loss. In a healthy individual this overload is usually well tolerated, but if excess administration of fluid continues for several days, the ability of the kidneys to secrete sodium may be exceeded and hypernatremia may result.

Answer: A, B, C, D

30. Which of the following statements regarding postoperative hyponatremia is/are true?

A. It may easily occur when water is used to replace sodium-containing fluids or when the water given exceeds the water loss
B. In the patient with head injury, hyponatremia despite adequate salt administration usually is due to occult renal dysfunction
C. Cellular catabolism with resultant metabolic acidosis increases cellular release of water and can contribute to hyponatremia

D. Bacterial sepsis may be a cause of hyponatremia
E. Hyperglycemia may be a cause of hyponatremia

Schwartz: 66
Sabiston: 83

Comments: Abnormalities of sodium concentration in the postoperative period usually don't occur if the functional extracellular fluid volume has been adequately replaced during operation. This is because, in the well-balanced patient, the kidneys retain the ability to excrete moderate excesses of water and solute administered in the early postoperative period. Hyponatremia does occur when water is given to replace losses of sodium-containing fluids or when the water given consistently exceeds water loss. • Patients with head injury may develop hyponatremia despite adequate salt administration because of excessive secretion of antidiuretic hormone with resultant increased water retention. • Patients with pre-existing renal disease and loss of concentrating ability may elaborate urine with a high salt concentration. This salt-wasting phenomenon is a problem commonly encountered in elderly patients. Often it is not anticipated since the BUN and creatinine are within normal limits. When there is doubt, determination of urine sodium concentration can help clarify the diagnosis. • Oliguria reduces the daily water requirement and can lead to hyponatremia if not anticipated. • Cellular catabolism in the patient without adequate caloric intake can lead to the gain of significant quantities of water released from the tissues. • Systemic bacterial sepsis is often accompanied by a drop in serum sodium concentration, possibly due to interstitial or intercellular sequestration. It is treated by withholding free water, restoring extracellular fluid volume, and treating the source of sepsis. • Hyperglycemia may produce a depressed serum sodium level by exerting an osmotic force in the extracellular compartment. As a result the serum sodium levels may be diluted. As a general rule each 100 mg/100 ml rise in the blood glucose level above normal is equivalent to a 3 mEq/liter fall in the apparent serum sodium concentration. As an example, the patient with a blood glucose of 500 mg/100 ml has a blood glucose level of 400 mg/100 ml above normal. This is equivalent to a 12 mEq/liter change in the serum sodium level. If, for example, this patient has a measured sodium concentration of 125 mEq/liter, he would have in reality a 137 mEq/liter concentration of sodium if the excess extracellular water were eliminated.

Answer: A, C, D, E

31. Which of the following statements regarding postoperative hypernatremia is/are true?

A. Hypernatremia may indicate a deficit of total body water
B. It may be caused by a high protein intake
C. Replacement of water loss with isotonic salt solutions can produce hypernatremia
D. A common cause is excessive extrarenal water loss

Schwartz: 67
Sabiston: 84

Comments: Hypernatremia can easily be produced when renal function is normal. In surgical patients hyperna-tremia most commonly arises from excessive or unexpected water loss, although it may result from the replacement of water loss with salt-containing solutions. Excessive extrarenal water loss is most often associated with loss of water due to excessive sweating and failure to humidify the air used to ventilate patients with a tracheostomy. Another source of loss is from granulating surfaces, which may be quite significant in the burn patient. Increased renal water loss results from hypoxic damage to the distal tubules and collecting ducts or from loss of antidiuretic hormone secondary to central nervous system injury. High protein intake produces an osmotic load of urea, which necessitates a secretion of large volumes of water. This can be avoided by allowing an intake of 7 ml of water per gram of dietary protein. Finally, isotonic salt solutions can produce hypernatremia if they are used to replace pure water loss.

Answer: A, B, C, D

32. Which of the following statements regarding high-output renal failure is/are true?

A. The condition is characterized by uremia without a period of oliguria and a daily urine output of 1,000 to 1,500 ml/day
B. Management requires serial measurement of blood urea nitrogen, serum electrolytes, and daily fluid outputs
C. Replacement fluid should be administered with sodium chloride to avoid alkalosis
D. Daily maintenance doses of potassium are given intravenously, since hyperkalemia is unlikely to develop because of the high urine output

Schwartz: 67
Sabiston: 84

Comments: High output renal failure is characterized by uremia that occurs without a period of oliguria and is accompanied by a daily urine output greater than 1,000 to 1,500 ml/day. It is managed by monitoring serial measurements of blood urea nitrogen and electrolytes, and the replacement of fluids based on these measurements as well as on accurate daily measurement of fluid output. Because of the kidneys' impaired ability to handle catabolic byproducts, mild metabolic acidosis occurs. Therefore, sodium-containing fluids should be administered as lactate to control this metabolic derangement. Severe acidosis may develop if gastrointestinal or renal losses of sodium are replaced as sodium chloride. Despite the high urine output, potassium salt should not be administered unless a precise dose is calculated on the basis of a measured deficit. As little as 20 mEq of potassium given intravenously may produce myocardial potassium intoxication. If this happens hemodialysis may be required. This type of renal dysfunction can occur in patients subjected to prolonged operative trauma or in patients following trauma who experience one or more episodes of hypotension. If the urine output continues after these episodes one may mistakenly assume normal renal function. It is for this reason that the administration of potassium during the first 24 hours postoperatively should be withheld unless a definite potassium deficit exists.

Answer: A, B

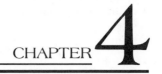

Shock

1. Which one of the following is considered to be the central physiologic event occurring in the various clinical states known as "shock"?

A. Inadequate blood volume
B. Inadequate tissue perfusion
C. Abnormal vascular resistance
D. Diminished cardiac output

Sabiston: 39
Schwartz: 115

Comments: There have been numerous attempts to define "shock." In the various clinical states that produce shock, there may be abnormally low or abnormally high total blood volume, there may be abnormally low or abnormally high vascular resistance, and there may be diminished or excessive cardiac output. Any of these abnormalities may be associated with a state of shock, depending on the status of the other parameters. The central concept of shock revolves around whether or not the circulating blood volume is effective in providing adequate tissue perfusion to permit normal organ function.

Answer: B

2. In which one or more of the following physiologic variables may alterations independently result in a state of shock?

A. Cardiac pumping action
B. Circulating blood volume
C. Arteriolar resistance
D. Venous capacitance

Sabiston: 40
Schwartz: 115

Comments: Shock has been considered in many categories (e.g., cardiogenic, neurogenic, septic, hypovolemic). These are useful considerations as they deal with the proposed etiology of the shock state. It is also useful, however, to consider shock in terms of the physiologic abnormalities that are actually occurring to produce shock. Abnormalities in any of the above physiologic pa-

rameters may produce shock, either independently or in combination. Neurogenic shock, for example, may result from many causes, including spinal trauma, severe pain, or spinal anesthesia; however, its final common pathophysiologic pathway is that of reduced peripheral vascular resistance, leading to a relative hypovolemia as a secondary event. Septic shock may be due to altered myocardial contractility as well as primary vascular events, including increased venous capacitance, decreased peripheral arterial resistance, and peripheral arteriovenous shunting. In such circumstances, the cardiac output may actually be increased. However, the effective circulating volume and tissue perfusion are clearly diminished.

Answer: A, B, C, D

3. Which one or more of the following may be commonly seen as clinical manifestations of shock?

A. Decreased core temperature
B. Apathy
C. Restlessness
D. Thirst
E. Vomiting
F. Diarrhea

Sabiston: 43
Schwartz: 116

Comments: The clinical manifestations of shock are many and varied depending on the etiology and severity of the shock state. The more obvious clinical manifestations relate to the sequelae of decreased circulating volume and include hypotension, tachycardia, and pale, cool skin. A fall in the body's core temperature is also seen, possibly due to a lowered metabolic rate. In the injured patient suffering from hemorrhagic hypovolemia, thirst is commonly seen. Obviously, administration of water by mouth in such circumstances may be quite hazardous. Also, in patients with hemorrhagic hypovolemic shock, one may initially see states of anxiety and restlessness giving way to apathy and somnolence as central nervous system perfusion falls. Nausea and vomiting from hypovolemic shock may be commonly seen. However, diarrhea is uncommon, and in fact intestinal ileus may be a common sequela of shock.

Answer: A, B, C, D, E

4. Which one or more of the following statements regarding the physiology of hemorrhagic or hypovolemic shock is/are correct?

A. A pulse rate of 120 in a patient admitted to the emergency room with a history of recent trauma is highly suggestive of underlying shock
B. Normal blood pressure effectively rules out the presence of shock
C. Blood pressure may initially be normal in a patient suffering from shock, but it may quickly fall to a dangerously low level until the compensatory mechanism of vasoconstriction takes effect
D. Hypotension is a late finding in hemorrhagic shock and suggests that other compensatory mechanisms have failed
E. When the source of bleeding causing hemorrhagic shock is controlled, the fall in hematocrit will stop within 15 minutes

Sabiston: 41
Schwartz: 117

Comments: The body's physiologic response to hemorrhagic or hypovolemic shock involves a complicated interplay of alterations in vascular resistance, heart rate, and blood pressure. In general, blood pressure tends to be maintained until the compensatory mechanisms of vasoconstriction, tachycardia, and shunting of blood are no longer effective. Preservation of blood pressure and flow to the heart and brain frequently occurs at the expense of other organs, such as the kidney and skin, owing to selective changes in local vascular resistance. Tachycardia clearly is a normal physiologic response to hemorrhagic shock; however, it may also be seen in states of pain and anxiety, and therefore is not in itself an indication of underlying shock. The alteration in pulse rate over a period of time of observation is a more reliable indicator of the cardiodynamic state of the patient. Early on in the course of hemorrhagic shock, the patient's hematocrit will probably be normal. According to the Starling hypothesis, a decrease in blood volume will be compensated for by an influx of extravascular fluid into the vascular space, resulting in hemodilution. This takes several hours to occur, and thus the hematocrit is not an accurate reflection of the presence or absence of active hemorrhage.

Answer: D

5. Which one or more of the following biochemical changes may be seen in patients in shock?

A. Negative nitrogen balance
B. Hypokalemia
C. Hyperkalemia
D. Increase in anaerobic metabolism
E. Hyperglycemia

Schwartz: 118

Comments: Shock almost invariably produces stimulation of adrenal medullary output of epinephrine, stimulation of the pituitary-adrenocortical axis, induction of a low flow state, and occasionally specific organ failure. These events in turn result in the relatively common biochemical changes seen in states of hemorrhagic shock. Increased circulating levels of epinephrine and cortisol result in glycogenolysis and frequently a sustained hyperglycemia. Additionally, they cause a change to a catabolic state, resulting in a negative nitrogen balance. The low flow state caused by hypovolemia results in a decreased oxygen delivery to skin and muscle, among other organs, and in an obligatory change in the metabolism of those organs from aerobic to anaerobic. Usually this is associated with a significant metabolic acidosis, due in part to the excess production of lactic acid. One of the compensatory mechanisms in hemorrhagic shock is the renal retention of sodium and water at the expense of increased potassium excretion. However, the intracellular stores of potassium are sufficient that hypokalemia is virtually never seen, even during maximum renal compensation. If hypoperfusion of the kidney persists for any significant length of time, the characteristic biochemical findings of renal failure, including metabolic acidosis and hyperkalemia, will be seen.

Answer: A, C, D, E

6. Which one or more of the following statements accurately characterize(s) fluid shifts that occur during hemorrhagic shock?

A. The loss of intravascular volume is usually fully compensated by movement of extravascular interstitial fluid into the vascular space
B. Intracellular fluid volume decreases as fluid shifts from the intracellular to the extracellular fluid compartment to compensate for the intravascular loss
C. There is movement of interstitial fluid into the intracellular space even though full compensation of intravascular losses has not yet occurred
D. There is a decrease in the transmembrane potential resulting in increased sodium permeability and influx of sodium into the cell

Sabiston: 42
Schwartz: 119

Comments: Numerous experiments on animals and humans have shed some light on the fluid shifts that occur in response to hemorrhagic shock. One of the important compensatory mechanisms in hemorrhagic shock is the movement of interstitial fluid into the intravascular space to compensate for the blood loss. However, full compensation is rarely obtained. Also, it has been found that the interstitial fluid loss exceeds that which passes into the intravascular space. Studies looking into the question of the movement of this interstitial fluid have resulted in the finding that in severe hemorrhagic shock there is an alteration in the transmembrane potential of cells (particularly muscle cells) associated with a decrease in the efficiency of the sodium-potassium pump. As a consequence, there is an increased permeability of the cell membrane to sodium with a subsequent influx of sodium and water into the cell. Thus, in states of hemorrhagic shock, intracellular volume may actually significantly increase at the expense of interstitial volume.

Answer: C, D

7. Which of the following statements is/are true regarding renal function during states of hemorrhagic shock?

A. Like the brain and heart, the kidneys are "favored" organs during hemorrhagic shock, to which adequate blood flow is usually preserved until late in the clinical picture
B. Renal ischemia for as long as 10 minutes will produce irreversible renal damage in most patients
C. Most patients tolerate renal ischemia for up to 100 minutes
D. Alteration in the BUN is as sensitive a measure of renal function as is osmotic, creatinine, or urea clearance
E. Furosemide does not effectively protect against renal failure

Schwartz: 125

Comments: Although the kidneys are clearly "vital" organs, blood flow to the kidneys is quickly diminished in states of hypovolemia and hemorrhagic shock in favor of flow to the brain and heart. Thus, like the skin and liver, compensatory reduction in blood flow to the kidneys is an early finding in hemorrhagic shock. Most kidneys tolerate ischemia for up to 15 minutes with full return of function; beyond 90 minutes of ischemia, virtually all patients will develop irreversible renal damage. There are numerous physiologic parameters that can be followed in monitoring the extent of renal damage sustained during hemorrhagic shock, including urine output, BUN, serum creatinine, and the clearance of creatinine and urea. The BUN does not appear to be a particularly sensitive parameter to follow. It may be normal even in states of significant renal parenchymal loss (e.g., unilaterally nephrectomized patients), or it may rise in response to prerenal azotemia, even though there may be no significant parenchymal renal damage. The clearance of creatinine, urea, and osmotic particles is a more sensitive indicator of renal function. Since these clearances are calculated based on the ratio of urine to plasma concentrations, it takes into account alterations caused by diminished urine output and therefore is a better measure of the physiologic activity of the kidneys. Obviously, the ideal initial management of the renal manifestations of hemorrhagic shock relate to the restoration of a proper effective circulating blood volume. Furosemide (a loop diuretic) alone, while increasing urine flow in many circumstances, is not effective in redistributing blood flow to the renal cortex, and in the absence of effective renal blood flow may worsen renal function by producing hypovolemia.

Answer: E

8. Which one or more of the following may occur in a patient with normal to elevated urine output following hemorrhagic shock?

A. Dehydration
B. Hyperkalemia

C. Progressive azotemia
D. The need for hemodialysis
E. Death due to renal failure

Schwartz: 127

Comments: Although the classic clinical presentation of renal failure is that of oliguria, possibly followed by a diuretic phase, one must recognize that "high-output renal failure" may occur with no antecedent oliguric phase. Excretion of water is only one of the kidney's numerous functions, and the ability to put out large volumes of urine in no way assures the appropriate clearance of solutes. Thus, one may see most of the characteristic findings of oliguric renal failure in the patient with high-output renal failure. The exact mechanism of high-output renal failure is not fully understood but is thought to be an intermediate form of renal failure representing a response to a less severe form of renal injury than that which is required to produce oliguric renal failure. Treatment of high-output renal failure includes providing sufficient water to prevent hypovolemia. Dialysis may be required.

Answer: A, B, C, D, E

9. Which of the following is/are among the major criteria for the diagnosis of adult respiratory distress syndrome (ARDS)?

A. Hypoxemia that is relatively unresponsive to elevations of inspired oxygen concentration
B. Decreased pulmonary compliance
C. Interstitial changes on chest x-ray, which usually precede clinical abnormalities
D. Decreased functional residual capacity
E. Increased dead-space ventilation

Sabiston: 61
Schwartz: 130

Comments: See Question 11.

10. Which one of the following is thought to represent the common pathophysiologic pathway in the adult respiratory distress syndrome?

A. Injury to the surfactant-producing cells of the alveoli
B. Injury to the alveolar-capillary interface
C. Edema of the terminal bronchioles
D. Plugging of the major lobar and segmental bronchi
E. Decompensation of the left ventricular pumping mechanism

Schwartz: 130

Comments: See Question 11.

11. Which of the following may be associated with adult respiratory distress syndrome?

A. Pulmonary infection
B. Aspiration
C. Excessive oxygen administration
D. Pulmonary contusion
E. Microembolization

Sabiston: 61
Schwartz: 132

Comments: The adult respiratory distress syndrome is a form of pulmonary pathology, the exact understanding of which is still in evolution. It may be seen following a number of events, including major trauma, sepsis, and aspiration. Although a number of ventilatory and gas exchange abnormalities coexist in ARDS, the final common pathophysiologic pathway is thought to relate to injury to the alveolar-capillary interface, allowing for intravascular fluid to leak into the interstitium and alveoli, resulting in a diffusion block. The major criteria for the diagnosis of ARDS include hypoxia, which is relatively unresponsive to an increase in the inspired oxygen concentration, decreased pulmonary compliance (stiff lung), decreased functional residual capacity, increased dead-space ventilation, and a diffuse interstitial pattern seen on chest x-ray. Of note is that the clinical and arterial blood gas abnormalities associated with ARDS may occur well before the radiographic changes are appreciated. Similarly, clinical improvement may occur at a time when the radiograph is still grossly abnormal.

Answer: Question 9: A, B, D, E
Question 10: B
Question 11: A, B, C, D, E

12. Which one or more of the following treatment modalities would be appropriate in the management of virtually all cases of ARDS?

A. Mechanical ventilation
B. Moderate-dose loop diuretics
C. PEEP (positive end-expiratory pressure)
D. Steroids
E. Broad-spectrum antibiotics

Sabiston: 61
Schwartz: 135

Comments: Since the principal physiologic problem in ARDS is hypoxemia refractory to increasing FIO_2, the therapy is centered upon the provision of mechanical ventilation. This nearly always includes the application of positive end-expiratory pressure (PEEP) which facilitates the maintenance of open alveoli and the diffusion of oxygen into the pulmonary capillaries. For a given FIO_2, the arterial pO_2 will usually increase upon administration of PEEP in cases of ARDS. Excessive PEEP can be hazardous, as it may result in pneumothorax and cause a decreased venous return to the heart. Diuretics (in cases of obvious fluid overload and cardiac decompensation), and broad-spectrum antibiotics (in the case of established pulmonary infection or other sources of sepsis) may be useful in patients with ARDS. However, their routine use, as well as that of steroids, in the absence of these complicating factors has not been shown to be beneficial and should be avoided.

Answer: A, C

13. Which one or more of the following may have a direct bearing on oxygen transport?

A. Cardiac output
B. Hemoglobin concentration

C. FIO_2
D. Peripheral vascular resistance
E. Blood pressure
F. Alveolar ventilation
G. Acid-base status

Schwartz: 138

Comments: Inasmuch as the fundamental abnormality in all states of shock is tissue hypoxia, it is important to appreciate the factors that play a role in oxygen transport. Considered very simplistically, oxygen gets to tissues by being present in the inspired air (FIO_2), reaching the alveoli and pulmonary capillaries (alveolar ventilation), and being transported in the blood (hemoglobin concentration) that is pumped (cardiac output) to the tissues, where the oxygen is then released to the tissue (oxygen-hemoglobin interaction). Any decrease in cardiac output, hemoglobin concentration, inspired oxygen, or alveolar ventilation and specific changes in the oxyhemoglobin dissociation curve, as may be seen in fluctuating acid-base status, will reduce the oxygen delivery to the tissues. Peripheral vascular resistance and blood pressure clearly play a role in cardiac output and oxygen delivery, albeit a more indirect one.

Answer: A, B, C, F, G

14. Which of the following statements regarding the oxyhemoglobin dissociation curve is/are correct?

A. This is a parabolic curve that describes the affinity of hemoglobin for oxygen
B. P_{50} is defined as the partial pressure of oxygen necessary to provide full hemoglobin saturation in 50% of patients
C. At high oxygen tensions, shifts of the curve have little impact on oxygen saturation of hemoglobin
D. A shift of the curve to the right is considered advantageous as regards oxygen delivery to tissues
E. The position of the curve is a factor in determining (a-v) O_2 difference

Schwartz: 139

Comments: See Question 15.

15. Which one or more of the following clinical states would normally result in a shift of the oxyhemoglobin dissociation curve to the right?

A. Acidosis
B. Increased body temperature
C. Carboxyhemoglobinemia
D. Hypercarbia
E. Increased levels of 2,3-diphosphoglycerate (DPG)

Schwartz: 140

Comments: The oxyhemoglobin dissociation curve is an S-shaped curve that describes the affinity of hemoglobin for oxygen at various oxygen tensions. Because of its shape, extremely high and extremely low oxygen tensions are found along relatively flat portions of the curve, and therefore, shifts of the curve to the right or left in such states of oxygen tension are associated with minimal changes in oxygen saturation. In the more vertical portion of the curve that occurs between oxygen tensions of 20 and 40 mm Hg, even small shifts of the curve to the right or left may be associated with dramatic increases in the affinity of hemoglobin for oxygen. P_{50} is defined as the oxygen tension at which hemoglobin is 50% saturated with oxygen and is therefore useful as a measurement of hemoglobin affinity for oxygen. Shifts of the curve to the right result in an increase in P_{50} and facilitate release of oxygen to the tissues (i.e., for a given oxygen tension, a shift of the curve to the right results in decreased affinity of hemoglobin for oxygen and hence increased delivery of oxygen to the tissues). From the standpoint of oxygen delivery to the tissues, a shift to the right is therefore seen as advantageous. Assuming a relatively normal arterial oxygen tension and saturation, a shift of the curve to the right results in an increased arteriovenous (a-v) O_2 difference (i.e., better extraction of oxygen from the hemoglobin), which would be useful in states of tissue hypoperfusion. Clinical states that shift the curve to the right include acidosis, hyperthermia, hypercarbia, and increased levels of DPG. Shifts of the curve to the left are caused by opposite trends in those parameters as well as the presence of carboxyhemoglobin and methemoglobin, among others.

Answer: Question 14: C, D, E
Question 15: A, B, D, E

16. Which of the following statements regarding fluid therapy in hemorrhagic shock is/are correct?

A. Fresh whole blood is probably the best fluid to be administered in hemorrhagic shock
B. Lactated Ringer's is useful in treating hemorrhagic shock but it must not exceed an administration rate of 500 ml/hour
C. Lactated Ringer's should be avoided in the management of shock, as the lactate present within it worsens the already existing lactic acidosis
D. Albumin is an excellent volume expander when blood is not available because most of it stays within the vascular space for relatively long periods of time
E. Low molecular weight dextran is of use as a volume expander but may be associated with increased bleeding

Sabiston: 44
Schwartz: 144

Comments: When available, properly cross-matched fresh whole blood is the ideal replacement fluid in a patient in hemorrhagic shock. It not only replenishes the intravascular volume, but does so with red blood cells, thereby preserving the oxygen-carrying capacity of the blood. In the absence of type-specific blood, type O Rh negative (preferably with a low anti-A titer) can be administered as the "universal donor" blood. Preparation of blood does require some time, and in the emergent situation when vascular volume must be replenished quickly, lactated Ringer's may be administered at a rate as high as 2,000 ml over a 45-minute period. Failure of the patient to stabilize despite this rapid crystalloid administration is usually a sign of life-threatening, ongoing hemorrhage. Many patients, however, will stabilize for variable periods of time during crystalloid administration, allowing for the proper preparation of type-specific

blood. Although lactic acidosis clearly occurs in states of hypoperfusion, the additional lactate present in lactated Ringer's does not appear to aggravate this metabolic situation. Much work has been done looking at the relative value of other forms of "volume expanders." Albumin has the theoretical advantage of being a protein and therefore more likely to stay within the intravascular space; however, it has been found that it rapidly equilibrates with all of the extracellular fluid compartment and its value as a blood volume substitute is transient. Low molecular weight dextran is probably more effective as a pure volume expander; however, it has been shown to interfere with the clotting mechanism and may worsen the hemorrhage.

Answer: A, E

17. Which of the following routes is the best for the administration of morphine to a patient in severe pain and hypovolemic shock?

A. Subcutaneous
B. Intramuscular
C. Intravenous
D. Oral
E. Per rectum (suppository)

Schwartz: 147

Comments: Perhaps paradoxically, pain is frequently not a problem in patients suffering from hypovolemic shock. When significant pain is present, however, administration of small doses of morphine intravenously is probably the preferred method of management. When narcotics are given by intramuscular or subcutaneous injection in states of hypovolemic shock, they frequently are not absorbed because of the low flow states in those tissues, and thus increasing doses are given in order to provide pain relief. When the patient finally reestablishes an adequate circulating blood volume, there may be a "washout" of the narcotics sitting within the subcutaneous and muscular tissues, resulting in a narcotic overdosage that may be lethal. The intravenous route provides immediate efficacy and is safe providing the patient's respiratory status is being carefully monitored. The oral and rectal routes of administration clearly would be inappropriate.

Answer: C

18. Which of the following statements is/are true regarding the use of vasopressors and vasodilators in the management of hemorrhagic shock?

A. Vasopressors usually result in an elevation of the blood pressure
B. Vasopressors achieve their goal of blood pressure support primarily through inotropic effects
C. Dopamine given in low to moderate doses may provide inotropic and chronotropic support to the heart as well as enhancing renal blood flow
D. In general, the use of vasopressors in hemorrhagic shock is discouraged
E. Vasodilators should be employed early in the management of hemorrhagic shock in order to promote tissue perfusion

Sabiston: 57
Schwartz: 149

Comments: The use of vasopressors in the management of hemorrhagic shock has been somewhat controversial, but the general tendency is toward the avoidance of their use. While they are effective in raising the blood pressure in patients in hemorrhagic shock, they do this primarily through increasing peripheral vascular resistance, which further reduces tissue perfusion (thus aggravating the principal problem in hemorrhagic shock). Different vasopressors work through different mechanisms, depending on their relative alpha and beta stimulating effects. Dopamine is an attractive vasopressor in that it provides beneficial inotropic and chronotropic support to the heart while selectively enhancing renal blood flow through its peripheral beta effects. Even so, dopamine and the other vasopressors should probably be avoided in the initial management of hemorrhagic shock, as the principal deficit is one of effective circulating blood volume and poor tissue perfusion. There is some evidence which suggests that after a proper circulating blood volume has been restored, the positive inotropic and chronotropic effects of vasopressors on the heart may lead to further improvement in the patient's status. Vasodilators have a theoretical advantage of promoting tissue perfusion by reduction of peripheral vascular resistance. However, this would only be appropriate once an effective circulating blood volume has been established, and the use of vasodilators in the initial management of hemorrhagic shock should be avoided.

Answer: A, C, D

19. Match each of the following clinical situations in the left-hand column with the most appropriate treatment listed in the right-hand column.

A. Adequate volume status; hypotension refractory to inotropic agents
B. Distended neck veins; distant heart sounds; equalization of pressures across the myocardium
C. Hypotension, appropriate volume, atrial fibrillation with ventricular response rate of 40
D. Hypotension, low right and left atrial pressures
E. Adequate volume, no mechanical defects, hypotension

a. Inotropic agents
b. Cardiac pacing
c. Pericardiocentesis
d. Fluid administration
e. Intraortic balloon counterpulsation

Sabiston: 46
Schwartz: 150

Comments: Cardiogenic shock may occur as a result of several mechanisms. Before assuming, however, that hypotension is due to a cardiogenic mechanism, one must be sure that there is adequate blood volume. Therefore, a patient who is hypotensive with low right and left atrial pressures should undergo fluid administration as the initial management. If cardiac performance improves with fluid administration, cardiogenic shock is probably not present. If adequate filling pressures are attained and hypotension persists in the absence of mechanical defects,

arrhythmia, and sepsis, a primary pump problem probably exists and should be managed with inotropic agents. One form of cardiogenic shock that may be seen in traumatized patients, in postoperative cardiac patients, and in those suffering from uremia and certain malignancies is cardiac tamponade. This presents clinically with evidence of venous hypertension, and on Swan-Ganz pressure determinations there appears to be a trend toward equalization of pressures in the right and left side of the heart. Appropriate treatment is initial pericardiocentesis to relieve the intrapericardial pressure and allow adequate heart filling. Abnormal heart rate and rhythm may alone produce cardiogenic shock, even if the myocardium contracts normally. Tachyarrhythmias are frequently due to atrial fibrillation or flutter and respond well to digitalis. In the patient who is overdigitalized or hypokalemic, a very low ventricular response rate to atrial fibrillation or flutter may result in hypotension and should be managed with cardiac pacing. When a patient remains in cardiogenic shock despite adequate volume, an appropriate rate, absence of a mechanical or valvular defect, and appropriate administration of inotropic agents, pressure and coronary blood flow support via intraortic balloon counterpulsation may be needed.

Answer: A–e; B–c; C–b; D–d; E–a

20. Which of the following statements regarding neurogenic shock is/are correct?

A. Neurogenic shock tends to be a milder and more easily treatable form of shock than are hypovolemic, cardiogenic, and septic shock
B. Neurogenic shock may be caused by acute gastric dilatation
C. The skin is usually cool and clammy
D. Fluid administration is usually indicated and may be the only treatment needed
E. Vasopressors are absolutely contraindicated in management

Sabiston: 50
Schwartz: 153

Comments: Neurogenic shock has as its final pathophysiologic pathway interference with the balance of vasodilator and vasoconstrictor functions of the arterioles and venules. This may be due to a number of factors, including spinal anesthesia or spinal trauma, sudden onset of severe pain, sudden exposure to unpleasant sights, the hearing of bad news, and the reflux interruption of autonomic impulses that may occur with acute gastric dilatation. What follows these inciting events is a peripheral vasodilatation with peripheral pooling of the blood, resulting in warm, dry skin rather than the cool, clammy skin seen in hypovolemic shock. With sudden peripheral pooling, however, there may be a relative central hypovolemia with decreased venous return and subsequent decreased cardiac output and hypotension. In many instances, such states of neurogenic shock may be self-limiting and may be corrected by removing the patient from the inciting stimulus. Additional forms of management may include fluid administration to restore appropriate venous return and the judicious use of vasoconstrictors (e.g., phenylephrine). In severe circumstances, a proper balance of vasopressor therapy and fluid administration may be warranted.

Answer: A, B, D

21. Of the following positions, which is preferred for the patient suffering from hypovolemic shock?

A. Head down and feet up (Trendelenburg's position)
B. Head up and feet down (reverse Trendelenburg's position)
C. Patient supine with elevation of legs only
D. Left lateral decubitus position
E. Both head and legs elevated (modified semi-Fowler's position)

Schwartz: 146

Comments: Traditional teachings regarding the management of shock have suggested a head-down, feet-up position as the most advantageous in promoting venous return and blood flow to the brain. While this has theoretical advantages, the head-down component of this position probably adds little to the venous "autotransfusion" that occurs simply by virtue of having the legs elevated. Furthermore, in Trendelenburg's position, there is some interference with the mechanics of respiratory exchange. It is generally felt that the patient should be kept in the supine position with the legs elevated. The lateral decubitus position is of value if one is concerned about vomiting and aspiration.

Answer: C

22. Which of the following treatment modalities may be appropriate in the management of a patient in severe septic shock?

A. Multi-drug antibiotic therapy
B. Aggressive volume administration
C. Steroid administration
D. Dopamine
E. Mechanical ventilation

Sabiston: 49, 55
Schwartz: 156

Comments: Of the various forms of "shock," septic shock is probably the most difficult to manage. In many instances, the source of sepsis may not be immediately apparent and therefore the correction of the underlying infectious process may be delayed. Appropriate antibiotic therapy of recognized or presumed infections is obviously central to the ultimate resolution of septic shock. While this is occurring, support of the patient's cardiopulmonary status is frequently warranted. In most cases of septic shock there is a peripheral vasodilatation leading to pooling of the blood volume and a need for aggressive fluid administration initially. Toxins produced in many infections are inhibitory to myocardial contractility, and thus once adequate volume has been achieved, inotropic agents may be warranted. Dopamine is one of the preferred such agents in that it provides inotropic and chronotropic support for the heart while augmenting renal blood flow when given in low to moderate doses. Sepsis is one of the common predisposing factors to the development of adult respiratory distress syndrome (ARDS), and as a consequence many patients in septic shock require mechanical ventilation. The use of pharmacologic doses of corticosteroids is somewhat controversial, but it is generally felt that short-term high-dose steroid therapy carries few risks and may be beneficial to patients who have not responded to initial fluid and antibiotic therapy. It is presumed that the steroid's beneficial effect is due to a stabilization of the cellular and lysosomal membranes, resulting in a protection against the deleterious effects of endotoxin release.

Answer: A, B, C, D, E

CHAPTER 5

Hemostasis and Transfusion

1. True statements regarding normal hemostasis and platelet function include:

A. Vascular disruption is followed by vessel constriction mediated by vasoactive substances released by platelets
B. Platelet adhesion depends on the pre-formation of fibrin monomers
C. Endothelial ADP release stimulates platelet adhesion
D. Heparin inhibits ADP-stimulated platelet aggregation
E. Platelet factor 3 is liberated when platelet aggregates fuse to form a platelet plug

Sabiston: 99
Schwartz: 82

Comments: Three physiologic reactions mediate initial hemostasis: (1) vascular response to injury, (2) platelet activity, and (3) activation of the coagulation cascade. Vasoconstriction independent of platelet participation is the initial response. In seconds, platelets adhere to subendothelial collagen. Adhesion stimulates release of platelet-ADP, which initiates platelet aggregation. This requires calcium and magnesium and is not affected by heparin. The platelets then begin to compact. Traces of thrombin are formed at the platelet surface, resulting in their destruction; the result is a platelet plug. Bleeding time measurements reflect the time it takes to form this plug. During plug formation, platelet factor 3 is released, which is necessary in the coagulation cascade. Platelets also contain platelet factor 4, which neutralizes heparin.

Answer: E

2. True statements regarding drug effects and platelet function include:

A. Vasoconstricting agents such as epinephrine, prostaglandin, PGG_2, PGH_2, and thromboxane A_2 cause platelet aggregation and lower cAMP levels
B. Vasodilators such as PGE_1, prostacyclin (PGI_2), and dipyridamole elevate cyclic AMP and block platelet aggregation

C. Aspirin and indomethacin interfere with platelet release of ADP and inhibit aggregation
D. Furosemide competitively inhibits PGG_2 and platelet aggregation
E. The effect of aspirin is reversible in 2–3 days

Sabiston: 100
Schwartz: 83

Comments: Aspirin and indomethacin are inhibitors of prostaglandin synthesis. They block the formation of PGG_2 and PGH_2 from platelet arachidonic acid and, as a result, inhibit platelet aggregation. The effect of aspirin is irreversible and lasts the 7- to 9-day lifespan of affected platelets. The result clinically is a prolonged bleeding time. Furosemide competitively inhibits ADP-induced platelet aggregation and reduces the response of platelets to PGG_2. Furosemide can also cause thrombocytopenia.

Answer: A, B

3. True statements regarding the coagulation cascade include:

A. The pathways of fibrin formation represent primary hemostasis
B. The extrinsic pathway leads to fibrin formation
C. The intrinsic pathway leads to platelet plug formation
D. Platelets play an important role in the coagulation cascade
E. The events of the intrinsic pathway consume the majority of time needed for blood to clot grossly

Sabiston: 100
Schwartz: 84

Comments: Primary hemostasis is the formation of the platelet plug. Secondary hemostasis, the result of the extrinsic and intrinsic pathways, leads to the formation of fibrin. Their paths join in the activation of Factor X. The intrinsic pathway begins with binding of kininogen and Factor XII to the subendothelial surfaces. Binding converts kininogen to kinin, which activates Factor XII. It, in turn, activates Factor XI, which then activates Factor IX. This step requires calcium. Activated Factor IX complexes with Factor VIII and, in the presence of calcium and platelet factor 3, activates Factor X. These events consume 90% of the time for blood to clot grossly. The extrinsic pathway activates Factor X by the combination of tissue lipoprotein derived from damaged tissue and calcium with Factor VII. Once Factor X is activated, it converts prothrombin (Factor II) to thrombin. This step is accelerated by Factor V, calcium, tissue lipoproteins, and platelet surface phospholipids. Thrombin in turn activates Factor XIII and cleaves fibrinogen (Factor I) to form a fibrin monomer. Activated Factor XIII cross-links these monomers to form a stable clot.

SCHEMATIC VERSION OF THE COAGULATION SYSTEM

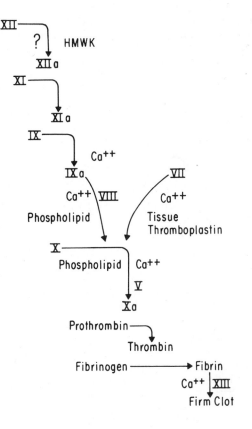

Answer: B, D, E

4. True statements regarding fibrinolysis include:

A. Plasmin is essential to fibrinolysis
B. Plasminogen kinase is the only enzyme that cleaves plasminogen to form plasmin
C. Plasmin acts on only cross-linked fibrin polymers
D. Ischemia is a potent activator of the fibrinolytic system
E. There is no such thing as "physiologic" fibrinolysis

Sabiston: 101
Schwartz: 84

Comments: Plasminogen is converted to plasmin by a number of kinases including blood-borne activators and tissue activators such as vascular endothelium, streptokinase, urokinase, and kallikrein. Ischemia is also a potent stimulator of its activation. Plasmin acts on fibrin, fibrinogen, Factor V, and Factor VIII. Physiologic fibrinolysis is the result of the natural affinity of plasminogen for fibrin. The two join during clot formation and result in locally controlled fibrinolysis. Pathologic fibrinolysis occurs when plasminogen that is free in plasma is activated, resulting in proteolysis of fibrin and other coagulation factors. Unrestrained fibrinolysis can result in bleeding owing to several factors: Small fibrin fragments are capable of interfering with normal platelet aggregation; large fibrin fragments join the clot instead of the normal monomers, producing an unstable clot; destruction of clotting factors other than fibrin contribute to the problem. Human blood and platelets contain antifibrinolytic substances capable of plasminogen inhibition.

Answer: A, D

5. True statements regarding the measurement of bleeding times include:

A. Spontaneous bleeding rarely occurs with platelet counts greater than 40,000
B. The Duke technique measures platelet aggregation in response to exogenous ADP
C. The upper limits of normal for the Ivy bleeding time is 5 minutes
D. Platelet counts greater than 75,000 are usually associated with normal bleeding time and adequate surgical hemostasis.

Schwartz: 86

Comments: Accurate platelet counts can be achieved by light microscopy examination of properly prepared peripheral smears or by electronic counters. Bleeding times can be measured by the Duke technique (using the ear lobe) or the Ivy technique (using the forearm with a proximal tourniquet inflated to 40 mm of mercury). Variability of bleeding time due to variation in the length and depth of the incision can be minimized by using a template or other device that produces a standard, reproducible incision. Normal values are 3.5 minutes for the Duke technique and 5 minutes for the Ivy technique and imply platelet counts of > 75,000. Bleeding time is prolonged in patients with normal platelet counts who have qualitative abnormalities present as a primary disorder or one secondary to uremia and liver disease or who have thrombasthenia (in which platelets fail to aggregate in the presence of ADP). Patients with defective platelets or capillaries, patients with von Willebrand's disease, and those with a history of recent aspirin ingestion also have prolonged bleeding times. Other tests of platelet function include assessment of ADP-stimulated release of platelet factor 4, platelet aggregation, and serotonin release.

Answer: A, C, D

6. Match the items in the two columns (any may be used more than once).

A. Measures function of intrinsic pathway
B. Measures function of extrinsic pathway
C. Detects deficiencies of Factors II, V, VII, X and fibrinogen
D. Detects deficiencies of Factors VIII, IX, XI and XII
E. Preferred method to monitor warfarin (Coumadin) anticoagulation
F. Prolonged by use of heparin

a. Prothrombin time (PT)
b. Partial thromboplastin time (PTT)
c. Both
d. Neither

Sabiston: 104
Schwartz: 86

Comments: The one-stage prothrombin time (PT) measures the events of the extrinsic pathway reflecting the function of Factors II, V, VII, and X and fibrinogen. The PTT screens for intrinsic pathway abnormalities reflecting the levels of Factors VIII, IX, XI, and XII, in addition to Factors II, V, and X. Both tests require comparison with normal control values obtained daily in the laboratory. Even trace amounts of heparin, because of its antithrombin effect, will prolong the PT. At least 5 hours must elapse after the last dose of intravenous heparin before the PT can be reliably interpreted. PT and PTT together can separate deficiencies into the first stage of coagulation or the second stage. A normal PT with an abnormal PTT suggests deficiences of Factors VIII, IX, XI, or XII or fibrin. A prolonged PT with a normal PTT suggests deficiencies of Factors II, V, or VII. The PTT is prolonged by heparin administration and can be used to monitor its efficacy. The PT is the preferred method of controlling anticoagulation with warfarin.

Answer: A–b; B–a; C–a; D–b; E–a; F–c

7. True or False: Thrombin times aid in detecting qualitative abnormalities of fibrin, circulating anticoagulants, and inhibition of fibrin polymerization.

Sabiston: 104
Schwartz: 87

Comments: The thrombin time is a measurement of the clotting time of plasma. In the absence of heparin or the byproducts of fibrinolysis, fibrinogen deficiencies may be detected. Pathologic fibrinolysis causes a prolonged thrombin time as well as rapid whole blood clot dissolution. Whole blood clot dissolution, which normally takes as long as 48 hours, may occur in as little as 2 hours in the face of increased fibrinolysis. An elevated hematocrit and thrombocytopenia may cause false-positive results of whole blood clot dissolution measurements.

Answer: True

8. True statements regarding the evaluation of the bleeding surgical patient include:

A. All wounds, no matter how small, must be evaluated
B. The most common cause of surgical bleeding is thrombocytopenia

C. ε-Aminocaproic acid is an excellent topical hemostatic agent
D. Isolated bleeding from the surgical wound implies poor local hemostasis

Sabiston: 104
Schwartz: 89

Comments: Bleeding from the surgical wound suggests ineffective local hemostasis, particularly if associated wounds (drain sites, tracheostomy wounds, I-V sites) are not bleeding. An exception is isolated bleeding from a resected prostatic bed where prostate-borne plasminogen activators can be activated by urokinase. Activation is inhibited by ε-aminocaproic acid. Blood transfusions can lead to bleeding by a number of mechanisms. Administration of 10 units or more of blood produces thrombocytopenia. Patients bleeding after a large number of blood transfusions should be considered thrombocytopenic and treated as such. Nonetheless, additional evaluation is indicated since an alternative explanation to transfusion-associated bleeding is a hemolytic transfusion reaction. In such an instance, disseminated intravascular coagulopathy is caused by the tissue thromboplastic activity liberated from the stroma of lysed red cells. Extracorporeal circulation may induce hemostatic failure on the basis of thrombocytopenia, inadequate reversal of heparinization, or the overadministration of protamine. Septic surgical patients may bleed because of endotoxin-induced thrombocytopenia. Defibrination and bleeding may occur with meningococcemia, *Clostridium welchii* sepsis, or staphylococcal sepsis. Uncommonly, an operation on tissues rich in fibrinolytic activity, such as the pancreas, liver, or lung, may lead to pathologic fibrinolysis and bleeding.

Answer: A, B, D

9. True statements regarding the assessment of the unsuspected bleeder include

A. The most reliable way to detect unsuspected bleeders is with a platelet count
B. Infants who do not bleed during circumcision have normal hemostatic function
C. An isolated episode of GI bleeding is often associated with generalized hemostatic disorders
D. Intermenstrual bleeding is common in patients with generalized hemostatic disorders
E. The presence of healthy parents and siblings does not exclude the possibility of a primary hemostatic disorder

Schwartz: 88

Comments: No single test to detect the unsuspected bleeder exists. The best way is a complete history and physical examination. Maternal Factor VIII crosses the placenta and protects infants with hemophilia who are circumcised immediately after birth. Only rarely will a patient with a bleeding disorder have tooth extractions or undergo tonsillectomy without encountering a bleeding problem; some patients with severe disease will experience bleeding with tooth eruption. Isolated GI bleeding without any associated non-GI bleeding or bruising is unusual in patients with bleeding disorders. Excessive menstrual flow, rather than intermenstrual bleeding, is common in patients with hemostatic disorders. Because inherited bleeding defects may be autosomal dominant, autosomal recessive, or sex-linked recessive, an inquiry into the family history should include grandparents, uncles, and cousins. A search for ecchymosis or petechiae, particularly near pressure points, is essential. The lesions of hereditary hemorrhagic telangiectasia are found on the lips, beneath the fingernails, and around the anus. Signs of liver disease suggest the presence of acquired deficiency of the prothrombin complex, not a predisposition to primary hemostatic disorders.

Answer: E

10. Match the items in the two columns

Hemostatic Abnormality	Mode of Inheritance
A. Factor XI deficiency (Rosenthal's syndrome)	a. Autosomal dominant
B. Factor X deficiency (Stuart-Prower syndrome)	b. Autosomal recessive
C. Factor V deficiency (parahemophilia)	c. Sex-linked recessive
D. Factor VII deficiency (proconvertin)	
E. Factor I deficiency	
F. Factor IX deficiency (Christmas disease)	
G. von Willebrand's disease (pseudohemophilia)	
H. Hereditary hemorrhagic telangiectasia	
I. Factor VIII deficiency (classic hemophilia)	

Sabiston: 101
Schwartz: 91

Comments: Autosomal dominant genes carrying hereditary disorders may be incompletely penetrant, which can explain why an apparently normal individual may have an offspring with von Willebrand's disease. Similarly, recessive autosomal genes are not necessarily an all-or-none phenomenon. For example, a heterozygote may demonstrate a measurable but clinically insignificant deficiency of Factor X. This variable expression may also be true with sex-linked genes. Occasionally, a female carrying the hemophilia gene will have a measurable, yet clinically insignificant deficiency of Factor VIII.

Answer: A–a; B–b; C–b; D–b; E–b; F–c; G–a; H–a; I–c

11. True statements regarding classic hemophilia include

A. The incidence in the general population is 1:10,000
B. A given patient's Factor VIII level remains constant
C. Muscle compartment bleeds are the most common orthopedic problem
D. Factor VIII component therapy is required before any elective surgery
E. Therapy with cryoprecipitate is free of risk for hepatitis

Sabiston: 101
Schwartz: 91

Comments: Bleeding in hemophiliacs usually appears in early childhood. Hemarthrosis is the most characteristic orthopedic problem. Epistaxis, hematuria, and intracranial bleeding may occur. Equinus contracture, Volkmann's contracture of the forearm, and flexion contracture of elbows or knees are sequelae of these bleeding episodes. Retroperitoneal or intramural intestinal bleeding may produce abdominal symptomatology. The level of Factor VIII depression (which tends to remain stable) determines the tendency to bleed (severe <10%, mild 10–30%). Using component therapy, levels of at least 30% must be achieved to control mild hemorrhage, 50% to control joint and muscle bleeding, and 80–100% to prepare patients for elective surgery. After elective surgery, levels of 30% should be maintained for 2 weeks. Preoperative preparation with cryoprecipitated plasma is preferred over whole plasma to avoid volume overload. Transmission of serum hepatitis, development of anti–Factor VIII antibodies, and development of abnormal platelet functions are possible complications of therapy with Factor VIII.

Answer: A, B, D

12. A 12-year-old boy with known Factor VIII deficiency presents with a painful, swollen, immobile right knee. You suspect a hemarthrosis; therapeutic options include:

A. Immediate aspiration and compression dressings to prevent cartilage necrosis
B. Compression dressings and immobilization to prevent further bleeding
C. Immediate aspiration after appropriate Factor VIII replacement therapy
D. Initial trial of Factor VIII therapy, cold packs, and active range of motion exercises

Sabiston: 101
Schwartz: 92

Comments: Treatment of soft-tissue bleeding is aimed at preventing the complications of an expanding hematoma in an enclosed space. Factor VIII therapy, bed rest, and cold packs constitute the usual initial therapy. Fasciotomy is avoided if possible. The goal of treatment of hemarthrosis is maintenance of range of motion. Aspiration is considered a major risk procedure. Maintenance of active range of motion, Factor VIII therapy, and cold packs often suffice. Intramural, intestinal, or retroperitoneal bleeding is best treated with Factor VIII, rest, and observation. Operation is avoided, if possible.

Answer: D

13. True statements regarding von Willebrand's disease include:

A. It is as common as true or classic hemophilia
B. It is best treated with purified Factor VIII
C. Levels of Factor VIII may vary over time, in a given patient
D. There is an associated platelet abnormality of 70% of patients

Sabiston: 101
Schwartz: 94

Comments: Von Willebrand's disease occurs once in 80,000 births, one eighth as commonly as hemophilia, and is associated with a variable deficiency of Factor VIII and the qualitative failure of platelets to aggregate. Bleeding manifestations are milder than with classic hemophilia. Treatment is with cryoprecipitated plasma, which contains Factor VIII R:WF (von Willebrand factor); purified Factor VIII lacks von Willebrand factor.

Answer: C, D

14. True statements regarding hereditary hemostatic disorders include:

A. Deficiencies of any of the four prothrombin factors (II, V, VII, or X) may be treated with aged plasma
B. Factor VII has the shortest intravascular half-life of any clotting factor
C. Factor IX deficiency is clinically indistinguishable from Factor VIII deficiency
D. Factor V is known as a labile factor
E. Factor XI deficiency is treated with fresh-frozen plasma

Schwartz: 94, 106

Comments: Factor VIII and IX deficiency are clinically indistinguishable. Minimal bleeding in patients with Factor IX deficiency (Christmas disease) can be treated with plasma. Severe bleeding is treated with prothrombin complex concentrates. Their use can be complicated by thrombosis and should be accompanied by prophylactic administration of low-dose heparin. Deficiency of Factor XI (Rosenthal's syndrome) is managed with fresh-frozen plasma. Factor V deficiency must be treated with fresh plasma or fresh-frozen plasma, since its activity is labile and is lost with storage. Factor VII, X (Stuart-Prower), or II deficiencies may be treated with stored plasma. Stored plasma (non–fresh-frozen) is not widely available, so its consideration for use in treatment is mostly theoretical. It is a possible treatment because the relevant factors are not labile at liquid stored temperatures, in contrast to Factors VIII and V, which are labile. Therefore, specific deficiencies of Factor VII, X, or II can be treated with liquid stored plasma if available.

Answer: B, C, D, E

15. True statements regarding acquired hypofibrinogenemia include:

A. Introduction of thromboplastic materials into the circulation is the most common cause of consumptive coagulopathy (DIC)
B. Release of excessive plasminogen activators causes pathologic fibrinolysis
C. Primary fibrinolysis can be differentiated from DIC on the basis of PT, PTT, and results of thrombin time
D. The most important aspect in the treatment of DIC is adequate heparinization

Sabiston: 103
Schwartz: 97

Comments: Consumptive coagulopathy (DIC) results from the introduction of thromboplastic materials into the circulation leading to activation of the coagulation system with secondary "protective" fibrinolysis. Transfusion reactions, hemorrhagic perinatal complications, disseminated cancer, and bacterial sepsis have all been implicated. The release of excessive plasminogen-activating substances leads to primary pathologic fibrinolysis. Shock, hypoxia, sepsis, disseminated prostate cancer, cirrhosis, and portal hypertension are possible causes. Differentiation between the two on laboratory grounds alone is difficult, although the thrombocytopenia of DIC is rarely seen with pure fibrinolysis. With both entities, treating the underlying medical or surgical problem is the most important single step. With DIC, maintenance of a patent microcirculation is important. Active bleeding should be appropriately treated and will not accelerate DIC. Heparin alone is not useful in the treatment of acute DIC. Fibrinolytic inhibitors may be useful in DIC after appropriate heparinization. Giving heparin to patients with primary pathologic fibrinolysis can be very dangerous, as is giving ε-aminocaproic acid to patients with secondary fibrinolysis. Correction of the underlying etiology is the most important part of treatment of DIC.

Answer: A, B

16. True statements regarding polycythemia vera include:

A. Spontaneous thrombosis is a complication of polycythemia vera
B. Spontaneous hemorrhage is a possible complication of polycythemia vera
C. The reason for bleeding is a deficit of platelet function
D. A hematocrit of less than 48% and a platelet count of less than 400,000 is desirable before an elective operation is performed on a patient with polycythemia vera

Schwartz: 99

Comments: An increased viscosity and platelet count and a tendency toward stasis may explain the spontaneous thrombosis seen in patients with polycythemia vera. Patients most likely to bleed are those with platelet counts greater than 1.5 million; it may be due to a qualitative defect in platelet function. When possible, operation should be delayed until the hematocrit and platelet count can be medically reduced. Phlebotomy may help in acute situations. Complication rates as high as 46% have been reported among patients with polycythemia vera undergoing operation. Hemorrhage, thrombosis, and infection are the major complications.

Answer: A, B, C, D

17. True statements regarding anticoagulation include:

A. Coumadin inhibits the production of vitamin K–dependent factors (II, VII, IX, X)
B. Heparin impairs the effect of thrombin on fibrinogen
C. Theoretically, 1.28 mg of protamine neutralizes 1 mg of heparin
D. The effects of vitamin K reversal takes 48 hours
E. A prothrombin time (PT) greater than 50% is considered safe for operation

Schwartz: 100

Comments: With meticulous hemostatic technique, many operations can be performed on patients with a PT of 20%. Exceptions include operations on the eye or the prostate, neurosurgical procedures, or a blind needle aspiration. In these cases, a PT greater than 50% is necessary. In patients who have recently received anticoagulant treatment with Coumadin and who require emergency surgery, vitamin K should be given parenterally, at least 6 hours preoperatively, to reverse the effect of Coumadin on vitamin K–dependent factors.

Answer: A, B, C, E

18. True statements regarding the storage of banked blood include:

A. CPD or CP2D-adenine stored blood kept at 4° C is suitable for transfusion for up to 3 months
B. Platelets in banked blood retain their function for only 3 days
C. Factors II, VII, IX, and XI are stable in banked blood
D. An increase in oxygen affinity occurs in stored blood due to a fall in 2,3-DPG levels
E. There is a significant rate of hemolysis in stored blood

Sabiston: 109
Schwartz: 104

Comments: Whole blood properly collected and stored at 4° C is "good" for 28 days in CPD and 35 days in CP2D adenine. The proportion of cells removed from the circulation within 24 hours of transfusion increases with the time the blood is in storage, reaching about 25–30% at 28 days in CPD (35 days in CP2D-adenine). The cells that survive the first 24 hours have a normal survival; cells can be detected for up to 120 days—the life span of the normal red cell! Red blood cell ATP and 2,3-DPG fall during storage. Factors II, VII, IX, and XI are stable in storage, whereas Factors V and VIII are not. Lactic acid concentrations increase and pH falls during storage. Potassium and ammonia concentrations steadily rise during storage. The citrate used for preservation may reduce plasma ionized calcium if large volumes are transfused. This is especially significant in pediatric patients.

Answer: C, D

19. True or False: A major cross-match compares donor cells with recipient serum, while a minor cross-match compares donor serum with recipient cells.

Schwartz: 104

Comments: Because the development of incompatibilities to "minor" antigens may occur after multiple transfusions, repeat recipient serum samples should be checked with the indirect antiglobulin test every 24 to 48 hours, if multiple transfusions are given.

Answer: True

20. True statements regarding blood components include:

A. Frozen red blood cells maintain their ATP and 2,3-DPG levels

B. Leukocyte and platelet-poor red blood cells are prepared by removal of plasma and the buffy coat
C. Platelets should be transfused within 6 hours of donation
D. Fresh frozen plasma retains Factor V and VII function
E. Dextran solution should not be used in place of plasma in hypovolemic patients

Schwartz: 105

Comments: A number of brief comments can be made: Fresh whole blood should be used within 24 hours of donation, since its platelets remain useful for only the first 6 hours. ● Factors V and VIII remain active through the entire 24 hours. ● Packed frozen red blood cells reduce the danger of volume overload. ● Leukocyte- and platelet-poor red blood cells are used in patients with demonstrated hypersensitivity to white blood cells or platelets and in patients whom you wish to protect from HLA antigen sensitization, such as transplant recipients and chronic transfusion patients. ● The recovery of platelets from a donor is less than 60% efficient. ● Platelet antibodies develop in 20% of patients after 10 to 20 platelet transfusions and can rise to close to 100% as the number of transfusions increases. ● Fresh-frozen plasma is needed for Factors V and VIII. ● Volume expansion with fresh-frozen plasma is rarely indicated. ● Dextran or Ringer's lactate and albumin are preferred for plasma expansion. ● Dextran volume should not exceed 1 liter per day so as to avoid bleeding complications.

Answer: A, B, D

21. True statements regarding hemolytic transfusion reactions include:

A. They are generally caused by ABO and Rh incompatibility
B. Urticaria and pruritus are the most common symptoms
C. Acidification of the urine prevents precipitation of hemoglobin
D. Intravenous diphenhydramine (Benadryl) should be given immediately
E. The laboratory findings include free hemoglobin concentrations greater than 5 mg/100 ml and serum haptoglobin concentrations less than 50 mg/100 ml

Sabiston: 110
Schwartz: 109

Comments: The most common cause of fatal hemolytic transfusion reaction is a clerical error that results in the transfusion of the wrong ABO type blood. Since the severity is proportional to the antigen dose, constant awareness, early recognition, and immediate intervention are important. Hemolytic transfusion reactions lead to the release of vasoactive amines through the activation of complement. This leads to shock, renal ischemia, tubular necrosis, and renal failure proportional to the depth and duration of hypotension. Hemolytic reactions lead to red cell destruction, hemoglobinemia, and hemoglobinuria. Haptoglobin can bind 100 ml of hemoglobin per 100 ml of plasma, but when free hemoglobin concentration exceeds 25 mg/100 ml, it is excreted in the urine and can cause tubular necrosis. Red cell lipid may initiate DIC in 8 to 30% of patients in whom a full unit of mismatched blood has been transfused. However, as little as 10 ml can produce serious hypotension and DIC. Typical signs and symptoms include chills, fever, lumbar and chest pain, pain at the infusion site, and hypotension. In anesthetized patients, diffuse bleeding and continued hypotension suggest the diagnosis. Laboratory criteria for this are hemoglobinuria with free hemoglobin concentrations over 5 mg/100 ml, serum haptoglobin concentrations less than 50 mg/100 ml, and serologic confirmation of incompatibility. Treatment includes stopping the transfusion, insertion of a bladder catheter, and administration of mannitol and bicarbonate to encourage excretion of an alkaline urine. This helps prevent precipitation of hemoglobin in the renal tubules. Should oliguria develop, appropriate fluid management and possibly dialysis are begun. The most important treatment is restoration of blood pressure and renal perfusion. A sample of recipient blood is compared to pre-transfusion samples to confirm incompatibility. The serum bilirubin can be monitored to follow the increase in level of indirect bilirubin caused by hemolysis.

Answer: A, E

22. True statements regarding complications of transfusion include:

A. Allergic reactions are rare
B. Gram-positive organisms are the most common contaminants of banked blood
C. Even small amounts of intravenous air are poorly tolerated
D. Transfusions lasting longer than 8 hours are often accompanied by thrombophlebitis
E. Malaria, Chagas' disease, brucellosis, AIDS, and hepatitis can be transmitted by blood transfusions

Sabiston: 111
Schwartz: 110

Comments: Allergic reactions to transfusion occur once per 100 units given. Fever and urticaria are the usual symptoms; if mild, these symptoms are treated with antihistamines, otherwise with epinephrine and steroids. Although unusual, gram-negative organisms capable of surviving at 4° C are the most common cause of bacterial contamination of banked blood. Air embolus has become rare since bottles have been replaced by collapsible plastic containers. Although air emboli as large as 200 ml may be tolerated by some adults, smaller volumes of air have the potential to cause fatal complications and should be avoided whenever possible. A mill wheel murmer, dizziness, loss of consciousness, and convulsions suggest air embolus. The patient should be placed on the left side with the head down to free the right ventricular outflow tract of air. The incidence of thrombophlebitis is greater when the leg is used for infusion.

Answer: A, D, E

CHAPTER 6

Physiologic Monitoring

1. Ideally, monitoring for surgical patients should include which of the following?

A. Automatic systems independently substituting for surveillance by health professionals
B. Assessment of oxygen transport
C. Central venous pressures (CVP)
D. Continuously recorded fundamental physiologic variables

Schwartz: 485

Comments: While useful adjuncts, monitoring systems can do no more than extend the senses of health-care professionals; close surveillance will remain a requirement for proper care of the surgical patient. Oxygen transport is essential to maintenance of homeostasis and serves as a model of essential physiologic function that ideally should be monitored. On the other hand, central venous pressure monitoring has two drawbacks: it is invasive and it is not reliably related to fundamental physiologic processes. Continuously recorded variables are useful in detecting unanticipated deteriorations as well as trends in physiologic processes. Pulse oximetry seems to satisfy the desire for a monitor capable of showing a trend of a physiologic variable that is practical for most surgical patients.

Answer: B, D

2. Which one of the following mechanisms is the body's most important defense in severe oxygen transport deficiency?

A. Hyperventilation
B. Reduction of oxygen consumption
C. Varying the organ distribution of cardiac output
D. Shift of the oxyhemoglobin dissociation curve

Schwartz: 488

Comments: See Question 3.

3. True statements regarding tissue utilization of oxygen include:

A. The brain requires 15% of the resting cardiac output and 20% of total basal oxygen consumption
B. The kidneys receive 25% of the cardiac output, but can tolerate a reduction to one third of their normal blood flow for up to 1 hour
C. The heart extracts 70% of available oxygen from its arterial supply
D. During acute hypoxia blood is preferentially shunted to the heart and brain
E. Arterial venous oxygen difference is a measure of the extent to which blood flow matches the metabolic demand for oxygen

Schwartz: 489

Comments: Increasing the proportion of cardiac output to satisfy the brain's and the heart's continuous high requirement for oxygen transport is crucial for survival during states of severe oxygen transport deficiency such as cardiac arrest. In general, organs with low oxygen extraction ratios tolerate decreased blood flow well. Since the kidney extracts only 10% of oxygen available in the arterial blood supply, it tolerates decreased blood flow far better than the heart or the brain. Organs other than the heart tend to compensate for decreased blood flow by extracting more oxygen from their blood supply. The extent of this extraction can be estimated by the arterial/venous oxygen content difference. Normally the body consumes only 25% of its total oxygen supply. The normal mixed venous blood is 75% saturated with a partial pressure of oxygen of 40 mm of mercury. These values decrease in response to a fall in cardiac output that can be detected before changes in blood pressure, pulse rate, or central venous pressure are noted. Increased extraction is made possible by the relaxation of precapillary sphincters that enlarge the available capillary beds for oxygen exchange.

Answer: Question 2: C
Question 3: A, B, C, D, E

4. True or False: Partial pressure of oxygen in the atmosphere is the same as that which reaches the alveoli and ultimately appears on the left side of the heart.

Sabiston: 1975
Schwartz: 486

Comments: The partial pressure of oxygen in the atmosphere is 160 mm Hg. As this air is humidified in the upper airways, partial pressure drops to 149 mm Hg owing to the effect of water vapor pressure at body temperature. Ultimately, arterial blood leaves the pulmonary capillaries with an oxygen tension of 100 mm Hg. This is diluted by unsaturated blood from the bronchial and coronary circulation that empties into the left side of the heart. The volume of this shunt is 3% of the output of the right side of the heart and results in an arterial partial pressure of 95 mm Hg as blood enters the left ventricle.

Answer: False

5. True or False: The normal pulmonary capillary bed can tolerate a two- to threefold increase in blood flow without a sacrifice in oxygenation.

Schwartz: 487

Comments: Only 90 ml of the right ventricular output is in the pulmonary capillaries at any one time. It takes approximately 0.8 second for a red blood cell to pass through the alveolar capillaries. As flow rate increases, the time spent in the capillaries is reduced. Only when this time is reduced to below 0.35 second does arterial desaturation occur, a phenomenon known as the "speed shunt."

Answer: True

6. True or False: The alveolar-arterial oxygen gradient "A-aDO$_2$" is useful as an early indicator of incipient respiratory failure.

Sabiston: 1975
Schwartz: 488

Comments: When the inspired oxygen concentration is 100% the normal alveolar-arterial oxygen gradient is 25 to 65 mm Hg. In circumstances causing serious venous admixture, this gradient may be more than 600 mm Hg, resulting in an arterial oxygen tension of 60 mm Hg or less. When arterial oxygen tension falls below 60 mm Hg in a patient without previous lung disease or intracardiac defects, a diagnosis of acute respiratory failure is made. An arterial oxygen tension below 30 mm Hg is incompatible with life if allowed to continue for more than a few hours. Several factors can cause this drop in oxygen tension: perfusion of sections of the lung containing closed or nonventilated airways or alveoli causes shunting of unsaturated blood into the arterial circulation. Injuries to pulmonary capillary endothelium or pulmonary vascular congestion leads to an increased diffusion distance for oxygen as well as collapse of alveoli. Pulmonary surfactant is depleted by the resultant hypoxemia, furthering the insult. As alveoli collapse, lung volume is reduced and there is an accompanying loss of compliance that contributes to further shunting. A number of insults can lead to this series of events, which is commonly known as adult respiratory distress syndrome (ARDS). The use of positive end-expiratory pressure (PEEP) helps correct this deficit by increasing the functional residual capacity of the lung, increasing compliance, and leading to alveolar re-expansion.

Answer: True

7. Which of the following is the most sensitive indication of a falling cardiac output during anesthesia?

A. Pulse rate
B. Central venous pressure
C. Systemic arterial blood pressure
D. Mixed venous oxygen tension

Schwartz: 489

Comments: Mixed venous oxygen tension changes in response to changes in any factor affecting the oxygen supply relative to demand. Decreases in cardiac output have a great influence on oxygen supply during anesthesia. When cardiac output is reduced, maintenance of oxygen consumption is achieved by removal of more oxygen from each milliliter of blood. The oxygen content of end-capillary blood is proportionately reduced within seconds, and the mixed venous oxygen tension reflects that decrease. Alterations in the other parameters listed may cause or be related to decreased cardiac output, but none are as sensitive.

Answer: D

8. Hemoglobin affinity for oxygen is decreased by which of the following?

A. Cooling
B. Diphosphoglycerate
C. Alkalosis
D. Anemia

Schwartz: 489

Comments: See Question 9.

9. The oxyhemoglobin dissociation curve:

A. May be shifted to the left when a patient receives massive transfusions of banked blood
B. May shift to the right, indicating an increase in the affinity of hemoglobin for oxygen
C. May be shifted to the left by hypoxic acidosis
D. May be shifted to the right with carbon monoxide poisoning

Schwartz: 489

Comments: The position of the oxyhemoglobin dissociation curve is determined by its P$_{50}$ value. The partial pressure of oxygen when hemoglobin is half saturated at 37° C, pH 7.4, at one atmosphere of pressure is 26 mm Hg. When the curve is shifted to the right, hemoglobin affinity for oxygen is decreased and oxygen is more easily released (as in the exercising muscle). When the curve is shifted to the left, affinity is increased and oxygen is less likely to be released. A shift to the right is caused by increasing temperature, increasing acidity, increasing carbon dioxide (Bohr effect), and an increase in red cell 2-3-diphosphoglycerate (DPG). This decreased affinity facilitates oxygenation of working muscle, including myocardium. DPG is depleted in banked blood more than 2 weeks old, causing a marked shift to the left. Carbon monoxide displaces oxygen from hemoglobin and becomes tightly bound to it, and shifts the oxyhemoglobin curve to the left.

Answer: Question 8: B
Question 9: A

10. In the healthy individual, the limiting factor of oxygen consumption is:

A. Oxygen delivery to tissue capillaries
B. Availability of cellular oxygen
C. Availability of mitochondrial oxygen
D. Availability of ADP

Schwartz: 491

Comments: Aerobic mitochondrial respiration is a process known as oxidative phosphorylation. The final step of this process involves the passage of two electrons from cytochrome C to an oxygen molecule. This oxygen molecule then combines with hydrogen to form one molecule of water. This is coupled to the conversion of adenosine diphosphate (ADP) to adenosine triphosphate (ATP). When ADP is not available, capillary oxygen is not consumed and it equilibrates with myoglobin, creating a reserve of intracellular oxygen that is released at low oxygen tensions. Normally, the intracellular oxygen tension is 6 mm Hg. Oxygen will not be consumed, a gradient will not be established, and oxygen will not enter the cell unless ADP is available for oxidative phosphorylation, making ADP the rate-limiting factor in the healthy individual. Only at very low mitochondrial oxygen tensions does oxygen delivery to the tissues become rate-limiting.

Answer: D

11. True or False: Arterial pH accurately reflects the intracellular acidosis associated with shock-induced anaerobic metabolism.

Schwartz: 491

Comments: When the oxygen needs of the body are not being met, oxidation of pyruvate is carried out anaerobically, leading to the creation of lactic acid. Acidosis and elevated lactate levels can be detected in arterial blood only if capillary perfusion is sufficient to wash these products into the venous circulation. This is why in some shock states, peripheral arterial pH may not accurately reflect intracellular pH.

Answer: False

12. Proper technique for radial artery cannulation includes:

A. Aseptic insertion technique similar to that employed for central venous cannulations
B. Assessment of the presence of a functioning ulnar collateral supply to the hand
C. Replacement of the catheter every 3 days
D. Intermittent flushing to keep the catheter free of clots

Schwartz: 495

Comments: The radial artery is the site most frequently used for arterial catheters. In the presence of a patent ulnar artery and palmar arterial arch, it is considered a safe and easily accessible site. Therefore, the Allen test, which checks for ulnar collateral flow to the palm, should be performed before radial artery catheterization. Catheters should be inserted using sterile technique and the site protected with a sterile occlusive dressing. The need for intermittent arterial catheter replacement is not established and indeed is controversial. Intermittent manual flushing with as little as 3 ml of fluid has been demonstrated to cause retrograde displacement of emboli from the radial artery cannula to the aortic arch and from there back into the cerebral circulation.

Answer: A, B

13. Regarding central venous pressure monitoring, true statements include:

A. The use of the femoral vein carries a high risk of contamination and thrombophlebitis
B. At the elbow, the cephalic vein is preferred, since it directs the catheter into the subclavian vein without having to negotiate passage at the shoulder
C. In subclavian catheterization, the catheter should never be withdrawn while the needle is in place
D. The safest and most reliable access site is the subclavian vein
E. Regardless of the access site chosen, correct placement of the catheter should always be verified radiographically at the completion of the procedure

Schwartz: 496

Comments: Central venous access sites in order of increasing risk include the median basilic vein, the external jugular vein, the internal jugular vein, and finally the subclavian vein. While the median basilic vein directs the catheter directly into the subclavian vein and superior vena cava, the cephalic vein often presents difficulty where it crosses the shoulder. Ease of access makes the subclavian route popular in emergency situations; it does, however, carry a greater risk of pneumothorax. When a plastic catheter is inserted directly through the access needle, it should never be withdrawn while the needle is in place because of the danger of shearing off the catheter tip. All central venous lines should be checked radiographically for proper position and for presence of pneumothorax (when using the subclavian or jugular access sites) after completion of the procedure.

Answer: A, C, E

14. True statements regarding the measurement of arterial blood gases and alveolar-arterial oxygen tension gradients include:

A. The Clark polarographic oxygen electrode uses a platinum probe to detect current that is proportional to the number of diffusing oxygen molecules
B. The Severinghaus potentiometric carbon dioxide electrode detects changes in pH caused by the diffusion of CO_2

C. Iced arterial blood gas samples suffer a 50% drop in oxygen tension within 1 hour

D. In normal individuals breathing room air, the alveolar-arterial oxygen tension gradient varies between 10 and 15 mm Hg

E. Radiographic changes usually precede abnormalities in the alveolar-arterial oxygen tension gradient

Schwartz: 493

Comments: The development of the Clark and Severinghaus electrodes in the 1950's has made the routine measurement of arterial and venous blood gases a standard procedure in the care of acutely ill patients. Iced heparinized blood samples can be kept for 1 hour with only a 1% drop in oxygen tension. In patients breathing room air, the alveolar-arterial oxygen tension gradient represents an admixture of true shunting of blood as well as desaturation caused by ventilation-perfusion imbalance. On breathing of 100% oxygen, this gradient is caused by true shunting and perfusion of totally nonventilated alveoli, eliminating the effects of alveolar-capillary diffusion barriers and ventilation-perfusion imbalances. On breathing of 100% oxygen, arterial oxygen tension is slightly above 600 mm Hg. An increase in the alveolar arterial oxygen gradient on 100% oxygen is an early warning sign for many pulmonary problems. This increase in gradient usually occurs before radiographic changes are evident.

Answer: A, B, D

15. Noncardiac factors that increase central venous pressure readings include:

A. The transducer being positioned too high
B. Positive-pressure ventilations
C. Vasodilator drugs
D. The transducer being positioned too low

Schwartz: 496

Comments: It is important to consider the pressure around the heart and great vessels when evaluating central venous pressure. This is because any extrinsic compression increases the intraluminal pressures. Normal values for central venous pressure assume normal values for transmural pressures. Thus, central venous pressures are elevated when pleural or mediastinal pressures are elevated, which is the case during positive-pressure ventilation. Correct transducer positioning is essential to central venous pressure measurements, since recording pressure is always the pressure above the transducer. Thus, too high a position would produce an incorrectly low central pressure reading. In general, vasodilators reduce central venous pressure.

Answer: B, D

16. True statements regarding interpretation of central venous pressure or pulmonary capillary wedge pressure measurements include:

A. They are best and most logically used in observing responses to volume and fluid infusion challenges
B. Strict adherence to expected normal values is the best guideline for their use

C. The central venous pressure (CVP) is a reliable index of left ventricular function
D. In the absence of pulmonary disease, the pulmonary capillary wedge pressure (PCw) is a reliable guide to left ventricular end-diastolic pressure
E. If an acceptable wedge position cannot be obtained, the pulmonary artery systolic pressure is an acceptable indicator of left atrial pressure

Sabiston: 2139
Schwartz: 496

Comments: The CVP reflects filling pressures of the right ventricle while the pulmonary capillary wedge pressure reflects filling pressures of the left ventricle. Elevated values reflect an inability of either ventricle to handle venous return. Nonmyocardial factors causing a rise in CVP include mechanical blockage or kinking of the catheter, vasoconstrictor drugs, positive-pressure ventilation, pneumothorax, flail chest, cardiac tamponade, or pulmonary embolism. Nonmyocardial causes of elevated pulmonary capillary wedge pressures include pulmonary vascular disease and mitral valve incompetency. Because of the interposed pulmonary vascular system, the CVP is not always a reliable index of left ventricular function. Left-sided pressures may rise sharply, and pulmonary edema may occur without a significant rise in the CVP. Both measuring devices are best used to assess response to fluid challenges rather than to measure absolute normal values. In the absence of an acceptable wedge position, the pulmonary artery end-diastolic pressure can be an alternative indicator of mean left atrial pressure.

Answer: A, D

17. Which of the following is the most reliable rise of central venous or pulmonary artery wedge pressure (PAw)?

A. PAw less than 5 mm Hg indicating the need for more fluids
B. Central venous pressure (CVP) increasing 5 mm Hg with 100-ml IV fluid bolus, indicating need to curtail fluid administration
C. PAw not increasing at all with 100-ml IV fluid bolus indicating the need for vigorous fluid administration
D. PAw greater than 15 mm Hg indicating the need to curtail fluid administration

Schwartz: 496

Comments: Although each answer could be correct in certain circumstances, only B is generally true. PAw and CVP are best used to attempt to infer venous volume and diastolic cardiac change per volume. A graph of pressure vs. volume is not linear, but markedly concave upward. When large veins are collapsed, volume increases rapidly with little pressure change. Once that "unstressed" volume is filled, further volume increases are impeded by the tensile strength of the elastic wall of the vessel. Therefore, additional "stressed" volume changes (after the vessel is filled) produce large increases in pressure, even when the volume increases are small. Clinically, whenever a small fluid bolus produces a large pressure change, one should beware of possible fluid overload. When no appreciable increase in pressure occurs with a small fluid bolus, one can legitimately infer that the patient is not fluid-overloaded. However, if the patient has adequate vital signs and circulatory function, he may be euvolemic. Therefore, a relatively low PAw may be consistent with euvolemia. Only if the patient is hypotensive, tachycardic, and oliguric (i.e., clinically hypovolemic) in conjunction with a low PAw would vigorous fluid administration be appropriate. Indeed, the most helpful use of a low PAw in a hypovolemic patient is to permit extremely rapid fluid resuscitation without overshooting since it can be relied upon to stay low until the unstressed circulatory volume fills. The PAw measures the intraluminal pressure only. The difference between the intraluminal and extraluminal pressures determines the volume in the unstressed part of the curve. Therefore, the intraluminal volume may be small (hypovolemia) but the pressure measurements appear high as when the extraluminal pressure is increased by the use of PEEP. Consequently, the 100-ml fluid challenge could, and frequently does produce no increase in PAw even when the baseline is elevated. In such a patient who otherwise appears hypovolemic, fluid administration, not curtailment, is appropriate.

Answer: B

18. Pulmonary artery catheters are useful for:

A. Measuring PAw
B. Measuring pulmonary artery (PA) pressures
C. Mixed venous blood sampling
D. Indicator dilution cardiac output determinations

Schwartz: 496

Comments: Pulmonary artery wedge pressure (PAw) is useful for evaluating volume status in conjunction with other clinical data and fluid challenges. Pulmonary artery pressures are useful for quantifying disorders of the pulmonary circulation. The diastolic PA pressure, in the absence of such disorders, approximates the left arterial pressure. As a matter of safety, it is also necessary to monitor the PA waveform continuously to ensure proper position of the PA catheter, because catheters can become displaced during use. Mixed venous blood sampling allows determination of mixed venous Po_2 ($P\bar{v}o_2$), which is a flow-weighted average of total body end-capillary Po_2. As such, this measurement reflects oxygen transport reserve. Measurement of mixed venous oxygen saturation ($S\bar{v}o_2$) allows determination of the intrapulmonary shunt. The use of mixed venous oxygen saturation to determine intrapulmonary shunt can reflect changes in cardiac output even before arterial pressure changes. Cardiac output determinations are central to all cardiopulmonary physiologic assessment. Indeed, the cardiac output appears in the equation of virtually every other cardiorespiratory variable except that for the intrapulmonary shunt.

Answer: A, B, C, D

19. Metabolic monitoring of patients by measurement of muscle surface pH takes advantage of which one or more of the following?

A. Muscle is more sensitive to ischemia than are other tissues

B. Muscle blood flow is reduced before the blood flow of other tissues in response to decreased cardiac output
C. Since they are charged particles, hydrogen ions and lactate are trapped within ischemic muscle cells
D. It is noninvasive

Schwartz: 501

Comments: Muscle is very resistant to hypoxia and returns to normal function promptly, even after hours of tourniquet ischemia. As such, it can be called upon without harm to donate its allotment of cardiac output to defend the central circulation. During ischemia, muscle readily makes use of anaerobic glycolysis to sustain energy levels. Lactate and hydronium are formed and diffuse rapidly into the interstitial fluid where they can be detected. Because bulk blood flow through ischemic muscle is low, local acidosis may not affect arterial pH. Indeed, muscle pH is for that very reason more sensitive than arterial pH for metabolic monitoring.

Answer: B

20. True statements regarding the physiology of blood flow include:

A. Cardiac output is an accurate indicator of myocardial contractility
B. Cardiac output varies directly with pulse rates up to 160 beats per minute
C. The Sarnoff ventricular function curve provides a good evaluation of myocardial contractility
D. Blood pressure is the best indicator of blood flow
E. Pulse pressure can be used as an indirect measure of total peripheral resistance

Schwartz: 488

Comments: Cardiac output alone is not an indicator of myocardial contractility. It is related to **preload** (the degree of muscle fiber stretch present in the ventricles during diastole), **afterload** (systemic vascular resistance, blood pressure, and blood viscosity), and pulse rate. Heart rates above 160 beats per minute do not allow sufficient time for complete ventricular filling, and cardiac output falls. The Sarnoff ventricular function curve plots stroke-work (stroke volume times mean aortic blood pressure) against ventricular end-diastolic pressure. Because it includes consideration of both afterload and preload, it provides a good evaluation of myocardial contractility. Systemic blood pressure varies with the product of total vascular resistance times the cardiac output and is not a direct measurement of blood flow. As total peripheral vascular resistance increases, systolic pressure falls, diastolic pressure rises, and a resultant narrowing of the pulse pressure is seen.

Answer: B, C, E

21. True statements regarding ventilatory mechanics include:

A. The work of breathing at rest consumes 2% of total body oxygen consumption
B. The work of breathing may increase to 50% of total body oxygen consumption in postoperative patients

C. COPD is associated with an increase in the work of breathing due to hindered inspiration
D. Compliance is measured as change in volume divided by change in pressure
E. Airway pressure reflects the compliance of the chest wall and diaphragm as well as that of the lung

Schwartz: 493

Comments: The work of breathing can be markedly increased in postoperative patients because of increased airway resistance and decreased compliance of lung, chest wall, and diaphragm. Patients with COPD have an increased work of breathing due to increased expiratory work. This can be assessed by preoperative pulmonary function testing and optimized by preoperative chest physical therapy, bronchodilators, and antibiotics, if infection is present. The proper use of volume-cycled ventilators can take over most of the work of breathing in the postoperative period. Measuring airway pressure reflects the compliance of the chest wall and diaphragm as well as lungs. In the relaxed patient, this is of little importance, but in restless patients, intraesophageal or intrapleural pressures provide a more accurate measure of compliance. Compliance is defined as the change in pressure associated with each milliliter increase in lung volume. Changes in blood pH and CO_2 tensions reflect changes in a patient's ventilation requirements. The most useful variable in this regard is the end-expiratory carbon dioxide tension.

Answer: A, B, D, E

22. Match the clinical and electrocardiographic findings with the most appropriate drug therapy.

Clinical and EKG Findings

A. Chest pain and dizziness; heart rate 100; blood pressure 140/70.

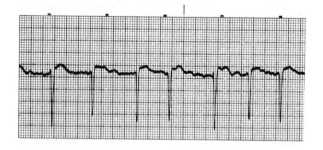

B. Asymptomatic

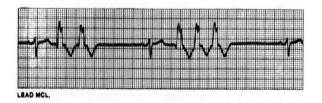

C. Patient confused; heart rate 50; blood pressure 90/65

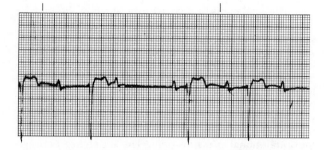

D. Dizziness; heart rate 160; blood pressure 155/70

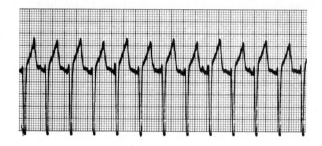

E. Sudden onset of coma

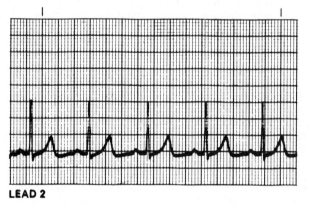

LEAD 2

Drug Therapy

a. Verapamil intravenously
b. Lidocaine
c. Digoxin intravenously, followed by quinidine or procainamide (Pronestyl)
d. Atropine intravenously
e. Quinidine followed by digoxin orally
f. No specific cardiac therapy

Sabiston: 2300, 2389
Schwartz: 465

Comments: A, Atrial fibrillation. The rhythm is irregularly irregular without P waves and narrow QRS complexes. The treatment is intravenous digoxin initially to control the ventricular rate, followed by quinidine or Pronestyl to convert the patient to sinus rhythm. The giving of quinidine first to be followed by digoxin orally is incorrect, since the rate may accelerate with quinidine if digoxin is not given first. Lidocaine and atropine are not used in the treatment of atrial fibrillation. Verapamil is not used as a primary treatment of atrial fibrillation, although it is occasionally used as an adjunct to digoxin for rate control. B, **Ventricular tachycardia.** Isolated premature ventricular contractions may not require treatment; however, runs of more than three beats should prompt a search for treatable causes of arrhythmia. Runs of six beats or more are more significant and can be treated with lidocaine, pending evaluation of potentially treatable causes such as hypokalemia, hypoxia, perioperative myocardial infarction, ischemia, and congestive heart failure. Verapamil, atropine, and digoxin do not have a role in the treatment of ventricular tachycardia. C, **Second degree AV block (Wenckebach or Mobitz type I).** Second degree AV block is characterized by intermittently nonconducted P waves (a P wave without a QRS). This tracing shows gradual PR prolongation followed by a nonconducted P. This prolongation of the PR is characteristic of Mobitz I (or Wenckebach) second degree block. It is most often due to excess vagal tones and responds to treatment with atropine. If the patient is stable hemodynamically (stable blood pressure, no evidence of con-

gestive heart failure, etc.), no treatment is necessary. In this case, however, the low systolic blood pressure and the confusion indicate that therapy is warranted. D, **Supraventricular tachycardia.** A rapid, regular rate with narrow QRS complexes and either absent or retrograde P waves suggests supraventricular tachycardia. Verapamil usually provides rapid conversion to sinus rhythm. The primary side effect is hypotension, which may be managed by placing the patient in a Trendelenburg position or by giving calcium intravenously. Lidocaine and atropine have no role in supraventricular tachycardia. Although digoxin can be used as chronic or subacute therapy, verapamil is superior for immediate conversion. E, The rhythm is **normal sinus** and the patient does not require any specific **cardiac** therapy. However, other causes of coma should be looked for and treated. For example, empiric therapy such as intravenous glucose to treat a possible hypoglycemia or naloxone (Narcan) to treat narcotic overdose might be appropriate. Other causes may be stroke, drug ingestion (intentional or accidental), or respiratory events causing some hypoxia or hypercardia.

Answer: A–c; B–b; C–d; D–a; E–f

CHAPTER 7

Nutrition

1. Which of the following statements regarding body fuel reserves is/are true?

A. Carbohydrates yield approximately 4 kcal/gm of wet weight
B. Protein, carbohydrate, and fat are equivalent energy sources when adjusted for energy available per gram of wet weight
C. The total protein mass is relatively fixed
D. Carbohydrate stores are capable of meeting basal caloric requirements for up to one week

Sabiston: 120
Schwartz: 69

Comments: Protein, carbohydrate, and fat are the three sources of fuel. The total protein mass is relatively fixed, and each gram of protein has a specific function. Therefore, protein loss represents loss of an essential body element. **Protein**, like carbohydrate, is an inefficient energy source relative to its wet weight since it exists in an aqueous environment. Protein stores, therefore, represent a potential source of energy but only at the cost of some essential function. Protein stores present in skeletal muscle and body cell mass represent 30,000 kilocalories of energy. When excess protein is consumed by an individual it is metabolized and stored as a fat. **Carbohydrates**, primarily in the form of liver and muscle glycogen, represent a very small source of energy and can supply basal caloric requirements for less than one day. However, it is an important source of energy in emergency situations during anaerobic glycolysis. As with protein, it is stored with water and yields only 1 or 2 kcal/gm of wet weight. **Fat**, on the other hand, is stored in a relatively anhydrous state and by weight is a rich source of energy, supplying 9 kcal/gm. Most of the fat in the body serves as a readily available energy source. Total fat stores equal 160,000 kilocalories.

Answer: C

2. Which of the following statements regarding starvation is/are true?

A. Carbohydrate stores are the first ones to be consumed
B. During the first several days of starvation 60 to 90 gm of protein per day are utilized
C. Daily obligatory nitrogen loss during starvation is approximately 10 to 15 gm
D. The majority of metabolized protein is converted to glycogen
E. Fat administration during starvation exerts a protein-sparing effect mediated by endogenous release of insulin

Sabiston: 29
Schwartz: 68

Comments: In the first days of starvation, energy needs are supplied by body fat and proteins. There is an obligatory 10 to 15 gm of nitrogen lost daily in the urine. Since each gram of nitrogen represents 6.25 gm of muscle protein, this represents a loss of 60 to 90 gm of protein, the majority of which is derived from skeletal muscle. This protein is converted in the liver to glucose (a process called gluconeogenesis), most of which is used by the brain. Some of this glucose is utilized by red and white cells and converted to lactate and pyruvate, which are then reconverted into glucose in the liver (the Cori cycle). The administration of 100 gm of glucose per day will reduce the nitrogen loss by a significant quantity because of its protein-sparing effect. This effect is regulated by insulin, which reduces the rates of amino acid release from muscle, amino acid extraction by the liver, and gluconeogenesis. During starvation the liver obtains its energy by oxidizing fatty acids to ketones; the rest of the body utilizes fatty acids and ketones to meet caloric requirements. After several days of starvation the brain begins to use fat as its fuel source. Since free fatty acids do not cross the blood-brain barrier, ketoacids that are produced from fatty acids by the liver are used by the brain in place of glucose. The net effect of conversion to ketone metabolism is protein sparing, with reduction of urinary nitrogen to approximately 4 gm/day. These 4 gm represent approximately 25 gm of protein (remember each gram of nitrogen equals approximately 6.25 gm of muscle protein). In addition to insulin, the blood level of alanine plays a role in protein sparing. A fall in the blood level of alanine seems to decrease gluconeogenesis and glucose production by the liver.

Answer: B, C

3. Which of the following statements regarding the metabolic and endocrine events that follow surgery, trauma, or sepsis is/are true?

A. The catabolic phase corresponds to the nitrogen consumption phase seen in simple starvation
B. In the catabolic phase exogenous glucose exerts a protein-sparing effect as during starvation
C. In the catabolic phase the extent of negative nitrogen balance is related to the magnitude of injury
D. After injury the early anabolic phase is characterized by a decline in nitrogen excretion and restoration of appropriate nitrogen balance
E. The late anabolic phase is associated with a gradual return to normal body weight

Sabiston: 34
Schwartz: 69

Comments: The metabolic and endocrine events that follow surgery, trauma, or sepsis can be divided into several phases. The first phase is the catabolic or adrenergic/corticoid phase. Following injury or trauma, metabolic demands and urinary excretion of nitrogen increase beyond levels associated with simple starvation. The effects of the endocrine changes make it impossible for the patient to use exogenous or endogenous fuels effectively to spare protein utilization. Instead, there is an obligatory mobilization of protein in an attempt to provide the energy for gluconeogenesis. Exogenous glucose has little or no effect on the rate of protein catabolism. The extent of negative nitrogen balance in injured patients is related to the magnitude of injury. Total starvation without injury in an adult produces a negative nitrogen balance of 12 gm. This is compared with a 20-gm negative nitrogen balance on day 3 following a rupture of the appendix with peritonitis. After the catabolic phase, the body turns to an early anabolic or corticoid withdrawal phase. This can occur within 3 to 8 days after uncomplicated surgery or after weeks in patients with extensive injury, sepsis, or burn. It is characterized by a sharp decline in nitrogen excretion and restoration of appropriate nitrogen balance. The transition lasts for approximately 2 days and often coincides with diuresis of retained water. After the transition, the early anabolic phase may last from weeks to months depending on the extent of protein loss during the acute period of injury. Positive nitrogen balance reaches a maximum of 4 gm/day, which represents synthesis of 25 gm of protein and a gain of 100 gm of lean body mass (remember, protein is stored in a hydrated form). The late anabolic phase is the final period of recovery from injury and may last from weeks to several months. It is associated with the restoration of adipose stores to levels present before injury. Eventually, normal body weight is restored.

Answer: C, D, E

4. Which of the following statements regarding the assessment of nutritional requirements is/are true?

A. Anthropometric data (weight change, skinfold thickness, and arm circumference over muscle area) are the single most accurate means of predicting nutritional requirements
B. Biochemical data (creatinine excretion, albumin and transferrin levels) are the single most important set of measurements in assessing nutritional requirements
C. Urinary nitrogen excretion is proportional to resting energy expenditure (REE) and can be used to estimate energy requirements
D. REE can be estimated by the equations of Harris and Benedict
E. The energy required for protein synthesis has been estimated as a calorie-to-nitrogen ratio of 100:1 to 150:1 (i.e., 100 to 150 nonprotein calories per gram of nitrogen)

Schwartz: 70
Sabiston: 120

Comments: Nutritional assessment is undertaken to determine the severity of the existing deficiencies and to aid in predicting nutritional requirements. There is no single or fixed combination of findings that accurately assess nutritional status or predict morbidity due to nutritional deficiency. Accurate assessment depends on a careful history (determining the presence of weight loss or of chronic illness), physical examination (looking for loss of muscle and adipose tissue, signs of organ dysfunction, changes in skin or hair, or changes in neuromuscular function), anthropometric data (weight change, skinfold thickness, and arm circumference over muscle area), and biochemical determinations (creatinine excretion, albumin and transferrin levels). The basal elemental requirements for nonstressed depleted patients have been determined and can be found in table form in most surgical texts. These should be used as guidelines when planning nutritional therapy for any given patient. It must be remembered that these guidelines are inadequate for patients who have undergone major surgery or who have suffered major trauma or sepsis. The goal in nutritional therapy is to meet energy requirements for metabolic processes, the maintenance of core temperature, and to allow for tissue repair. These requirements can be measured by indirect calorimetry or estimated from urinary nitrogen excretion, which is proportional to resting energy expenditure (REE). As an example of how this proportionality can be used, elective major surgery is associated with a 24% increase above baseline REE. Basal energy expenditure (BEE) may also be estimated by the equations of Harris and Benedict, which are as follows: BEE (men) $= 66.47 + 13.75$ (W) $+ 5.0$ (H) $- 6.76$ (A) kilocalories per day; BEE (women) $= 65.51 + 9.56$ (W) $+ 1.85$ (H) $- 4.68$ (A) kilocalories per day, where W = weight in kilograms, H = height in centimeters, and A = age in years. These equations estimate the energy requirements for up to 80% of hospitalized patients. Adjustments are made for the degree of trauma or stress present using the same proportionality that relates urinary nitrogen excretion to energy expenditure. In addition to providing for maintenance of baseline metabolic processes, the second objective of nutritional support is to meet the substrate requirements for protein synthesis. In the absence of severe renal or hepatic dysfunction, approximately 0.25 to 0.35 gm of nitrogen per kilogram of body weight should be provided daily. The energy required for protein synthesis is a calorie-to-nitrogen ratio of approximately 100:1 to 150:1 (nonprotein calories per gram of nitrogen). This ratio should be carefully monitored, since deleterious effects of glucose when given in excess include fatty infiltration of the liver.

Answer: C, D, E

5. Which of the following statements regarding amino acid formulations is/are true?

A. Branched-chain amino acids are used to promote muscle protein synthesis
B. The combination of branched-chain amino acids with reduced aromatic amino acid concentrations is used to reduce the incidence of encephalopathy
C. Providing intact essential amino acids or their keto-analogues is useful in the nutritional management of patients with acute renal failure
D. Appropriate use of amino acids supplements eliminates the need for fatty acid supplementation

Schwartz: 71

Comments: There are several amino acid formulations available to manage different clinical situations. Solutions enriched in branched-chain amino acids are used to preserve or enhance muscle protein synthesis. Branched-chain amino acids combined with reduced aromatic amino acid concentrations may reduce the incidence of encephalopathy secondary to hepatocellular dysfunction. Formulations that provide intact, essential amino acids or ketoanalogues of them are proving useful in the nutritional management of patients with acute renal failure. • Patients maintained on either elemental or parenteral hyperalimentation require complete vitamin and mineral supplementation. Many commercial vitamin preparations do not contain vitamin K, and some do not contain vitamin B_{12} or folic acid. These supplements, along with trace minerals and essential fatty acids, must be given to patients receiving long-term intravenous feedings in order to prevent the development of deficiencies.

Answer: A, B, C

6. Which of the following statements regarding the indications for the implementation of nutritional support is/are true?

A. It has been shown that the majority of surgical patients benefit from nutritional supplementation
B. A well-nourished individual having an elective operation optimally requires complete nutritional support after the second postoperative day
C. The parenteral route of administration is the preferred method of nutritional support because of its simplicity and low incidence of complication
D. Unconsciousness and absence of laryngeal reflexes are the major contraindications to nasoesophageal or gastric tube feedings

Sabiston: 124
Schwartz: 72

Comments: The majority of surgical patients do not require special nutritional supplementation. Well-nour-

ished healthy individuals undergoing uncomplicated major surgical procedures have sufficient fuel reserves to withstand the catabolic insult and partial starvation of elective surgery for at least one week. Fluids with appropriate electrolyte composition and a minimum of 100 gm of glucose daily (to minimize protein catabolism) is sufficient in most cases. Accordingly, in an uncomplicated postoperative course, enteral feeding or parenteral hyperalimentation is unnecessary and inadvisable because of the associated risks. Contrariwise, preoperative patients who are chronically debilitated because of their disease or because of malnutrition or patients who have suffered trauma, sepsis, or surgical complications are candidates for specialized nutritional support. Choices for this support include enteral, enteral plus peripheral vein, and central venous routes. The enteral route is generally considered first because of its simplicity, reasonable cost, and relatively low risk of complication. Nasopharyngeal, gastrostomy, or jejunostomy tubes are the usual routes used to provide enteric feedings. Parenteral alimentation is used in patients in whom use of the gastrointestinal tract is not feasible. Tolerance of enteric feedings is determined by the rate of infusion, the osmolarity, and the composition of the fluid administered. A standard approach is to begin with half-strength feedings at a rate of 50 ml/hr and increasing this by 10 to 25 ml/hr each day until the desired volume is reached. Then the concentration is increased slowly to the desired strength. If the route of administration is esophageal or gastric, residual gastric volume must be monitored intermittently to decrease the risk of aspiration. These fluids are best administered by bedside infusion pumps that deliver a constant rate and volume over each 24-hour period. Use of these pumps avoids complications of too rapid delivery and minimizes gastric distension. If abdominal cramping or diarrhea occurs, the rate of administration or the concentration should be decreased. When these symptoms occur with patients being fed by tubes placed distally in the small intestine, intussusception around the tube should be considered as a possible cause of cramping. The main contraindications to the use of nasogastric or gastrostomal tube feedings are unconsciousness and lack of protective laryngeal reflexes. This is true even in patients with a tracheostomy, since feedings can often be recovered during tracheostomy suction; this is evidence of aspiration of gastric contents. Although hyperosmolarity can be a problem with feedings administered into the small bowel, the osmolarity of the administered fluid usually is not a problem if given by a gastric tube in a patient whose pylorus is intact.

Answer: D

7. Which of the following statements regarding jejunal tube feedings is/are true?

A. Unlike nasoesophageal or nasogastric tubes, placement of a jejunal feeding tube requires a laparotomy
B. The Witzel type jejunostomy allows simple reinsertion of the tube at any time should it be removed inadvertently
C. Audible peristalsis must be present before jejunostomy tube feedings can be safely begun
D. The development of diarrhea is an indication to begin parenteral hyperalimentation

E. Refeeding of aspirated gastric juice may cause jejunal irritation and diarrhea

Schwartz: 73

Comments: Feeding by jejunostomy tube is indicated in comatose patients or patients without laryngeal reflex, in patients with high gastrointestinal fistulas or obstruction, and in patients in whom nasoesophageal, nasogastric, or nasojejunal tubes cannot be placed. A laparotomy to place a jejunostomy can sometimes be avoided by passing a mercury-weighted tube through the duodenum to a level past the ligament of Treitz. Occasionally, this positioning can be achieved by fluoroscopic or endoscopic guidance. Jejunostomy requiring laparotomy may be of the Roux-en-Y or of the Witzel type. The Witzel type is accomplished by inserting a feeding tube into the jejunum 12 inches distal to the ligament of Treitz followed by inversion of the jejunum over the tube for approximately 3 cm proximal to the point where it emerges from the bowel. Alternatively a small-bore polyethylene catheter may be placed into the lumen of the jejunum with the point of entry sutured to the anterior abdominal wall. Unless a Roux-en-Y stoma is present, a jejunostomy tube removed inadvertently should not be reinserted if more than a few hours have passed. If reinsertion is attempted, it should be done under fluoroscopic control and the patient observed for signs of peritonitis for 12 to 18 hours after feedings are resumed. After placement of a jejunostomy, feedings can often be safely started 12 to 18 hours postoperatively even in the absence of audible peristalsis. About 85% of jejunostomy patients tolerate their feedings well. Diarrhea often can be controlled by temporarily reducing the concentration and volume of feeding. If diarrhea persists, feeding should be stopped for 24 hours and then resumed (as in the beginning of the feeding regimen discussed in the previous question). If mild diarrhea persists, 8 to 10 drops of tincture of belladonna or a crushed Lomotil tablet can be given through the tube prior to infusion of the formula. Occasionally 5 ml of paregoric before the formula administration is begun may be necessary to control cramping and diarrhea. Proximal small bowel or biliary fistula drainage can be refed into the jejunostomy tube throughout each day. It usually is not possible to refeed more than 2 liters per day. Aspirated gastric juice should not be refed since it may cause jejunal irritation and diarrhea.

Answer: E

8. Match the type of elemental diet listed in the left column with its indication for use listed in the right column.

Elemental Diet	Indicated for Use
A. Carnation Instant Breakfast	a. Useful in severe liver deficiency
B. Meritene	b. Useful in renal failure
C. Ensure	c. For lactose-tolerant patients
D. Isocal	d. For lactose-intolerant patients
E. Vital	e. Hydrolyzed protein content useful where absorption is impaired
F. Vivonex	
G. Amin-Aid	
H. Hepatic Aid	

Sabiston: 126
Schwartz: 74

Comments: Nutritionally complete liquid diets that contain no bulk and produce minimal residue are referred to as chemically defined or elemental diets. They are useful in patients who have a portion of their small bowel available for absorption of simple sugars and amino acids. These supplements are designed to contain baseline requirements of electrolytes, water-soluble and fat-soluble vitamins, and trace minerals. • **Carnation Instant Breakfast** and **Meritene** are derived from milk products and eggs and are designed for oral consumption in lactose-tolerant patients. **Ensure** and **Isocal** contain protein from milk, soybean, or egg; they do not contain lactose, and they are better tolerated in patients with lactose deficiency. **Vital** and **Vivonex** contain protein that is either partially or completely hydrolyzed, which may make absorption of amino acids more efficient in patients with compromised absorptive function. **Amin-Aid** contains essential amino acids and histidine and is useful in patients with renal failure. **Hepatic Aid** is enriched with branched-chain amino acids and deficient in aromatic amino acids and is useful in patients with liver insufficiency. • Most of these preparations contain long-chain fats derived from corn oils, soy oil, or safflower oil. In patients with malabsorption, a diet low in fat or a diet supplemented with medium-chain triglycerides such as Precision-LR and Vital may be useful. When administering these diets to patients with fistulas, additional sodium and potassium may be added to the mixture. Additional fluids to be given intravenously should be considered in patients with high-output fistulas. • The most common complications from the use of elemental diets include nausea, vomiting, and diarrhea. These usually are controlled by decreasing either the rate or the concentration of the mixture being administered. Hypertonic, nonketotic coma can occur if the diets are administered at concentrations above those recommended.

Answer: A–c; B–c; C–d; D–d; E–e; F–e; G–b; H–a

9. True or False. In parenteral alimentation, the source of nonprotein calories and the source of nitrogen can be given at different times without compromising ultimate utilization of nitrogen.

Schwartz: 74

Comments: Parenteral alimentation is the continuous infusion of a hyperosmolar fluid that contains carbohydrates, protein, fats, and other nutrients necessary to maintain metabolic balance. Because of its hyperosmolarity, it is administered into a large vein, preferably the superior vena cava. As stated in Question 4, the calories-to-nitrogen balance must be at least 100 to 150 kcal/gm of nitrogen. The source of nonprotein calories and nitrogen must be given simultaneously, otherwise there is a significant decrease in nitrogen utilization.

Answer: False

10. Which of the following statements regarding the preparation and administration of parenteral hyperalimentation is/are true?

A. The solution should be designed to contain a concentration of 20 to 25% dextrose and 3 to 5% crystalline amino acids
B. Using commercially available kits, these preparations can be reconstituted at the bedside
C. Fatty acid deficiency is clinically apparent as dry, scaly dermatitis and loss of hair
D. Once hyperalimentation is begun, electrolytes should be drawn every day until stable and every 2 to 3 days thereafter
E. Unless the patient is diabetic, blood glucose or urine sugars need not be checked
F. The glucose that is infused with hyperalimentation may cause a shift of potassium from the extracellular to the intracellular space, resulting in hypokalemia

Schwartz: 76

Comments: Parenteral hyperalimentation is indicated in patients who are malnourished or who suffer from severe septic, surgical, or traumatic episodes, and in whom the gastrointestinal tract is unavailable for such use. It should be restated that in severely malnourished or traumatized patients who have functional gastrointestinal tracts, enteral routes for administration of nutrition should be used, if possible. There are several contraindications to the use of hyperalimentation: (1) the lack of a specific goal for patient management or where inevitable death is postponed by the start of hyperalimentation; (2) cardiovascular or metabolic instability requiring control or correction before beginning parenteral hyperalimentation; (3) patients with an accessible, functional gastrointestinal tract; (4) patients in good nutritional status in whom nutritional support is required for a short time; (5) infants with less than 8 cm of small bowel are usually not considered for hyperalimentation, since very few adapt to a point where enteral feedings can replace parenteral nutrition. Solutions today are reconstituted from commercially available kits in the pharmacy under laminar flow conditions. This helps reduce the incidence of bacterial contamination. The final solution carries a concentration of 20 to 25% dextrose and 3 to 5% crystalline amino acids. A patient on hyperalimentation should have vital signs, urinary output, and weight monitored daily. At the start of hyperalimentation, a full complement of biochemical studies and electrolytes should be determined. Electrolytes should be drawn daily until stable, and every 2 to 3 days thereafter. The infusion rate of parenteral hyperalimentation is usually increased over 2 to 3 days until the desired rate is reached. Also, at the start of hyperalimentation, urine glucose levels are checked every 6 hours and the blood sugar concentration is checked daily until stable. If hyperglycemia or glycosuria develops, the dextrose concentration in the administered solution can be decreased, the infusion rate can be slowed, or regular insulin can be added to each bottle. To maintain positive nitrogen balance, an adequate amount of potassium must be administered. Because the uptake of infused glucose requires potassium, this glucose infusion may lead to a shift of potassium from the extracellular to the intracellular space, producing hypokalemia, metabolic alkalosis, and decreased glucose utilization. If glycosuria is detected, therefore, serum potassium levels must be checked. In some cases, glycosuria associated with hypokalemia is best treated by administering potassium rather than insulin. ● Intravenous vitamin preparations (vitamin B complex and ascorbic acid) should be given on a daily basis; vitamin A, vitamin D, vitamin E, thiamine, riboflavin, pyridoxine, niacin, vitamin K, and folic acid should be administered weekly; vitamin B_{12} should be given intramuscularly once monthly. Liver functions, phosphate, magnesium, and coagulation studies should be determined once or twice weekly. ● Periodic infusion of fat emulsions at a rate equal to 4 to 5% of total calories will prevent essential fatty acid deficiency, which is clinically apparent as a dry, scaly dermatitis and loss of hair.

Answer: A, C, D, F

11. Which of the following statements regarding fat emulsions is/are true?

A. They are derived from unsaturated animal fat sources
B. In the nonstressed patient, fat emulsion, dextrose, and amino acid combinations are as effective as dextrose and amino acid solutions
C. Administration of fat emulsion is usually enhanced by premixing with solutions of crystalline amino acids
D. Barring allergic reaction, there is no contraindication to the use of fat emulsions
E. Administration of fat emulsions should be limited to between 2.0 and 2.5 gm/kg of body weight per day

Schwartz: 77

Comments: To avoid the complications of essential fatty acid deficiency during hyperalimentation, fat emulsions should be administered on a regular basis. They are derived from soybean or safflower oils, not animal fat. In nonstressed patients, it appears that a nonprotein calorie source composed of fat emulsion and dextrose is as effective as is dextrose alone. The effectiveness of this combination in the traumatized, hypermetabolic patient is not well documented. Fat emulsions are incompatible with amino acid solutions and cannot be mixed together prior to administration. Therefore, fat emulsions are delivered by separate tubing, joined to the intravenous catheter at skin level using a "Y" connector. Patients with abnormal fat metabolism, lipoid nephrosis, coagulopathy, or serious pulmonary disease should not receive fat emulsions. The infusion rate should be limited to between 2.0 and 2.5 gm/kg of body weight per day.

Answer: B, E

12. Which of the following statements is/are true?

A. The most common and serious complication associated with long-term parenteral hyperalimentation is catheter sepsis
B. Fluid contamination is a rare complication when proper pharmacy techniques are observed
C. The sudden development of glucose intolerance is one of the earliest signs of systemic sepsis
D. Clinically evident thrombophlebitis or thrombosis of the superior vena cava is a relatively uncommon complication
E. Hyperosmolar nonketotic hyperglycemia occurs only in patients with impaired glucose tolerance
F. Abnormality of the serum transaminases, alkaline phosphatase, and bilirubin are uncommon but when

present are indications for the withdrawal of parenteral hyperalimentation

Sabiston: 141
Schwartz: 77

Comments: Most complications associated with parenteral hyperalimentation relate either to catheter placement or to difficulties with fluid administration. The complications of catheter placement include pneumothorax, hemothorax, hydrothorax, subclavian artery injury, air embolism, catheter embolism, and rarely, cardiac perforation with tamponade. If the catheter is placed too far into the atrium, cardiac arrhythmia may occur. One of the most common complications of long-term parenteral hyperalimentation is catheter sepsis. Contamination of the solutions themselves is unusual if proper preparation technique has been used. The sudden development of glucose intolerance is one of the earliest signs of systemic sepsis, arising either from an infected catheter or from some other site. Although catheter infection should be suspected, a complete search for other foci is indicated. If the catheter site looks clean, the catheter may be replaced over a J-wire and the patient observed for 24 to 48 hours. If fever persists, the catheter should be replaced in the opposite subclavian vein or in one of the internal jugular veins. Some advise waiting a day or two before reinserting the catheter. ● Hyperosmolar nonketotic hyperglycemia can develop in patients with impaired glucose tolerance receiving normal rates of infusion. It can also develop in any patient if the parenteral solutions are infused too rapidly. Patients most prone to develop this complication after rapid infusion are those with latent diabetes or those who are in the immediate recovery period following severe stress or trauma. Careful daily observation of fluid balance and frequent determinations of urine and blood sugar levels help avoid this complication. The treatment consists of the administration of insulin, correction of electrolyte abnormalities, and volume replacement. ● It is possible to overfeed the patient maintained on parenteral feeding. Excessive calorie administration may result in carbon dioxide retention and respiratory insufficiency. Hepatic steatosis and glycogen deposition may occur in some patients. It is not unusual to see mild abnormalities of serum transaminases, alkaline phosphatase, and bilirubin in patients receiving parenteral hyperalimentation. These abnormalities should plateau or return to normal over 7 to 14 days. Failure to do so raises the possibility of other causes of these abnormalities.

Answer: A, B, C, D, F

CHAPTER 8

Wound Healing

1. Arrange the following in the sequence of healing of an uncomplicated wound.

A. Epithelialization
B. Inflammation
C. Contraction
D. Collagen synthesis

Sabiston: 194
Schwartz: 300

Comments: The process of wound healing is not a simple sequence of events, but an array of simultaneously oc-curing metabolic and physiologic changes that are initi-ated at the time of injury and continue long after the pro-cess appears to have been completed. The basic processes are similar for sutured wounds, which heal by primary intention, and wounds with tissue loss, which heal by secondary intention. In general terms, the initial event in wound healing is an inflammatory response, which begins almost immediately, followed by epithelia-lization, which begins at 12 to 24 hours. The morphologic changes of wound contraction (a dynamic term), carried out by myofibroblasts, are subsequently noted after 4 or 5 days. Collagen synthesis is biochemically evident by the second to fourth day, but an increase in tensile strength begins around the fourth to sixth day.

Answer: B, A, C, D

2. Wound contraction depends upon:

A. Dehydration of wound tissue
B. Collagen contraction
C. Myofibroblasts
D. Changes in ground substance

Sabiston: 206
Schwartz: 291, 296

Comments: Wound contraction is a characteristic phe-nomenon of the wound healing process that is not en-tirely understood. Nevertheless, experimental evidence suggests that movement of wound edges requires living

cells—in particular, myofibroblasts, which contain con-tractile protein similar to muscle. Experimental observa-tions have disproved the hypothesis that wound dehy-dration is responsible for contraction. Although collagen is a dynamic substance undergoing constant change dur-ing the healing process, contraction is not related to col-lagen content and is not inhibited by suppression of col-lagen synthesis or its cross-linking. Mucopolysaccharide ground substance plays a role in wound healing because of its relation to collagen synthesis and remodeling.

Answer: C

3. Clinical implications of wound contraction include:

A. Proper coaptation of wound edges will prevent con-traction
B. Skin grafting of open wounds will prevent contrac-tion
C. Full thickness skin grafts inhibit contraction more than thin grafts
D. Skin defects on the face or hands of children result in little deformity if allowed to heal by contraction, be-cause of the elasticity of growing skin

Sabiston: 206
Schwartz: 290

Comments: Although the signals that initiate and termi-nate the contraction process have not been fully eluci-dated, wound contraction is a very reproducible biologic phenomenon. It occurs in all wounds and does not al-ways stop immediately with wound closure. Closure of an open wound by skin grafting or with a flap may re-duce the amount of contraction; however, some correc-tion still persists, especially since the process has already started. The cosmetic and functional deformities that may result from contraction of wounds over the face or joints can pose difficult problems and highlight the fact that wound contraction is not merely a biologic phenom-enon without clinical impact. In children, usually there is not an excess of skin to the degree found in older indi-viduals; as a consequence, the accompanying contraction can produce significant distortion, especially in growing structures.

Answer: C

4. Select the true statement(s) about epithelialization.

A. It produces a watertight seal of surgical incisions within 24 hours
B. It contributes significant tensile strength to early wounds
C. It is a process normally inhibited by surface contact with other epithelial cells
D. Occurrence along suture tracks can be prevented by use of absorbable suture material
E. Chronic healing injury in a wound may produce malignancy

Schwartz: 292

Comments: Migration of epithelial cells is one of the earliest events in wound healing. Meticulously coapted surgical incisions seal rather promptly and thus are protected from the external environment; epithelialization of large wounds, of course, requires a longer period of time. Early tensile strength is a result of blood vessel ingrowth, epithelialization, and protein aggregation. If the wound is not under excessive tension, this allows approximation until adequate fibrous protein has been synthesized to provide significant structural strength. The control of the cellular processes in wound epithelialization is not completely understood but appears to involve contact inhibition with similar cells. Certainly, derangements in the control of this process can result in epidermoid malignancy. This has particularly been observed in wounds resulting from ionizing radiation or chemical injury, but can occur in any wound when the healing process has been chronically disrupted, such as in chronic burn wounds or osteomyelitis (Marjolin's ulcer).

Answer: A, C, E

5. Select the true statement(s) regarding the role of collagen in wound healing.

A. Thermal shrinkage temperature and solubility both correlate with age of collagen
B. Collagen synthesis and destruction continues for life
C. There is little quantitative change in collagen after 6 weeks
D. There is no qualitative change in collagen after 6 weeks

Sabiston: 203
Schwartz: 296

Comments: Collagen synthesized by fibroblasts is responsible for the structural integrity of wounds. Collagen synthesis begins by the second to fourth day and collagen content of wound tissue increases rapidly until approximately the 17th day and then more slowly until the 42nd day. After 6 weeks, there is no measurable increase in net collagen content; however, synthesis and turnover is ongoing for life. Historical accounts of sailors with scurvy who developed reopening of previously healed wounds serve to further emphasize this fact. The saline solubility and thermal shrinkage of collagen reflect intra-

molecular and intermolecular cross-links, which are directly proportional to collagen age.

Answer: A, B, C

6. Select the true statement(s) regarding tensile strength of wounds.

A. Tensile strength correlates with collagen content until maximal wound strength is attained
B. Tensile strength increases for 2 years
C. Final strength equals that of unwounded tissue
D. Tensile strength is synonymous with burst strength

Sabiston: 201
Schwartz: 301

Comments: Tensile strength correlates with total collagen content for approximately the first 3 weeks of wound healing. After this time, there is a plateau in the content of collagen, but tensile strength continues to increase as the result of intermolecular bonding of collagen and changes in the physical arrangement of collagen fibers. Although the most rapid increase in tensile strength is early, there is a slow gain for at least 2 years. The ultimate strength, however, never equals that of unwounded tissue. Tensile strength itself is measured as the strength per unit area of tissue; the term burst strength signifies the strength of the entire wound as a whole independent of area.

Answer: B

7. Which of the following is/are associated with inhibition of collagen synthesis?

A. Ascorbic acid deficiency
B. Beta-aminopropionitrile
C. Penicillamine
D. Ehlers-Danlos syndrome

Sabiston: 210
Schwartz: 297

Comments: All of the above agents impair wound healing through different mechanisms. The hydroxylation of proline is a metabolic process unique to collagen synthesis. Proline hydroxylase activity requires ascorbic acid and ferrous iron and is inhibited in their absence. Osteolathyrogens, such as beta-aminopropionitrile and penicillamine, do not inhibit collagen synthesis per se, but impair wound healing by interfering with formation of intramolecular and intermolecular cross-links. There has been limited clinical experience with the use of these agents in situations in which scar formation is undesirable. In one type of Ehlers-Danlos syndrome, failure to cleave terminal ends of the collagen molecule impairs subsequent fibril aggregation.

Answer: A

8. Normal healing is accelerated by which one or more of the following?

A. Ascorbic acid
B. Vitamin A

C. Zinc
D. Increased local oxygen tension
E. Scarlet red

Sabiston: 210
Schwartz: 304

Comments: Surgeons have long sought substances that might accelerate the wound healing process. Increased local oxygen tension stimulates healing; it produces only a 15 to 20% increase in wound strength at 7 days, however, which is not enough to be of clinical significance. Although normal healing requires sufficient quantities of vitamins and minerals such as vitamin C or zinc, greater than physiologic amounts do not improve healing. Vitamin A may prevent the inhibition of epithelialization resulting from steroid therapy, but does not accelerate the normal healing process. It was once thought that scarlet red or other substances incorporated in dressings might stimulate epithelial growth, but they do not.

Answer: D

9. If a patient requires reoperation 1 month after a vertical midline abdominal incision has been made, the most rapid gain in strength of the new incision will occur if:

A. A separate transverse incision is used
B. The midline scar is excised
C. The midline incision is reopened without scar excision
D. Rate of strength gained will not be affected by incision technique

Sabiston: 209
Schwartz: 301

Comments: When a normally healing wound is disrupted after approximately the fifth day and then reclosed, the return of wound strength is more rapid than with primary healing. This is termed secondary healing effect and appears to be due to elimination of the lag phase present in normal primary healing. If skin edges more than about 7 mm around the initial wound are excised, however, this accelerated secondary healing does not occur.

Answer: C

10. Match the following characteristics with the type of skin graft that is most appropriate.

Characteristic	Graft
A. Epidermis only	a. Split thickness skin graft
B. Dermis and epidermis	b. Full thickness skin graft
C. Donor site requires closure	c. Neither
D. Pigmentation and contraction after transfer	d. Both
E. Nourished primarily by nutrient diffusion through graft bed	

Sabiston: 1575
Schwartz: 304

Comments: Split thickness skin grafts involve the entire epidermis and a portion of the dermis; full thickness skin grafts involve the entire epidermis and dermis. Selection of the appropriate type of skin graft for wound coverage must take into consideration the type and location of the wound to be covered as well as available donor sites. When a full thickness skin graft is harvested, the donor site (such as the groin or postauricular region) must be closed. Full thickness grafts are, therefore, usually reserved for smaller wounds, where a more normal final appearance takes precedence. The final appearance of the recipient and donor sites from a split thickness skin graft is determined by the amount of dermis present at each site. The thicker the graft, the less contraction and more normal texture and pigmentation, with split thickness skin grafts developing more pigmentation and contraction than do full thickness grafts. During the first several days after grafting, skin grafts survive by plasmatic imbibition; later both types of free grafts primarily derive their sustenance from capillary ingrowth rather than simple diffusion.

Answer: A–c; B–d; C–b; D–a; E–c

11. Situations in which a full thickness skin graft is preferred to a split thickness skin graft include which one or more of the following?

A. Contaminated wounds
B. Small facial wounds
C. Wounds in an irradiated field
D. Burn wounds
E. None of the above

Schwartz: 305

Comments: In any situation in which a wound is more likely to be compromised by vascular insufficiency, hematoma, or infection, thicker grafts will have a higher rate of failure. Thinner split thickness skin grafts are therefore generally preferred for any situation that may be suboptimal for graft take. In extensive burn injury, multiple grafts are often required from limited donor sites and split thickness skin techniques may increase the availability of donor tissue. For wounds in which the most normal final appearance and less contraction is desired, as in the face or hands, full thickness skin grafts are preferred.

Answer: B

12. The vessels most important to survival of a random pedicle flap are:

A. Epidermal capillary network
B. Epidermal-dermal plexus
C. Subdermal plexus
D. Development of arteriovenous shunts

Schwartz: 307

Comments: Random pedicle flaps maintain vascular connection through their base and are useful when wound coverage requires more tissue than just skin. The subdermal vascular plexus between the dermis and underlying fat is felt to provide the critical blood supply. When flaps are designed, great care must be taken to avoid a flap that has inadequate blood supply at its base. This varies with anatomic location. Utilizing an axial blood supply with specific cutaneous vessels nourishing the flap, longer flaps will survive (e.g., deltopectoral or groin), as will musculocutaneous flaps, which are supplied by the underlying musculature.

Answer: C

13. Delay of random pedicle flaps is useful because it:

A. Increases germinal cells in the dermal layer
B. Stimulates new capillary in-growth at the dermal-subdermal junction
C. Stimulates new vessel in-growth at the base of the flap
D. Increases blood flow through existing vessels

Sabiston: 1577
Schwartz: 307

Comments: Flap delay is a technique by which a planned random pedicle flap is partially elevated at its native site and then resutured into its original position for a period of time prior to actual transfer. This technique improves blood supply of the flap and permits subsequent transfer on a base that may initially have been inadequate. The principle is that reduced blood supply along the distal edges of the flap, probably through metabolic alterations and release of vasoactive amines, increases blood flow through existing vessels at the base.

Answer: D

14. Necrosis of a pedicle flap is usually due to:

A. Arterial thrombosis
B. Venous thrombosis
C. Arterial spasm
D. Venous spasm
E. Trauma from manipulation of a compromised flap

Schwartz: 307

Comments: All flaps must be observed closely following transfer because of possible ischemic compromise, which will produce death of the flap. Initial dusky coloration may be due to venous spasm or excess tension with compromised venous return. Development of a sharp line of color demarcation portends venous thrombosis, which is the most common cause of flap necrosis. Arterial insufficiency is not commonly responsible for flap failure. Complications such as excessive tension, infection, or hematoma can eventually lead to venous thrombosis. Treatment of a seriously compromised flap requires immediate attention and may involve taking down a dressing, removing tight sutures, return of a flap to its donor site, use of heparin, aspirin, or low molecular weight dextran, and (experimentally) use of hyperbaric oxygen.

Answer: B

15. Scar revision:

A. Should be performed within 3 months to minimize fibrosis
B. Should be performed earlier in children than in adults
C. Corrects undesirable pigmentation
D. Should be delayed approximately 1 year to allow for maturation

Schwartz: 303

Comments: Changes in pliability, pigmentation, and configuration of a scar are known as scar maturation. This continues for many months following an incision, and it is generally recommended that revision should not be carried out for approximately 12–18 months since natural improvement can be anticipated. In general, scar maturation occurs more rapidly in adults than in children. The majority of erythematous scars will show little improvement after revision, so surgery should not be undertaken for correction of undesirable scar color alone.

Answer: D

CHAPTER **9**

Anesthesia

1. Which of the following properties is/are common to inhalational anesthetics?

A. Controllable duration of action
B. Equivalent potency
C. Reproducible dose-response curves
D. Depression of neuronal excitability

Sabiston: 160
Schwartz: 437

Comments: Control of reversibility is one of the principal advantages of inhalational anesthetics. Duration of action depends upon ventilation and not on biotransformation or excretion. All inhalational agents depress neuronal excitability; the physiologic effects of specific agents are otherwise variable. Potency of inhalational anesthetics is measured by minimum alveolar anesthetic concentration (MAC) and is widely variable. Among the commonly used agents, halothane is the most potent, followed by enflurane and isoflurane, which are roughly equivalent, and by nitrous oxide, which is the weakest. Dose-response curves differ, and no reliable dose-response relationship exists on a weight per kilogram basis. It is the partial pressure of inhalational agents, not the tissue concentration, that determines anesthetic effect; differences in molecular weight and coefficients of distribution can produce different concentrations at the same partial pressure.

Answer: A, D

2. Relative contraindications to use of halothane include which of the following?
A. Simultaneous use of nitrous oxide
B. Hepatic cirrhosis
C. Head trauma with increased intracranial pressure
D. Term pregnancy during labor
E. Renal failure

Sabiston: 160
Schwartz: 439

Comments: Halothane is a potent inhalational anesthetic that causes cardiovascular depression, vasodilation, sen-

52

sitization of ventricular pacemakers to arrhythmogenic stimuli, and depression of myometrial tone. Simultaneous use of nitrous oxide decreases the anesthetic requirements of halothane and provides a sympathetic cardiovascular effect that ameliorates hypotension and decreased cardiac output. The vasodilation accompanying halothane anesthesia increases cerebral blood flow and intracranial pressure; this can be partially compensated for by prior hyperventilation. Although halothane is metabolized by hepatic microsomal enzymes and is a halogenated hydrocarbon, it by itself is not a true hepatotoxin, and the risk of an adverse hepatic response is not greater in patients with pre-existing liver disease. The metabolism of methoxyflurane and enflurane increases plasma levels of inorganic fluoride, which can be nephrotoxic in high dosages. Methoxyflurane has been associated with high-output renal failure and is now infrequently used. Fluoride elevations following enflurane anesthesia are not clinically significant except in very prolonged usages. Isoflurane undergoes no significant metabolism.

Answer: C, D

3. Which of the following statements is/are true about halothane hepatitis?

A. The use of halothane is contraindicated in patients with a history of infectious hepatitis
B. It is an idiosyncratic reaction, most commonly seen in males following a single exposure to halothane
C. It is clinically similar but histologically separable from viral hepatitis
D. It can be minimized by the preoperative administration of phenobarbital to induce hepatic enzymes
E. None of the above

Sabiston: 161
Schwartz: 440

Comments: Halothane hepatitis describes a clinical syndrome characterized by fever, eosinophilia, and jaundice that occurs 2 to 5 days following exposure to halothane anesthesia. It has been described more frequently following multiple exposures to halothane, in female patients, in hypoxic patients, and in animal studies with hepatic enzyme induction as seen with chronic phenobarbital therapy. Histologically, it is difficult to differentiate from viral hepatitis (centrilobular necrosis). Whether the syndrome is actually caused by halothane is controversial; the National Halothane Study demonstrated that hepatic dysfunction following administration of halothane was rare and no greater than with other anesthetics. Past evidence has suggested that halothane hepatitis may represent an allergic, hypersensitivity reaction, but today it is believed to be caused by reductive breakdown products of halothane.

Answer: E

4. Which of the following statements is/are true about nitrous oxide?

A. It has been reported to cause bone marrow suppression after prolonged exposure
B. It depresses myocardial contractility primarily by its effect on medullary centers
C. When combined with halothane, it decreases arterial oxygen content as compared with the use of halothane and oxygen alone
D. Its solubility characteristics may produce diffusion hypoxia during induction
E. It may be hazardous in patients with pneumothorax or intestinal obstruction

Sabiston: 160
Schwartz: 438

Comments: Nitrous oxide is primarily an analgesic agent and usually is used in combination with more potent inhalational or intravenous drugs to decrease their dose requirements and side effects. Sympathetic activity is increased through action on medullary vasomotor centers, thereby offsetting the depressant effects of agents such as halothane. When nitrous oxide is combined with halothane, however, less oxygen is administered and arterial oxygen content decreases. Since the net effect may still be some degree of cardiac depression due to halothane, this situation may not be beneficial. Nitrous oxide is approximately 30 times more soluble than nitrogen in blood. At the conclusion of anesthesia when the patient begins to breathe room air, nitrous oxide diffuses into the alveoli more rapidly and displaces oxygen; this may contribute to producing a period of diffusion hypoxia. This effect is transitory and is prevented by increasing alveolar oxygen tension. The high solubility may also produce rapid increases in the volume of gas collections, as in patients with pneumothorax or intestinal obstruction. If N_2O is to be used in the presence of a pneumothorax, consideration should be given to insertion of a chest tube or to the avoidance of N_2O. N_2O has been shown to inhibit the enzyme methionine synthetase, which is important for bone marrow proliferation and function of parts of the nervous system.

Answer: A, C, E

5. Epinephrine administration should particularly be restricted with which of the following anesthetic agents?

A. Halothane
B. Enflurane
C. Methoxyflurane
D. Cyclopropane

Schwartz: 439

Comments: Halothane increases the sensitivity of the ventricular pacemakers to epinephrine and other arrhythmogenic stimuli. During halothane anesthesia in a 70 kg patient, for example, it has been recommended that epinephrine be restricted to 10 ml of a 1:100,000 solution every 10 minutes. Enflurane and isoflurane do not increase ventricular irritability to the extent that halothane does, and methoxyflurane protects against epinephrine-induced arrhythmias (methoxyflurane is nephrotoxic, however). Cyclopropane is highly explosive and infrequently used. It produces a centrally mediated increase in sympathetic activity and elevation of catecholamines, thereby predisposing to ventricular arrhythmias, particularly if exogenous epinephrine is also administered.

Answer: A, D

6. Appropriately match the items in the two columns.

A. Short duration of action
B. Metabolized by pseudo-cholinesterase
C. Duration of action dependent upon redistribution
D. Muscle fasciculation
E. Reversible with anticholinesterase
F. Neomycin may prolong effect
G. Nondepolarizing (competitive) type block
H. Malignant hyperthermia

a. Nondepolarizing muscle relaxants (curare, pancuronium, atracurium, and vecuronium)
b. Depolarizing muscle relaxants (succinylcholine)
c. Both
d. Neither

Sabiston: 163
Schwartz: 445

Comments: Muscle relaxants can be divided into two categories: nondepolarizing agents (such as curare and pancuronium), which interfere with transmission at the myoneural junction by competing with acetylcholine, and depolarizing agents (such as succinylcholine), which depolarize the motor end-plate. The two are not mutually exclusive, however; following prolonged administration of succinylcholine, a nondepolarizing type of block occurs. Depolarizing agents are short-acting and are metabolized by pseudocholinesterase; the above-mentioned nondepolarizing relaxants have a longer duration of action depending upon metabolism and excretion. Decreased pseudocholinesterase activity or conversion to a nondepolarizing block may prolong succinylcholine effect; in the case of nondepolarizing agents, prolongation of action can occur from hypothermia, electrolyte imbalance, water intoxication, or with certain antibiotics such as neomycin or kanamycin. Muscle fasciculation, hyperkalemia, and postanesthesia muscle pain are associated with the use of succinylcholine. These effects may be attenuated by the initial administration of a small dose of nondepolarizing agent. Malignant hyperthermia has occurred with succinylcholine as well as with halothane and other inhalational anesthetics.

Answer: A–b; B–b; C–a; D–b; E–a; F–a; G–c; H–b

7. Because of specific effects, the use of succinylcholine may be detrimental in which of the following conditions?

A. A patient with closed-angle glaucoma
B. A patient with a space-occupying intracranial lesion
C. An emergency laparotomy on an unconscious victim of a motor vehicle accident
D. A patient with a severe crush injury of the lower extremity
E. A patient with a history of epilepsy

Schwartz: 446

Comments: The initial depolarization produced by succinylcholine results in skeletal muscle fasciculation and myoclonic contraction. Fasciculation of the extrinsic muscles of the eye increases intraocular pressure, which is an undesirable side effect in patients with glaucoma or open orbits. Similarly, intra-abdominal pressure is increased, predisposing to regurgitation and aspiration of gastric contents. This risk is minimized by the use of cricoid pressure to occlude the esophagus before the airway is protected with a cuffed endotracheal tube. Depolarization also results in efflux of potassium from skeletal muscles. Significant hyperkalemia may occur in patients with burns, crush injury, or conditions associated with denervation of skeletal muscles.

Answer: A, B, C, D

8. A crop farmer from northern Illinois has prolonged apnea following anesthesia during which succinylcholine was used. Potential etiologies include (one or more):

A. Residual effect of an inhalational anesthetic
B. Residual narcotic effect
C. Insecticide exposure
D. Genetic cholinesterase defect
E. All of the above

Schwartz: 447

Comments: Prolonged apnea following the use of succinylcholine can occur for several reasons, including residual effect of inhalational anesthetics or narcotics. Normally, the duration of action of succinylcholine is short because of its metabolism by pseudocholinesterase. The farmer (likely exposed to insecticides containing succinylcholine-like agents) may be depleted of pseudocholinesterase and require longer periods of time for the metabolism of administered succinylcholine. Rarely, patients have a genetically transmitted abnormal form of pseudocholinesterase incapable of metabolizing succinylcholine. Treatment consists of prolonged ventilation until available pseudocholinesterase is able to metabolize the succinylcholine. Transfusion of plasma with normal amounts of pseudocholinesterase is reserved for instances in which there is little or no metabolism evident after prolonged support.

Answer: E

9. Fifteen minutes after the administration of a spinal anesthetic, severe hypotension would be most likely to occur with the patient in which of the following positions?

A. Jackknife
B. Reverse Trendelenburg
C. Trendelenburg
D. Lithotomy

Sabiston: 166
Schwartz: 449

Comments: Spinal anesthesia is accomplished by the injection of a local anesthetic agent into the subarachnoid space with resultant blockade of somatic motor and sensory fibers as well as preganglionic sympathetic fibers. The level of sympathetic block extends approximately two spinal segments above the sensory level, while the level of the somatic motor block extends approximately two spinal segments caudally. Preganglionic fibers are affected at the lowest concentrations of the anesthetic agent, and physiologic changes associated with spinal anesthesia are the result of sympathetic denervation. Peripheral arterial and arteriolar dilatations produce a modest reduction in peripheral vascular resistance. The most significant hemodynamic effect, however, is the ablation of venous tone with a variable decrease in venous return depending upon the patient's position. Severe decreases in cardiac output occur with venous pooling below the level of the right atrium as occurs in patients in the head-up position. If a patient is placed in the Trendelenburg position, just after placement of a hyperbaric spinal anesthetic, hypotension can occur because of ascending levels of neural blockade, with greater degree of sympatholysis.

Answer: A, B

10. Concerning malignant hyperthermia, which of the following is/are true?

A. Testing for elevated CPK is a useful screening method
B. It often affects young, muscular males
C. Treatment includes administration of dantrolene
D. It may be triggered by local anesthetics
E. Family history is the most valuable screening tool

Schwartz: 446

Comments: Malignant hyperthermia (MH) is a rare, potentially lethal condition, characterized by muscular rigidity, fever, tachycardia, respiratory and metabolic acidosis, severe hypermetabolism, arrhythmias, and eventually hypotension and cardiovascular collapse. It can occur at any time after the administration of anesthetic agents such as succinylcholine, inhalational anesthetics, or some local anesthetics. Treatment involves the cessation of anesthesia, the administration of dantrolene, and general supportive measures. Dantrolene is administered prophylactically to patients at risk, as determined by a muscle biopsy or by a prior episode of documented MH. Although the biochemical basis is not fully known, there is a genetically transmitted susceptibility; a family history, therefore, is most useful in detecting patients at risk. The diagnosis may be substantiated by contractility studies of muscle biopsy specimens. Patients with a susceptibility to MH may have elevated CPK levels, but the test is not useful for screening because it has poor specificity and is abnormal in patients with other myopathies.

Answer: B, C, D, E

11. Which of the following is/are true about epidural anesthesia as compared with spinal anesthesia?

A. Epidural anesthesia results in spinal headaches more frequently
B. It is more likely to produce systemic effects of local anesthetics
C. It produces minimal sympathetic denervation
D. It is more advantageous for continuous administration
E. It requires larger anesthetic doses

Sabiston: 166
Schwartz: 451

Comments: Injection of a local anesthetic into the epidural space and subsequent transfer across the dura produces sympathetic denervation, and the physiologic response is similar to that evoked by spinal anesthesia. Larger amounts of anesthetic must be used, however, and subsequent absorption may produce systemic cardiovascular effects. Spinal headaches are less frequent, although they may occur if the dura is inadvertently punctured. Potential advantages of epidural over spinal anesthesia include its use for a caudal block during rectal surgery in the prone position and the continuous administration of epidural anesthesia when prolonged regional effect is desired. Continuous epidural administration of narcotics with or without small amounts of local anesthetics is now becoming a popular method of postoperative pain relief.

Answer: B, D, E

12. Match the local anesthetics with their characteristic feature(s).

Characteristic Feature	Local Anesthetic
A. Safest maximal dose	a. Procaine
B. Marked central effect	b. Tetracaine
C. Naturally occurring	c. Lidocaine
D. Long duration of action	d. Bupivacaine
E. Marked vasodilation	e. None
F. Topical for tracheobronchial tree	
G. Agent of choice for continuous epidural anesthesia	

Sabiston: 165

Comments: The availability of the ideal local anesthetic remains elusive, something hardly surprising considering the desired characteristics: short latency, potent, controllable duration of action, penetrating, reversible, nontoxic, water-soluble, heat-sterilizable, nonirritating, nonantigenic, and not interfering with the healing of the tissue into which it is injected. Available local anesthetic agents are either amino-amide (lidocaine and bupivacaine) or amino-ester (procaine and tetracaine) compounds, which act to block neural transmission, probably by blocking sodium channels in nerve cell membranes. All the compounds are synthetically produced (except cocaine). They produce systemic effects that depend on serum levels. These range from vasodilation to tremulousness, seizures, CNS depression, and finally, cardiovascular collapse due to myocardial depression at high serum levels. Procaine requires the highest maximal dose before toxicity is seen (tetracaine the lowest). Lidocaine can produce a marked CNS effect, especially in elderly or critically ill patients. Duration of action depends on metabolism, elimination, lipid solubility, protein binding, and site of injection. Of the listed compounds, the order from shortest to longest duration is procaine, lidocaine, tetracaine, and bupivacaine. Because of its long duration of action, bupivacaine is commonly used for lumbar epidural anesthesia. Procaine is used essentially only for local infiltration and spinal anesthesia. The tracheobronchial mucosa is commonly anesthetized for airway procedures by using nebulized lidocaine.

Answer: A–a; B–c; C–e; D–d; E–a; F–c; G–d

Trauma

1. A 22-year-old man presents with a stab wound along the anterior border of the sternocleidomastoid muscle at the level of the cricoid cartilage with violation of the platysma; there are no other significant findings. The vital signs are normal. The most appropriate management would be:

A. Admission of the patient to the intensive care unit to observe closely for airway obstruction
B. Performance of a carotid arteriogram; if this is negative, observe patient
C. Performance of a carotid arteriogram, bronchoscopy, and barium swallow; if these are negative, observe patient
D. Formal exploration of the left neck
E. Intubation, intravenous antibiotics, and close observation in the intensive care unit

Sabiston: 299
Schwartz: 221

Comments: For purposes of managing penetrating neck trauma, the neck is divided in three zones. Zone I extends below the level of the head of the clavicle and involves the thoracic inlet. Zone II extends from the head of the clavicle to the angles of the mandible and anterior to a perpendicular line drawn from the mastoid process. Zone III is superior to the angle of the mandible. In managing penetrating Zone II injuries that involve significant structures (major vascular, laryngotracheal, or pharyngoesophageal injuries), the physical examination may be negative in as many as 30 per cent of patients. A full diagnostic work-up, including arteriography, bronchoscopy, and barium swallow, has a significant number of false positive and negative findings in addition to being costly. Neck exploration is a very safe procedure, with minimal complications, no missed injuries, and no prolongation of hospital stay. For these reasons, mandatory exploration of Zone II injuries that penetrate the platysma remains the treatment of choice.

Answer: D

2. Which of the following are essential steps in managing rectal injuries?

A. Presacral drainage
B. Proximal, completely diverting colostomy
C. Irrigation of the distal segment with saline solution
D. Primary repair of the rectal injury if it is accessible
E. Insertion of a rectal tube if the injury cannot be repaired

Sabiston: 311
Schwartz: 240

Comments: Rectal injuries continue to be a significant problem facing the trauma surgeon, with mortality rates averaging 10 to 15%. This mortality is a reflection of the particularly dangerous soilage that occurs in the pelvis, which is a relatively hypovascular area, poor in combatting sepsis. A high index of suspicion and prompt performance of proctoscopy are necessary to diagnose these injuries in a timely fashion. Any blood on the examining finger and any penetration that crosses the midline in the pelvis should prompt a proctoscopy. ● The **first principle** in managing rectal injuries is the formation of a proximal colostomy that is completely diverting. The colostomy should be placed as close to the peritoneal reflection as is possible. Classic teaching is to form a double-barrel colostomy, although a generously opened loop colostomy probably functions just as well. The **second principle** in managing rectal injuries is the insertion of presacral drains. This is done through a curvilinear incision midway between the anal verge and coccyx. The surgeon must take care to dissect the entire retrorectal space and ensure that the drains are placed high enough to communicate with the rectal injury. For most civilian injuries, passive drains will suffice, although in the face of extensive contamination and/or devitalization active suction drainage is preferable. The **third principle** in the management of rectal injuries is primary repair of the rectal injury itself, if it is accessible. This can be accomplished transperitoneally for high rectal injuries (i.e., 9 cm or more above the anal verge) or transanally for low rectal injuries (i.e., 5 cm or less above the anal verge). Midrectal injuries are usually inaccessible. Distal colonic segment irrigation was found to be beneficial in treating victims in the Vietnam conflict. Civilian studies, however, have failed to demonstrate any effect on mortality or morbidity rates using this modality. It should be used only for wounds that are high-velocity in nature or those associated with extensive contamination and/or devitalization. The majority of civilian-type rectal injuries can be managed without distal segment irrigation. Insertion of a rectal tube can enlarge existing wounds and is of no benefit if the colostomy is completely diverting.

Answer: A, B, D

3. A 24-year-old man is the unrestrained driver in a head-on collision. He presents to the emergency room with a blood pressure of 110/80, pulse of 110, and a respiratory rate of 40 with noisy respirations. He has an obvious LeFort III fracture bilaterally, bilateral mandibular fractures, and a laceration of the tongue with a small amount of oral bleeding. The remainder of his physical examination is normal. An oropharyngeal airway inserted by the paramedics failed to improve ventilation. The correct method of establishing an airway in this patient is:

A. Oral endotracheal intubation
B. Blind nasotracheal intubation
C. Percutaneous needle cricothyroidotomy with jet insufflation of oxygen
D. Tracheostomy
E. Cricothyroidotomy

Sabiston: 297

Comments: The establishment of a patent upper airway is always the first priority in the management of any trauma victim. The risk and difficulty in airway management in the trauma patient is the potential presence of an associated cervical spine injury and its aggravation while performing the intubation. Patients who should be considered at risk for a cervical spine injury include any patient who is unconscious, has sustained head or neck trauma, was involved in a deceleration/acceleration accident, or has signs or symptoms of a cervical spine injury. **Oral endotracheal intubation** can be accomplished only with some hyperextension of the neck. Therefore, it should be performed only if a cervical spine fracture has been excluded radiographically or, in an apneic patient, where the risk is offset by the benefits of obtaining an airway as soon as possible. **Blind nasotracheal intubation** in a trauma victim who is breathing is likely to be successful over 90 per cent of the time. One contraindication to nasotracheal intubation is significant maxillofacial trauma. **Needle cricothyroidotomy** with jet insufflation is a useful technique for obtaining direct control of the airway in small children. In adults, however, because of the limited size of the catheter that can be placed using this technique, CO_2 retention occurs quickly. **Cricothyroidotomy** is the preferred technique for emergency airway control in the patient with significant maxillofacial trauma. Its advantages over tracheostomy include the following: the speed with which an airway can be established, lesser amounts of bleeding during the procedure, and the fact that it can much more easily be performed without hyperextension of the cervical spine. The one disadvantage to cricothryoidotomy is that it will not suffice as a permanent airway because of the associated higher incidence of subglottic stenosis. The length of time required to develop this complication is not clearly established. It is generally recommended that the crico-

thyroidotomy be converted to a formal tracheostomy in 5 to 7 days if airway control is still required.

Answer: E

4. The indications for peritoneal lavage in evaluating a patient with blunt abdominal trauma include which of the following?

A. Peritonitis
B. An unconscious patient
C. Equivocal abdominal findings
D. Spinal cord injury
E. Pregnancy

Sabiston: 307
Schwartz: 230

Comments: Since its introduction by Root in 1965, peritoneal lavage has become the standard in evaluating blunt abdominal trauma. Peritoneal lavage has an accuracy rate as high as 98% and is associated with very few complications. There are two techniques for performing peritoneal lavage: the closed or percutaneous technique and the open technique, which is currently recommended. This involves an infraumbilical midline incision performed with the patient locally anesthetized. The fascia is divided in the midline, the peritoneum is opened, and the catheter is placed under direct vision. One liter of crystalloid solution is instilled, and the fluid is returned using the syphon effect. The fluid that is returned is examined for red blood cells (RBC), white blood cells (WBC), bile, feces, or bacteria. A positive lavage is indicated by an RBC count of >100,000 cells/μl, a WBC count of >500 cells/μl or the presence of bile, feces, or bacteria. The indications for peritoneal lavage to evaluate blunt abdominal trauma include the following: an altered level of consciousness secondary to head injuries, alcohol, or drugs; a spinal cord injury; equivocal abdominal findings; and an indication for general anesthesia to treat associated injuries. Relative indications used by some traumatologists include lower rib fractures and unexplained hypotension. The only absolute contraindication to peritoneal lavage is an indication for exploratory laparotomy, such as peritonitis. Relative contraindications include previous abdominal incisions, pregnancy, and significant pelvic fractures. A positive lavage result is an absolute indication for abdominal exploration.

Answer: B, C, D

5. Which of the following statements regarding duodenal hematomas is/are true?

A. The common presentation is that of a high small bowel obstruction occurring 12 to 72 hours after abdominal trauma
B. Patients with duodenal hematomas generally present with peritonitis
C. An upper gastrointestinal series will demonstrate extravasation of contrast into the retroperitoneum
D. Nonoperative management with nasogastric decompression and parenteral alimentation is usually successful
E. Associated injuries must be excluded prior to undertaking conservative management

Sabiston: 847
Schwartz: 239

Comments: Duodenal intramural hematomas generally result from blunt upper abdominal trauma. The mechanism of injury is thought to be a force that crushes the third portion of the duodenum against the vertebral column. This causes disruption of submucosal vessels and the development of an enlarging hematoma that occludes the duodenal lumen. Generally, the patient presents with signs of high small bowel obstruction, including nausea, vomiting, and upper abdominal pain without significant tenderness. The signs and symptoms usually develop in the 12 to 72 hours following the trauma episode. Once associated injuries are excluded through physical examination, peritoneal lavage, and other ancillary diagnostic tests, an upper gastrointestinal tract series using water-soluble contrast material should be obtained. The demonstration of a "coiled spring" or "stacked coins" sign confirm the diagnosis. This study must be obtained to ensure there is no extravasation. Conservative management including nasogastric decompression, electrolyte repletion, and parenteral alimentation is likely to be successful in 80 to 90% of cases. The process of resorption of the hematoma may take as long as 2 or 3 weeks. If no resolution occurs over this period of time, surgical intervention must be undertaken. The operation can include evacuation of the intramural hematoma with careful inspection of the mucosa for areas of disruption and reapproximation of the seromuscular coat. The overall prognosis for this injury is excellent.

Answer: A, D, E

6. The most reliable finding on a chest x-ray that indicates a transected thoracic aorta is:

A. Apical pleural cap
B. Right-sided deviation of the trachea
C. Widened mediastinum
D. Blurring of the aortic knob
E. Left hemothorax

Sabiston: 1810
Schwartz: 201

Comments: Aortic transections are fatal at the scene 90% of the time. However, the majority of patients who arrive at the hospital with vital signs have few or no signs or symptoms indicating the presence of this injury; a high index of suspicion is necessary if one is to detect it. The mechanism of injury is a sudden deceleration that leads to shear forces developing between the mobile aortic arch and the fixed descending aorta. These shear forces lead to intimal disruption at the ligamentum arteriosum distal to the left subclavian artery, which is the first point of fixation. The most reliable finding on a chest x-ray indicating a potential aortic transection is a widening of the superior mediastinum. Other findings that may indicate a thoracic aortic injury include apical pleural cap, deviation of the trachea or nasogastric tube to the right, and obliteration of the aortic knob. Any patient who has sustained a significant deceleration injury should be considered at risk for an aortic transection. While many diagnostic tests, including ultrasonography and computerized tomography, have been used, a formal arch aortogram remains the most reliable test for this injury. Operation on an emergency basis is indicated to repair this injury, since about half the patients will suffer rupture of the contained injury and die within the first 6 hours if it is not repaired. In such favorable circumstances the operative mortality is 8%.

Answer: C

7. A 30-year-old man has an exploratory laparotomy for a gunshot wound to the right upper quadrant. An injury to the common bile duct is discovered with a loss of 2 cm of the wall of the duct. Appropriate management of this injury would be:

A. Débridement and primary anastomosis without stent
B. Débridement and primary anastomosis with stent
C. Roux-en-Y choledochojejunostomy without stent
D. Roux-en-Y choledochojejunostomy with stent
E. Ligation of the common bile duct with formation of a cholecystojejunostomy

Schwartz: 248

Comments: Ninety-five percent of injuries to the extrahepatic biliary tree are secondary to penetrating trauma. The diagnosis is generally made by a thorough surgical exploration of the entire tract of a penetrating injury. If the diagnosis cannot be established on the basis of exploration, as may be the case with injuries to the intrapancreatic portion of the common bile duct, an intraoperative cholangiogram should be performed via a needle introduced into the gallbladder. The danger in repairing injuries to the common bile duct is the development of stricture at the site of repair. The blood supply to the common bile duct in most patients comes primarily from two vessels that run parallel to the duct and opposite to each other. An injury that completely transects the duct interrupts this blood supply. Consequently, primary repair of a completely transected duct is likely to result in a stricture. Partial transections that are clean may be repaired primarily over a T-tube stent. Complete common bile duct transections necessitate the formation of a Roux-en-Y choledochojejunostomy. This anastomosis should also be stented, because the common bile duct is generally normal in caliber. All anastomoses to the common bile duct should be drained externally, since about 10% of them will leak.

Answer: D

8. A 42-year-old man strikes his upper abdomen on the steering wheel during a motor vehicle accident. Because of a positive peritoneal lavage he has an exploratory laparotomy, at which time a transection of the pancreas at the neck is located. Appropriate management of this injury could be:

A. Distal pancreatectomy with oversewing and drainage of the proximal pancreatic stump
B. Primary repair and drainage of the pancreatic duct
C. Roux-en-Y pancreaticojejunostomy to the distal pancreas with oversewing and drainage of the proximal pancreatic stump
D. Roux-en-Y pancreaticojejunostomy to both proximal and distal pancreatic stumps
E. Total pancreatectomy

Sabiston: 316
Schwartz: 250

Comments: Eighty percent of pancreatic injuries are secondary to penetrating trauma, almost all being diagnosed during exploratory laparotomy. Care must be taken to thoroughly explore all hematomas within the lesser sac or at the root of the small bowel mesentery so as not to overlook such an injury. Blunt pancreatic injuries are more difficult to diagnose. If there is an associated intraperitoneal injury, the peritoneal lavage will be positive. Isolated pancreatic injuries usually are missed on peritoneal lavage. These patients will have signs and symptoms similar to acute pancreatitis, including nausea, vomiting, abdominal distension, upper abdominal pain, and increased fluid requirements. While the initial amylase is unreliable, even if elevated, demonstration of persistent hyperamylasemia can be a significant finding. Computerized tomography, unfortunately, is associated with too many false positive and negative results in evaluating pancreatic trauma. The operative management of pancreatic injuries centers on débridement of devitalized tissue, hemostasis, assessment and treatment of the pancreatic duct, and adequate external drainage utilizing active and passive drains. When the pancreatic duct is not injured, no internal drainage procedure is required. If the main pancreatic duct is injured to the left of the mesenteric vessels, the standard treatment is to perform a distal pancreatectomy with adequate drainage of the proximal stump. The pancreatic injury described in this question is the typical blunt pancreatic injury that results from a crushing blow against the vertebral body. This likewise may be treated by distal pancreatectomy. Some surgeons would perform a Roux-en-Y pancreaticojejunostomy to the distal pancreas and oversew the proximal pancreas, in an effort to preserve as much functioning pancreatic tissue as possible. Internal drainage of the proximal pancreas is not indicated, since the proximal pancreatic duct is not obstructed. Major pancreatic resection such as total pancreatectomy or pancreaticoduodenectomy (Whipple) are reserved for injuries that involve extensive devitalization of the duodenum and head of pancreas. These procedures are associated with a high mortality rate and should be performed only when no other procedure will suffice.

Answer: A, C

9. Regarding peripheral arterial injuries, which of the following statements is/are true?

A. All patients with peripheral arterial injuries will have diminished or absent pulses distal to the injury
B. If the injury cannot be primarily repaired, prosthetic material should be used
C. Arteriography is indicated in any penetrating trauma that threatens the path of a major vessel
D. Evidence of compartmental hypertension is a contraindiction to arteriography
E. All patients with posterior knee dislocations should have popliteal arteriography

Sabiston: 326
Schwartz: 927

Comments: Peripheral arterial injuries may be a source of significant morbidity and disability if not appropriately managed. About 20% of patients with significant arterial injuries have normal pulses distal to the site of the injury. Consequently, any penetrating injury that threatens the path of a major artery should be evaluated with an arteriogram. Other signs that may be associated with arterial injuries include an expanding or pulsatile hematoma, a thrill or bruit in the area of the injury (usually associated with an arteriovenous fistula), a neurologic deficit, or evidence of compartmental hypertension. While in general most peripheral arterial injuries are caused by penetrating trauma, certain blunt injuries are associated with a high incidence of vascular damage. These include posterior knee dislocation, supracondylar femoral or humeral fractures, and first or second rib fractures. These likewise demand routine arteriography. The only contraindications to arteriography are exsanguinating hemorrhage, limb-threatening ischemia, or compartmental hypertension. In these cases, immediate surgical intervention must be undertaken. The principles of surgical repair of major vascular trauma include the following: proximal and distal control of the vessel prior to approaching the hematoma associated with the injury; repair of major venous as well as arterial injuries, if possible; the use of autogenous material in the form of vein patch or vein bypass graft, when primary repair cannot be accomplished; and adequate soft tissue coverage to protect the site of vascular repair. Associated compartmental hypertension should be treated by fasciotomy.

Answer: C, D, E

10. Intraperitoneal colon injuries:

A. Should never be closed primarily
B. Can appropriately be treated with exteriorization and formation of a colostomy
C. Are often diagnosed based on the presence of pneumoperitoneum on an upright chest x-ray
D. May be treated with resection and primary anastomosis
E. Have an intra-abdominal abscess rate of 10 to 15%

Sabiston: 308
Schwartz: 240

Comments: Colon injuries remain a significant source of morbidity and mortality in the patient with trauma because of an abscess formation rate of 10 to 15%. The diagnosis of colon injuries usually is made on the basis of peritoneal signs on physical examination. Free air can be demonstrated on chest x-ray only 10% of the time. Care must be taken to explore all hematomas involving the wall of the colon or the mesocolon in order to identify relatively occult perforations. The mortality rates for colon injuries were significantly reduced when exteriorization as a colostomy became the mainstay of surgical treatment during the Korean War. This form of treatment remains the cornerstone of management in colonic injuries. However, primary repair of colon injuries in civilian practice can be safely accomplished provided certain criteria are met. These criteria include: no preoperative or intraoperative hypotension; less than 2000 ml of blood loss; a colon injury that is less than 2 cm in diameter after débridement; no compromise of the blood supply to the colon; less than 8 hours between time of injury and repair; minimal or no fecal contamination; and no need for prosthetic material to reconstruct either abdominal wall or any vascular injuries. If any of these criteria are violated the injury should be treated with exteriorization, with a few exceptions. Cecal injuries that cannot undergo primary repair must be treated with resection and ileostomy, because cecal exteriorization does not allow for an adequate stomal appliance to be fitted. Injury to a distal sigmoid that cannot be exteriorized because it cannot be mobilized adequately to reach the abdominal wall must be treated by repair and proximal diverting colostomy, if the criteria for primary repair cannot be met. Injuries that involve more than one anatomic area of the colon are usually treated by exteriorization of the proximal injury with repair of the distal injury. Drains are never placed at the site of a repaired colon because there seems to be a higher incidence of anastomotic leak. If drains are indicated for treatment of another injury, they should be separated from a colostomy site as much as possible to avoid contamination of the peritoneal cavity. Antibiotics are started preoperatively and should be continued postoperatively, although the exact duration of treatment is controversial.

Answer: B, E

11. A 22-year-old woman presents with a single stab wound to the left fifth intercostal space in the midclavicular line. The blood pressure is 80 systolic, the pulse 130, and the respiratory rate 24. There is jugular venous distension, a midline trachea, muffled heart tones, and slightly decreased breath sounds over the left chest. The most likely diagnosis is:

A. Massive left hemothorax
B. Pericardial tamponade
C. Tension pneumothorax
D. Open pneumothorax
E. Ruptured left mainstem bronchus

Comment: See Question 12.

12. The initial management could be:

A. Pericardiocentesis
B. Needle decompression of the left chest in the second intercostal space, midclavicular line
C. Left tube thoracostomy
D. Subxyphoid pericardial window
E. Median sternotomy and repair of the cardiac injury

Sabiston: 300
Schwartz: 201

Comments: All of the possible injuries listed are immediately life-threatening thoracic injuries that must be identified and treated during the primary survey and resuscitation of the trauma victim. The triad of systemic hypotension, distended neck veins, and muffled heart tones is known as Beck's triad and is diagnostic of pericardial tamponade. Tension pneumothorax may frequently mimic tamponade because both conditions result in obstruction to venous return to the heart and low cardiac output because of inadequate filling. The presence of a midline trachea and breath sounds on the affected side essentially excludes the diagnosis of tension pneumothorax. A massive left hemothorax (i.e., greater than 1500 ml of blood in the left pleural space) may also exhibit systemic hypotension and decreased but present breath sounds over the left chest. In such a case, however, the neck veins would be flat and the heart tones

normal. Patients with an open pneumothorax will be in respiratory distress because of total collapse of the affected lung and an obvious "sucking" chest wound. Because the pericardium is relatively noncompliant, relatively small amounts of blood in the pericardial sac (e.g., 100 to 150 ml) can produce a hemodynamically significant tamponade. The initial step in managing such a patient is to reduce the intrapericardial pressure by removing some of the blood. Pericardiocentesis will usually accomplish this with a significant tamponade. The subxyphoid approach is used because the anterior approach is associated wtih a much higher incidence of complications, such as left pneumothorax and coronary artery injuries. Because the pericardium is inelastic, the withdrawal of small amounts of blood (10 to 20 ml) will often result in a significant decrease in intrapericardial pressure and improved ventricular filling. Pericardiocentesis is useful to stabilize the patient's status, but must be followed by prompt surgical intervention to treat the underlying cardiac injury. Many experts are now creating subxyphoid pericardial windows as an initial stabilizing measure. This can be performed relatively quickly using local anesthesia and has the advantage of being effective even if a large amount of the pericardial blood is clotted. If the patient's condition is stable there is no need to perform either of these maneuvers. The surgeon in such a case can proceed directly to median sternotomy and repair of the cardiac injury. In the unstable patient, however, this takes too much time and requires the induction of general anesthesia.

Answer: Question 11: B
Question 12: A, D

13. Indications for resection of a segment of injured small bowel include:

A. Loss of more than 50% of the bowel wall
B. Multiple injuries in a short segment
C. Compromise of the blood supply of a segment
D. Injuries within 3 feet of the ileocecal valve
E. Injuries within 3 feet of the ligament of Treitz

Sabiston: 308
Schwartz: 239

Comment: Small bowel injuries can be surprisingly lethal if not dealt with promptly. The mortality of blunt small bowel injuries treated more than 24 hours after trauma ranges from 30 to 70%. The majority of small bowel injuries are secondary to penetrating trauma and are found during routine abdominal exploration. One must be certain during a laparotomy for abdominal trauma to inspect the small bowel and its mesentery, segment by segment, from the ligament of Treitz to the ileocecal valve. Blunt trauma can give rise to small bowel injuries by one of three mechanisms: sudden deceleration that causes shear forces to develop near a point of fixation (i.e., ileocecal valve, ligament of Treitz, adhesion from previous surgery); a crushing force that traps the small bowel against the vertebral body; or a blow to a fluid-filled loop of small bowel causing a burst injury. All three of these mechanisms are probably operational. Isolated jejunal or ileal injuries frequently do not cause peritonitis immediately because the succus entericus that is spilled is chemically neutral and relatively sterile. It is only after bacterial growth occurs, over a period of hours, that peritoneal signs develop. Aggressive use of peritoneal lavage may help one diagnose the presence of these injuries, but frequently the lavage is positive only for white blood cells. There is recent evidence that alkaline phosphatase can be demonstrated in the lavage effluent of patients with small bowel injuries. The majority of small bowel injuries are managed by débridement and primary closure in one or two layers. The indications for segmental resection with primary closure include: a loss of more than 50% of the bowel wall, in which primary closure will lead to stricture; multiple injuries in a short segment, when a great deal of operative time can be saved by resection with one reanastomosis; and any compromise to the blood supply of a segment of small bowel.

Answer: A, B, C

14. Regarding neck injuries, which of the following statements is/are true?

A. The internal jugular vein may be ligated unilaterally without unfavorable sequelae
B. Unilateral ligation of the common carotid artery will result in neurologic deficiency in 80% of cases
C. Esophageal injuries should be drained externally only when extensive devitalization is present
D. Injuries to the thyroid gland must be drained externally
E. Tracheostomy is indicated in dealing with most laryngeal or tracheal injuries

Sabiston: 299
Schwartz: 222

Comments: The management of patients with penetrating neck trauma requires a surgeon capable of performing vascular, general surgical, and otolaryngologic procedures. Internal jugular venous injuries should be repaired if the patient's condition allows and the injury is amenable to repair. The internal jugular vein can be ligated unilaterally without adverse consequences, and this treatment is advised in unstable patients. ● The management of carotid artery injuries is somewhat controversial. In the patient who has no neurologic deficit preoperatively, every effort should be made to repair carotid artery injuries. This may include the use of a temporary shunt and vein grafting. In the patient who has a dense neurologic deficit established preoperatively, repair of the carotid artery injury may worsen the neurologic condition by converting an ischemic into a hemorrhagic injury. The carotid artery may be ligated in these patients. If the patient is unstable, carotid artery ligation might also be employed. It has been shown that only 20% of adults will develop a neurologic deficit as a result of carotid artery ligation. ● Esophageal and hypopharyngeal injuries should be débrided and repaired primarily if possible. If damage is extensive or if the injury has been neglected, it may be advisable to perform cutaneous esophagostomy for purposes of feeding and drainage, with a planned second-stage procedure once sepsis subsides. All esophageal repairs must be adequately drained externally, since anastomotic leaks occur as often as 20% of the time. ● Simple laryngeal or tracheal injuries can be repaired with mucosal-to-mucosal apposition. Cartilage fragments should be sutured in place to provide support for the airway. If cartilage is lost or shattered, a flap using strap muscles can be used to provide airway support. A tracheostomy should be performed on

the majority of patients with these injuries to allow edema to subside and to assess for stricture formation. ● Injuries to the thyroid gland are managed by débridement, hemostasis, and adequate external drainage with excellent results.

Answer: A, D, E

15. Which of the following statements is/are true regarding splenic trauma?

A. Splenic injuries in children can usually be managed successfully without operation
B. The organism most commonly responsible for postsplenectomy sepsis is *Escherichia coli*
C. Hypotension is a contraindication to splenic salvage
D. The risk of postsplenectomy sepsis is present only during the first 2 years following splenectomy
E. Only 30 to 40% of patients with splenic injuries are hypotensive

Sabiston: 311
Schwartz: 254

Comments: The spleen is the organ most commonly injured in patients with blunt abdominal trauma. The management of splenic trauma has changed a great deal with the recognition of the postsplenectomy sepsis syndrome. This is an overwhelming infection (with a 60-fold increased incidence over the general population) that occurs in patients who have had their spleen removed for trauma. The organisms most often responsible for postsplenectomy sepsis are pneumococcus, *Haemophilus influenzae*, and meningococcus. The risk of this syndrome is greatest during the first 2 years following splenectomy, but actually continues throughout the patient's entire life span. If splenectomy is performed, the patient must be educated regarding the signs and symptoms of postsplenectomy sepsis and the need to seek medical attention promptly. Pneumococcal and meningococcal vaccines should be administered. The use of lifelong prophylactic antibiotics is controversial and is not advocated by most authorities in the field. Once sepsis is established, the mortality rate is on the order of 50%. Because of the syndrome, trauma surgeons have developed methods aimed at dealing with these injuries that stop short of splenectomy. In children, about two thirds of splenic injuries can be managed conservatively. For this to be possible the following conditions must be present: a normal blood pressure can be achieved; absence of major associated injuries; and less than 50% of the child's circulating volume is transfused over the first 24 hours. Contraindications to splenic salvage procedures include: hypotension, because of the greater time and blood loss involved in the procedure; massive associated injuries; and a shattered or avulsed spleen that is not amenable to salvage. ● The results in adults using the same management protocol have not been good; consequently, splenic injuries in adults should be treated with prompt surgical intervention. The diagnosis of splenic injury is often suspected on clinical grounds. About 30 to 40% of patients will be hypotensive, and half the patients will have abdominal guarding and distension. Peritoneal lavage is very accurate in the diagnosis of splenic injuries and is the main diagnostic test in adults. In children, more specific information is necessary to make a decision regarding nonoperative management; for this reason, computerized tomography of the splenic area is the diagnostic test of choice. Splenic salvage can be performed successfully 50 to 80% of the time in adults.

Answer: A, C, E

16. A 22-year-old man has an exploratory laparotomy for a gunshot wound to the abdomen at which time a through-and-through injury to the infrarenal inferior vena cava is encountered. Appropriate management might consist of:

A. No management is necessary, since a low-pressure venous injury will tamponade itself
B. Primary repair of the injuries if the resultant stenosis is less than 50%
C. PTFE patch graft
D. Saphenous vein patch graft
E. Ligation of the infrarenal inferior vena cava

Schwartz: 257

Comments: Injuries to the inferior vena cava most often result from gunshot wounds to the abdomen. A major determinant of survival is the presence of hemorrhagic shock, which, if present, is associated with a mortality rate as high as 80%. Inferior vena caval injuries are diagnosed by a thorough exploration of retroperitoneal hematomas. The Cattell maneuver, involving mobilization of the right colon and small bowel mesentery, is very useful for this purpose as it provides rapid exposure of the entire infrarenal inferior vena cava. Proximal and distal control is most easily achieved by direct pressure on the inferior vena cava above and below the injury. Complete encirclement and application of vascular clamps frequently makes repair difficult because it leads to complete collapse of the vessel on itself. Primary venorrhaphy is the simplest and quickest method of repair and can be accomplished with a running monofilament nonabsorbable suture. Repair of injuries to the posterior wall can be accomplished through the anterior injury or by mobilizing the inferior vena cava sufficiently to "roll it over." A resultant stenosis of up to 50% of the cross-sectional area is acceptable; vein patch graft should be utilized if greater than 50% stenosis is to result from a primary venorrhaphy. Prosthetic material should never be used because of the potential for infection, especially when there are associated gastrointestinal injuries. In patients who are unstable, the infrarenal inferior vena cava can be ligated, although the incidence of late complications with this treatment exceeds 50%. This form of treatment should be used only as a life-saving measure. Ligation can never be used to treat suprarenal inferior vena caval injuries.

Answer: B, D, E

17. In resuscitating a trauma patient from hemorrhagic shock:

A. At least two large-bore intravenous lines should be established
B. The initial 2 liters infused should be in the form of a balanced crystalloid solution
C. External hemorrhage should be controlled using direct pressure
D. Hypotension that does not resolve after 2000 ml of crystalloid should be treated with the addition of blood products and surgical control of blood loss
E. Central lines serve primarily to monitor volume replacement

Sabiston: 295
Schwartz: 200

Comments: Hemorrhagic shock remains the most common cause of preventable death from trauma. Effective resuscitation of major trauma victims must involve a team approach, so that multiple procedures can be performed simultaneously. Prompt surgical intervention to control exsanguinating hemorrhage is also critical. The initial step is the establishment of at least two large-bore intravenous catheters with the infusion of 2000 ml of a balanced crystalloid solution. Peripheral catheters are more effective than longer central venous catheters because the resistance to flow is inversely proportional to the fourth power of the radius, but directly proportional to the length of the catheter. Central venous catheters are primarily useful in monitoring fluid replacement. Equally important to volume infusion is the control of ongoing external hemorrhage. This can be most safely accomplished using direct digital pressure. Tourniquets are contraindicated because they obstruct venous return and eliminate collateral flow to the extremity. Hemostats, when applied deep within a wound, may injure associated structures such as peripheral nerves and, thus, are contraindicated. A pneumatic antishock garment (PASG) may be useful if there are multiple sites of external hemorrhage in the lower extremities. During this initial infusion of volume, an effort should be made to locate sources of blood loss by performing a brisk, targeted physical examination including a chest x-ray, and possibly by peritoneal lavage. If after 2000 ml of crystalloid infusion the patient remains in hemorrhagic shock, an immediate operation should be undertaken to control internal sources of blood loss. In such cases, the operation is part of the resuscitation; digital control of the internal bleeding is accomplished, and nothing further is done until the blood pressure is stabilized. At this point, blood products should be added to the volume resuscitation because of the relatively larger degree of blood loss incurred. The one exception to the general need for prompt surgical intervention is the case in which the patient has major blood loss associated with a pelvic fracture and no other identified source of bleeding. In such instances, PASG application, external pelvic fixation, and transcatheter arterial embolization may be useful techniques.

Answer: A, B, C, D, E

18. During laparotomy on a trauma patient, an actively bleeding injury in the right lobe of the liver is found. Which of the following five sequences of maneuvers to control the bleeding is correct?

1. Point ligation of bleeding vessels	A. 1, 3, 5, 4, 2
	B. 5, 1, 3, 4, 2
2. Hepatic lobectomy	C. 3, 1, 5, 4, 2
3. Temporary compression	D. 3, 4, 5, 1, 2
4. Finger fracture with point ligation and omental packing	E. 3, 1, 4, 5, 2
5. Right hepatic artery ligation	

Sabiston: 314
Schwartz: 243

Comments: Hepatic trauma causes mortality by two different mechanisms. Acutely, patients die because of uncontrolled hemorrhage. In the late phase, patients succumb to sepsis because of inadequately débrided injuries or uncontrolled bile leakage. The initial approach to hepatic injuries is predicated on the need to control life-threatening hemorrhage. About one half of all liver injuries have stopped bleeding prior to operation. Because the incidence of rebleeding is almost nil, no active intervention is required for these wounds. When a bleeding hepatic injury is encountered, the initial step is to temporarily compress the injury with sponge-packs while the remainder of the abdomen is explored. This will stop the hemorrhaging in the majority of wounds. After removal of these temporary packs, vessels that are actively bleeding should be point-ligated. If these vessels are plainly visible, this is a simple matter. If the bleeding vessels are not plainly visible, the liver should be finger-fractured so as to open the wound and expose the bleeding vessels, which can then be ligated. Packing such an open wound with a viable omental flap may be very helpful following this maneuver, as it helps control oozing from the raw surface that has been created in the liver. If the injury is still actively bleeding after these maneuvers, temporary compression of the portal triad (Pringle maneuver) should be employed. This can be accomplished either digitally or with a noncrushing vascular clamp. The Pringle maneuver may be valuable therapeutically by slowing the rate of hemorrhage and allowing resuscitation. It is also a valuable diagnostic maneuver to differentiate hepatic arterial bleeding from hepatic venous bleeding. If the bleeding is controlled with the Pringle maneuver, the appropriate hepatic lobar artery should be isolated and occluded temporarily. If this controls the hemorrhage, the artery may be ligated. If the bleeding is of hepatic venous origin, then steps that must be taken to control this include vascular isolation and extensive mobilization of the liver, possibly with a thoracic extension of the laparotomy incision. Hepatic lobectomy is a formidable undertaking in the unstable trauma patient. This is reserved as a last resort or when extensive devitalization of the liver has occurred. Intraperitoneal packing of the bleeding area with a planned "second-look" operation in 24 hours can be a proper alternative in the patient who requires lobectomy but has developed hypotension, hypothermia, and coagulopathies. All major liver injuries should be drained externally. The use of T-tube decompression of the biliary tree is no longer practiced because of the lack of effectiveness and the high incidence of associated complications.

Answer: E

19. Which of the following statements is/are true regarding the management of abdominal arterial injuries?

A. Severe stretching of any artery can cause injury to the different layers of the arterial wall; the intima is the layer most susceptible to stretch injuries
B. Prosthetic vascular graft material should not be used for repair in a contaminated field because of the risk of infection
C. Primary arterial reanastomosis rather than interposi-

tion grafting is the preferred method of repair, provided it can be performed without undue tension
D. The renal vascular pedicle is at particular risk for stretch injuries in cases involving acute deceleration

Sabiston: 319
Schwartz: 256

Comments: Severe stretching of an artery without actual transection of the vessel can cause injury to its wall. Usually arterial stretching first causes intimal fractures, which can be followed by thrombus formation. The media is the layer injured next most frequently, and the adventitia is least susceptible because of its relative flexibility. Sudden deceleration and shearing are the most frequent causes of a stretch-type injury. While any blood vessels are at risk, the renal, splenic, and superior mesenteric vascular pedicles are particularly vulnerable. Primary reanastomosis of an arterial injury is the treatment of choice if it can be performed without undue tension. If this is not possible, a reversed saphenous vein makes an excellent graft. Composite vein grafts and femoral or iliac artery grafts can be used in the repair of large-diameter arteries when it is not possible to repair with a simple interposition of the saphenous vein. A prosthetic graft, if it is placed in a clean extraperitoneal site, is acceptable but should never be used for repair of an injury in a contaminated field.

Answer: A, B, C, D

20. Regarding open pneumothorax wounds, which of the following statements is/are true?

A. If the chest wall opening is greater than two-thirds the diameter of the trachea, on inspiration air will pass preferentially through the chest wall defect into the pleural cavity
B. A flutter-valve type of dressing may be used temporarily if formal surgical closure is not immediately available
C. Tube thoracostomy is not indicated in such an injury because the pleural cavity already freely communicates with the atmosphere
D. Ventilation by the contralateral lung is unaffected by this injury since the two sides are separated by the mediastinum

Sabiston: 302
Schwartz: 201

Comments: An open pneumothorax or "sucking chest wound" occurs when the soft tissue components of the chest wall do not seal the defect. If the defect is greater than two-thirds the diameter of the trachea, on inspiration air passes preferentially through the chest wall. A flutter-valve type of dressing theoretically acts as a barrier to entry of air into the pleural cavity during inspiration but allows air to escape on expiration. Such a dressing is rarely if ever a substitute for operative closure of the chest wall defect and should only be used as a temporary measure. Tube thoracostomy is still indicated because of the possibility of air trapping in the pleural space. If air is drawn into the pleural space on inspiration, but becomes trapped because of a one-way valve mechanism of the wound, a tension pneumothorax may develop. Intermittent shifts of the mediastinum during respiration can cause ineffective ventilation in the contra-lateral lung, impairment in venous return because of bending of the vena cava, and cardiac arrhythmias.

Answer: A, B

21. A 21-year-old woman with blunt trauma to the head sustained in a motor vehicle accident presents with a history of loss of consciousness for approximately 10 minutes at the scene of the accident. She is presently fully awake, alert, oriented, and responsive. Which of the following statements is/are true regarding the appropriate care of this woman?

A. In this setting, a fully awake patient who has a normal neurologic examination does not require hospital admission for observation
B. If skull x-rays show no fracture, then the likelihood of a significant intracranial injury is low, such that hospital admission is not warranted
C. If funduscopic examination of this patient shows no signs of papilledema, elevated intracranial pressure can be excluded
D. The initial effects of elevated intracranial pressure are bradycardia and hypertension
E. If this patient were to show a sudden fall in blood pressure and alteration in mental status, spinal cord shock or brain stem injury would be the most likely cause

Sabiston: 323, 1382
Schwartz: 201

Comments: Any patient sustaining blunt trauma to the head with an associated loss of consciousness for 5 minutes or more should be admitted to the hospital for at least a 24-hour period for reassessment of neurologic function. Routine hospitalization of patients with loss of consciousness for less than 5 minutes alone, however, is controversial. Blunt trauma to the head can cause significant intracranial injury without an associated skull fracture. Papilledema is a late and unreliable indicator of an elevated intracranial pressure, taking on average 24 hours to develop. The initial effects of an elevated intracranial pressure are bradycardia and hypertension. Hypotension in such a patient rarely is due to brain injury; a source of hemorrhagic shock must be sought.

Answer: D

22. A 40-year-old man presents with a single stab wound to the left chest in the seventh intercostal space in the anterior axillary line. His vital signs are normal and he has bilaterally normal breath sounds. On abdominal examination there is no tenderness or mass. An upright chest x-ray shows no sign of hemothorax or pneumothorax. Which of the following statements is/are true regarding this patient's further management?

A. The absence of a hemo/pneumothorax on chest x-ray indicates that the pleural cavity was not entered during injury
B. The absence of a hemo/pneumothorax effectively excludes a significant intra-abdominal injury
C. Further evaluation must be carried out for a possible intra-abdominal injury

D. If this patient is to have general anesthesia, he must first have a left-sided tube thoracostomy

Sabiston: 302
Schwartz: 201

Comments: In penetrating trauma, violation of the pleural cavity can occur without the development of a hemothorax or pneumothorax. Also, hemo/pneumothorax may later develop as a delayed complication of penetrating injuries to the chest, especially if the patient is given positive-pressure ventilation during general anesthesia. It is advisable, therefore, to perform prophylactic tube thoracostomy in these patients before general anesthesia is begun in order to avoid the life-threatening complication of a tension pneumothorax. On moderate expiration, the diaphragm rises to the level of the fifth intercostal space on the left and to the fifth rib on the right. Injury to intra-abdominal organs or to the diaphragm alone can occur in any penetrating injury to the lower chest. For this reason, further studies should be done to exclude such injuries; a diagnostic peritoneal lavage is frequently advocated as the study of choice.

Answers: C, D

23. Which of the following is/are appropriate management steps to reduce septic complications in an open pelvic fracture involving a perineal wound?

A. A diverting colostomy with distal colon and rectal washout
B. Diverting colostomy only if there is an associated rectal injury
C. Intravenous hyperalimentation and strict enforcement of no oral feeding
D. Frequent débridement and irrigation of the open wound and cleansing of the perineum
E. Primary suture closure of the open perineal wound after débridement and irrigation

Sabiston: 1468

Comments: The mortality rate associated with an open pelvic fracture is reported to be as high as 50%. Early mortality is largely the result of uncontrollable hemorrhage or concomitant head and thoracic injuries. Late mortality usually is due to sepsis. Steps designed to avoid perineal and pelvic sepsis include diversion of the fecal stream by a colostomy and washout of any stool that is present in the distal colon and rectum. A concomitant rectal injury must be examined for and dealt with appropriately, if present. The perineal wound should be adequately débrided and irrigated frequently, with the patient under general anesthesia if necessary, and packed open for continued wound care.

Answer: A, D

24. Regarding duodenal injuries, which of the following statements is/are true?

A. In trauma patients, the most frequent site of duodenal injury is the second portion of the duodenum
B. During abdominal exploration for blunt trauma, a retroperitoneal hematoma in the area of the duodenum does not need to be explored provided it is small in

size and the peritoneum overlying the hematoma is intact

C. Approximately 75 to 85% of all duodenal injuries can be managed by simple débridement and closure

D. In dealing with associated pancreatic injuries, it is not possible to resect the entire head of the pancreas without significant risk of devascularization of the remaining duodenum

E. Some form of tube decompression following duodenal repair is advisable to reduce the incidence of duodenal leak and fistulization

Sabiston: 318
Schwartz: 235

Comments: Duodenal injuries are associated with a high rate of morbidity and mortality. The most frequent site of injury is the second portion of the duodenum, followed in decreasing order by the third, fourth, and first portions. During exploration of the abdomen, any retroperitoneal hematoma in the area of the duodenum must be thoroughly explored in order to avoid a missed duodenal injury, which carries a mortality rate of up to 50%. Approximately 75 to 85% of all duodenal injuries can adequately be dealt with by simple acute débridement and closure. In cases of duodenal injuries involving 75% of the circumference or in those with large tissue loss or with devascularization, surgical therapy tailored to the particular circumstances of the injury is required; usually, this is more than simple closure of the defect. Because the pancreas and duodenum share a common blood supply, it is not possible to resect the entire head of the pancreas alone, since the pancreaticoduodenal arteries are within the substance of this portion of the gland and give off perforating arteries to the duodenum. If, therefore, one is to avoid devascularizing the mid-duodenum, a rim of pancreatic tissue must be preserved around the inner sweep of the second and third portions of the duodenum. Other principles of management in the repair of duodenal injuries can include re-establishment of gastrointestinal continuity, internal decompression and diversion of the flow of gastric contents, external drainage in the area of duodenal repair, and provision for continued nutritional support.

Answer: A, C, D, E

25. A 30-year-old man is brought into the emergency room after being involved in a motor vehicle accident. His blood pressure is 100/60, pulse 120. He complains of pelvic pain that is increased when pressure is applied to his iliac crest. He is unable to void urine freely; you suspect a pelvic fracture. To monitor his urine output during resuscitation, the next step should be:

A. Wait for the patient to void urine freely before attempting transurethral bladder catheterization

B. Initially attempt gentle transurethral bladder catheterization but stop if resistance is encountered

C. Perform a urethrogram before attempting a transurethral bladder catheterization

D. Insert a suprapubic cystostomy tube

Sabiston: 321
Schwartz: 1722

Comments: Genitourinary injuries are frequently associated with pelvic fractures. The membranous portion of the urethra is particularly at risk for transection in the male. If urethral transection is suspected, a urethrogram should be performed to exclude such an injury before transurethral catheterization is performed. If a urethral injury is present and bladder catheterization is attempted, a partial transection can be converted to a complete one or bacteria can be introduced into a false passage with the catheter. Inability to void is one of the classic signs of urethral transection. Other signs are blood at the urethral meatus, a free-flowing or high-positioned prostate on rectal exam, and scrotal or perineal hematoma. A suprapubic cystostomy tube is usually required if a urethral transection is present.

Answer: C

26. Regarding myocardial contusion, which of the following statements is/are true?

A. Appropriate management of a suspected myocardial contusion includes serial electrocardiograms and cardiac enzyme determinations, correction of hypovolemia and hypoxia, continuous monitoring of cardiac electrical activity, and control of arrhythmias

B. The most common arrhythmias associated with myocardial contusion are ventricular arrhythmias

C. The most common time period for arrhythmias to occur is within the first 24 hours after injury

D. Anticoagulants are contraindicated when there is a myocardial contusion

E. Patients with myocardial contusion who do not have associated arrhythmias within 3 days of injury do not need long-term follow-up

Sabiston: 304

Comments: Management of a suspected myocardial contusion includes cardiac monitoring as well as treatment directed at correcting factors such as hypotension or hypoxia that may precipitate arrhythmias. The most common arrhythmias associated with myocardial contusion are supraventricular tachycardia, atrial flutter, and atrial fibrillation, although ventricular arrhythmias can occur. The first 24 hours after injury is the time period when patients are at greatest risk for these arrhythmias to occur. Delayed complication may develop months to years after injury, however, and so long-term follow-up is necessary even if early arrhythmias do not occur. Systemic anticoagulation is contraindicated in the presence of this injury because of the increased risk of bleeding into the myocardium.

Answer: A, C, D

27. Regarding ureteral injuries, which of the following statements is/are true?

A. A significant ureteral injury from penetrating abdominal trauma can safely be excluded if no red blood cells are seen on microscopic urinalysis

B. An excretory urogram is indicated in any patient with penetrating abdominal injury that may pass over the course of the ureter, unless the patient is unstable

C. The procedure of choice for injuries of the lower third

of the ureter near the bladder is primary repair over a stent and with external drainage

D. An excretory urogram after ureteral repair may be omitted only if the patient is asymptomatic

Sabiston: 322
Schwartz: 1722

Comments: In 10% of patients with ureteral injuries, red blood cells are not seen on urinalysis. Therefore, all stable patients who have sustained penetrating abdominal trauma over the course of the ureter require an excretory urogram to search for such an injury, which may be visualized as a total obstruction or a narrowing of the ureter or as extravasation of the contrast material. Injuries to the lower one third of the ureter are best managed by re-implantation of the ureter into the bladder, since the rates of leakage and stenosis are lower with this repair than with direct ureteroureterostomy. Because late stenoses or obstructions following ureteral repair may be clinically silent, urograms should be done in all patients for proper follow-up.

Answer: B

28. Regarding flail chest injuries, which of the following statements is/are true?

A. Initial therapy involves external splinting of the chest wall with sand bags, taping of the chest wall, or traction with sterile towel clips
B. Immediate endotracheal intubation with ventilatory support should be performed as soon as a flail chest is diagnosed
C. Paradoxical motion of the flail segment is due to loss of bony continuity of that segment with the rest of the thoracic skeleton
D. Vigorous pulmonary hygiene along with intercostal nerve blocks and other analgesics may obviate the need for tracheal intubation and ventilatory support in some cases
E. Pulmonary complications of flail chest are the result of inadequate ventilation secondary to an inability to develop an adequate negative intrathoracic pressure because of the inward movement of the chest wall segment on inspiration

Sabiston: 301
Schwartz: 633

Comments: A segment of chest wall that loses bony continuity with the rest of the thoracic skeleton will move paradoxically in accordance to the differences in intrathoracic and extrathoracic pressure. This "free floating" segment of chest wall requires that at least two (and usually more) elements of the thoracic skeleton are disrupted. Pulmonary complications associated with flail chest injuries are due largely to injury of the underlying lung in the form of pulmonary contusions or to tears in conjunction with poor ventilation secondary to pain and reactive splinting from rib fractures. The direct effect on intrathoracic pressure by motion of the flail segment is not of great importance in the development of pulmonary complications. Therefore, external splinting of the chest wall is of little help in the management of flail chest and may be deleterious in that it may limit chest wall expansion in the normal segments of chest wall. Vigorous respiratory care and pain control may obviate the need for ventilatory support in some cases.

Answers: C, D

CHAPTER 11

Burns

1. Match the burn classification with the appropriate morphology.

Burn Classification	Morphology
A. First degree	a. Epidermal coagulation necrosis, blister formation
B. Second degree	b. Only superficial epidermis devitalized
C. Third degree	c. Coagulation of subdermal plexus

Sabiston: 215
Schwartz: 271

Comments: See Question 3.

2. Match the burn classification with the clinical appearance.

Burn Classification	Clinical Appearance
A. First degree	a. Weeping, painful, remaining skin elements waxy, blister formation
B. Second degree	b. Dry, hard, inelastic, translucent
C. Third degree	c. Blanches on pressure, no blisters

Sabiston: 215
Schwartz: 271

Comments: See Question 3.

3. Match burn classification with the most likely lettered cause of the burn.

Burn Classification	Likely Cause
A. First degree	a. Ultraviolet light exposure
B. Second degree	b. Electrical current
C. Third degree	c. Spill scald

Sabiston: 215
Schwartz: 271

Comments: **First degree** burns involve only the epidermis, present as blanching erythema, and are most often caused by excess sunlight or exposure to ultraviolet light. **Second degree** (partial thickness) burns are due to injury to the dermis and may be considered to be either superficial or deep. Superficial partial thickness burns present with weeping blisters. Skin elements are usually viable, and from these, re-epithelialization can occur. Deep partial thickness burns, however, result in so few skin appendages remaining within the dermis that re-epithelialization is unlikely or occurs so slowly that grafting is advisable. Partial thickness burns are most often caused by a short flash or a spill of scalding liquid. **Third degree** (full thickness) burns involve coagulation necrosis of all skin elements down to the subdermal plexus and present as a dry, firm wound. Electrical current, prolonged flame exposure, immersion in scalding liquid, and chemical contact are the most common causes. Such burn classification is useful in determining the overall prognosis of a burn wound, including the likelihood of infection, need for skin grafting, and need for fluid resuscitation.

Answer: Question 1: A–b; B–a; C–c
Question 2: A–c; B–a; C–b
Question 3: A–a; B–c; C–b

4. Which of the following statements is/are true regarding burns?

A. Full thickness chemical burns are recognized easily
B. "Port wine" colored urine is not unusual following major electrical injury
C. Escharotomy/fasciotomy may be required to restore peripheral perfusion
D. Electrical injury results in a deceptively small amount of skin destruction

Sabiston: 231
Schwartz: 269

Comments: Severe full thickness **chemical** burns, when compared with **thermal** burns, may appear to be superficial in the first several days. Injury from an **electrical** burn is also distinct from that of a thermal burn in that significant deep muscular injury can occur in the presence of only minimal skin destruction. This is due to the fact that electric current passes more easily through tissues of lesser resistance than skin (nerve, blood, and muscle). Because of this extensive muscular injury, "port wine" colored urine due to myoglobinuria is not uncommon in patients with electrical burns. In all forms of burns, impaired perfusion due to increased fluid pressure within the compartments of an extremity may require escharotomy or fasciotomy.

Answer: B, C, D

5. True or False: Patients with only 25% total body surface area burns do not require gastric decompression.

Sabiston: 223
Schwartz: 274

Comments: Patients with body surface area burns greater than 20% usually develop a reflex paralytic ileus. This can result in vomiting and aspiration in patients who may already be sedated or obtunded. Periodic examination of gastric contents may allow for earlier diagnosis of hemorrhagic gastritis, which is a significant risk. For these reasons, nasogastric decompression is advisable in such patients.

Answer: False

6. Which of the following statements is/are true regarding administration of antibiotics to burn patients?

A. Gram-negative organisms are responsible for the initial bacterial colonization of a burn wound
B. Systemic antibiotics should be given for the first 8 days following the burn, regardless of any specific bacterial infection
C. Penicillin should be administered prophylactically for a period of 3 to 4 days to patients with major burns
D. Systemic administration of antibiotics after the fourth post-burn day has resulted in decreased morbidity from infection
E. None of the above

Sabiston: 223
Schwartz: 273

Comments: Gram-positive organisms are responsible for the initial bacterial colonization and proliferation in burn wounds. Systemic antibiotics do not penetrate the avascular burn eschar. Their use following the fourth post-burn day has not decreased the morbidity from infection and generally is not recommended unless a specific bacterial infection has been identified. Recent studies have not shown any benefit of prophylactic penicillin during the first days after major burn injury.

Answer: E

7. Which of the following fluid administration plans should be utilized in the first 24 hours vs. the second 24 hours following a major burn?

Fluid Administration Plan	Time Utilized
A. Colloid solution to maintain plasma volume in patients with more than a 40% second and third degree burn	a. First 24 hours
B. D5/W to replace evaporative water loss, maintaining normal sodium concentration	b. Second 24 hours
C. Lactated Ringer's 4 ml/kg body weight/percent second and third degree burns/24 hours	
D. Administration rate: half during first 8 hours, remainder during the last 16 hours	

Sabiston: 218
Schwartz: 272

Comments: There is no uniform agreement on the ideal fluid management of patients with burns. In general, however, it is recognized that during the first 24 hours a balanced salt solution should be administered according to body weight and percent burn area, with the rate of administration more rapid in the immediate post-burn period (first 8 hours). In the second 24 hours, evaporative water loss and plasma volume depletion remain as significant potential problems and should be corrected with administration of dextrose in water and colloid. The goal of fluid resuscitation in the severely burned patient is to maintain adequate tissue perfusion and urine output.

Answer: A–b; B–b; C–a; D–a

8. The "smoke inhalation syndrome" is characterized by which of the following statements?

A. Carboxyhemoglobin levels are most accurate when determined 4 hours after injury
B. Manifestations are always present within the first 24 hours after exposure
C. The severity of the syndrome relates to the type and amount of smoke inhaled and the magnitude of accompanying thermal injuries
D. Xenon scanning is easy to perform but is notoriously inaccurate
E. Specific treatment includes the administration of humidified air, oxygen as required, and steroids.

Sabiston: 221
Schwartz: 281

Comments: The "smoke inhalation syndrome" is a potentially lethal complication of thermal injury, the clinical manifestations of which (dyspnea, alveolar edema, impaired gas exchange) may occur as late as 72 hours after exposure to the gaseous products of incomplete combustion. The components and volume of smoke inhaled as well as the magnitude of accompanying injuries determine the severity of the syndrome. In the asymptomatic individual, carboxyhemoglobin testing immediately upon arrival at the hospital is beneficial if positive, as it suggests that there has been inhalation of a significant amount of smoke. Normal carboxyhemoglobin levels, however, do not exclude the diagnosis of "smoke inhalation syndrome." Measuring the pulmonary washout of peripherally administered xenon is highly accurate in determining a significant lower respiratory tract injury. It is rarely used, however, because of the need to transport these usually critically ill patients to special nuclear medicine facilities. Specific treatment includes humidified air and oxygen as well as mechanical ventilation, positive end-expiratory pressure, and systemic bronchodilators as needed. The routine use of steroids, however, should be avoided, as it significantly increases the risk of infectious complications.

Answer: C

9. Which of the following statements accurately characterize(s) the morbidity and mortality from burn injury?

A. 25 years ago, survival following a 30% body surface area burn was rare
B. Patients over the age of 65 have a 50% mortality with a 25% body surface area burn
C. The size of a burn injury capable of producing a 50% mortality has steadily risen over the past three decades
D. More than 90% of survivors of significant burn injury are able to return to gainful employment

Schwartz: 284

Comments: The development of special burn centers and multidisciplinary teams for the management of patients with major burns, as well as improvements in nutritional and antibiotic support, have resulted in a steady improvement in the outlook for such patients over the past 30 years. The extremes of age and associated chronic diseases continue to worsen the prognosis for patients with major burns.

Answer: A, B, C, D

10. Which of the following statements is/are true regarding burn wound sepsis?

A. Host resistance to infection is markedly diminished following major thermal injury
B. Burn wound sepsis is a major cause of death following massive thermal injury
C. Septic complications at sites uninvolved with the initial burn injury are frequent
D. Pneumonia occurring after major thermal injury most often results from hematogenous spread

Sabiston: 235
Schwartz: 282

Comments: Major thermal injury significantly reduces host resistance to infection, both at the burn wound site and at distant sites. The burn wound itself is often the origin of hematogenously disseminated infection; however, fewer than one third of pneumonias occurring in burn patients are thought to originate hematogenously. The inability of topical antibiotics to penetrate the eschar and of the systemic antibiotics to reach these avascular wounds allows for uncontrolled proliferation of bacteria within the wounds of many burn patients and can be a major cause of death.

Answer: A, B, C

11. Match the items in the two columns.

Topical Agent	Disadvantage
A. Sodium mafenide (Sulfamylon)	a. Painful application; excessive drying of eschar
B. Silver nitrate 0.5%	b. Skin allergy; resistant organisms
C. Silver sulfadiazine (Silvadene)	c. Hyponatremia, hypochloremia, methemoglobinemia
D. Povidone-iodine (Betadine)	d. Painful application; carbonic anhydrase inhibition; resistant organisms

Sabiston: 225
Schwartz: 277

Comments: Topical antibacterial therapy for burn wounds was introduced in the early 1960's and has resulted in the development of numerous agents with varying clinical spectra of activity and varying potential complications. There is no uniform opinion as to the optimal topical agent. The purpose of topical therapy is not to sterilize the wound, but rather to reduce the bacteria thereon. This in turn reduces the likelihood of invasive burn wound sepsis and helps prevent conversion of partial thickness necrosis to full thickness necrosis.

Answer: A–d; B–c; C–b; D–a

12. Which of the following statements is/are true regarding tetanus prophylaxis in burn injury?

a. All burn wounds should be considered as being contaminated
b. A patient who has received a tetanus booster within the preceding 10 years should receive 250 to 500 units of human tetanus immunoglobulin simultaneously with 0.5 ml of absorbed tetanus toxoid
c. Tetanus prophylaxis is mandatory except in those patients who have been actively immunized within the preceding 12 months
d. Administration of tetanus immune globulin and adsorbed toxoid is more effective if both are given at the same site

Sabiston: 223
Schwartz: 273

Comments: Based on the assumption that all burn wounds are contaminated, tetanus prophylaxis is indicated in all patients who have not been actively immunized within the preceding year. Absorbed tetanus toxoid (0.5 ml) is sufficient if there has been active immunization within the preceding 10 years. Otherwise, the toxoid should be administered simultaneously with 250 to 500 units of human tetanus immunoglobulin to provide passive as well as active immunization. These should be administered at separate sites in order to prevent inactivation of the immunoglobulin by the toxoid.

Answer: A, C

13. The rule of 9's:

A. Was developed to estimate the body surface area of burns in children
B. Assigns a value of 18% each to the anterior and posterior trunk and each lower extremity and 9% each to the upper extremities and head
C. Includes an estimate of first degree burn area
D. Has no real practical value in patient management because of the anatomic variability among patients

Sabiston: 216
Schwartz: 271

Comments: The rule of 9's was developed to estimate the body surface area burned in adults. It is not applicable to children because they have proportionately larger heads and smaller legs. It is applicable only in patients with second and third degree burns and is clinically important in determining the requirement of fluids for initial resuscitation. It should not be adhered to rigidly after the initiation of fluid resuscitation, as changes in subsequent therapy should relate more to the patient's response to initial fluid therapy.

Answer: B

14. Which of the following statements accurately characterize(s) the appropriate management of a second degree burn wound?

A. The blister covering the wound should not be unroofed, as it provides a natural sterile dressing
B. Unroofing and débridement of the wound should be performed, but usually requires general anesthesia
C. Topical antibiotic therapy is usually indicated
D. Second degree wounds can convert to third degree wounds as a result of local infection

Sabiston: 228
Schwartz: 275

Comments: Unless they are very small (less than 1 to 2% of body surface), the blisters associated with second degree burn wounds should be punctured and the nonviable skin removed. Although painful, this débridement can usually be performed on a lightly sedated patient without the need for general anesthesia. Such débridement permits the application of topical antibiotic agents. Their application is effective in reducing the likelihood of burn wound infection, which otherwise, by means of local vascular thrombosis, can convert a partial thickness to a full thickness wound.

Answer: C, D

15. Which of the following statements is/are true regarding escharotomy and fasciotomy?

A. Escharotomy should generally be avoided because of the risk of introducing infection through the open wound
B. Escharotomy should never cross the major joint line (elbow-knee) for fear of future scar contracture
C. Fasciotomy is more often indicated in electrical rather than in thermal burns
D. The primary indication for escharotomy is vascular compromise within the extremity

Sabiston: 220
Schwartz: 274

Comments: Third-degree burns of the extremities, particularly those that are circumferential, may result in vascular compromise owing to the inelastic eschar and the underlying swelling. When indicated by virtue of the clinical setting, escharotomy should be performed on the lateral and medial aspects of the extremity, with the inci-

sion carried through the full depth of the skin and across joint lines where the skin is most adherent to the underlying fascia. If impaired perfusion persists after adequate escharotomy, the patient's cardiodynamic status should be reassessed. Fasciotomy, which involves opening of the deep muscular fascia to relieve increased compartmental pressures, is more often required in electrical injuries, in which there can be significant muscle necrosis. It is less often used in thermal burns in which the injury is confined to the skin and subcutaneous tissues. Escharotomy may also be indicated for respiratory compromise in patients with deep burns of the chest wall, which may limit respiratory excursion.

Answer: C, D

16. Which of the following statements is/are true regarding airway management in the early post-burn period?

A. Carbon monoxide is a frequent cause of death in burn patients because of its severe pulmonary toxicity
B. Upper airway obstruction may occur as late as 48 hours after the burn injury
C. Fiberoptic bronchoscopy has no role in the assessment of the airway in burn patients
D. Tracheostomy is the preferred method of initial airway intubation because of the hazards associated with endotracheal intubation through an inflamed, edematous pharynx

Sabiston: 214
Schwartz: 270

Comments: Carbon monoxide is a common cause of death in burn victims; however, this is due to the tissue hypoxia brought about by the strong affinity of carbon monoxide for the hemoglobin molecule. There is no direct toxic effect of carbon monoxide on the pulmonary parenchyma. Soft tissue swelling leading to airway obstruction can occur anytime during the first 48 hours after injury, and careful monitoring of airway patency is important during this time. Assessment of the airway can be done through indirect or direct laryngoscopy, or by fiberoptic bronchoscopy, which has the added advantage of providing assessment of the lower airway in cases of "smoke inhalation syndrome." Impending airway obstruction should be treated by endotracheal intubation if at all possible because of the risk of infection with tracheostomy. Initial tracheostomy is indicated only if endotracheal intubation is impossible or contraindicated because of other head and neck injuries.

Answer: B

CHAPTER 12

Surgical Infection—Principles

1. Following the repair of a perforated colon secondary to diverticulitis, a patient receives a 10-day course of clindamycin and gentamicin. He then develops bloody diarrhea, and the presence of *Clostridium difficile* toxin is detected. Which is the drug of choice to treat this problem?

A. Erythromycin
B. Penicillin
C. Tobramycin
D. Vancomycin
E. Tetracycline

Sabiston: 272
Schwartz: 178

Comments: One of the risks of broad-spectrum systemic antibiotic therapy is the development of enterocolitis due to a necrotizing toxin produced by *Clostridium difficile*. This has been closely associated with the use of clindamycin and other broad-spectrum antibiotics to which this organism is resistant. Endoscopically, one may find an adherent membrane, which has led to the designation of this entity as "pseudomembranous enterocolitis." Vancomycin, administered orally, is not absorbed systemically and is highly effective in the treatment of this entity.

Answer: D

2. Review of a patient's clinical course reveals that at approximately 4 o'clock every afternoon, the patient develops a chill and an abrupt temperature elevation to 39.5° C. The best time to draw blood cultures from this patient would be:

A. During the febrile period
B. One hour before the anticipated temperature elevation and chill
C. One hour after the return of the temperature to normal
D. At random

Sabiston: 267
Schwartz: 168

Comments: The systemic manifestations of bacteremia, which include abrupt temperature elevations and chills, may occur as many as 30 to 90 minutes subsequent to the bacteria entering the blood stream. Since circulating phagocytes usually are quite effective in removing these bacteria from the circulation, blood cultures drawn during the chill are frequently negative. If there is a time pattern to the chill and fever, one's likelihood of obtaining a positive blood culture increases if it is obtained approximately 1 hour before the anticipated fever.

Answer: B

3. Which of the following treatment modalities is contraindicated in the management of surgical wound infection?

A. Specific antibiobic
B. Drainage
C. Débridement
D. Moist heat
E. None of the above

Sabiston: 267
Schwartz: 169

Comments: Surgical wound infections may take the form of a localized abscess, a soft tissue cellulitis, or a combination of the two. In the case of discrete abscess cavities, the most effective treatment is drainage of the abscess and débridement of devitalized tissue. In the majority of instances, this will result in resolution of the infection. Specific antibiotic therapy may facilitate treatment of localized abscesses; however, its primary role in the management of surgical infection is in the treatment of cellulitis and in the prevention or treatment of the bacteremia associated with localized infections. Moist heat applied to accessible areas of infection may also be beneficial by increasing local blood flow, facilitating exudation, and hastening the sloughing of necrotic tissue.

Answer: E

4. In which of the following surgical procedures are prophylactic antibiotics unnecessary?

A. Gastric resection
B. Nissen fundoplication
C. Common bile duct exploration for obstruction
D. Hemicolectomy for carcinoma
E. None of the above

Sabiston: 266
Schwartz: 172

Comments: The value of prophylactic perioperative antibiotic therapy has been studied in many clinical settings. It is generally acceptable to use perioperative antibiotics in operations on the colon or the stomach, or on the biliary tract in instances of acute cholecystitis, obstructive jaundice, or stones in the common bile duct. Its value remains debatable in instances of biliary tract surgery when common bile duct stones and acute infection are absent. Abdominal procedures in which the gastrointestinal and genitourinary tracts are not entered have not been shown to benefit from perioperative antibiotic therapy. Operations that are anticipated to be lengthy or that are performed in elderly, debilitated, or immunosuppressed patients **may** be appropriate exceptions to this generalization.

Answer: B

5. Which of the following is the best time to begin the administration of prophylactic antibiotic therapy for abdominal surgery?

A. Two days prior to the operation
B. One hour prior to the operation
C. As the incision is being made
D. When and if contamination is found during the operation
E. After closure of the abdomen

Sabiston: 266
Schwartz: 172

Comments: Debate persists over the optimal choice of antibiotic(s) for perioperative chemoprophylaxis as well as over the length of time in the postoperative period that antibiotics should be administered. There is general agreement, however, that the effective use of perioperative antibiotics depends upon having tissue levels of the drug present when the opening incision is made. This is best achieved by administering the drug just prior to the operation. Beginning antibiotic therapy after contamination has been detected, or after the operation is completed, does not appear to alter the risk of postoperative wound infection.

Answer: B

6. Which of the following statements is/are true regarding bacteremia?

A. Bacteremia seldom, if ever, occurs in the absence of a pre-existing clinical infection
B. Bacteria usually persist in the blood stream for several hours, allowing colonization of numerous organs and subsequent disseminated sepsis
C. Bacteremic patients who are not on appropriate antibiotics will show clinical signs of toxemia or septicemia

D. One should consider bacteremia from an occult source as a possible etiologic factor in isolated infections arising in internal organs

Schwartz: 170

Comments: Bacteremia is defined simply as the presence of bacteria in the circulating blood. Although the release of bacterial toxins or bacteria in sufficiently large numbers may produce signs of septicemia, it is likely that the majority of bacteremic episodes are asymptomatic. Normal individuals probably have frequent episodes of asymptomatic bacteremia. In the immunocompetent patient, humoral and cellular immune mechanisms are quite effective in ridding the blood of bacteria within a very short time. Dental procedures, traumatic wounds, and even breaks in the anal skin during defecation may lead to transient episodes of bacteremia, which usually have no clinical significance. Occasionally, blood-borne bacteria may colonize and infect internal organs, causing serious clinical infections (e.g., osteomyelitis, brain abscess, pyelonephritis, bacterial endocarditis).

Answer: D

7. Match the form of infection with its one or more appropriate characteristics.

Form of Infection	Characteristics
A. Cellulitis	a. Suppuration
B. Lymphangitis	b. Erythematous streaking
C. Abscess	c. Antibiotics almost always indicated
	d. Surgical treatment alone frequently sufficient

Sabiston: 273
Schwartz: 169

Comments: It is useful to consider surgical infections in terms of their being suppurative or nonsuppurative. Abscesses are localized suppurative collections that may or may not be associated with surrounding cellulitis. In the absence of cellulitis, surgical drainage alone is frequently sufficient treatment. To the contrary, cellulitis is a nonsuppurative, poorly localized infection of soft tissues which in its late stages may go on to necrosis and abscess formation. Group A beta-hemolytic streptoccocci and *Straphylococcus aureus* are the most common bacteria causing non-nosocomial cellulitis. Appropriate initial treatment involves antibiotic therapy, which usually results in significant improvement within 48 to 72 hours. If this does not occur, one must search for an associated abscess, resistant organism, unusual pathogen, or failure of drug absorption. Lymphangitis is an infection of the lymphatic vessels and usually occurs in association with another focus of cellulitis or abscess. It is characterized by erythematous streaking of the skin and is appropriately managed with rest and antibiotics. Lymphadenitis (inflammatory swelling of the lymph nodes) may be seen in association with any of these forms of surgical infection.

Answer: A–c; B–b, c; C–a, d

8. Match each of the following forms of superficial infection with its one or more appropriate characteristics.

Superficial Infection	Characteristics
A. Furuncle	a. Primarily cellulitic
B. Carbuncle	b. Primarily abscess
C. Erysipelas	c. Usually Group A beta-hemolytic streptococci
D. Impetigo	d. Usually staphylococci
	e. Surgery is primary therapy

Schwartz: 170

Comments: A **furuncle,** or boil, is an abscess that begins in the area of a hair follicle or sweat gland. There is usually an intense inflammatory response leading to central necrosis as well as to a peripheral zone of cellulitis. A **carbuncle** is a furuncle that has extended into the surrounding subcutaneous tissues in a multilocular fashion. Both of these infections are usually caused by staphylococci and, as they represent localized areas of suppuration, are primarily treated by surgical drainage. Antibiotic therapy is indicated in the management of furuncles and carbuncles when the associated cellulitis is severe. **Erysipelas** is an acute cellulitis, usually caused by Group A beta-hemolytic streptococci. It may be of abrupt onset and is usually associated with systemic symptoms of chills, fever, and prostration. It is usually effectively treated with appropriate antibiotics. **Impetigo** is a contagious skin infection characterized by small intraepithelial abscesses. Both streptococci and staphylococci are commonly cultured. Although these are considered to be small abscesses, appropriate treatment usually involves systemic and/or topical antibiotics.

Answer: A–b, d, e; B–b, d, e; C–a, c; D–c, d

9. Which of the following factors are important in determining the likelihood of the development of a clinical infection and the severity of the infection?

A. Size of bacterial inoculum
B. Bacterial virulence
C. Bacterial capacity to invade tissue
D. Bacterial capacity to produce toxin
E. Host defenses

Sabiston: 260
Schwartz: 166

Comments: Despite one's best efforts, absolute sterility is rarely achieved in surgical practice, and patients are constantly exposed to bacteria in the environment. The likelihood of clinical infection developing from bacterial exposure of colonization depends on an interplay of all of the factors listed above. The larger the number of bacteria involved, the greater the likelihood that some will survive the host defense mechanisms. Bacteria that have been successful in doing this can go on to cause clinical infection by way of invading tissues locally or producing toxins, which may have both local and systemic effects. Some bacteria (e.g., *Staphylococcus aureus*), although capable of producing exotoxins, cause infections primarily by their local invasiveness. Others (e.g., *Clostridium tetani*) are almost solely toxigenic. Still others (e.g., *Streptococcus pyogenes*) have both invasive and toxigenic capacities. Even small inocula of relatively nonvirulent bacteria may cause clinical infection in patients whose defense mechanisms (humoral and/or cellular) are deficient. Such deficiencies may relate to specific immunologic abnormalities or may be a more generalized impairment due to underlying conditions such as diabetes, malnutrition, malignant disease, or chronic alcoholism.

Answer: A, B, C, D, E

10. Which of the following clinical or laboratory signs effectively rules out the presence of significant infection?

A. Normal pulse rate
B. Normal leukocyte count
C. Leukopenia
D. Normal body temperature
E. None of the above

Sabiston: 267
Schwartz: 168

Comments: The classic clinical and laboratory presentation of a patient with a significant infection is that of localized redness, swelling, heat, and pain associated with fever, tachycardia, and leukocytosis. One must be alert, however, to the possibility that any or all of these manifestations may be absent in a patient with infection. In the elderly and debilitated, the capacity of the body to mount a significant inflammatory response to infection may prevent the development of the classic rubor, tumor, calor, and dolor (see above). Patients with abscesses that are well walled-off may not show the systemic signs of infection. Furthermore, severe infections may result in bone marrow depression and exhaustion of the supply of leukocytes, resulting in leukopenia. Hypothermia and leukopenia may in fact be signs of life-threatening sepsis.

Answer: E

11. Match the agent with one or more of its mechanisms of antimicrobial action.

Agent	Mechanism of Antimicrobial Action
A. Amphotericin B	a. Inhibition of cell wall synthesis
B. Penicillin	b. Disruption of membrane barrier function
C. Cephalosporins	c. Disruption of ribosomal protein synthesis
D. Gentamicin	d. Disruption of chromosome DNA replication
E. Griseofulvin	

Sabiston: 270
Schwartz: 171

Comments: All of the antimicrobial agents listed are bactericidal (i.e. their associated mechanism of action results in actual bacterial death). Bacteriostatic agents (e.g. tetracyclines, chloramphenicol, erythromycin, clindamycin) act by preventing bacterial growth, but do not result in bacterial death. These agents work primarily through inhibition of ribosomal protein synthesis. Appreciation of the mechanism of action of antimicrobials may have a bearing on the selection of alternative therapies when bacterial resistance to the drug of choice develops.

Answer: A–b, c; B–a; C–a; D–c; E–d

12. Which of the following statements is/are true regarding intestinal antisepsis?

A. In the presence of adequate systemic antimicrobial prophylaxis, mechanical bowel cleansing adds little to reducing the incidence of postoperative infection
B. In the presence of adequate mechanical cleansing of the bowel, oral antibiotic bowel preparation adds little to reducing the incidence of postoperative infection
C. Mechanical bowel preparation effectively reduces the number of bacteria per gram of stool
D. There is yet to be general agreement as to the ideal oral antibiotic agent(s)
E. Appropriate intestinal antisepsis allows some added measure of protection against infection, should there be an anastomotic leak

Sabiston: 266
Schwartz: 173

Comments: It is generally agreed that proper intestinal antisepsis involves a combination of mechanical cleansing of the bowel and intraluminal antibiotic therapy. This has resulted in a decrease in the incidence of postoperative wound infections. Mechanical cleansing may be achieved by a combination of appropriate cathartics and enemas or by the oral administration of large volumes of balanced salt solutions to flush the colonic contents effectively. Whatever stool remains, however, continues to contain large numbers of bacteria (approximately 10^{11}/gm stool). Although there is not general agreement as to which antibiotic agents are most effective, commonly employed regimens include oral kanamycin for several days prior to surgery and oral neomycin/erythromycin base the afternoon before surgery. Regardless of one's method of achieving mechanical or antibiotic preparation of the bowel, neither alone appears to result in the same reduction in postoperative wound infections as both combined. All the above notwithstanding, proper mechanical and antimicrobial bowel preparation does not protect against infections due to technical operative errors. Although done commonly, the addition of systemic antibiotic therapy to mechanical preparation has not been shown to further reduce the incidence of postoperative infection.

Answer: D

13. Match each of the following gram-positive cocci with one or more of the antibiotics that would be therapeutic choices.

Gram-Positive Cocci	Appropriate Antibiotics
A. Lactamase-producing *Staphylococcus aureus*	a. Methicillin
	b. Penicillin G
B. Non–lactamase-producing *Staphylococcus aureus*	c. Ampicillin
	d. Oxacillin
C. *Streptococcus pyogenes*	
D. *Streptococcus pneumoniae*	
E. *Streptococcus faecalis*	

Sabiston: 268
Schwartz: 174

Comments: Most gram-positive cocci are sensitive to penicillin G, which is the drug of choice if there is no history of allergy to it. Exceptions to this general rule include beta-lactamase-producing *Staphylococcus aureus* (>95% of today's isolates), which is able to destroy the penicillin G. Alterations in penicillin structure have led to a number of related drugs (methicillin, nafcillin, oxacillin) that are highly effective against these species of *Staphlycoccus*. *Streptococcus faecalis* may on occasion be resistant to penicillin G. Ampicillin is more active than penicillin G on a weight basis.

Answer: A–a, d; B–a, b, c, d; C–a, b, c, d; D–a, b, c, d; E–b, c

14. Which of the following statements is/are true regarding the relationship of the penicillins to the cephalosporins?

A. Both are bactericidal
B. Both are effective against almost all strains of *Staphylococcus*
C. Cephalosporins are recommended in the management of streptococcal infections in patients who have had anaphylactic reactions to penicillin
D. Although the biochemical structures of the cephalosporins and penicillins are similar, their mechanisms of action against bacteria are different

Sabiston: 270
Schwartz: 176

Comments: The cephalosporins and penicillins share many properties. In addition to their similar biochemical structures, they both produce their bactericidal effects by inhibition of bacterial cell wall synthesis. Both antibiotics are effective against pneumococci and most streptococci; however, cephalosporins are more effective than penicillin against staphylococci that produce beta lactamases. Semisynthetic isoxazolyl penicillins have been developed that are effective against these strains of *Staphylococcus aureus* and are actually more active on a weight basis than cephalosporins. There is significant cross-resistance of these strains of staphylococci to the penicillins and the cephalosporins. Approximately 10% of patients with allergy to penicillin are also allergic to cephalosporins. This should be considered before treatment of penicillin-allergic patients with cephalosporins.

Answer: A

15. Which of the following characterize the use of tetracyclines?

A. Bactericidal
B. Activity against *Mycobacterium tuberculosis*
C. Discoloration of teeth
D. Risk of superinfection
E. Narrow spectrum of activity

Sabiston: 271
Schwartz: 177

Comments: The tetracyclines are a family of closely related antibiotics that exert their bacteriostatic effect by altering ribosomal protein synthesis. These antibiotics have a broad spectrum of activity against most gram-positive species and many gram-negative species as well as *Treponema pallidum* and *Mycobacterium tuberculosis.* Tetracyclines may be deposited in developing teeth during the early stages of calcification and will result in a yellowish-brown discoloration. For this reason, these drugs should be avoided in children less than 8 years old. As with most broad-spectrum antibiotics, alteration in the normal flora may result in superinfection by a number of other organisms including *Candida, Staphylococcus, Proteus,* and *Pseudomonas.* The injudicious use of broad-spectrum antibiotics should be avoided.

Answer: B, C, D

16. Chloramphenicol is characterized by which of the following?

A. Broad-spectrum
B. Possible bone marrow aplasia
C. Useful in perioperative antimicrobial prophylaxis
D. Useful in the treatment of typhoid fever

Sabiston: 271
Schwartz: 177

Comments: Chloramphenicol is a broad-spectrum antibiotic that can be very useful in selected clinical situations. In patients allergic to penicillin or ampicillin, it is considered the drug of choice in the treatment of typhoid fever, other severe *Salmonella* infections, and severe infections caused by *Haemophilus influenzae.* Potential lethal toxic effects of the drug include an idiosyncratic aplastic anemia and circulatory collapse in infants. Because of these potential problems, chloramphenicol is not indicated for prophylactic therapy. When used in selected clinical situations, white cell counts should be monitored carefully.

Answer: A, B, D

17. Which of the following is/are characteristic of aminoglycosides?

A. Active against broad spectrum of gram-negative aerobes
B. Emergence of resistant strains does not occur
C. Nephrotoxicity
D. Ototoxicity

Sabiston: 271
Schwartz: 177

Comments: The aminoglycosides are a family of bactericidal antibiotics with a broad spectrum of activity against gram-negative aerobic organisms. They are the antibiotics of choice for established infections by *Pseudomonas aeruginosa,* but therapeutic options are rapidly changing. Because of the dose-related toxicity of these drugs to the auditory branch of the 8th cranial nerve as well as to the kidney, their use in prophylaxis has been discouraged. Resistant strains have been identified, and this is particularly true of *Pseudomonas aeruginosa* resistance to gentamicin.

Answer: A, C, D

18. Match the following antibiotics with one or more associated characteristics.

Antibiotic	Characteristic
A. Clindamycin	a. A causative factor of pseudomembranous enterocolitis
B. Vancomycin	b. Is used to treat pseudomembranous enterocolitis
C. Metronidazole	c. Excellent anaerobic activity
	d. Ototoxicity
	e. Peripheral neuropathy

Sabiston: 270
Schwartz: 178

Comments: The above three drugs do not easily fit into other broader categories of antimicrobials but are similar in that they have fairly specialized and specific indications for their use. Vancomycin and metronidazole, given orally, are both highly effective in treating pseudomembranous enterocolitis due to toxin production from an overgrowth of *Clostridium difficile.* Use of clindamycin in the management of other infections has been commonly associated with the development of this type of enterocolitis. Both clindamycin and metronidazole have excellent activity against anaerobic organisms. Vancomycin is used primarily as a reserve antibiotic in the treatment of infections due to methicillin-resistant staphylococci and *Staphylococcus epidermidis.* As with many of the other "mycin" drugs, ototoxicity is a potential dose-related complication. Metronidazole is associated with a number of side effects including vomiting, diarrhea, skin rash, peripheral neuropathy, and convulsions and may occasionally cause pseudomembranous enterocolitis.

Answer: A–a, c; B–b, d; C–a, b, c, e

19. Which of the following statements is/are true regarding amphotericin B?

A. It is the best currently available antifungal agent for the treatment of systemic mycotic infections
B. It is effective only against systemic candidiasis
C. It may cause fever and chills
D. It may cause permanent renal damage

Sabiston: 271, 281
Schwartz: 179

Comments: A number of antifungal antibiotics (griseofulvin, nystatin, flucytosine, imidazole derivatives) are available for oral and/or topical administration in the treatment of superficial fungal infections. However, ketoconazole and miconazole have some activity against certain systemic fungi. Amphotericin B is the current best and most predictable antifungal agent for the treatment of systemic mycotic infections including candidasis, mucormycosis, cryptococcosis, histoplasmosis, coccidioidomycosis, sporotrichosis, and aspergillosis. Its numerous potential toxic effects include fever, chills, vomiting, anemia, hypokalemia, and renal impairment.

Answer: A, C, D

20. Match the following clinical characteristics with their streptococcal infections.

Clinical Characteristics	Infection
A. May be polymicrobial	a. Necrotizing fasciitis
B. Frequently significant overlying skin involvement	b. Myonecrosis
	c. Both
C. Seen following trauma and abdominal surgery for peritonitis	d. Neither
D. Treatment consists of appropriate surgical drainage, débridement, and antibiotics	

Sabiston: 273
Schwartz: 181

Comments: As their names imply, these severe infections are distinguished by whether the infection involves primarily the superficial fascia or the underlying muscle. Both infections may be polymicrobial. **Necrotizing fasciitis** is usually caused by beta-hemolytic streptococci, which may be found in association with coagulase-positive staphylococci or gram-negative enteric pathogens. Necrotizing fasciitis involves superficial and widespread fascial necrosis, and the overlying skin frequently shows a pale, red discoloration which may progress to a distinct purple color in association with the development of blisters and bullae. **Myonecrosis** is caused by clostridia, aerobic streptococci, and other anaerobes which may be found in association with *Staphylococcus aureus* or gram-negative rods. Although both of these entities may occur following operation, they most often occur following trauma outside the hospital. Both are potentially life-threatening infections, which must be treated immediately with wide surgical débridement and appropriate antibiotic therapy.

Answer: A–c; B–a; C–c; D–c

21. Which of the following statements is/are true regarding staphylococcal infections?

A. The skin is the most common site
B. The pattern of antiobiotic sensitivity has been stable over the last four decades
C. *Staphylococcus epidermidis* should be considered a contaminant only and is not associated with clinically significant infections
D. Invasive staphylococcal enterocolitis is a self-limiting process and does not require a specific therapy.

Sabiston: 273
Schwartz: 183

Comments: Staphylococci are permanent bacterial inhabitants of normal skin and nasopharynx. Although the skin is the most common site of staphylococcal infections, hematogenous spread of this organism has resulted in metastatic abscesses in the lungs, heart, kidneys, liver, bone, and brain. Fulminating lethal septicemia may also result from staphylococcal skin infections. Most clinically significant infections are caused by *Staphylococcus aureus;* however, *Staphylococcus epidermidis* is associated with infections occurring in the setting of central venous catheters, or prosthesis implantations and have been a source of endocarditis and septicemia following

heart surgery. Staphylococcal enteritis in its mild, noninvasive form usually produces only mild to moderate symptoms, which nonetheless require discontinuance of the predisposing oral antibiotic therapy. In its invasive form, however, staphylococcal pseudomembranous enterocolitis may lead to a fulminating septic course and death. Numerous strains of staphylococci resistant to commonly used antibiotics have developed and are of particular significance in hospital-acquired staphylococcal infections.

Answer: A

22. Which of the following statements is/are true regarding clostridial infections?

A. The presence of clostridial organisms in a surgical or traumatic wound warrants immediate antibiotic and surgical intervention
B. The oxidation-reduction potential in contaminated tissues is a significant factor in the development of a clostridial infection
C. Despite its potentially fulminant course, the skin overlying clostridial cellulitis may not be discolored or edematous
D. Clostridial myonecrosis (gas gangrene) should be treated with immediate surgical débridement, antibiotics, clostridial antitoxin, and hyperbaric oxygenation

Sabiston: 278
Schwartz: 184

Comments: Clostridial organisms are ubiquitous and are a common contaminant of traumatic wounds. In most wounds, however, the high oxidation-reduction potential of the surrounding healthy tissues prevents colonization and invasion of these tissues. In such cases, the presence of clostridia is clinically insignificant. When colonization occurs in the presence of necrotic tissue, proliferation and invasion of clostridia can occur, leading to clostridial cellulitis. This form of clostridial infection is confined to the superficial fascial planes and, although it may spread rapidly, systemic effects may be mild and the skin of normal color. Clostridial myonecrosis occurs when the deeper muscular compartments are invaded, usually by *Clostridium perfringens*. The inaccessibility of systemic antibiotics to this ischemic, necrotic tissue, coupled with the low oxidation-reduction potential of such wounds, permit the rapid dissemination of the clostridia through the muscular compartments. An innocuous appearance of the postoperative wound does not exclude the possibility of clostridial sepsis in the appropriate clinical setting. Treatment should be immediate surgical débridement and antibiotic therapy (penicillin G). Adjunctive hyperbaric oxygenation has been helpful, but horse antitoxin therapy is of no proven value and may be followed by serum sickness.

Answer: B, C

23. Match the following clinical situations with their appropriate tetanus prophylaxis (select the single best answer).

Clinical Situation	Tetanus Prophylaxis
A. A previously unimmunized child under 5 years of age without wounds	a. No treatment
B. Previously unimmunized adult without wounds	b. 0.5 ml adsorbed toxoid
C. Previously immunized patient, booster 7 years ago, non–tetanus-prone wound	c. 0.5 ml adsorbed toxoid and 250 units of human tetanus immune globulin-now; two additional injections of toxoid over the next year
D. Previously immunized patient, booster 7 years ago, tetanus-prone wound	d. Three injections of toxoid over approximately a 1-year period with booster every 10 years
E. No prior immunization, non–tetanus-prone wound	e. Series of four injections of tetanus toxoid with diphtheria and pertussis vaccine
F. No prior immunization, tetanus-prone wound	

Sabiston: 279
Schwartz: 188

Comments: Tetanus is a severe, progressive syndrome caused by the neurotoxin released by *Clostridium tetani*. In ideal therapeutic circumstances, the mortality rate usually exceeds 30%. As with most diseases, the best treatment is prevention. Fortunately, active immunization with adsorbed tetanus toxoid and passive immunization with human tetanus immunoglobulin have been very effective in preventing this clinical syndrome. The principles of prophylactic immunization and the appropriate active and passive immunization of patients with wounds are outlined above.

Answer: A–e; B–d; C–a; D–b; E–d; F–c

24. Which of the following statements accurately characterize(s) infections with common aerobic gram-negative bacilli?

A. Most of these organisms are pathogenic to humans, even with small inocula
B. Infections with these organisms occur only within the abdomen or in abdominal wounds
C. Pending results of cultures and sensitivities, broad-spectrum antimicrobial therapy is necessary when infection with gram-negative bacilli is suspected
D. These organisms may infect prosthetic surgical implants.

Sabiston: 278
Schwartz: 189

Comments: Most of the aerobic gram-negative bacilli responsible for clinically significant infections (*Escherichia coli, Klebsiella pneumoniae, Enterobacter aerogenes,* and others) are facultative organisms usually found colonizing the intestinal tract. *Pseudomonas aeruginosa* is ubiquitous in the environment and becomes bowel flora in hospitalized patients. Although the majority of infections caused by these organisms occur postoperatively in wounds following surgery on the gastrointestinal tract, abdominal cavity, or genitourinary tract, these bacteria may be responsible for pneumonia, endocarditis, and other extra-abdominal infections in hospitalized patients. All these organisms act opportunistically and can cause serious infections in debilitated or immunosuppressed patients or in those receiving foreign implants or prosthetic vascular grafts.

Answer: C, D

25. Which of the following statements is/are true regarding anaerobic bacterial infections?

A. Anaerobic bacteria are common inhabitants of skin and mucous membranes
B. *Bacteroides* species are the most frequent isolates in anaerobic infections
C. If appropriate cultures are obtained, anaerobes are found in only 20% of intra-abdominal abscesses
D. Proper treatment of anaerobic infections consists of surgical drainage, débridement of necrotic tissue, and appropriate antibiotic therapy

Sabiston: 279
Schwartz: 190

Comments: Anaerobic bacteria are found as normal flora on the skin and mucous membranes and in fact outnumber aerobic organisms by greater than 10:1 in the oral cavity and by greater than 1,000:1 in the colon. It is not surprising, therefore, that anaerobes are cultured from intra-abdominal abscesses in up to 90% of cases. The most common pathogens in this group are the *Bacteroides* species. As with most serious infections, proper treatment involves appropriate drainage of abscesses and débridement of devitalized tissue when present, as well as appropriate antibiotic therapy

Answer: A, B, D

26. Match the following:

A. All microorganisms are killed	a. Antiseptic
B. Pathogenic organisms on the body are killed or their growth inhibited	b. Disinfectant
C. Pathogenic organisms on inanimate objects are killed	c. Sterilization

Schwartz: 195

Comments: The safety of modern surgery is enhanced by the ability to reduce the number of bacteria in the vicinity of the operative field. An **antiseptic** is a chemical agent that either kills or inhibits the growth of pathogenic organisms. By custom and law, this term refers only to agents applied to the body. A **disinfectant** is a chemical used on inanimate objects to kill pathogenic organisms. Not all organisms are necessarily killed by these two classes of chemicals. **Sterilization,** on the other hand, is the process of killing all microorganisms (bacteria, viruses, parasites, fungi, and spores). This can be achieved through pressurized steam, dry heat, chemicals, or radiation.

Answer: A–c; B–a; C–b

27. Match the following:

Clinical Characteristics	Infecting Organisms
A. Not a true fungus	a. *Actinomyces israelii*
B. Amphotericin B is the drug of choice for severe infection	b. *Nocardia asteroides*
	c. *Histoplasma capsulatum*
C. Common inhabitant of oral mucosa	d. *Cryptococcus neoformans*
	e. *Candida albicans*
D. Pulmonary manifestations are common	
E. Central nervous system manifestations are common	

Sabiston: 280
Schwartz: 191

Comments: Pseudomycotic infections, actinomycosis and nocardiosis, are caused by organisms that are true bacteria but behave morphologically and clinically like fungi. *Actinomyces israelii* is an inhabitant of normal oral flora and causes burrowing, tortuous abscesses in the cervicofacial, thoracic, and abdominal areas. Appropriate treatment includes surgical drainage and penicillin G as the drug of choice. **Nocardiosis** is an opportunistic infection occurring either as pulmonary infection or as subcutaneous and brain abscesses and is difficult to treat. Sulfonamides are used in combination with other antimicrobials. **Histoplasmosis** is predominantly a pulmonary infection caused by *Histoplasma capsulatum,* which is endemic to the Mississippi and Ohio valleys and along the Appalachian Mountains. Infection may be quite mild or may go on to a severe form with pulmonary cavitation; pulmonary and extrapulmonary disease may mimic tuberculosis. **Cryptococcosis** is caused by a yeast. Its most frequent form of disseminated disease is meningitis, although cavitary and nodular pulmonary disease is also seen. *Candida albicans* is a common inhabitant of the mucous membranes. In debilitated patients, or those whose normal flora has been altered by antibiotic therapy, superficial candidal infections (e.g., thrush) may develop and are usually effectively treated with topical agents (e.g., nystatin). Severe systemic candidiasis is a life-threatening infection commonly associated with severe debilitation, immune suppression, other chronic infections, and intravenous lines. The foundation of therapy for systemic candidiasis and the other true systemic mycotic infections is amphotericin B.

Answer: A–a, b; B–c, d, e; C–a, e; D–a, b, c; E–b, d

CHAPTER 13

Peritonitis and Intra-abdominal Abscesses

1. True statements regarding the peritoneal cavity include:

A. The peritoneal cavity consists of a greater and a lesser sac that communicate through the foramen of Winslow
B. The peritoneum consists of a flat layer of epithelial cells reinforced externally by the endoabdominal fascia
C. The peritoneal cavity is a completely enclosed sac in males and females
D. The parietal peritoneum is innervated by both somatic and visceral nerves and is quite sensitive, while the visceral peritoneum receives only autonomic innervation and is relatively insensitive
E. Visceral peritoneal irritation often produces a somatic response

Sabiston: 786
Schwartz: 1391

Comments: The peritoneum is a single layer of mesothelial cells that is reinforced externally by the endoabdominal (transversalis) fascia. It forms a completely enclosed sac in males; in females it is open at the ends of the fallopian tubes. The parietal peritoneum is supplied by both somatic and visceral afferent nerves and is quite sensitive. The anterior parietal peritoneum is the most sensitive area, while that in the pelvis is the least sensitive. Because of its somatic innervation, irritation of the parietal peritoneum produces pain that can be localized to its site of origin. Irritation of the parietal peritoneum also leads to voluntary guarding, and severe irritation can lead to involuntary muscular spasm. In contrast, the visceral peritoneum is innervated only by the autonomic nervous system and is relatively insensitive; these visceral afferent nerves respond primarily to traction or distension and less well to pressure. The visceral peritoneum at the root of the small bowel and over the biliary tree is somewhat better innervated, accounting for the more pronounced symptoms produced by irritation in these areas. Although autonomic responses to visceral peritoneal stimulation are uncommon, severe stimulation

will occasionally lead to bradycardia and hyportension; it is not unusual for visceral irritation to produce ileus.

Answer: A, D

2. Which of the following statements is/are true regarding peritoneal function?

A. The surface area of the peritoneum is larger than the filtering surface area of the renal glomeruli
B. The peritoneum is a semipermeable membrane allowing bidirectional movement of water, electrolytes, and small molecules
C. The peritoneum is incapable of active transport of agents of high molecular weight
D. Absorption of particulate matter (including bacteria) occurs only through stomata on the parietal surface of the diaphragmatic peritoneum
E. Sympathetic pleural effusions can originate anywhere from the parietal pleura in response to irritation

Sabiston: 782
Schwartz: 1392

Comments: The peritoneum covers nearly 2 m^2 of surface area, this being larger than the filtering surface area of the renal glomeruli. It is a semipermeable membrane and allows bidirectional passive movement of water, electrolytes, and very small molecules. Normally, these interactions produce 100 ml of fluid that acts as a lubricant between the viscera and the abdominal wall. There is evidence that the peritoneum is also capable of active absorption requiring expenditure of energy. Many components of plasma, including albumin, electrolytes, and urea, rapidly equilibrate with the blood volume when placed in the abdominal cavity. This is also true for many antibiotics and endogenous and exogenous toxic substances (including bacterial toxins). Absorption of particulate matter from the peritoneal cavity occurs only through stomata on the peritoneal surface of the diaphragm. Material absorbed by the diaphragm passes unidirectionally to the retrosternal and mediastinal lymphatics. These lymphatics play a role in the transport of fluid from the peritoneal cavity and account for the sympathetic pleural effusion that develops in response to inflammation of the diaphragmatic peritoneum. These lymphatics also allow transport of amylase-rich abdominal fluid into the pleural space.

Answer: A, B, D

3. True statements regarding the peritoneal response to injury include:

A. Denuded peritoneum regenerates slowly over the course of 5 to 7 days as a result of mesothelial ingrowth from the edge of the defect
B. Fibrin is elaborated from underlying connective tissue after the peritoneum is destroyed
C. In most instances, once fibrin is deposited, adhesions will form
D. Nonabsorbed fibrin is invaded by fibroblasts between 5 and 10 days after injury, resulting in fibrous adhesions
E. Once formed, fibrous adhesions do not disappear

Sabiston: 784
Schwartz: 1392

Comments: The peritoneum heals rapidly after injury, often within a matter of hours. This occurs as a result of differentiation of stem cells within the subperitoneal tissues, transperitoneal migration of shed mesothelial cells, and the ingrowth of mesothelial cells from the intact edges of the defect. Adhesions form when peritoneal healing is delayed or incomplete. Fibrin is elaborated from peritoneal mesothelial cells as a result of inflammation. Most deposited fibrin is absorbed, but when it is not, fibroblast invasion between 5 and 10 days after injury leads to organization of the fibrin into true fibrous tissue. Continued intraperitoneal irritation, necrosis extending through the mesothelium to the subperitoneal tissues, and a predisposition to adhesion formation in certain individuals all favor the development of fibrous adhesions. With time, fibrous adhesions can become attenuated and may disappear.

Answer: D

4. Which of the following statements is/are true regarding the primary response to peritonitis?

A. The initial response is vascular dilatation and fluid transudation
B. There is immediate cessation of bowel activity, producing a profound ileus
C. Parietal engorgement secondary to inflammation allows transmigration of leukocytes and bidirectional passage of large molecules such as intra-abdominal toxins and byproducts of necrosis
D. The inflammation that produces ileus also leads to increased secretion into the bowel lumen as well as to decreased resorption and therefore sequestration of luminal contents
E. "Third-spacing" is primarily a function of the bowel rather than the peritoneum

Sabiston: 783, 797
Schwartz: 1392

Comments: The peritoneum reacts to irritation by vascular dilatation and outpouring of fluid. The initial fluid is a transudate with low protein content from the extracellular interstitial compartment. It is accompanied by large numbers of white blood cells, and during this phase toxins and other materials within the peritoneal fluid are easily absorbed into the blood stream. Later in the process, the fluid becomes a protein-rich exudate that is capable of clotting, leading to adherence of loops of bowel in the area of inflammation, helping to confine the extent of peritoneal contamination. Quantitative changes that occur include a decrease in the RNA-DNA ratio and an increase in uronic acid concentrations within the peritoneal membrane. The bowel's initial response to peritonitis is transient hypermotility followed by varying degrees of adynamic ileus. Fluid secretion by the bowel increases, while at the same time resorption decreases, promoting sequestration of fluid within its lumen. The lumen is further distended by swallowed air. The outpouring of fluid from the irritated peritoneum combined with sequestering of fluid within the loops of adynamic bowel leads to significant "third space" sequestration. The rate of sequestration is proportional to the surface area of peritoneum involved with inflammation; 4 to 6 liters of fluid can be "third spaced" by the inflamed peritoneum within 24 hours.

Answer: A, C, D

5. Regarding the secondary responses to peritonitis, which of the following statements is/are true?

A. Peritonitis produces an almost immediate adrenomedullary response of increased production of epinephrine and norepinephrine
B. Hyponatremia often results, owing to excessive loss of sodium into the peritoneal cavity
C. The cardiac output increases as the result of increased production of catecholamine
D. The respiratory rate increases, while tidal volume decreases
E. The acidosis of peritonitis is due to mitochondrial inhibition by a circulating factor produced by inflamed peritoneum

Sabiston: 48, 797
Schwartz: 1394

Comments: Peritonitis in its more severe form can lead to a series of interrelated secondary events which eventually may result in multisystem organ dysfunction as follows: There is an immediate increased production of epinephrine and norepinephrine by the adrenal medulla in response to peritonitis, leading to vasoconstriction, tachycardia, and sweating. This effect can persist for up to 72 hours. The hypovolemia of peritonitis causes increased aldosterone and ADH production that often leads to water retention in excess of sodium retention, producing hyponatremia. Cardiac output decreases because of the hypovolemia; the usual cardiac compensations for this are less than optimal, because contractility is impaired by the progressive acidosis. Respiratory volume is decreased as a result of abdominal distension and of splinting due to diaphragmatic irritation. These cardiac and pulmonary changes may lead to a severe compromise of delivery of oxygen to the peripheral tissues. The hypovolemia and decreased cardiac output may lead to decreased renal blood flow with associated compromise of the renal handling of solutes and acid byproducts. The metabolic rate is increased during episodes of peritonitis; in the face of decreased oxygen delivery, this leads to a shift from aerobic to anaerobic metabolism, further contributing to the development of acidosis. As a result of the decreased cardiac output, compensatory vasoconstriction occurs, further compromising oxygen delivery and increasing acid production that cannot be cleared properly because of pulmonary and renal insufficiency. Glycogen stores are rapidly utilized, but insulin resistance due to circulating catecholamines interferes with utilization of glucose by the muscles. Lipolysis is increased, but the fatty acids are not efficiently utilized. Protein catabolism of muscle mass develops early and can result in a 25 to 30% loss of lean body mass. Plasma synthesis does continue, but a considerable amount is lost into the peritoneal cavity.

Answer: A, D

6. Which of the following statements is/are true regarding the clinical presentation of peritonitis?

A. Patients with peritonitis frequently shift position in order to relieve their pain
B. Most patients with peritonitis are anorectic
C. High-pitched bowel sounds become prominent as bowel wall edema leads to progressive compromise of the intestinal lumen
D. Peritonitis is usually associated with marked elevations of the white blood cell count
E. There may be only minimal temperature elevation in infants and debilitated elderly patients
F. Before the diagnosis can be confirmed, there must be x-ray evidence of ileus and obliteration of the psoas shadow

Sabiston: 798
Schwartz: 1395

Comments: Steady, unrelenting abdominal pain aggravated by motion is the predominant symptom of peritonitis. The pain may develop acutely (as with perforation) or insidiously. Generally, patients lie very still with knees bent, and breathe in a shallow manner in order to minimize peritoneal motion (and thus, pain). A decrease in the severity and extent of pain over time implies localization of the offending process, whereas increasing severity and extent implies spreading peritonitis. Most patients are anorectic; nausea with or without emesis is frequently present. The temperature is usually markedly elevated (38 to 40° C), but infants and debilitated elderly patients may have only moderate fever. The abdomen frequently is distended, is tender to palpation over the area of inflammation, and demonstrates direct and referred rebound tenderness. Rigidity—initially voluntary to prevent pain from motion during palpation, and later involuntary due to reflex muscle spasm—may ultimately lead to the typical boardlike abdomen. Bowel sounds are present only in the earliest stages of peritonitis; the abdomen is silent once adynamic ileus occurs. Because white blood cells enter the peritoneum in large numbers during transudation, the peripheral white blood cell count may be paradoxically low. Therefore, the differential count (demonstrating a left shift) is more important than the absolute white blood cell count. X-ray films of the abdomen may demonstrate small and large intestine dilatation, increased space between bowel loops due to inflammatory exudate and edema, obliteration of the peripheral fat lines and psoas shadows, and, if a viscus has perforated, free air on upright or decubitus films. It cannot be overemphasized that the diagnosis is made mainly on clinical grounds and that laboratory studies should play a supportive rather than a major diagnostic role. This also holds true for evaluation of a patient's response to therapy.

Answer: B, E

7. The most dangerous site of spillage from the gastrointestinal tract is the:

A. Stomach
B. Jejunum
C. Ileocecal area
D. Sigmoid colon

Sabiston: 993
Schwartz: 1398

Comments: See Question 8.

8. True statements regarding acute suppurative peritonitis include:

A. The virulence of the contaminants, the extent and duration of contamination, the presence of an adjuvant, and the appropriateness of initial therapy determine the magnitude of peritonitis
B. Abdominal contents must be cultured as soon as the peritoneum is opened to avoid missing anaerobic contamination
C. The most common offending organisms include aerobic coliforms, anaerobic *Bacteroides* species, aerobic and anaerobic streptococci, enterococci, and clostridia
D. Anaerobes or their degradation products may be responsible for evolution toward abscess formation as opposed to complete healing

Schwartz: 1396

Comments: Most patients with acute suppurative peritonitis have a polymicrobial infection. The mortality is dose-related and the mixed flora acts synergistically. Even normally nonpathogenic bacteria act in the synergism. Aerobes consume oxygen and elaborate nutrients, thus enhancing anaerobes, while anaerobes can elaborate antibiotic-destroying enzymes, thus enhancing aerobes. Anaerobes are responsible for formation of abscesses rather than the expected complete healing when peritonitis is resolved. Massive sudden contamination, as in cecal rupture, overwhelms the peritoneal mechanisms of localization, and the entire peritoneal cavity can become contaminated. Intestinal and diaphragmatic motion and the effects of gravity can spread an inoculum throughout the peritoneal cavity in 3 to 6 hours. Perforations of the distal ileum or cecum (where the bowel content is liquid and rich in mixed flora) produce the highest morbidity, while those of the proximal gastrointestinal tract (containing few bacteria) and distal colon (where the contents are solid and less likely to spread widely) are better tolerated. The virulence of peritonitis is enhanced by the presence of adjuvants that act to retard the clearance of bacteria from the peritoneal cavity. Because adjuvants are indiscriminately phagocytized by white blood cells, this dilutes the efficiency of phagocytosis normally devoted to clearance of bacteria. Hemoglobin is the most potent adjuvant, but others include bile salts, talc, gastric mucin, and proteinaceous debris. The injudicious use of laxatives and enemas may stimulate an otherwise quiescent bowel, thus increasing spillage and/or interfering with the normal processes of localization.

Answer: Question 7: C
Question 8: A, B, C, D

9. Match the choices in the two columns.

Characteristics	Toxin
A. Lipopolysaccharide elaborated by gram-negative organisms	a. Endotoxin
B. Protein elaborated by gram-positive organisms	b. Exotoxin
C. Acts primarily on blood vessels	c. Both
D. Hemolysis of red cells, interference with cellular processes	
E. Produces arteriolar dilation	
F. Causes intraorgan shunting, capillary leakage, loss of endothelial integrity, "third-spacing"	

Schwartz: 1398

Comments: See Question 10.

10. True statements regarding the pathophysiology of sepsis include:

A. The vasoconstricting effect of hypovolemia may mask the vasodilating effect of endotoxin
B. The appearance of mild hyperventilation, respiratory alkalosis, and an altered sensorium associated with a diffuse patchy pulmonary infiltrate may be the earliest sign of gram-negative sepsis
C. Endotoxin-induced intrarenal shunts at the corticomedullary level preserve renal glomerular perfusion
D. One system organ failure produces 30% mortality, which increases to 100% when four organ systems have failed

Sabiston: 39, 48
Schwartz: 1398

Comments: The interaction of endotoxemia and hypovolemia in acute suppurative peritonitis presents a profound physiologic insult. In normovolemic patients, septic shock presents as a hyperdynamic state with increased cardiac output, low peripheral vascular resistance (due to endotoxin-induced vasodilatation), low blood pressure, warm extremities, hyperventilation, and respiratory alkalosis. When these effects are superimposed on hypovolemia (secondary to peritonitis), there is compensatory peripheral vasoconstriction, cardiac output is depressed, blood pressure is low, and the extremities are cold. The hypovolemia of peritonitis is augmented by peripheral third-spacing due to endotoxin-

induced endothelial leakage at the capillary level. If the compensatory vasoconstriction of hypovolemia yields to endotoxin-induced vasodilatation, profound shock results that may not respond to fluid replacement. Capillary leakage in the lung leads to loss of compliance and creates a physical barrier to gas diffusion. Hypoxemia results that stimulates compensatory hyperventilation and respiratory alkalosis. Hyperventilation, alkalosis, and an altered sensorium secondary to hypoxemia may be the earliest signs of gram-negative sepsis. At this stage, the chest x-ray appears normal. In the lung, continued sepsis leads to protein leakage, loss of surfactant, and alveolar collapse further decreasing compliance. Perfusion of collapsed alveoli creates a ventilation-perfusion mismatch that is augmented by the opening of pulmonary arteriovenous shunts secondary to excessive beta-adrenergic stimulation brought about by sepsis. The resultant hypoxemia may be profound. It is at this point that the chest x-ray may demonstrate a diffuse patchy white infiltrate characteristic of the adult respiratory distress syndrome. Endotoxin-induced opening of intrarenal shunts aggravates the decreased glomerular perfusion caused by hypovolemia. As a result, the medulla is perfused at the expense of the cortex, producing "corticomedullary disconnection," a greatly diminished urine output, and decreased excretion of acid. At this point, metabolic acidosis rather than respiratory alkalosis predominates. To further compound the problem, sepsis impairs macrophage and leukocyte bactericidal activity and causes platelet and white blood cell aggregation (due to release of complement fractions) that can plug the small vessels of the lung and kidney. The ultimate result of this process is multiple system organ failure. The most effective treatment in acute suppurative peritonitis is eradication of the underlying infection as soon as possible.

Answer: Question 9: A–a; B–b; C–a; D–b; E–c; F–a
Question 10: A, D

11. True or false: Delay of operation for the purpose of fluid resuscitation in patients with acute peritonitis is contraindicated because of the hazards of ongoing abdominal sepsis.

Sabiston: 48
Schwartz: 1401

Comments: In considering the diagnosis of acute suppurative peritonitis, several nonabdominal causes must also be considered and excluded. Pneumonia, particularly in the very young or very old, has the potential to induce ileus, distension, and irritation of the diaphragm that can produce abdominal pain mimicking peritonitis. Uremia is another condition that has the potential to produce ileus and abdominal distension. A number of other conditions can produce pain suggesting acute peritonitis, including acute gastroenteritis, renal calculus, and gynecologic disorders such as torsion of an ovarian cyst, ruptured ovarian follicle, and ectopic pregnancy. Once the diagnosis of acute suppurative peritonitis is made, fluid resuscitation and clinical stabilization should be attempted prior to operation. While it is true that certain causes demand immediate intervention (such as intestinal infarction), generally there are several hours during which initial resuscitative measures can be started to correct hypovolemia and any accompanying cardiovascular, pulmonary, and renal dysfunction. Measures that may be required include fluid resuscitation, appropriate antibiotics, oxygen therapy, ventilatory support, nasogastric intubation, urinary catheterization, central venous catheterization, and establishment of baseline biochemical and hemodynamic parameters.

Answer: False

12. Which of the following statements is/are true regarding preoperative management of patients with acute suppurative peritonitis?

A. Albumin is more effective than crystalloid in replacing interstitial fluid loss
B. Crystalloid should be given slowly, because of the risk of heart failure, even when the patient is otherwise healthy
C. Both crystalloid and colloid leak from endotoxin-damaged pulmonary capillaries
D. Albumin has been clearly shown to cause greater pulmonary damage than crystalloid

Schwartz: 1401

Comments: A common error during the initial resuscitation of patients with peritonitis is to infuse fluid too slowly. Rapid resuscitation with crystalloid is not likely, in itself, to precipitate heart failure, particularly in patients whose CVP is normal. Patients with a history of heart failure still require large volumes of crystalloid to replace interstitial fluid loss, and in this setting, monitoring with a Swan-Ganz catheter is appropriate. There is controversy regarding the relative role of crystalloid vs. colloid in fluid resuscitation. Interstitial fluid losses are best replaced with crystalloid, preferably Ringer's lactate. Crystalloid can replace intravascular deficits as well, but up to three times the volume is required compared with the amount of albumin needed to provide the same intravascular effect. Albumin presents a smaller salt load, and edema and weight gain are less likely; it is extremely expensive, however. The development of pulmonary interstitial edema is more a function of endotoxin-induced capillary dysfunction than of the type of fluid used in resuscitation. Both crystalloid and colloid are prone to leakage from damaged capillaries. Crystalloid resuscitation, however, is more likely than colloid resuscitation to be associated with pulmonary edema due to volume overload. Although there is some evidence that large doses of albumin given to patients with sepsis can produce greater pulmonary dysfunction, there are no reports comparing moderate doses of albumin with crystalloid. It seems reasonable to use crystalloid as the main resuscitative fluid and to add colloid in those who develop signs of volume overload or have a history of underlying heart disease.

Answer: C

13. Which of the following statements is/are true regarding preoperative preparation of patients with acute suppurative peritonitis?

A. Antibiotics effective against *Escherichia coli* include the cephalosporins, cephamycins, aminoglycosides, and chloramphenicol
B. Antibiotics effective against *Bacteroides fragilis* include clindamycin, chloramphenicol, metronidazole, erythromycin, cephalomycins, and the newer penicillin derivatives

C. Patients with an arterial pO$_2$ of less than 70 mm Hg should be considered as candidates for intubation
D. Nasogastric suction prevents aspiration during induction of anesthesia
E. Alpha-adrenergic agents are frequently used as first-line therapy in the treatment of sepsis-related hypotension

Sabiston: 267
Schwartz: 1402

Comments: Antibiotics should be started empirically, once the diagnosis of peritonitis is made. It is desirable to obtain adequate tissue levels prior to operation. The early mortality in experimental models of fecal peritonitis is reduced by the use of agents effective against *E. coli*, while the late mortality associated with subsequent abscesses is reduced with agents effective against *B. fragilis*. Septic peritonitis is often associated with hypoxemia. Measurement of arterial blood gases provides the most accurate index of the need for oxygen therapy and ventilatory support. Patients may require oxygen supplementation (by mask or nasal cannula) prior to the induction of anesthesia. Those patients with an arterial pO$_2$ of less than 70 mm Hg may require ventilatory support, and PEEP should be considered in any patient with an arterial pO$_2$ less than 60 mm Hg. First-line treatment for sepsis-associated hypotension is fluid replacement, not vasopressors. The use of alpha-adrenergic agents compounds the problem of peripheral vasoconstriction and should be avoided if possible. When volume replacement fails to restore blood pressure and circulation, dopamine or dobutamine may be helpful. When sepsis occurs in patients with a history of heart failure or limited cardiac reserve, the judicious use of digitalis may be helpful. Attention to serum potassium levels is important when digitalis is used, since potassium wasting is one of the renal derangements associated with early sepsis. Analgesia should be withheld until the diagnosis is made, to avoid potential confusion caused by the masking of pain. Once the diagnosis of acute septic peritonitis is made or the patient is scheduled for operation, pain should be relieved with intravenous narcotics. A nasogastric tube is inserted to empty the stomach, prevent further emesis, and prevent the accumulation of swallowed air. It does not guarantee protection from aspiration during induction of anesthesia.

Answer: A, B, C

14. Which of the following statements is/are true regarding the use of steroids in patients with sepsis?

A. Prospective randomized trials have established the usefulness of steroids in the treatment of shock
B. Steroids are indicated in patients with a history of adrenal insufficiency
C. Steroids may be useful in patients with a prolonged history of symptoms prior to the development of sepsis
D. If there is no response to steroids after two doses, they should be discontinued

Sabiston: 49
Schwartz: 1402

Comments: The usefulness of steroids in sepsis is a matter of debate. Although some studies support the impression that steroids can reduce the mortality in patients with sepsis, no prospective, randomized clinical trial has established their precise role. Steroids should, of course, be used in patients with adrenal insufficiency. If no response is seen after several doses of intravenous steroids, they should be discontinued.

Answer: B, C, D

15. Which of the following statements is/are true regarding the operative therapy for acute suppurative peritonitis?

A. The incision of choice is in the midline
B. Débridement of fibrin and proteinaceous debris following aspiration of any pus is associated with increased morbidity due to dissemination of infection
C. Lavage solutions containing antibiotics are superior to those that do not contain antibiotics
D. Interrupted closures reduce the risk of dehiscence
E. Drainage of generalized peritonitis reduces the risk of postoperative abscess formation

Comments: In adults, a vertical midline incision is the most advantageous for exploration of an abdomen with diffuse peritonitis. Transverse incisions are used in patients under 2 years of age. When the peritonitis is localized (as in appendicitis), an incision directly over the inflammatory process may avoid contamination of the uninvolved abdomen. The goal of operation is to control the source of contamination and to provide peritoneal toilette (débridement, lavage). Peritoneal débridement and gentle dissection of mesenteric and bowel adhesions and cleansing of the pelvic, subhepatic, and subdiaphragmatic recesses decreases morbidity and does not increase mortality as long as significant bleeding is avoided. After débridement, irrigation with saline until the return is clear aids in reducing the mortality of generalized peritonitis. It has not been shown that lavage disseminates peritoneal contamination in such patients. When systemic antibiotics are given preoperatively, antibiotic lavage solutions do not offer a clear benefit. When systemic antibiotics are not used, antibiotic lavage solutions decrease the incidence of wound infection. Sump drainage of localized abscesses is useful, but offers no advantage when dealing with generalized peritonitis; in fact, in that setting, drainage may be harmful in that it interferes with normal peritoneal defense mechanisms, provides a route for exogenous contamination, and promotes formation of adhesions. Closure with a continuous stitch of monofilament suture is quick and effective. Dehiscence after suppurative peritonitis is due mainly to wound infection, and the use of interrupted sutures does not diminish its rate of occurrence. The skin and subcutaneous tissue should be left partially or completely open and lightly packed. Delayed closure is undertaken after the wound begins granulating without evidence of infection. Leaving the wound entirely open to allow bedside abdominal exploration and to break up loculations in cases of severe peritonitis offers no advantage over conventional fascial closure.

Answer: A

16. Which of the following statements is/are true about aseptic peritonitis?

A. It occurs when the peritoneal irritant is sterile or nearly sterile
B. Unlike in acute suppurative peritonitis, pain and guarding are minimal
C. In the absence of trauma or gastrointestinal leakage, the process remains aseptic
D. Early improvement of symptoms indicates resolution of the process

Sabiston: 784
Schwartz: 1405

Comments: Aseptic or chemical peritonitis differs from acute suppurative peritonitis in that the peritoneal irritant is sterile or nearly so. The soilage results in the signs and symptoms of peritonitis as described previously. Secondary bacterial invasion commonly occurs, even if there is no evidence of trauma or contamination from the intestinal tract, as a result of transient bacteremia from remote sites. The onset of symptoms usually is sudden, the pain is severe, and the degree of tenderness and abdominal rigidity is indistinguishable from that caused by acute suppurative peritonitis. Early improvement of symptoms can occur because of dilution and neutralization of the irritant secondary to the outpouring of peritoneal fluid. This does not eliminate the risk of secondary bacterial infection. Principles of surgical management are the same as in suppurative peritonitis and include the use of antibiotics to combat the risk of secondary infection.

Answer: A

17. Which of the following statements is/are true regarding the cause of aseptic "chemical" peritonitis?

A. Patients on H2 blockers have an increased risk for bacterial contamination of gastric contents
B. Nonactivated pancreatic secretions can produce massive ascites without peritoneal irritation
C. In the absence of secondary infection, sterile bile is not a peritoneal irritant
D. In the absence of secondary infection, sterile urine is not a peritoneal irritant
E. Endotoxic peritonitis cannot occur unless there is a bowel perforation
F. Barium produces peritonitis because of bacterial contamination associated with visceral perforations

Sabiston: 784, 797
Schwartz: 1405

Comments: **Gastric juice** is highly irritating because of its hydrochloric acid and mucin content. It is normally sterile, but with increasing gastric pH (as in those on H2 blockers) increasing numbers of bacteria can be encountered, particularly those originating from swallowed saliva. Operation performed within 6 hours of perforation is associated with less peritoneal contamination than operation performed beyond this period of time. **Pancreatic juice** that leaks from an injury of the pancreatic duct can produce pancreatic ascites. The degree of dilution of the pancreatic fluid produces variable degrees of peritoneal irritation. Activated pancreatic secretions released because of pancreatitis are diluted to a lesser degree, and secondary infection occurs in a high proportion of patients with pancreatitis. **Sterile bile** is a peritoneal irritant, the effect of which is compounded by frequently occurring secondary infection. Bile leakage can occur from an apparently intact gallbladder if the wall is severely ischemic. **Sterile urine** is extremely irritating and usually enters the peritoneal cavity secondary to trauma. Spontaneous leakage can occur in patients with neurologic conditions producing an atonic, massively distended bladder. **Blood** in itself is not irritating, but acts as a potent adjuvant should secondary infection occur. **Mucus** released from the small bowel, appendix, or ruptured ovarian cyst has the capacity to induce a sterile peritonitis and, when encountered, should be removed. **Endotoxic** peritonitis can occur during peritoneal lavage owing to contamination of the dialysate fluid by preformed coliform endotoxin. It can also occur when the bowel wall becomes ischemic, allowing transudation of preformed endotoxin, producing the signs and symptoms of gram-negative sepsis. **Barium** is extremely irritating and induces a granulomatous peritoneal reaction that is augmented by the frequent presence of bacterial infection at the time of soilage. Barium crystals are difficult to remove at operation; the best treatment is prevention. In radiographic studies for suspected perforations, the initial x-ray should be made with water-soluble contrast media.

Answer: A, B

18. Which of the following statements is/are true regarding granulomatous peritonitis?

A. That caused by tuberculosis is usually due to reactivation of a latent peritoneal infection
B. Iatrogenic granulomatous peritonitis can be due to a hypersensitivity response to surgical glove lubricants
C. In both tuberculous and iatrogenic granulomatous peritonitis, reoperation should be avoided if possible
D. Cultures are rarely useful in making the diagnosis of tuberculous granulomatous peritonitis

Sabiston: 783
Schwartz: 1407

Comments: Granulomatous peritonitis is a disease characterized by the formation of granulomas and a propensity to form adhesions that exceed those seen in other forms of peritonitis. **Tuberculous peritonitis** was formerly quite common, but is now usually seen only in patients who are severely malnourished or who are cirrhotic. Most cases are due to reactivation of a latent peritoneal tuberculosis established by previous hematogenous spread from a pulmonary source. Clinically, its presentation is insidious and includes fever, anorexia, and weight loss. Classically, the abdomen in tuberculous peritonitis has been described as "doughy." Ascites is almost always present and, when cultured, will be positive for tuberculosis in 80% of cases. "Blind" peritoneal biopsy is positive in 60% of cases. If laparotomy is performed for diagnosis, the placement of drains or the exteriorization of bowel should be avoided. Appropriate antituberculous therapy started early in the course of the disease is associated with a good prognosis. This therapy should continue for 2 years after the patient becomes asymptomatic. **Iatrogenic granulomatous peritonitis** is a hypersensitivity response to common surgical glove lu-

bricants, including lycopodium, mineral oil, cornstarch, rice starch, or cellulose fibers from gauze pads. Findings include migratory abdominal pain, fever, and evidence of peritonitis developing within 3 weeks of a routine abdominal operation. Occasionally, an eosinophilia is identified on the peripheral blood smear. Reoperation should be avoided. Treatment is supportive and may include the administration of corticosteroids. Eventually, the peritonitis should resolve. The most important aspect of management is prevention and includes washing the surgical gloves before placing them into the abdominal cavity. **Candidal infection** can be another cause of granulomatous peritonitis. This etiology most often is seen in immunosuppressed patients or those who have been on prolonged antibiotic therapy. Oral antifungal agents may reduce the incidence of intestinal overgrowth by *Candida* and help reduce the incidence of candidal peritonitis in these patients.

Answer: A, B, C

19. Which of the following statements is/are true regarding spontaneous (primary) peritonitis?

A. It is a diffuse bacterial peritonitis without any apparent intra-abdominal source of infection
B. It occurs in 3% of hospitalized cirrhotic patients without ascites and in 8% of those with ascites in precoma or coma
C. It is a polymicrobial infection, with coliforms being the predominant organism in over 50% of cases
D. The clinical picture is the same as in suppurative peritonitis
E. A peritoneal tap is the most useful diagnostic test; greater than 300 polymorphonuclear cells/ml suggests the presence of peritonitis
F. Laparotomy should be avoided whenever possible

Sabiston: 783
Schwartz: 1408

Comments: Spontaneous or primary peritonitis is a diffuse bacterial peritonitis without an apparent intra-abdominal source of infection. It is more common in adults, and the incidence does not vary by sex. Children with nephrosis and adults with cirrhosis or systemic lupus erythematosus are the populations usually affected. In adults ascites appears to be a predisposing factor, but this is not so in children. Spontaneous peritonitis is a monomicrobial infection, with coliforms being the chief pathogens in over half of the cases. Pneumococci formerly were the most common pathogen; now streptococcal infections occur but are uncommon. Transmural migration of bacteria from the intestine and infection during bacteremia are the two most likely sources of contamination. The onset of symptoms is usually insidious and is never as severe as with suppurative peritonitis. A peritoneal tap is a useful diagnostic test; more than 300 polymorphonuclear cells/ml indicate that a bacterial peritonitis is present. While a Gram stain of this fluid may demonstrate the presence of a monomicrobial gram-positive or gram-negative infection, this cannot exclude the possibility of a surgically correctable intra-abdominal problem. When the diagnosis is in doubt, exploratory laparotomy is useful since the risk of exploration is small compared with the risk of neglecting a problem requiring an operation. In nephrotic children or in cirrhotic adults with advanced hepatic decompensation who have clinical and diagnostic findings suggestive of spontaneous peritonitis, antibiotic therapy alone rather than laparotomy is sometimes used. Appendectomy in the presence of spontaneous peritonitis does not increase morbidity and eliminates appendicitis as a diagnostic consideration should recurrent episodes occur. Drains should not be used since their presence retards the resolution of peritonitis.

Answer: A, B, E

20. Which of the following statements is/are true regarding peritonitis related to peritoneal dialysis?

A. It occurs more frequently in patients undergoing continuous ambulatory rather than intermittent peritoneal dialysis
B. The infective agent usually is monomicrobial
C. Most patients with positive cultures have a gram-positive coccus, usually *Staphylococcus aureus* or *Staphylococcus epidermidis,* as the causative organism
D. These patients rarely have positive blood cultures, in contrast to patients with other causes of peritonitis, who have a 30% incidence of bacteremia
E. The presence of anaerobic bacteria indicates intestinal perforation and carries a very poor prognosis
F. The initial treatment is administration of broad-spectrum antibiotics and heparin in the dialysate accompanied by increases in the dwell time

Schwartz: 1409

Comments: Peritonitis is the major cause of morbidity in patients undergoing peritoneal dialysis. It is more common in patients undergoing continuous ambulatory peritoneal dialysis than in those undergoing intermittent peritoneal dialysis. The diagnosis is made when two of three of the following are found: (1) positive culture from the peritoneal fluid; (2) cloudy dialysate effluent; (3) clinical signs of peritonitis. The infection is usually monomicrobial, and two thirds of the patients have cultures positive for gram-positive cocci, usually *Staphylococcus aureus* or *Staphylococcus epidermidis*. Gram-negative organisms suggest intestinal perforation or changes in flora related to chronic antibiotic administration. Anaerobic bacteria are rarely cultured, and when present indicate intestinal perforation and a very poor prognosis. Blood cultures are rarely positive in this group of patients compared with those having other causes of peritonitis, of whom up to 30% may have positive blood cultures. The initial treatment is the addition of broad-spectrum antibiotics and heparin to the dialysate, which is allowed to dwell in the peritoneal cavity for longer than the customary period. Persistence of peritonitis after 4 to 5 days of treatment is an indication for removal of the catheter and possible operative therapy.

Answer: A, B, C, D, E, F

21. Which of the following statements is/are true regarding intra-abdominal abscesses?

A. Often they are polymicrobial
B. They tend to localize along the spine because of the effect of gravity
C. The usual pattern of fever is low-grade and persistent

D. The use of antibiotics may interfere with the diagnosis
E. Pain, if present, usually is diffuse and difficult to localize

Sabiston: 338
Schwartz: 1410

Comments: Intra-abdominal abscesses arise during resolution of generalized peritonitis or in areas where there has been localization of a perforation. Abscesses in solid viscera are usually due to hematogenous spread from a distant site. Infected material can rapidly spread throughout the peritoneal cavity, but gravity tends to localize the material in the dependent areas of the pelvis and in the subphrenic and subhepatic spaces. Intra-abdominal abscesses are polymicrobial, anaerobic organisms predominate, and *Bacteroides* and anaerobic streptococcal species are the most commonly isolated bacteria. Fever is seen in most patients, often "spiking" initially but then becoming persistently elevated as the abscess matures. The frequent association of temperature "spikes" with chills and tachycardia is due to episodes of transient bacteremia. When present, pain is often localized to the site of the abscess. Abdominal tenderness and pain is often associated with visceral and midabdominal abscesses, but less so with subphrenic or retroperitoneal abscesses. Pelvic abscesses rarely cause anterior abdominal wall tenderness. In addition to having fever and pain, patients often have an ileus, distension, and anorexia and sometimes vomit. Suppression of infection with antibiotics tends to mask these signs and symptoms and may hamper early diagnosis.

Answer: A, D

22. True statements regarding the diagnostic work-up of intra-abdominal abscesses include:

A. Elevation of the WBC is not a reliable test
B. Abdominal ultrasound, especially in thin patients, may be useful in localizing upper abdominal or retroperitoneal abscesses
C. Abdominal CT scanning, particularly in the obese patient, is the most useful test for localizing intra-abdominal abscesses
D. The indium-111–labeled white blood cell scan is the most sensitive test for localizing intra-abdominal abscesses
E. Discontinuation of antibiotics may play an important role in the diagnosis of intra-abdominal abscesses

Schwartz: 1411

Comments: Diagnostic tests are ordered on the basis of clinical suspicion. The **white blood cell** count will be elevated and show a shift to the left in most patients with an intra-abdominal abscess. **Plain x-ray films** of the abdomen may show localized gas bubbles or air-fluid levels in the area of abscess formation. A **CT scan** is the most useful test in localizing intra-abdominal abscesses. It is particularly useful in obese patients, whose intra-abdominal fat helps delineate normal anatomic structures. **Ultrasound** may be useful in localizing abscesses in thin patients, but its most important application is in following resolution of an abscess after it has been drained. **Gallium** scans are limited by the fact that the radioisotope is excreted into the colon, a problem compounded by associated ileus. Indium-111–labeled white blood cell scans may be better than gallium, but do not approach the accuracy of a CT scan. **Barium** studies can demonstrate organ displacement due to abscess formation and occasionally will identify a causative fistula or sinus tract. **IVP** can demonstrate ureteral displacement due to retroperitoneal abscesses. Antibiotics are rarely curative after the formation of liquid pus and may hamper the diagnosis by modifying the underlying symptoms; discontinuation of antibiotics for a short period of time may help clarify the clinical picture. Once localized liquid pus is formed, it must be drained; attempts at treating it noninvasively with antibiotics are not correct. Failure to drain an intra-abdominal abscess prolongs the course of the illness and is associated with a high risk for rupture, recurrent peritonitis, and even death.

Answer: B, C, E

23. Which of the following statements is/are true regarding percutaneous drainage of intra-abdominal abscesses?

A. The technique decreases the risk of spreading contamination to uninvolved tissue planes
B. It is best applied to well-organized uniloculated collections in contact with the abdominal wall
C. In properly selected patients, it has several distinct advantages over surgical drainage
D. A disadvantage is the relatively long period of time needed to obtain complete resolution of the abscess

Sabiston: 268
Schwartz: 1412

Comments: An important principle in drainage of intra-abdominal abscesses is the avoidance of unnecessary contamination of the uninvolved peritoneal cavity. The advantages of percutaneous drainage are precisely this avoidance of unnecessary contamination, the fact that it can be done using local anesthesia, and, in properly selected cases, its ability to provide adequate drainage. Finally, and most importantly, it can eliminate the need for a formal operation. Criteria for successful percutaneous drainage include: (1) the presence of a well-established unilocular collection of appropriate viscosity; (2) the presence of a safe "window" through which a catheter can be passed without damaging interposed viscera; and (3) the availability of surgical back-up. The success rate of percutaneous drainage is as high as 80% and, in properly selected cases, compares favorably with surgical management. Disadvantages include the longer period usually needed for complete drainage and an occasional catheter erosion into adjacent structures. The frequent failure in patients in whom abscesses are related to underlying bowel fistulas can be considered as resulting from improper patient selection.

Answer: A, B, C, D

24. Which of the following statements is/are true regarding right subphrenic abscesses?

A. They are most frequently secondary to either rupture of a hepatic abscess or operations on the stomach
B. They are most commonly secondary to operations on the biliary tract

C. They classically produce right upper quadrant pain with radiation to the right flank and back
D. Because the triangular and coronary ligaments arise from the dome of the diaphragm, operatively they are best approached posteriorly through the bed of the 12th rib

Sabiston: 338
Schwartz: 1413

Comments: The right subphrenic space lies between the liver and the diaphragm and extends from the costal margin anteriorly to the coronary and triangular ligaments that attach posteriorly. These abscesses are most frequently secondary to rupture of a hepatic abscess or to operations on the stomach or duodenum. Less frequently, they are related to operations on the appendix or biliary system. Clinical signs and symptoms are minimal, but pain in the upper abdomen or lower chest, sometimes referred to the right flank and back, does occur. Most patients will demonstrate a pleural effusion or platelike atelectasis in the right lower chest; reduced motion of the diaphragm is seen in 75% of patients. These abscesses preferably are drained using a lateral subcostal approach; the dissection begins at the tip of the 11th rib and continues extraperitoneally until the abscess is reached. This method avoids operative contamination of the peritoneal cavity. They cannot be drained via a posterior approach unless the pleural space is crossed.

Answer: A

25. Which of the following statements is/are true regarding right subhepatic abscesses?

A. The space is bounded inferiorly by the hepatic flexure and the transverse mesocolon, medially by the duodenum, and laterally by the body wall
B. The deepest portion of this space is called "Morison's pouch"
C. They are most commonly the result of infection following gastric or biliary tract procedures
D. They usually produce right upper quadrant pain exacerbated by coughing
E. They should be approached transabdominally because of the high incidence of synchronous abscesses elsewhere in the abdomen

Schwartz: 1413

Comments: Abscesses in the right subhepatic space most frequently are complications of gastric and biliary tract operations, although their incidence is increasing after colonic operations as well. These abscesses usually produce tenderness in the right upper abdomen that is exacerbated by coughing or by any activity that produces motion of the viscera in this area. While there is the risk of unrecognized synchronous abscesses elsewhere in the abdomen, current imaging and localizing techniques have markedly reduced this; a well-localized subhepatic abscess is best drained either through a lateral subcostal incision or posteriorly through the bed of the 12th rib. If, of course, associated abscesses in the midabdomen or lesser sac are suspected prior to exploration, a transabdominal approach is more appropriate.

Answer: A, B, C, D

26. Which of the following statements is/are true regarding left subphrenic abscesses?

A. They are the commonest variety of upper abdominal abscesses after resolution of generalized peritonitis
B. These abscesses sometimes produce Kehr's sign
C. The left subdiaphragmatic space is one contiguous area, unlike the situation on the right
D. These abscesses may be approached through either a lateral subcostal or posterior incision

Sabiston: 338
Schwartz: 1414

Comments: Left subphrenic abscesses are the most common upper abdominal abscess after resolution of a generalized peritonitis. They may also result following splenectomy or pancreatitis. Physical signs may include costal tenderness, pain in the shoulder (Kehr's sign), a left pleural effusion, and limitation of left-sided diaphragmatic excursion. Unlike the subdiaphragmatic space on the right, the left subdiaphragmatic space is not divided into two separate areas. The area can be approached through a lateral subcostal incision or posteriorly through the bed of the 12th rib. During exploration of this space, loculations are broken by having the exploring finger gently reach the aorta, the esophagus, the esophageal hiatus, the caudate lobe of the liver, and the anterior margin of the left lobe of the liver.

Answer: A, B, C, D

27. Which of the following statements is/are true regarding lesser sac abscesses?

A. They are a type of left subphrenic abscess and are approached in the same fashion
B. They are usually complications of diseases of the stomach, duodenum, and pancreas
C. They are easy to diagnose since they cause extreme irritation of the transverse colon
D. Because of their location, extraperitoneal drainage is impossible

Schwartz: 1415

Comments: Lesser sac abscesses are unusual complications of diseases of the stomach, duodenum, and pancreas. The clinical diagnosis is difficult; vague tenderness in the midepigastrium may be present but is usually nonspecific. Ultrasound is particularly useful in identifying this type of abscess. Although the lesser sac lies in the subdiaphragmatic space, the operative approach to drain this form of abscess is different than for those under the right or the left hemidiaphragm. Lesser sac abscesses should be approached through an upper abdominal incision that avoids dividing the rectus muscle. Because of the dense adhesions between the stomach and the pancreas that are encountered, the commonly utilized route of drainage is along the superior border of the antrum. Adequate drainage is difficult to obtain and, as a consequence, these abscesses are associated with a poorer prognosis.

Answer: B, D

28. Which of the following statements is/are true regarding interloop "midabdominal" abscesses?

A. They arise as loculations between loops of bowel, the mesentery, the abdominal wall, and the omentum
B. The transverse colon prevents involvement of the upper part of the abdomen
C. There are no reliable signs or symptoms
D. They are frequently multiple
E. The insertion of drains is not indicated

Schwartz: 1415

Comments: Abscesses in this location are seen in patients with generalized peritonitis and are the result of loculations between loops of bowel, mesentery, the abdominal wall, the omentum, and occasionally the right and left colic gutters. The transverse colon appears to prevent involvement of the upper abdomen. There are no reliable signs and symptoms, and large abscesses may be present without significant physical findings. Their presence can be suspected when peritonitis does not resolve completely or promptly and there is supportive laboratory evidence of sepsis. Occasionally, abdominal x-rays will demonstrate bowel wall edema or separation of visible loops of bowel. Interloop abscesses are usually multiple and need to be explored and drained transabdominally. Unless the abscess is discrete and in contact with the abdominal wall, the use of drains is not indicated. Appropriate surgical therapy includes a thorough débridement and irrigation of the peritoneal cavity followed by the administration of systemic antibiotics. These abscesses commonly recur, so these patients demand close attention postoperatively.

Answer: A, B, C, D, E

29. Which of the following statements is/are true regarding pelvic abscesses?

A. The findings on examination of the abdomen often are unremarkable
B. Often they are directly palpable by rectal or vaginal examination
C. Drainage is accomplished transabdominally with the placement of appropriate suction catheters
D. They are best drained through the rectum or vagina followed by daily dilatation of the drainage tract

Sabiston: 1626
Schwartz: 1415

Comments: Pelvic abscesses most often follow ruptured colonic diverticula, pelvic inflammatory disease, a ruptured appendix, or drainage into the pelvis during resolution of a generalized peritonitis. They do not produce significant findings on examination of the abdomen unless they involve the anterior abdominal wall. Patients occasionally complain of poorly localized, dull lower abdominal discomfort; irritation of the bladder and rectum produces urgency, diarrhea, and tenesmus. The pelvic space is easily felt through the rectum or vagina, and the diagnosis of these abscesses is made by direct palpation. Pelvic inflammatory problems without abscesses do not bulge into the rectum, an important point in the differential diagnosis during examination. Drainage is best accomplished either through the rectum or vagina and is performed when the abscess is palpable as a discrete bulge. Incisions placed prior to this run the risk of injuring the small bowel and other intra-abdominal viscera.

Answer: A, B, D

14

Principles of Oncology

1. Regarding neoplastic disease in general, which of the following statements is/are true?

A. Malignant neoplasms are composed of a group of cells that proliferate excessively
B. Malignant neoplasms are characterized by cells that may invade locally or metastasize to distant sites
C. There has been a slow, steady increase in the overall death rates from cancer
D. The overall 5-year survival for women with cancer is significantly greater than for men

Schwartz: 313

Comments: Malignant neoplasms are composed of a population of cells that proliferate in an excessive and uncontrolled manner. They may invade locally and/or metastasize to distant sites, or they may behave in a benign manner and neither invade nor metastasize. ● Cancer is the second most common cause of death in the United States: one of every four persons living today has or will develop it. ● Although the mortality from some cancers has decreased, there has been a slow, steady increase in the overall cancer death rates. For example, the death rate from cancer of the stomach has decreased while that from pancreatic cancer has increased. This is especially true of lung cancer, which has increased alarmingly in both sexes. ● Although the reasons are unclear, women with cancer have an overall 5-year survival of 50% compared with 30% for men.

Answer: A, B, C, D

2. Match each of the following carcinogens with its associated neoplasm(s).

Carcinogen	Neoplasm
A. Beta-naphthylamine	a. Acute leukemia
B. Benzene	b. Cancer of the larynx and bronchus
C. Coal tar	c. Bladder cancer
D. Asbestos	d. Mesothelioma
E. Epstein-Barr virus	e. Skin cancer
F. Ultraviolet radiation	f. Nasopharyngeal cancer and Burkitt's lymphoma

Sabiston: 512
Schwartz: 315

Comments: Carcinogenic agents may be chemical, physical, viral, or genetic and have in common the ability to induce malignant neoplasms. The first description of a causal relation between a carcinogen and the development of cancer was written in 1775, when Pott described cancer of the scrotum in chimney sweeps. Coal tar has been associated with cancer of the skin, larynx, and bronchus. Exposure to beta-naphthylamine, an aromatic amine used in the dye industry, has been associated with tumors of the urinary tract. Benzene exposure has been associated with the development of acute leukemia, and asbestos exposure with the development of mesothelioma. Physical carcinogens include ionizing and ultraviolet radiation. Both are associated with the development of skin cancer, while ionizing radiation additionally may lead to the development of neoplasms of the thyroid, bone, and blood. There is clear-cut evidence that both RNA and DNA viruses are carcinogenic in several animal species. There is increasing evidence to link viruses with certain human neoplasms; the Epstein-Barr (EB) virus has been associated with the development of Burkitt's lymphoma and nasopharyngeal cancer.

Answer: A–c; B–a; C–b, e; D–d; E–f; F–e

3. Regarding the biology of malignant neoplasms, which of the following statements is/are true?

A. Malignant neoplasms seem to arise from a single cell that has undergone transformation to form a malignant clone
B. Cancer cells proliferate faster than normal cells, the rate of proliferation increasing as the tumor mass grows
C. Characteristics of malignant cells include a reversion to more primitive cell types, cellular pleomorphism, and loss of contact inhibition
D. Tumors double in size at least every 20 days, so that essentially all human neoplasms are clinically detectable within 1 year after the inception of neoplastic transformation

Schwartz: 319

Comments: Although most cancers are believed to arise from a single cell that has undergone malignant transformation to a malignant clone, some cancers (e.g., neurofibromas in von Recklinghausen's disease) may develop from multiple clones of cells. • Cancer cells generally proliferate faster than normal cells; notable exceptions are leukocytes and intestinal mucosal cells. • This rate of proliferation, however, tends to decrease as the tumor increases in size. • Changes characteristic of malignant cells include the production of various polypeptides and hormones not normally produced, reversion to a more primitive cell type, cellular pleomorphism, frequent mitoses, hyperchromatism, and the loss of contact inhibition. • Tumor doubling time may be used to assess the aggressiveness of a tumor and therefore the patient's prognosis following therapy. Most tumors double in volume every 20 to 100 days, although this can vary from 8 to 600 days. Most tumors, therefore, have been present at least 1 year, and many for as long as 10 to 15 years, before they are clinically detectable. A l-cm tumor requires 30 exponential divisions and is made up of approximately one billion cells.

Answer: C

4. Regarding the immune response to neoplasms, which of the following statements is/are true?

A. Tumor-specific antigens induced by chemical and physical carcinogens are distinct for each tumor, while tumor-specific antigens induced by viral carcinogens are common to all neoplasms induced by the same virus
B. Immunized mice are able to inhibit tumor growth even when challenged with large numbers of tumor cells (i.e., greater than one million)
C. Thymus-derived (T) lymphocytes are thought to play a role in immune surveillance independent of major histocompatibility antigens
D. Host-immune effectors are many times more effective against primary tumors than against metastatic deposits

Sabiston: 507
Schwartz: 320

Comments: Tumor-specific antigens are cell surface antigens distinctly different from those antigens normally found on the cell surface of tissue from which the tumor originates. Furthermore, these antigens are not found on cell surfaces of this tissue during embryonic development, nor on other tissue, be that tissue malignant or benign. In general, chemical and physical carcinogens induce tumor-specific antigens distinct for each tumor, while viral carcinogens induce common antigens that may cross-react. A challenge with large numbers of tumor cells (greater than one million) overwhelms the immunologic defense in immunized mice and allows tumor growth. Thymocyte-derived lymphocytes or T cells may be separated into subsets based on phenotype determined by specific monoclonal antibodies. These subsets include inducer cells, helper cells, cytotoxic cells, and suppressor cells. T cell–mediated lysis of neoplastic cells is dependent on major histocompatibility (MHC) interactions and is complement-independent. Natural killer

(NK) cells have spontaneous reactivity to tumor cells. They are not MHC-restricted and may play a role in immune surveillance as a natural defense of a host against neoplastic cells. Besides T cells and NK cells, host defenses against tumors include circulating antibody, antibody-dependent cellular cytotoxicity (ADCC), and the macrophage. In vitro studies demonstrate that these effectors are many times more effective against the primary tumor than against metastatic deposits.

Answer: A, D

5. Regarding oncofetal antigens, which of the following statements is/are true?

A. Alpha-fetoglobulin is diagnostic of hepatoma as it is found in virtually 100% of patients with hepatoma
B. Alpha-fetoglobulin is found in patients following liver resection, in those with cirrhosis, or in those with other tumors
C. Oncofetal antigens are thought to be expressed as a result of selective repression of genes
D. Carcinoembryonic antigen elevation is diagnostic of adenocarcinoma of the colon
E. Carcinoembryonic antigen is not significantly elevated with liver metastases, limiting its usefulness as a test for recurrent cancer

Schwartz: 326

Comments: Fetal antigens are produced by normal fetal organs during embryonic development. Their expression in adulthood is thought to represent selective repression of genes secondary to dedifferentiation of tumor cells. **Alpha-fetoglobulin** is found in approximately 70% of patients with primary hepatoma. It is found occasionally in patients with gastric, prostate, and testicular tumors; it is not found in patients with rapidly dividing cells, liver regeneration following hepatic resection, or cirrhosis. **Carcinoembryonic antigen** is found in fetal gut, liver, and pancreas. It is often elevated in the blood of patients with adenocarcinoma of the colon; it may be increased in cirrhotics, smokers, and patients with pancreatitis, cholecystitis, diverticulitis, or ulcerative colitis. The highest levels are found in patients with liver metastases. Measurement of carcinoembryonic antigen levels, therefore, is of little help in diagnosis but is most useful as a follow-up test to detect recurrence of cancer.

Answer: C

6. Regarding monoclonal antibodies, which of the following statements is/are true?

A. A monoclonal antibody is defined as an antigenic determinant in the variable region of an immunoglobulin
B. Monoclonal antibodies have the ability to react with an indefinite number of different antigenic determinants
C. Monoclonal antibody–producing hybridomas are made by fusing a plasma cell to a myeloma cell
D. Since a given monoclonal antibody reacts with many different antigenic specificities, its usefulness as a diagnostic or therapeutic tool is limited

Sabiston: 507
Schwartz: 327

Comments: Hybridomas are made by fusing a plasma cell to a myeloma cell. A given hybridoma cell line produces a monoclonal antibody with specificity against only one set of antigenic determinants or epitopes. An antigenic determinant in the variable region of an immunoglobulin is defined as an idiotype. An anti-idiotype is an antibody to the idiotype which may suppress or augment host response to different antigens. The potential applications of monoclonal antibodies seem limitless and include immunodiagnosis, immunotherapy, tests for the follow-up after cancer treatment, and research.

Answer: C

7. Regarding the spread of neoplasms, which of the following statements is/are true?

A. Carcinoma-in-situ is a lesion with histopathologic characteristics of malignancy but without detectable invasion into deeper cell layers or adjacent tissue
B. Lymph node metastases permeate the sinusoids of the node and later spread throughout it to involve the subcapsular space
C. Lymphatic involvement is common with sarcomas, while most epithelial neoplasms metastasize hematogenously
D. Cancer cells reach the blood stream mainly through the thoracic duct

Schwartz: 329

Comments: Carcinoma-in-situ is a neoplasm with cytologic characteristics of malignancy but without detectable invasion into surrounding tissue or deeper cell layers. • There are essentially four mechanisms for the dissemination of cancer cells: infiltration into surrounding tissue planes, lymphatic invasion, vascular invasion (capillaries and veins frequently and arteries rarely), and direct implantation. • Metastatic cells generally first enter the lymph node via the subcapsular space; later the tumor cells permeate the sinusoids, gradually replacing the parenchyma of the node. Lymph nodes are commonly involved in epithelial neoplasms, while sarcomas rarely metastasize to them.

Answer: A

8. Regarding the biopsy of a tumor mass, which of the following statements is/are true?

A. Fine needle aspiration biopsy rarely is able to diagnose a malignancy and runs the significant risk of leaving tumor deposits along the needle track
B. Excisional biopsy is the procedure of choice for large soft tissue sarcomas
C. Incisional biopsy involves removal of a small portion of a tumor and is useful for thyroid nodules so as not to compromise curative resection
D. Cervical lymph node biopsy should not be performed until a careful search for a primary tumor has been made

Schwartz: 333

Comments: **Fine needle aspiration biopsy** of a tumor can be a simple office procedure with minimal risk. Although it requires expertise in interpretation by a cytopathologist, needle aspiration biopsy is a very reasonable method of making a diagnosis of malignancy with considerable frequency and reliability. A false negative biopsy, however, occurs sufficiently often that, with most tumors, further investigation is necessary. **Incisional biopsy** involves removal of a small portion of tumor. It suffers the same problem as needle biopsy in that the specimen obtained may not represent all of the involved tissue. It is appropriate for large soft tissue sarcomas so as to not compromise adequate curative resection. An incisional biopsy should be performed in such a fashion as not to compromise any subsequent operation. Excisional biopsy is used for total removal of small masses (2 to 3 cm) as is frequently performed for breast masses. Biopsy of cervical lymph nodes requires a prior search for a primary tumor. This search may include indirect laryngoscopy, pharyngoscopy, esophagoscopy, bronchoscopy, and thyroid scan in addition to the careful physical examination.

Answer: D

9. Which of the following statements is/are true regarding the surgical management of malignant neoplasms?

A. Enucleation is the usual treatment of choice for malignant neoplasms
B. Radical local resection is required when surgery alone is used to treat soft tissue sarcomas
C. En bloc regional lymphadenectomy should not be performed in patients having clinically involved lymph nodes
D. Lymph node dissection is thought to decrease the host's immune system and therefore should not be routinely performed

Schwartz: 338

Comments: Malignant neoplasms are not usually well encapsulated but instead are often covered by a pseudocapsule composed of a compression zone of neoplastic cells. Simple enucleation, therefore, is never adequate treatment of the tumor, and the surgeon must attempt to achieve a margin of normal tissue around the tumor during its removal. • When excision alone is used to treat a sarcoma, radical local resection is required, as these lesions tend to infiltrate beyond the palpable limits of the tumor. • Lymphadenectomy does not decrease the host's immune system. It is generally agreed that a regional lymph node dissection for clinically involved nodes should be done as an en bloc procedure when it is clinically feasible. When regional lymph nodes without clinical evidence of involvement are excised, microscopic examination reveals metastatic spread in 20 to 40% of carcinomas and melanomas.

Answer: B

10. Regarding the general principles of surgical management of metastatic and/or advanced malignancies, which of the following statements is/are true?

A. Pelvic exenteration can be curative for certain well-differentiated and locally extensive invasive adenocarcinomas of the rectum
B. The routine "second look" operation (within 6

months) is indicated to "search and destroy" early recurrence of colon cancer before it manifests itself physically or biochemically

C. Contraindications to hepatic resection of metastatic colon cancer include multiple metastases limited to one lobe of the liver, synchronous metastases, and a solitary but large (7 cm) metastasis

D. Multiple hepatic metastases from colon cancer to both lobes of the liver but with no obvious other involvement is best treated by hepatic transplantation

E. Pulmonary metastases have a rapid doubling time, effectively limiting their resection to palliative operations

Schwartz: 340

Comments: Pelvic exenteration is an uncommon operation that can be useful when applied within narrow proscriptions; it can result in a 25% 5-year survival rate when performed for radiation-treated recurrent cancer of the cervix and in certain well-differentiated and locally extensive adenocarcinomas of the rectum. • The routine "second look" operation, popularized by Wangensteen, was an effort to search for colon cancer in its very earliest stages and then perform resection for cure. The operation was repeated (a third and an even fourth time) until no more cancer could be found or until it was too extensive or metastatic. The considerable morbidity and the questionable improvement in results forced the operation into disfavor. Now, of course, markers such as carcinoembryonic antigen are helpful in selecting patients for reoperation. • An approximately 25 to 40% 5-year survival may be expected in patients having partial hepatectomy for solitary or multiple liver metastases from cancer of the colon limited to one lobe. Multiple liver metastases discovered at the time of primary resection or a large liver metastasis does not preclude resection with intent to cure. Nevertheless, only 5% of patients with colon cancer metastatic to the liver are candidates for such treatment. • Resection of a solitary lung metastasis from some primary tumors results in a 5-year survival rate at least as good as that for resection of primary lung cancer in general, which supports the practice of resecting metastases to the lung from some other site in selected cases. Patients with a tumor doubling time of greater than 40 days receive significant palliation and an increase in survival from resection of metastatic pulmonary nodules.

Answer: A

11. Which of the following statements is/are true regarding infusion and/or perfusion of malignant neoplasms with chemotherapeutic agents?

A. Chemotherapeutic agents may be infused into an artery supplying a malignant neoplasm at a greatly increased concentration

B. Hepatomas are resistant to intra-arterial infusion of 5-fluorouracil (5-FU)

C. The isolated extremity perfusion method entails an excessively high risk of extremity ischemia

D. Hyperthermic perfusion dramatically increases the risk of complications without significant increase in effectiveness

Sabiston: 520, 528
Schwartz: 341

Comments: The infusion of chemotherapeutic agents into an artery supplying a neoplastic lesion allows administration of a concentration of drug to that lesion far greater than that which can be given systemically. Portable infusion pumps allow continuous infusion over a prolonged time period. Some success has been reported in treating patients with hepatoma with hepatic arterial infusion of 5-FU. • With the isolated perfusion technique, the artery and vein supplying a tumor-bearing extremity are cannulated and isolated from the systemic circulation. The tumor is then perfused by means of a pump-oxygenator with cancericidal drugs in concentrations prohibitive in the systemic circulation. • Hyperthermia may increase the effectiveness of the isolation-perfusion technique; it has been successful in the treatment of malignant melanoma and primary or recurrent soft tissue sarcomas of the extremity.

Answer: A

12. Regarding the radiotherapy of malignant neoplasms, which of the following statements is/are true?

A. The newer supervoltage machines (1,000 to 50,000 kv) penetrate to a greater depth and therefore cause essentially no damage to adjacent normal tissue

B. Gamma rays are electrons that penetrate only a few microns

C. Osteosarcomas and melanomas are very sensitive to radiation, while seminomas and hematologic malignancies are relatively insensitive

D. Radiation causes the release of hydroxy and peroxide radicals, which results in breaks in both tumor and normal cellular DNA

Sabiston: 962
Schwartz: 342

Comments: Radiation penetrates to varying degrees and collides with tissue atoms, resulting in the release of hydroxy and peroxide radicals. These radicals cause breaks in the DNA of both tumor and normal cells. It is thought that the difference in toxicity may be related to a more adequate repair mechanism in normal cells. A rad is the unit of measurement used to express the amount of radiation absorbed. Alpha particles penetrate only a few microns; beta particles or electrons penetrate only a few millimeters. Electromagnetic radiation such as gamma rays can penetrate even several centimeters of metal. The newer supervoltage machines penetrate to a greater depth; they cause less ionization and so less skin damage than 250-kv machines used in the past. The effects of radiation, however, may be seen both within minutes and months to years after exposure. The following are listed in decreasing order of radiosensitivity from most to least sensitive: hematologic malignancies, seminoma, basal cell carcinoma, adenocarcinoma of breast, intestine and endocrine organs, soft tissue sarcoma, osteosarcoma, and melanoma.

Answer: D

13. Which of the following statements is/are true regarding radiation injury of the gastrointestinal tract?

A. Total body irradiation of 400 rads is relatively well tolerated by most patients

B. Acute changes seen in radiation injury include

edema, ulceration, and diarrhea; chronic changes include stricture and perforation

C. Radiation-induced small intestinal and rectovaginal fistulas are most frequently self-healing

D. Free perforation of the intestine should be managed by a bypass procedure

Sabiston: 964
Schwartz: 344

Comments: Large areas of irradiation such as 400 rads to the total body, which may occur in accidental overexposure, constitutes an LD_{50} in humans. With smaller portals, larger doses are generally well tolerated. Nevertheless, acute radiation injury to the bowel may result in edema, ulceration, and diarrhea; chronic changes include stricture, ulceration, and perforation. Late injury results from progressive vasculitis and diffuse fibrosis. The best treatment for radiation injury of the gastrointestinal tract includes prevention by such means as reperitonealization and positioning of the omentum as a buffer or pelvic sling. Obstructed bowel should initially be managed conservatively with intestinal decompression and fluid replacement. If laparotomy is necessary, wide resection of diseased bowel is the treatment of choice. Though a bypass procedure may be required, perforated bowel requires proximal defunctionalization, drainage, and exteriorization of the perforation. Radiation-induced small intestinal fistulas rarely heal spontaneously and will require operative correction. However, prior to this, a period of parenteral nutrition usually is necessary. Rectovaginal fistulas frequently require biopsy to differentiate them from recurrent cancer. Treatment includes a proximal diverting colostomy of the sigmoid or descending colon.

Answer: B

14. Which of the following statements is/are true regarding the chemotherapy of malignant neoplasms?

A. Alkylating agents produce breaks in the DNA molecule and are therefore called "radiomimetic"
B. Neoplastic cell growth is initially slow and increases later as the tumor increases in size
C. The most frequent cause of treatment failure is insufficient administration of a phase-specific drug
D. Partial response to chemotherapy is defined as a single log kill of a neoplasm

Schwartz: 346

Comments: Chemotherapeutic agents are divided into five groups as follows: **antimetabolites** (e.g., methotrexate, 5-FU), which act by inhibiting the enzymes of nucleic acid synthesis; **alkylating** agents (e.g., cyclophosphamide, nitrogen mustard), which act by substituting an alkyl group for hydrogen atoms of nucleic acids, producing the radiomimetic effect of breaks in the DNA molecule; **antibiotics** (e.g., adriamycin, actinomycin D, bleomycin), which act by forming relatively stable complexes with DNA, thereby inhibiting further synthesis; **vinca alkaloids** (e.g., vincristine, vinblastine), which bind microtubular proteins necessary for cell division; and **miscellaneous** (e.g., nitrosoureas, DTIC). Both normal and neoplastic cell growth follow a gompertzian curve, which initially is exponential with a high growth fraction followed later by lengthening of doubling time

and a decreasing growth fraction. Chemotherapeutic agents are divided into **phase-specific drugs,** which kill only during specific phases of the cycle, and **phase-nonspecific drugs,** which kill during all or most phases of the cell cycle. According to the log–cell kill hypothesis, chemotherapeutic agents kill in logarithmic terms with no more than a one log–cell kill per exposure. Partial response to treatment is defined as a 50% reduction in the product of the greater and lesser diameters of any given tumor. Treatment failure is most commonly the result of development of drug resistance by the tumor cells.

Answer: A

14. Which of the following statements is/are true regarding the various chemotherapeutic protocols?

A. Combinations of drugs such as cyclophosphamide, methotrexate, and 5-FU have had little success in improving the survival of premenopausal women with breast cancer and positive axillary nodes
B. Despite intensive treatment with methotrexate, metastatic choriocarcinoma is uniformly fatal
C. The most effective single agent against melanoma is imidazole carboxamide (DTIC)
D. Little increase in survival is seen in multimodality treatment of Wilms' tumor, supporting operation only as the appropriate therapy

Sabiston: 520, 527, 568
Schwartz: 353

Comments: The cure rate of certain tumors (e.g., Wilms' tumor) has been dramatically improved by the use of combined modality therapy. Similar improvement has been seen in localized retinoblastoma and sarcomas in children and adults. Combination chemotherapy has certain theoretical advantages over single agents. As an example, administration of a phase-nonspecific drug may lead to a 2 log–cell kill. During recovery, only dividing cells will repopulate the tumor, and thus repopulation may be inhibited by a phase-specific drug. Alternating courses would be expected to lead to progressively increased killing of tumor cells. Combinations such as cyclophosphamide, methotrexate, and 5-FU have resulted in significant increases in survival in premenopausal women with breast cancer and positive axillary nodes. Despite the theoretical advantages of multi-drug regimens, single-agent therapy such as methotrexate for metastatic choriocarcinoma can lead to dramatic increases in survival. Chemotherapy for melanoma has met with very limited success; nevertheless, the single agent most effective is imidazole carboxamide (DTIC).

Answer: C

16. Which of the following statements is/are true regarding the immunotherapy of malignant neoplasms?

A. Immunotherapeutic modalities have the advantage of specificity against a tumor, and therefore should be effective even in patients with advanced disease
B. Immunotherapy should be avoided in combination with irradiation and chemotherapy, as all are immunosuppressive
C. Greater efficiency of antitumor responses could be expected if the immunogenicity of the tumor cells could be decreased

D. Surgery may be thought of as immunotherapy because it removes the immunosuppressive effect of a large tumor mass

Sabiston: 508
Schwartz: 353

Comments: Various immunotherapeutic modalities have the theoretical advantage of achieving a greater specific antitumor effect. Nevertheless, immunity against cancer is limited, and the presence of greater than 10 million neoplastic cells almost always nullifies immunotherapy. Since a l-cm tumor has approximately one billion cells, immunotherapy alone would not be expected to be adequate treatment of patients with advanced disease. Immunotherapy is a logical adjunct to radiotherapy and chemotherapy, as the aim of immunotherapy is to improve immune function while the latter two are immunosuppressive. Greater efficiency of antitumor responses could be expected if the immunogenicity of the tumor cells could be increased. An operation may be thought of as an immunotherapeutic modality which removes the immunosuppressive effect of a large tumor bulk, potentially allowing the host to better mount an immune response against subclinical foci of tumor cells.

Answer: D

17. Which of the following statements is/are true regarding the immunotherapy of malignant neoplasms?

A. Passive immunotherapy involving transfer of sensitized lymphoid cells is a type of adoptive immunotherapy
B. An example of active specific immunotherapy includes the administration of bacillus Calmette-Guérin (BCG) vaccine directly into melanomas
C. Interferons induce an antiviral state and therefore inhibit activity of cytotoxic T cells and NK cells
D. Active nonspecific immunotherapy involves the ad-

ministration of antisera with high titers of antitumor antibody

Sabiston: 510
Schwartz: 355

Comments: Numerous trials of immunotherapy for malignant neoplasms have been attempted. Although hopes were and still are high for its potential, results to date have, in general, been disappointing. Immunotherapy may be divided into active specific, active nonspecific, and passive. The greater effectiveness of active immunization, as compared with passive immunization, against microbial disease led to high expectations for active immunotherapy against cancer. **Active specific immunotherapy** attempts to increase the host's immune response to a tumor by administration of a vaccine of specific tumor cells that has been altered in some way by chemical or radiation treatment. **Active nonspecific immunotherapy** is based on the ability of certain substances, such as mixed bacterial toxins and fractions of tubercle bacillus, to stimulate immune responses to a wide variety of antigens, including tumor antigens. As an example, local injection of BCG into melanoma nodules has led to local and occasionally distant regression of nodules. **Passive immunotherapy** may be divided into the transfer of antisera containing high titers of antitumor antibody and administration of sensitized lymphoid cells, also called adoptive immunotherapy. Recently a great deal of investigation has been directed to looking at the administration of lymphoid cells cultured in the lymphokine interleukin-2, the so-called lymphokine activated (LAK) cell, to patients with advanced cancer. Passive immunotherapy may also involve the transfer of interferon, transfer factor, immune RNA, thymic hormones, levamisole, and various lymphokines. Interferons are glycoproteins produced by lymphocytes, macrophages, and fibroblasts. They appear to induce an antiviral state and induce cytotoxic T cell and NK cell activity.

Answer: A

CHAPTER 15

Complications

1. A higher incidence of wound dehiscence has been associated with:

A. Older patients
B. Vertical incisions
C. Ascites
D. Anemia
E. Obesity

Sabiston: 339
Schwartz: 456

Comments: Dehiscence of an abdominal incision involves separation of the anterior fascial closure. Local factors that predispose to infection, technical errors in suture selection or placement, and systemic factors that impair wound healing can all contribute to this development. A higher incidence has been reported in older patients and in those with malnuturition, hypoproteinemia, carcinoma, ascites, increased intra-abdominal pressure, wound infection, and obesity. The presence of anemia alone does not correlate with wound dehiscence. Vertical incisions generally have been reported to have a higher incidence of dehiscence than have transverse incisions.

Answer: A, B, C, E

2. Abdominal wound dehiscence:

A. Usually is caused by suture breakage
B. Invariably results in evisceration
C. Characteristically presents with serosanguinous wound drainage
D. Has a low incidence of postoperative hernia if recognized early

Sabiston: 339
Schwartz: 456

Comments: The usual mechanism in dehiscence involves sutures tearing through tissue. Partial dehiscence results in ventral hernia; total dehiscence leads to evisceration. Late hernias occur in at least 30% of these patients.

Answer: C

3. Preoperative factors associated with an increased risk of wound infection include:

A. Alcoholism
B. Diabetes mellitus
C. Concomitant urinary tract infection
D. Longer preoperative hospitalization
E. Shock

Sabiston: 336
Schwartz: 456

Comments: Anything that causes local hypoxia or impairs immunologic defenses increases the risk of infection. A longer preoperative hospitalization predisposes to colonization of the skin with pathogenic bacteria. A distant infection triples the rate of wound infection. Diabetes mellitus is associated with a higher rate of wound infection, although not when there is adjustment for the age of the patient.

Answer: A, B, C, D, E

4. Preoperative factors that decrease the rate of wound infection include:

A. Prophylactic antibiotics in "clean" cases
B. Preoperative skin shaving
C. A shower using hexachlorophene
D. Combination of oral and systemic prophylactic antibiotics in colon surgery

Sabiston: 338
Schwartz: 456

Comments: Systemic antibiotics administered before the incision is made decrease the infection rate of "clean-contaminated" cases. Prophylactic antibiotics are not indicated in "clean" cases unless prosthetic materials are used. A combination of systemic and oral antibiotics prior to colon surgery has not been shown to be superior to the use of nonabsorable oral antibiotics and mechanical bowel cleansing alone. Preoperative skin shaving, especially when performed 24 hours before operation, provides serous substrates for colonizing bacteria and actually increases the rate of wound infection.

Answer: C

5. Appropriate treatment of a wound infection might include, in addition to drainage, antibiotic coverage with a second generation cephalosporin if:

A. The infecting organism is a hemolytic streptococcus
B. The infecting organism is a gram-negative rod
C. Bacteremia is present
D. The infection invovles the mid-face
E. Antibiotics are never indicated when there is adequate drainage

Sabiston: 338
Schwartz: 456

Comments: The primary treatment of wound infections is surgical drainage. Additional antimicrobial therapy is indicated with bacteremia, spreading cellulitis, infection with hemolytic streptococci, and infections around the central face which pose the risk of intracranial extension.

Answer: A, C, D

6. In "clean-contaminated" cases, wound infection is most frequently the result of:

A. Preoperative contamination by exogenous bacteria
B. Intraoperative contamination by endogenous bacteria
C. Intraoperative exogenous contamination from operating room personnel
D. Intraoperative airborne contamination
E. Postoperative hematogenous seeding or direct contamination

Sabiston: 338
Schwartz: 456

Comments: In "clean-contaminated" cases, bacterial wound infection is caused by endogenous organisms and the giving of antibiotics prophylactically is an important preventive measure. Exogenous sources of bacteria have a more imortant role in "clean" cases, emphasizing the role of asepsis. Postoperative factors are relatively unimportant.

Answer: B

7. Postoperative parotitis:

A. Is usually caused by oral anaerobic bacteria
B. Can be prevented by prophylactic antibiotics
C. Can be treated with irradiation
D. Should initially be treated by frequent massage of the gland to stimulate sailvary flow and promote drainage
E. Should not be surgically drained unless fluctuance is apparent because drainage risks injury to the facial nerve

Sabiston: 339
Schwartz: 458

Comments: Postoperative parotitis is most often associated with the following: elderly patients, poor oral hygiene, dehydration, anticholinergic drugs, and nasogastric intubation. Staphylococci are the usual responsible organisms, and antibiotics given prophylactically are of no benefit. In the presence of infections, however, treatment involves administration of antibiotics and early surgical drainage if there is no improvement; massage is contraindicated. Irradiation in the early stages may alleviate pain by decreasing the rate of salivary secretion.

Answer: C

8. Which of the following suggest(s) the need for ventilatory support on the basis of inadequate ventilation:

A. Respiratory rate greater than 35
B. $PaCO_2$ grater than 60 mm Hg
C. Arterial alveolar oxygen difference greater than 350 mm Hg
D. Dead space to tidal volume ratio greater than 0.6

Sabiston: 1973
Schwartz: 460

Comments: The indications for respiratory support include inadequate parameters of **ventilation** (respiratory rate VD/VT, $PaCO_2$), **oxygenation** (AaO_2 difference, PaO_2) and **respiratory mechanics** (vital capacity, inspiratory force). In the absence of chronic hypercapnia, a $PaCO_2$ greater than 60 is abnormal.

Answer: A, B, D

9. Positive end-expiratory pressure (PEEP):

A. Effectively increases functional residual capacity, thereby improving physiologic shunting
B. Is especially useful in relieving the physiologic shunt associated with emphysema
C. May be detrimental in patients with high cardiac output because of associated increases in pulmonary vascular resistance
D. Has been particularly useful in the management of respiratory failure associated with massive chest wall injuries

Sabiston: 301, 1987
Schwartz: 461

Comments: The physiologic effects of PEEP include increased functional residual capacity, increased pulmonary compliance, decreased shunting, increased pulmonary vascular resistance, and decreased cardiac output. PEEP is useful in the management of respiratory failure associated with adult respiratory distress syndrome, atelectasis, and chest-wall injury. The associated increased intrathoracic pressures, however, can have potentially deleterious effects because of the resultant sequence of decreased venous return, diminished cardiac output, and hypotension. Direct barotrauma to the lungs by PEEP can produce pneumothorax, particularly in patients with chronic pulmonary emphysema. PEEP therapy should be monitored by sequential assessment of PaO_2, cardiac output, shunt fraction, pulmonary compliance, and parameters of oxygen delivery such as mixed venous oxygen concentration and arterial–venous oxygen content difference.

Answer: A, D

10. Postoperative atelectasis:

A. Is characterized by decreased PaO_2 and increased $PaCO_2$
B. Is more common with vertical rather than with transverse abdominal incisions
C. Is best prevented by constant volume ventilation with normal tidal volumes
D. Can be treated effectively with the use of intermittent positive pressure breathing (IPPB)
E. Treatment may require the use of bronchodilators, mucolytic agents, antibiotics, bronchoscopy, or tracheostomy

Sabiston: 331
Schwartz: 461

Comments: Multiple factors contribute to postoperative atelectasis; the common pathophysiologic causes are hypoventilation, tracheobronchial obstruction, and decreased surfactant activity. Patients who smoke, have underlying pulmonary disease, or are handicapped by factors that are mechancially unfavorable to optimal breathing, such as obesity or kyphoscoliosis, are at increased risk. The incidence of atelectasis is higher with upper abdominal or thoracic operations and with vertical abdominal incisions. The usual clinical signs within the first 24 to 48 hours postoperatively are fever and tachycardia; the PaO_2 is decreased and the $PaCO_2$ may be normal or decreased. The success of therapy depends on the effectiveness of mechanical measures in increasing lung volume and in clearing the lungs of their secretions; antibiotics are indicated for treatment of specific infections. IPPB is not an effective method for pulmonary re-expansion; it can, however, be useful for nebulization.

Answer: B, E

11. Concerning perioperative cardiac complications:

A. Halothane anesthesia is usually associated with bradycardia and artrioventricular dissociation
B. Cardiac arrhythmias more commonly occur after thoracic operations
C. An elective operation should be delayed at least 6 months following myocardial infarction
D. Most perioperative myocardial infarctions occur within the first 3 days postoperatively and are associated with shock
E. Chest pain is characteristic of postoperative myocardial infarction

Sabiston: 94, 2448
Schwartz: 464

Comments: Cardiac arrhythmias, congestive heart failure, and myocardial infarction are the most common cardiac complications postoperatively. Arrhythmias are related to underlying heart disease, electrolyte and acid-base status, type of operation, and anesthetic agents. Halothane and cyclopropane are the agents most frequently associated with arrhythmias; halothane sensitizes the myocardium to catecholamines. Most myocardial infarctions in these patients are precipitated by shock during the intraopertive or immediate postoperative period. Chest pain is often absent or not perceived. The risk of postoperative infarction in a patient with a previous infarction is related to the time from the initial episode; if less than 3 months previously, the risk is greater than 30%; 3 to 6 months, 15%; greater than 6 months, 5%. Patients with congestive heart failure, ventricular ectopy, or elevated left ventricular filling pressures are at increased risk. The mortality of reinfarction is 30 to 50%.

Answers: A, B, C, D

12. In the surgical management of patients with diabetes, the following is/are true.

A. Anesthetic agents that release catecholamines should be avoided
B. Severe hyperglycemia is best managed with regular insulin administered intravenously
C. Patients on oral hypoglycemic agents should take their medication with a sip of water preoperatively
D. Continuous administration of balanced solutions containing glucose and insulin is not recommended for routine use in uncomplicated cases
E. Patients on long-acting insulin require conversion to regular insulin for effective perioperative control

Sabiston: 152
Schwartz: 467

Comments: The choice of anesthetic is not influenced critically by the presence of diabetes mellitus. Nitrous oxide, trichloroethylene, and halothane, however, have the least effect on carbohydrate metabolism. The release of epinephrine and glucocorticoids can produce hyperglycemia by hepatic glycogenolysis and insulin antagonism. There are several effective methods for controlling diabetes in the perioperative period. Oral hypoglycemic agents are generally discontinued the day prior to operation, and administration of a fraction of the daily dose of insulin as regular insulin or in the form that the patient usually takes can be effective; continuous intravenous insulin infusions likewise are safe and effective. Severe hyperglycemia (including nonketotic hyperosmolar coma, and diabetic ketoacidosis are best managed with intravenous insulin. All methods of management in the perioperative period require serial assessment of serum glucose levels and of glycosuria.

Answer: B

13. Concerning the fat embolism syndrome:

A. In a patient with extensive trauma, an elevated serum amylase within the first 48 hours strongly suggests the diagnosis and indicates a poor prognosis
B. Emboli may originate from coalescence of circulating blood lipids
C. The principal symptoms are related to cerebral involvement
D. A diagnosis may be established by biopsy of petechial hemorrhages
E. Treatment may include intravenous heparin in doses to achieve therapeutic anticoagulation

Sabiston: 1768
Schwartz: 470

Comments: Fat embolism most commonly occurs in association with trauma and fractures of major long bones.

Emboli may originate from the bone marrow or from circulating lipids, which may explain its occurrence in non-traumatic conditions such as severe infection and with the use of extracorporeal circulation. The predominant clinical manifestations are pulmonary; cerebral fat embolism usually does not occur without pulmonary involvement. Classic petechial hemorrhages may occur in the shoulders, chest, axillae, palate, and subconjunctival regions. Biopsy and frozen-section examination can be diagnostic. Elevation of serum lipase occurs in about half the cases, usually beginning on the third day after injury, a sequence associated with a better prognosis. Early lipase elevations are more suggestive of pancreatitis. Low doses of intravenous heparin (5,000 units q 6 hours) accentuate lipase activity and may help clear lipemic plasma. Low molecular weight dextran, aprotinin (Trasylol), and ethyl alcohol have also been utilized in treating this syndrome.

Answer: B, D

14. A 40-year-old man has had a Billroth II gastrectomy, and on the third postoperative day develops signs and symptoms of mild shock. On the sixth day, he has a purulent foul-smelling drainage from the wound, which subsequently opens widely. At this time, he complains of left shoulder pain. The likely cause of all this is:

A. Intra-abdominal hemorrhage
B. Wound infection
C. Pancreatitis
D. Dehiscence of the duodenal stump
E. Cholecystitis

Comments: See Question 15.

15. In the patient above, the most appropriate treatment would be:

A. Immediate operation and sump-suction drainage of the abscess
B. Immediate operation and resuturing of the duodenal stump
C. Nonoperative care with gastric aspiration, antibiotics, and intravenous fluid and electrolyte replacement
D. Observation to see if a local abscess will form
E. Application of suction to the draining wound

Sabiston: 842
Schwartz: 479

Comments: Leakage of the duodenal stump is a serious complication and is most commonly seen after gastric resection for duodenal ulcer. Predisposing factors include a scarred, inflamed duodenum, obstruction of the afferent loop, and pancreatitis. Potential complications from this include intra-abdominal sepsis, pancreatitis, and fluid and electrolyte disturbances due to external losses through the fistula. During the operation, the surgeon must decide whether the duodenal stump can be closed safely. For difficult situations, a catheter duodenostomy is an appropriate alternative. Once dehiscence of the duodenal stump occurs, treatment consists of prompt drainage utilizing sump catheters, the control of sepsis, and fluid and nutritional support. With such treatment and if there is no distal intestinal obstruction, closure of the fistula may be anticipated within several weeks.

Answer: Question 14: D
Question 15: A

16. Concerning postoperative complications of gastric resection with Billroth II reconstruction, the following is/are true.

A. Suture line hemorrhage on the first postoperative day usually is from an arterial source and most often requires reoperation
B. With a retrocolic gastrojejunostomy, the transverse mesocolon may cause stomal obstruction
C. The episodic symptoms of afferent loop obstruction most often are the result of intermittent jejunogastric intussusception
D. A Roux-en-Y reconstruction relieves symptoms in the vast majority of patients with alkaline reflux gastritis
E. Necrosis of the gastric remnant is unusual because there is an abundant vascular supply to the stomach.

Sabiston: 842
Schwartz: 477

Comments: Suture line bleeding is usually minimal or moderate and generally responds to nonoperative measures. Delayed gastric emptying may result from stomal or efferent loop obstruction due to edema, a bulky transverse mesocolon or omentum, or torsion of the jejunum, or it may occur as a result of vagotomy. Jejunogastric intussusception is an unusual cause of obstruction. Roux-en-Y reconstruction relieves symptoms in approximately one half of patients with alkaline reflux gastritis. Necrosis of the proximal gastric remnant is unusual; it may occur following high subtotal gastrectomy, however, if the left gastric artery and short gastric vessels have been divided.

Answer: B, E

17. Afferent loop syndrome:

A. Usually becomes apparent several months following gastrectomy
B. Classically presents with persistent abdominal pain and diarrhea
C. Can usually be diagnosed by the appearance of the afferent loop on barium x-ray studies of the stomach
D. Constitutes a surgical emergency when obstruction is complete
E. May be associated with hyperamylasemia

Sabiston: 842
Schwartz: 477

Comments: The afferent loop syndrome is caused by acute or chronic obstruction of the duodenum and jejunum proximal to the site of a Billroth II gastroenterostomy. In most cases, it occurs within the first postoperative week, although its presentation may be delayed. The classic symptoms of partial obstruction are postprandial epigastric fullness and pain, relieved by vomiting of bilious material. X-ray contrast studies with a barium swallow may demonstrate delayed gastric emptying but often fail to visualize the afferent loop. The serum amylase may be elevated because of stasis of pancreatic secretions in the obstructed loop; chronic baterial overgrowth may produce vitamin B_{12} deficiency. Complete obstruction requires treatment urgently as it may cause duodenal necrosis and perforation.

Answer: D, E

18. Match the items in the two columns.

A. Fluid and electrolyte problems are common
B. Incidence of infection is high
C. Skin irritation is significant
D. Patient almost always can be maintained on oral diet

a. Small bowel fistula
b. Colonic fistula
c. Both
d. Neither

Schwartz: 479

Comments: The successful treatment of external intestinal fistulas requires appropriate fluid and electrolyte replacement, nutritional support, control of infection, and elimination of distal obstruction. Also, the fistulous discharge must be controlled; generally this entails skin protection, collection of the discharge, and sometimes sump-suction. Fluid and electrolyte losses from proximal high-output jejunal fistulas can be particularly difficult to correct. Infection in the form of intra-abdominal abscess, peritonitis, or systemic sepsis can be a problem with fistulas at any level; intra-abdominal sepsis is an indication for early operation. Patients with distal small bowel or colonic fistulas may be maintained on elemental or low-residue diets; those with proximal, high-output fistulas frequently require parenteral nutritional support.

Answer: A–a; B–c; C–a; D–b

CHAPTER 16

Skin

1. True statements regarding the physical properties of skin include:

A. Tension allows skin to regain its original shape after distortion
B. Elasticity is the property that resists stretching
C. The striae of Cushing's syndrome are due to loss of tensile strength and elasticity
D. Langer's lines indicate the direction of elastic forces in the skin
E. None of the above

Sabiston: 1571
Schwartz: 507

Comments: Tension is the property of skin that resists stretching. It is reduced in infants, in the elderly, and in patients with Ehlers-Danlos syndrome. Elasticity is the property that allows skin to regain its original shape after distortion. It, too, is decreased in the elderly. The direction of tension varies anatomically. In 1861, Langer described the direction of these lines of tension in the skin, a description still useful today when planning skin incisions.

Answer: C

2. True statements regarding percutaneous absorption of some materials include:

A. The major barrier to diffusion is the stratum corneum
B. Electrolytes applied to the skin in aqueous solution are rapidly absorbed
C. Lipid-soluble substances are rapidly absorbed
D. Substances in gaseous form cannot penetrate the skin

Schwartz: 508

Comments: The skin allows selective absorption of some materials, enabling them to appear in detectable amounts in the blood. Water is absorbed in vapor or in liquid form. Electrolytes applied in aqueous form are not absorbed, except in small quantities that enter via skin appendages. Iodine may enter the blood by skin appendage absorption or by increase in the negative charge of

skin. Lipid-soluble substances, particularly those partially water-soluble, are rapidly absorbed. Phenol and steroid hormones rapidly penetrate the skin, whereas protein hormones do not. Lipid-soluble but not water-soluble vitamins are rapidly absorbed. With the exception of carbon monoxide, substances in gaseous form (O_2, N_2, CO_2) easily enter via the skin.

Answer: A, C

3. Match the items in the two columns.

A. Contributes to the color of skin
B. Caused by local capillary dilatation and increased permeability
C. Causes vasoconstriction of cutaneous arteries and arterioles
D. Prolonged exposure to cold water

a. Sympathetic nervous system
b. Wheal
c. Subpapillary plexus
d. "Trenchfoot"

Schwartz: 508

Comments: The blood supply to the skin is complex and capable of multiple vascular reactions. Arteriovenous anastomoses in the digital skin (glomus end-organ apparatus) contribute to temperature regulation. Skin color and temperature depend upon the amount of blood flowing through the subpapillary plexus, flow increasing as ambient temperature rises. Cold produces vasoconstriction and pallor. Prolonged cold causes paresis of skin capillaries and arteriolar dilatation, producing livid discoloration. If, after prolonged exposure to ice-cold water, the skin is rapidly brought to normal temperature, reactive hyperthermia and even blistering may result. Vigorous scratching of the skin causes vasodilatation and leakage of capillary plasma, producing a wheal. Sympathetic stimulation of skin vessels causes vasoconstriction, while sympathectomy results in dilatation of small cutaneous arteries and arterioles, forming the basis of the therapeutic usefulness of sympathectomy.

Answer: A–c; B–b; C–a; D–d

4. Match the items in the two columns.

A. Modulates cold sensation
B. Modulates sensitivity to warmth
C. Modulates sensation of pressure
D. Modulates pain
E. Modulates tactile sensation
F. Increased pain and vasodilatation after traumatic peripheral nerve injury

a. Ruffini's endings
b. Krause's end-bulbs
c. Free nonmyelinated nerve endings
d. Meissner's corpuscles and Merkel's discs
e. Pacinian corpuscles
f. Causalgia

Sabiston: 1570
Schwartz: 508

Comments: A variety of structures are responsible for modulating the skin's various sensory functions. The numbers of these structures vary with the region of the body. Sympathectomy at the appropriate level may relieve the symptoms of causalgia.

Answer: A–b; B–a; C–e; D–c; E–d; F–f

5. True statements regarding sweat secretion include:

A. There are three types of sweat glands: apocrine, eccrine, and holocrine
B. The highest concentration of sweat glands is in the axilla
C. Direct application of heat is the major stimulus for sweat formation
D. Eccrine sweat is an ultrafiltrate of plasma
E. The eccrine sweat glands are distributed over the entire body and produce aqueous sweat for thermal regulation

Schwartz: 508

Comments: There are two types of sweat glands: eccrine glands and apocrine glands. The eccrine glands secrete aqueous sweat and the apocrine glands secrete a milk-like substance. Sweat glands are distributed over the entire body, the highest concentration per square inch being on the palms and soles. Most sweat is the result of nervous stimulation carried over sympathetic nerves and mediated by acetylcholine. It is inhibited by atropine. Hyperhidrosis is a condition of increased sweating that can be corrected by sympathectomy performed at the appropriate level. The production of sweat is an active process. Normally, sweat is hypotonic but can approach isotonic concentrations at high rates of production. Sodium secretion parallels that of chloride, the concentration being less than that of plasma. Potassium concentration approaches that of plasma. Urea and ammonia are excreted in concentrations much higher than that in plasma. Lactic acid is actively secreted and provides the skin with an acid mantle. Evaporative water loss does not contain electrolytes and is insensitive to atropine. Total cutaneous water loss as the result of evaporation at rest without visual sweating is about 500 to 700 ml/day.

Answer: E

6. True statements about decubitus ulcers include:

A. Pressure must be continuous for at least 4 hours to cause a decubitus ulcer
B. Decubitus ulcers usually occur over bony prominences
C. Correction of nutritional deficiency and anemia is important in treatment
D. The use of rotation flaps in treatment is contraindicated

Schwartz: 510

Comments: Decubitus ulcers result from prolonged pressure applied over bony prominences. In the nutritionally impaired, pressure for as short as 2 hours can produce ischemia, leading to ulcer formation. Special mattresses, routine positional changes, nutritional support, and correction of anemia are important adjuncts to surgical débridement. Surgical therapy includes excision of all necrotic tissue, resection of obvious bony prominences, covering exposed bone with muscle, and providing cover for the skin. Skin cover is achieved by primary epithelialization over a granulation base, split thickness skin graft, or occasionally rotation flaps of subcutaneous tissue and skin.

Answer: B, C

7. True statements about hidradenitis suppurativa include:

A. It is an infection of apocrine glands, subcutaneous tissue, and fascia
B. Staphylococci and streptococci are the predominant organisms isolated
C. The axilla, areola, groin, perineum, and perianal and periumbilical areas are usually involved
D. The lesions begin with slight subcutaneous induration and progress to suppuration and cellulitis
E. Treatment can vary from improved hygiene to radical excision with split thickness skin graft

Schwartz: 510

Comments: Hidradenitis suppurativa is an acneiform infection involving the apocrine glands in several areas. The presenting symptoms are an acute episode with suppuration and cellulitis or a chronic condition characterized by coalescing cutaneous nodules surrounded by fibrous reaction. Treatment is individualized. Some patients are cured with improved hygiene and incision and drainage, some respond to high doses of tetracycline, and occasionally in extensive chronic cases radical excision and reconstruction with split thickness skin grafts are required.

Answer: A, B, C, D, E

8. Match the items in the two columns.

A. Lined by glandular epithelium, filled with sebum
B. Cystic mass occurring over a tendon sheath
C. Epidermal-lined cysts filled with keratin
D. Congenital lesion occurring in the midline
E. Congenital coccygeal sinus

a. Epidermal inclusion cyst
b. Ganglion
c. Sebaceous cyst
d. Dermoid cyst
e. Pilonidal cyst

Sabiston: 1545, 1580, 1596
Schwartz: 510

Comments: A number of cystic lesions occur in the skin. Complete excision of each of these lesions listed above is curative; lesser procedures often lead to recurrence. When infection is present, primary incision and drainage with secondary excision is preferred. The diagnosis often can be determined from the history and location of the cyst. **Epidermal inclusion cysts** are caused by trauma leaving epithelium trapped in subcutaneous tissue. A **ganglion** consists of a wall of collagenous tissue occurring commonly over the wrist and tendons of the hands and feet and may be related to trauma. **Sebaceous cysts** are found almost anywhere on the body but most commonly on the face and midline of the trunk. They slowly increase in size and can become secondarily infected. **Dermoids** usually occur over the midline abdominal and sacral regions, over the occiput, and on the nose. Malignant degeneration has not been reported. **Pilonidal cysts** result from penetration of a congenital coccygeal sinus by an ingrown hair, setting the stage for infection and cyst formation.

Answer: A–c; B–b; C–a; D–d, E–e

9. Match the items in the two columns.

A. Wart	a. Hypertrophy of epidermis
B. Keratosis	b. Viral etiology, contagious, autoinoculable
C. Keloid	c. Dense accumulation of fibrous tissue
D. Lipoma	d. Occurs commonly on the back, between the shoulders, and on the back of the neck
E. Neuroma	e. Can be associated with von Recklinghausen's disease

Sabiston: 1580
Schwartz: 511

Comments: **Warts** (verruca vulgaris) can occur anywhere on the body, but are most common on the hands and feet. Those occurring on the plantar surface of the foot can become very painful. Treatment options include cryotherapy, caustic agents (salicylic acid), or electrodesiccation. Surgical excision is associated with a high incidence of recurrence. There are several types of **keratoses,** some considered premalignant, others not. Senile keratoses may be premalignant and occur in older persons with a fair complexion. Treatment options in addition to excisional biopsy include freezing, application of trichloroacetic acid, topical 5-fluorouracil, or electrocautery. Seborrheic keratoses are not premalignant and develop mainly on the trunk in older persons. They can be darkly pigmented and be mistaken for melanomas. Treatment can be by electrocautery, excision, or curettage. A third type of keratosis is the arsenical keratoses frequently associated with degeneration to squamous cell carcinoma. **Keloids** are the result of exuberant scar formation after trauma and occur commonly in blacks, with a predilection for skin of the face, neck, and sternum. Treatment includes excision with primary closure combined with pressure dressings, intradermal steroids, or low-dose radiation therapy. **Lipomas** are extremely common, often

encapsulated, and cured by excision. Malignant degeneration is uncommon. **Neuromas** can be either neurilemmomas arising from Schwann's cells or subcutaneous masses of neurofibromatous tissue. **Pheochromocytoma, meningioma,** or **glioma** can develop in patients with neurofibromatosis. Sarcomatous degeneration can occur in 10% of these patients.

Answer: A–b; B–a; C–c; D–d; E–e

10. The concerned mother brings her 2-month-old daughter to your office and points out a reddish, raised lesion, 2 cm in diameter, with irregular borders on the child's right lateral chest. There are no bruits, and there is no accompanying subepidermal component. Your diagnosis is

A. Capillary (port-wine) hemangioma
B. Immature hemangioma (strawberry mark)
C. Cavernous hemangioma
D. Dermatofibroma
E. Glomus tumor
F. Lymphangioma

Sabiston: 1589
Schwartz: 512

Comments: A number of vascular lesions occur at birth. Their appearance and behavior vary. A **capillary hemangioma** is an abnormal capillary located in the skin and appears as a reddish, nonraised stain. **Cavernous hemangiomas** contain immature blood vessels with multiple arteriovenous communications. When these communications are multiple and large, a bruit may be auscultated. **Dermatofibromas** are areas of subepidermal nodular fibrosis usually related to trauma. They occur chiefly on the extremities and often dimple when compressed. **The glomus tumor** is a painful lesion of the glomus end-organ occurring most commonly in the nailbeds. Pain is a consistent finding and is due to a nonmyelinated nerve supply. **Lymphangiomas** are cystic collections of anatomically abnormal lymphoid channels. When occurring in the neck, axilla, and mediastinum, they are called cystic hygromas.

Answer: B

11. Treatment of the lesion identified in Question 10 includes

A. Reassurance of the parent, since most of these lesions spontaneously regress within the first 24 months of life
B. Immediate excision, since malignant degeneration is frequent
C. A course of high-dose steroids to avoid subsequent formation of arteriovenous anastomoses
D. Compression dressings to avoid possible bleeding complications

Sabiston: 1589
Schwartz: 512

Comments: Immature hemangiomas appear in infancy, change in character during the first 12 months of life, and then regress. Occasionally, larger lesions bleed; when this occurs, it is easily controlled with pressure.

The majority of these lesions spontaneously regress. Capillary hemangiomas, however, do not regress and often present a cosmetic problem. Small lesions can be excised, but larger lesions present a therapeutic dilemma. Laser therapy seems to hold promise. Cavernous hemangiomas can sometimes be large, involving deep muscular and fascial structures. Steroids sometimes can induce regression in childhood, but most lesions persist into adulthood. When possible, established lesions are treated by excision. Embolization may be useful in selected cases. Dermatofibromas are simple fibrous tumors that are treated by simple excision. The glomus tumor is benign, and excision is curative. Lymphangiomas are treated with excision and rarely recur, even if excision is incomplete.

Answer: A

12. True statements regarding basal cell and squamous carcinomas include

A. Basal cell carcinomas grow more slowly than squamous cell carcinomas; they can be darkly pigmented, resembling melanomas, and produce little sign of inflammation or induration
B. Basal cell carcinomas grow more rapidly than squamous cell carcinomas, metastasize to regional lymph nodes more readily, and induce significant induration
C. Ulceration without induration or inflammation is characteristic of squamous cell carcinomas and has been referred to as "rodent ulcer"
D. Squamous cell carcinomas induce induration, are often surrounded by satellite nodules, lead to ulceration with rolled edges, and metastasize more frequently than basal cell carcinomas
E. Squamous cell carcinomas can develop in post-irradiation dermatitis or in old, burn-scar ulcers (Marjolin's ulcer)

Sabiston: 1583, 1586
Schwartz: 514

Comments: **Basal** cell carcinomas grow slowly and rarely metastasize, but are capable of extensive local invasion. Although most common in the head and neck, they can occur in any location. They are often waxy or translucent with underlying telangiectasia, but with time can produce a flat ulcer with little induration or reaction that can become quite deep (rodent ulcer). Superficial nonrecurrent basal cell carcinomas can be treated with curettage or cryosurgery, but surgical excision is preferred. **Squamous** cell carcinomas grow more rapidly and can and do metastasize. They are common at the vermilion border, paranasal areas, and maxilla. They tend to occur in blondes with light, thin, dry, irritated skin. Central ulceration with marked induration is common. They arise often in actinic keratosis, xeroderma pigmentosum, and atrophic epidermis and in persons exposed to arsenicals, nitrates, and hydrocarbons. Excision of both lesions should include a frozen section evaluation of the surgical margins. Both lesions are radiosensitive, and in some cases radiotherapy offers better cosmetic results. Operation is preferred in areas that have a burn scar or that have been irradiated. Large lesions may require a combination of radiotherapy and surgical excision. Mohs' chemosurgery involves the application of zinc chloride paste

followed by histologic examination of excised tissue; this is repeated until all tumor margins are clear. Lymph node excision for squamous cell carcinoma is performed therapeutically, not prophylactically.

Answer: A, D, E

13. Match the items in the two columns.

A. Fibrosarcoma
B. Lymphangiosarcoma
C. Hemangiopericytoma
D. Kaposi's sarcoma

a. Reddish-purple plaques; more common in men
b. Radioresistant; more common in women
c. Malignant counterpart of the glomus tumor
d. Associated with chronic lymphedema

Sabiston: 522, 1591, 1905, 2051
Schwartz: 515

Comments: Skin is the site of 6% of all sarcomas. **Fibrosarcomas** occur most commonly in the buttock, thigh, and inguinal region of women. Fibrosarcomas are radioresistant, and wide excision is the treatment of choice. Metastases occur in 25% of patients. **Hemangiopericytoma** is highly malignant. Radiotherapy is considered the treatment of choice. **Kaposi's sarcoma** occurs most commonly in Mediterranean men and recently in patients with acquired immune deficiency syndrome (AIDS) or other types of immune deficiency. It usually begins on the feet or hands and can become extensive. Excision, sometimes even amputation, and radiation are current therapies with merit in each. Florid lesions may respond to intravenous actinomycin D. **Lymphangiosarcoma** occurring in the postmastectomy edematous extremity is known as Stewart-Treves syndrome. Although amputation offers the best result, the prognosis is poor.

Answer: A–b; B–d; C–c; D–a

14. Match the items in the two columns.

A. Intradermal nevus
B. Junctional nevus
C. Compound nevus
D. Freckle
E. Hutchinson's freckle

a. Precancerous melanosis of the face
b. Pigments located in the basal layer of the epidermis and upper dermis
c. Melanocytes confined to the dermis
d. Melanocytes confined largely to the basal layer of the epidermis
e. Epidermal and intradermal melanocytes

Sabiston: 513
Schwartz: 516

Comments: Melanocytic nevi have been classified as congenital or acquired. Classification into intradermal, compound, or junctional nevi is based on location of melanocytes as described above. **Compound** nevi are smooth, raised, and hairless. **Intradermal** nevi are often associated with hairs. **Junctional** nevi are smooth, flat, and often on the genitalia, soles, palms, nailbeds, and mucous membranes. **Hutchinson's freckle,** or lentigo maligna, occurs more often in the elderly and is less aggressive when located on the face. The indications for excision include change in pigmentation, size, or shape, scaling, oozing, bleeding, pain, burning, numbness, or itching. **Dysplastic** nevi are unusual melanocytic nevi whose occurrence may be familial. In some individuals it is believed that these represent true precursors of malignant melanoma. They are reddish to brown in color and have scalloped edges and variegated pigmentation. Most melanomas, however, seem to arise de novo or from preexisting "nondysplastic" nevi. **Freckles** pose no threat and are found mostly in persons with light complexions. The pigment is in the basal layer and upper dermis.

Answer: A–c; B–d; C–e; D–b; E–a

15. True statements regarding melanomas include:

A. Lesions of the head, neck, and trunk have the best prognosis
B. Depth of invasion measured in millimeters, ulceration, anatomic location, and sex of the patient are the most important prognostic criteria
C. Nodular melanomas have a poorer prognosis than do superficial spreading melanomas of the same thickness
D. Melanomas in blacks are frequently subungual or on the palms and soles

Sabiston: 514
Schwartz: 516

Comments: The incidence of melanoma is increasing and may be related to increasing exposure to solar radiation in fair-skinned people. Melanomas are rare in darkly pigmented people. Nodular melanomas tend to have a poorer prognosis than superficial spreading melanomas, but only because they are thicker. Acrolentiginous melanomas may be more aggressive level for level. Ulcerated melanomas, located on the trunk, head, or neck, and melanomas in men have a poorer prognosis. Two thirds of melanomas arise from a pre-existing mole with junctional activity, and one third arise de novo.

Answer: B, D

16. Relative to malignant melanoma, indicate by the letter on the left side of the illustration the minimal depth of extension for each Clark level.

A. Clark level I
B. Clark level II
C. Clark level III
D. Clark level IV
E. Clark level V

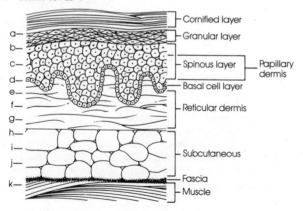

Sabiston: 516
Schwartz: 516

Comments: Microstaging, either by level of penetration (Clark) or by tumor thickness in millimeters (Breslow), is used to predict the likelihood of regional and distant metastasis. Breslow's measurements are considered more reliable in predicting biologic behavior. **Clark's** levels are as follows: I—above the basement membrane; II—into the papillary but not reticular dermis; III—to an ill-defined interface between papillary and reticular dermis; IV—in reticular dermis; V—into subcutaneous fat. **Breslow's** method makes use of an occulomicrometer in which several slides are examined and the measurement is taken from the top of the granular layer to the deepest point of penetration. In ulcerated lesions, the base of the ulcer over the deepest point of penetration is used instead of the granular layer. These determinants often are divided as follows: 0.75 mm or less; 0.76 to 1.5 mm; 1.51 to 3.0 mm; greater than 3.0 mm. Relative to clinical staging, Stage I indicates a lesion isolated to the skin, Stage II involvement of regional lymph nodes, and Stage III distant metastasis.

Answer: A–c; B–d; C–e; D–f; E–h

17. Which of the following is/are true regarding the treatment of melanoma?

A. Wide excision with 5-cm margins is the treatment of choice for primary melanoma
B. Prophylactic regional lymph node dissection improves survival
C. Isolated regional hyperthermic profusion is superior to wide excision
D. Thickness of the tumor, location, ulceration, and the age of the patient must be considered when planning treatment

Sabiston: 517
Schwartz: 517

Comments: Superficial melanomas less than 0.76 mm have an excellent prognosis when treated with local excision. Deep melanomas greater than 4 mm thick have a high incidence of distant metastases and treatment is limited to local excision, unless palpable regional lymph nodes are present. Melanomas of an intermediate thickness (0.76 mm to 4.00 mm) are the subject of controversy regarding the usefulness of prophylactic vs. therapeutic regional lymph node dissection and its influence on cure. Results of studies supporting each therapeutic approach have been reported, and the question is presently being examined by the Inter-group Melanoma Study Program in a prospective, randomized fashion. The traditional practice of a 5-cm margin of excision has been modified. In general, a 2- to 3-cm margin for lesions greater than 1 mm in thickness and a 1- to 2-cm margin for lesions less than 1 mm in thickness are appropriate when anatomically possible. Hyperthermic regional perfusion has been used in an effort to control advanced unresectable tumor in an extremity. Its use as a prophylatic adjunct following resection of intermediate thickness melanomas remains controversial. The inconstancy of lymph nodal drainage patterns for lesions on the head and neck or trunk can be difficult and may account for their poor prognosis.

Answer: D

CHAPTER 17

Breast

1. Which of the following statements is/are true regarding the incidence of breast cancer?

A. There are approximately 115,000 new cases annually in the United States
B. There are approximately 37,000 deaths from breast cancer annually in the United States
C. Breast cancer is slightly less common than lung cancer in adult American women
D. Twenty percent of women will develop some form of breast cancer in their lifetime
E. The age-adjusted incidence of breast cancer has been constant over the past 40 years
F. Breast cancer prevalence rates show very little difference from country to country, world-wide

Sabiston: 541
Schwartz: 530

Comments: There are an estimated 115,000 new cases of breast cancer in the United States annually, making it the most common malignancy (other than skin) in American women. This correlates with a lifetime risk of 6 to 8% among American women for the development of breast cancer. Approximately 37,000 deaths annually are due to breast cancer in this country. The age-adjusted incidence of breast cancer has been slowly rising for the past 40 years for reasons that are unclear. There is a wide variability of breast cancer prevalence in different countries, the Dutch having the highest national mortality from breast cancer (24.2 patients per 100,000 population) and the Japanese having the lowest (3.8 patients per 100,000 population).

Answer: A, B

2. Which of the following statements is/are true regarding risk factors for breast cancer?

A. Incidence does not appear to be age-related among those over 35 years old
B. Family history is a major predictor of risk for developing breast cancer
C. Late first pregnancy increases the risk of breast cancer

D. Diet and weight have no association with breast cancer risk

Sabiston: 542
Schwartz: 530

Comments: Breast cancer is clearly age-related, with its incidence being very low in women under the age of 20. It then rises gradually up to the mid-40's, after which there is a plateau, followed by a sharp increase in incidence after the age of 55. A positive family history is a significant risk factor for the development of breast cancer and is associated with a diagnosis at an earlier age and an increased incidence of bilaterality. Late first pregnancy (a greater than 20-year interval between menarche and first pregnancy) is associated with a higher incidence of breast cancer, particularly in the younger age group. In the older population, diets that are high in cholesterol and obesity appear to be related to a higher incidence of breast cancer.

Answer: B, C

3. Which of the following statements is/are correct regarding the natural history of breast cancer?

A. On the average, a 1-cm breast cancer has been subclinically present for approximately 1 year
B. Dimpling of the skin occurs as a result of glandular fibrosis and shortening of Cooper's ligaments
C. Skin edema in breast cancer results only from direct skin invasion by tumor
D. Vertebral metastases result from arterial dissemination of cancer cells
E. Ipsilateral lung involvement occurs most often as a result of direct lung invasion

Schwartz: 532

Comments: The majority of breast cancers are estimated to have volume-doubling times of between 2 and 9 months, suggesting that the average 1-cm tumor has been present in the range of 5 years prior to its clinical detection. Neither skin dimpling nor edema require direct skin invasion; these conditions result respectively

105

from fibrosis and lymphatic blockage in the subdermal tissues. The axial skeleton is a favored site for distant metastases from breast cancer, and this is thought to be due to access of cancer cells to the paravertebral venous plexus. All other forms of distant metastases, including ipsilateral lung involvement, are due to hematogenous spread as well.

Answer: B

4. Which of the following statements is/are correct regarding the natural history of breast cancer?

A. Virtually all patients with untreated breast cancer will die within 2 years of their diagnosis
B. The likelihood of distant metastasis is related to primary tumor size and inolvement of axillary nodes
C. Among patients dying of disseminated breast cancer, the lung is the most common site of metastasis
D. Liver and bone metastases occur with essentially equal frequency throughout the entire time course of a given cancer
E. Appropriate surgical therapy for breast carcinoma has been shown to increase overall survival

Sabiston: 544
Schwartz: 532

Comments: Breast cancer is a disease of wide biologic variability, and although the median survival among untreated patients is 2.7 years, nearly 20% of patients survive 5 years and some as long as 15 years without treatment. The increased likelihood of distant metastases occurring in the presence of large tumors and/or axillary nodal metastases has led to the current studies on the efficacy of adjuvant chemotherapy in these high-risk patients. Among patients dying of disseminated breast cancer, lung is the most common site of distant disease, with liver and bone involvement occurring equally less frequently. However, as the initial sites of distant disease, lung and bone predominate and liver involvement is less often seen. Appropriate local-regional therapy including surgery and radiation therapy has definitely improved the cure rate and cancer-free interval of patients with breast cancer over those in patients who are untreated. Beyond a certain point, however, improved local regional control of tumor does not necessarily translate to the same benefits.

Answer: B, C, E

5. Each of the patients depicted below has a breast cancer and normal chest X-ray and blood chemistries; none has bone pain. Complete the preoperative TNM designation and the stage of each cancer.

Sabiston: 550
Schwartz: 533

Comments: The correct staging of breast cancer is important as a prognostic indicator. **T** is for **tumor size:** T1 is for tumors less than 2 cm; T2 between 2 and 5 cm; T3 greater than 5 cm. Chest wall or direct skin involvement (T4) should also be assessed. **N** is for **lymph nodes;** suspicious mobile nodes (N1), matted or fixed nodes (N2), and periclavicular involvement or ipsilateral arm edema (N3) should be specifically described. **M** is for **metasta-**

ses; evidence of lung (chest x-ray) or liver or bone involvement (serum chemistries or scans) should be sought in each patient.

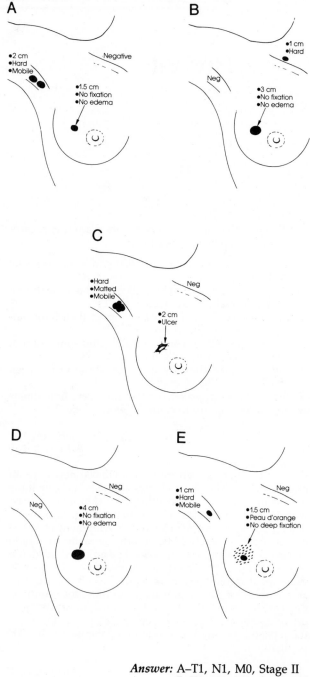

Answer: A–T1, N1, M0, Stage II
B–T2, N3, M0, Stage IIIB
C–T4, N2, M0, Stage IIIB
D–T2, N0, M0, Stage II
E–T4, N1, M0, Stage IIIB

6. Which of the following statements is/are true regarding Paget's disease of the nipple?

A. It appears as an eczematoid skin lesion on the nipple
B. It represents a primary carcinoma of the skin of the breast

C. It represents a primary ductal carcinoma with secondary skin involvement
D. It is a cutaneous manifestation of Paget's disease of the bone
E. It can be effectively treated by topical 5-FU

Sabiston: 546
Schwartz: 537

Comments: Paget's disease of the nipple is considered a primary ductal carcinoma that secondarily invades the skin of the nipple. It is unrelated to Paget's disease of the bone. As it represents a primary breast carcinoma with a significant incidence of invasive features, it should be managed aggressively, with a modified radical mastectomy being the treatment of choice.

Answer: A, C

7. Match the following histologic types of breast cancer with the features with which they are associated.

Histologic Type

A. Infiltrating duct carcinoma
B. Intraductal carcinoma
C. Lobular carcinoma in situ
D. Cystosarcoma phylloides
E. Medullary carcinoma
F. Inflammatory carcinoma

Features

a. Lymphocytic infiltrate and better-than-average prognosis
b. Often very large in size but quite mobile
c. Highest likelihood of multicentric ipsilateral disease
d. Highest likelihood of bilateral disease
e. Dermal lymphatic invasion
f. Most common breast carcinoma

Sabiston: 546
Schwartz: 538

Comments: The clinical presentation, natural history, and biological aggressiveness of breast cancer depend in part upon its histologic type. **Inflammatory carcinoma,** characterized by clinical inflammation and dermal lymphatic invasion, carries the worst prognosis. **Infiltrating duct carcinoma,** the most common type of breast cancer, carries an intermediate prognosis. **Medullary carcinoma** characterized by a lymphocytic infiltrate carries a better-than-average prognosis. **Lobular carcinoma** and **intraductal carcinoma** have a higher-than-average likelihood of multicentric disease within the involved breast (intraductal predominating) as well as bilateral breast involvement (lobular carcinoma in situ predominating). The in situ forms (intraductal and lobular carcinoma in situ) carry an excellent prognosis because of their noninvasive nature. **Malignant cystosarcoma** may achieve very large size and yet remain mobile within the breast. Lymph node metastases are uncommon from this tumor.

Answer: A–f; B–c; C–d; D–b; E–a; F–e

8. Which of the following treatment plans is/are contraindicated in the management of lobular carcinoma in situ?

A. Careful clinical and mammographic follow-up
B. Bilateral total mastectomy
C. Modified radical mastectomy on the involved side with careful follow-up of the contralateral breast

D. Mastectomy on the involved side with random biopsy of the contralateral side with mastectomy later performed if the biopsy reveals carcinoma
E. Subcutaneous mastectomy with reconstruction (unilateral or bilateral)
F. None of the above

Schwartz: 543

Comments: There is a great deal of controversy over the proper management of lobular carcinoma in situ. This has been generated by differences of opinion as to whether this entity is, in fact, carcinoma or a form of dysplasia. Its recognized association with multicentric ipsilateral and bilateral breast cancers has led some clinicians to adopt an aggressive approach to management. On the other hand, the extremely low likelihood of aggressive local behavior and regional lymph node metastases has led some to adopt principles of conservative management. All of the treatment options listed above have advantages and disadvantages and any one of them may be appropriate in a given clinical situation, depending to a great extent on the patient's desires. • Careful clinical and mammographic follow-up enables the patient to avoid mastectomy and makes it quite likely that any future cancer that may develop will be diagnosed at an early stage. Total mastectomy avoids the morbidity of the axillary dissection, which, when performed, reveals the presence of nodal metastases in only 2% of cases. Modified radical mastectomy enables those few patients with axillary nodal metastases to be appropriately treated and considered for adjuvant chemotherapy; however, this is at the cost of the added morbidity of axillary dissection. • Subcutaneous mastectomy with reconstruction preserves the nipple and increases the likelihood of an excellent cosmetic reconstructive result. This form of mastectomy, however, usually leaves some breast tissue behind, which may be hazardous in a disease process that is noted for its multicentric behavior. Management of the contralateral breast can range from careful follow-up to random biopsy (looking for occult contralateral disease) to "prophylactic" mastectomy. The rationale for these varying approaches again depends on one's view of the natural history and biologic behavior of this tumor.

Answer: F

9. Which of the following treatment modalities may be appropriate in the management of patients with recurrent breast cancer that is estrogen-receptor-positive?

A. Bilateral oophorectomy
B. Anti-estrogen drugs (tamoxifen)
C. High-dose estrogen or progesterone
D. Androgenic steroids
E. Aminoglutethimide

Sabiston: 564
Schwartz: 550

Comments: The presence of a significant amount of estrogen/progesterone receptor protein on breast cancer cells suggests that the tumor is more likely to respond to endocrine manipulation. Indeed, patients with high ER/PR levels fare better than those with low or absent values, when other discriminants are comparable. The mechanism of this more favorable course or response is not well understood, and various types of endocrine manipulation including anti-estrogen therapy (both surgical and chemical, as with aminoglutethimide) and hypophyseal ablation have been successful in receptor-positive patients. The most accepted initial endocrine manipulation has been oophorectomy or tamoxifen according to the patient's menopausal status.

Answer: A, B, C, D, E

10. Which of the following statements is/are true regarding needle aspiration biopsy of breast tumors?

A. It is performed easily in the office setting with minimal morbidity
B. Its results are inferior to those of needle-core biopsy technique
C. A negative needle aspiration biopsy effectively excludes the diagnosis of carcinoma
D. The success of needle aspiration biopsy depends to a great degree on the experience of the cytologist

Sabiston: 554
Schwartz: 537

Comments: Needle aspiration biopsy with a No. 20 or No. 22 needle is an effective and safe way of initially assessing suspicious masses within the breast. An aspirate that is cytologically positive for carcinoma is highly accurate, depending on the skill and experience of the cytologist; a negative aspirate may result from sampling error and necessitates further biopsy intervention. Although a smaller volume of tissue is obtained with needle aspiration than with needle-core biopsy, needle aspiration biopsy frequently yields results that are equal to or superior to those of core biopsy.

Answer: A, D

11. Which of the following statements is/are true regarding adjuvant chemotherapy for breast cancer?

A. Only patients with more than three positive nodes are appropriate candidates
B. To date, no significant improvement in survival has been seen with the use of adjuvant chemotherapy
C. Multiple-agent therapy seems to be more effective than single-agent therapy
D. The longer the treatment is taken, the more effective it is

Sabiston: 558
Schwartz: 543

Comments: Although most patient populations tested in prospective, randomized studies have shown some benefit from adjuvant chemotherapy (not always statistically significant), premenopausal women with up to three positive nodes have derived the greatest survival advantage. These successes in early studies have lead to broadening of the criteria for adjuvant treatment to include all patients with positive nodes. Controlled studies by multiple centers have shown that multiple-agent therapy is more effective than single-agent therapy and that 6 months of therapy is probably as effective as 12 months.

Answer: C

12. Which of the following statements is/are true regarding adjuvant radiotherapy for breast cancer?

A. Local recurrence rate is reduced
B. Disease-free survival is improved
C. There are few, if any, significant side effects from chest wall irradiation
D. It should be offered routinely to all patients whose primary tumors are larger than 2 cm

Sabiston: 558
Schwartz: 543

Comments: Adjuvant radiation therapy does decrease the local recurrence rates; however, this has not been found to translate into longer overall or relapse-free survival. Although relatively uncommon with modern techniques, skin ulceration, arm edema, rib fracture, radiation pneumonitis, and the potential for radiation-related chest wall sarcomas represent some of the potential side effects from chest wall irradiation. As a consequence of the above, adjuvant radiotherapy should be reserved for patients who are at high risk for local recurrence (very large tumors, skin involvement, multiple node involvement).

Answer: A

13. Which of the following 5-year survival rates by stage for treated breast cancer is/are correct?

A. Stage I: 90–95%
B. Stage II: 50–80%
C. Stage III: 30–50%
D. Stage IV: 15–20%

Sabiston: 559
Schwartz: 546

Comments: The wide range in rates of survival among patients with the same stages of cancer reflects the criteria by which that staging designation was made and, more importantly, the wide variability in the biologic behavior of breast cancer. In general, any follow-up of patients with breast cancer that is shorter than 10 years is considered inadequate, because of the ability of breast cancer to recur even after long disease-free intervals. In reporting breast cancer follow-up data, one must differentiate between "survival" and "disease-free interval."

Answer: A, B, C, D

14. Match the estrogen/progesterone receptor value of the recurrent cancer with its expected rate of response to hormonal therapy.

Receptor Status	Expected Response to Hormonal Therapy
A. ER positive/PR negative	a. 80%
B. ER positive/PR positive	b. 45%
C. ER negative/PR positive	c. 25%
D. ER negative/PR negative	d. 10%

Schwartz: 550

Comments: The exact mechanism by which hormonal therapy is influenced by receptor status is unclear. However, the trend of increasing response rates being associated with increasing receptor positivity appears to hold true for all types of endocrine manipulation, both additive and ablative.

Answer: A–c; B–a; C–b; D–d

15. Which of the following statements is/are true regarding chronic cystic mastitis?

A. It is a well-defined abnormality of the breast with specific and consistent histologic features
B. It is of primarily bacterial etiology
C. It is rarely seen in women under 45 years of age
D. The cyst must be at least 1 cm in size to provide clinical confirmation of the diagnosis
E. None of the above

Comments: See Question 16.

Sabiston: 539
Schwartz: 533

16. Which of the following does not belong to the chronic cystic mastitis group?

A. Papillomatosis
B. Blunt duct adenosis
C. Sclerosing adenosis
D. Apocrine metaplasia
E. Mondor's disease

Sabiston: 539, 1719
Schwartz: 533

Comments: Chronic cystic mastitis is a poorly defined group of histopathologic processes within the breast that relate in a broad way to variations in the stromal vs. epithelial architecture of the breast and are unrelated to previous bacterial or traumatic insults. It can be seen in patients in their 20's, although its incidence does increase throughout the reproductive years. Gross cysts need not be present. Mondor's disease, which is a superficial thrombophlebitis of the breast, does not belong in this category.

Answer: Question 15: E
Question 16: E

17. Biopsy-proven chronic cystic mastitis in a patient is associated with what, if any, increase in the likelihood of that patient subsequently developing breast cancer?

A. None
B. 3 times
C. 10 times
D. 25 times

Schwartz: 535

Comments: While the overall cancer risk conferred by the presence of chronic cystic mastitis may be 3 times that of the general population, the majority of lesions associated with subsequent cancer are the more proliferative types of papillary and epithelial hyperplasia, particularly those with atypical cytology.

Answer: B

18. Which of the following statements is/are true regarding breast infections?

A. Acute bacterial infections occur most often as a result of pre-existing chronic dermatitis
B. Bacterial infections are usually indolent, taking up to several weeks to become clinically apparent
C. Surgical drainage, once suppuration has occurred, is the treatment of choice for acute infections
D. Chronic infections of the breast are rare and most often caused by tuberculosis

Sabiston: 538
Schwartz: 550

Comments: Acute bacterial breast infection most often occurs during lactation within the first several months following delivery. Because the lactating breast is such an excellent culture medium, these infections usually develop quite rapidly and their size is often underestimated on clinical examination. When there is just a cellulitis, antibiotics may abort the infection. Once suppuration has occurred, however, surgical drainage is required, usually with the patient under general anesthesia.

Answer: C, D

19. Which of the following statements is/are true regarding breast development?

A. Breast enlargement in male infants is a finding indicative of an underlying estrogen-secreting adrenal tumor
B. Accessory nipples can be found anywhere from the axilla to the groin
C. Extramammary breast tissue is not under the influence of the hormonal status of the patient
D. Inverted nipples in children suggest underlying breast cancer

Sabiston: 531
Schwartz: 523

Comments: If the embryologic mammary ridge extending from the axilla to groin fails to involute fully, accessory nipples can appear along this route. Accessory breast tissue may also be seen (frequently in the axilla) and may enlarge during pregnancy and lactation in response to the changes in the patient's hormonal status. • Shortly after birth, both males and females may exhibit unilateral or bilateral breast enlargement, which is thought to relate to high levels of circulating maternal estrogens; these changes spontaneously regress. • In female infants failure of one or both nipples to evert following birth and into adulthood will lead to functional problems with attempted breast feedings; however, all this is unrelated to breast cancer.

Answer: B

20. Regarding mammography in the evaluation of breast disease, which of the following is/are true?

A. It can detect many cancers that are too small to be palpated
B. It is equally accurate in detecting lesions in all breasts regardless of age or glandular architecture
C. It delivers 2 rads of radiation to the middle of the breast being studied, and therefore should not be used for routine screening
D. Although it can occasionally miss very small cancers, a positive reading for carcinoma on mammography is virtually always accurate

Sabiston: 536
Schwartz: 529

Comments: Mammography is an important aid in the overall evaluation of breast disease. Current technology allows as little as 0.1 rad of radiation to the mid-breast per study, making it quite safe for routine annual mammography. Although it can frequently detect cancers that are not recognized on physical examination, it still has a false-negative and a false-positive rate on the order of 10%. The accuracy of mammography decreases in the extremely dense breast and increases in the more fatty older breast.

Answer: A

21. Which of the following statements is/are true regarding the current therapy of Stage I and Stage II breast cancer?

A. The Halsted radical mastectomy has resulted in a cure rate that is superior to that of other treatment options
B. The modified radical mastectomy involves preservation of the nipple in order to improve cosmesis following reconstruction
C. Wide local excision with axillary dissection and radiation therapy to the remainder of the breast is reserved for patients too debilitated to undergo the more radical mastectomy
D. The NSABP has shown equivalent 5-year disease-free survivals for selected patients randomized to receive either modified radical mastectomy or wide local excision, axillary dissection, and breast radiation therapy

Sabiston: 554
Schwartz: 541

Comments: The two most commonly employed modalities of definitive therapy for Stage I and Stage II breast cancer are (1) modified radical mastectomy, which preserves the pectoralis muscles but removes the entire breast, including the nipple, and the axillary lymph nodes, and (2) wide local excision of the breast tumor with axillary dissection and radiation therapy to the remainder of the breast. Studies with long-term follow-up have shown no significant disease-free survival advantage for the more radical (pectoralis removing) Halsted mastectomy. The NSABP (National Surgical Adjuvant Breast Project) has conducted a multi-institutional study with more than 1,800 patients with Stage I and Stage II breast cancer randomized to undergo either modified radical mastectomy or wide local excision and axillary dissection with and without breast radiation therapy. At an average of 5 years from treatment, there appeared to be no statistically significant differences in disease-free

survival between the mastectomy and the wide local excision, axillary dissection, and radiation therapy groups. Those undergoing wide local excision with axillary dissection but without radiotherapy had a higher local recurrence rate. Since all of these treatment modalities involve axillary dissection, which usually requires general anesthesia, consideration of anesthetic risk is not a major factor in the selection of the treatment modality.

Answer: D

22. Which of the following physical characteristics of breast masses are more suggestive of carcinoma than of benign disease?

A. Indistinct borders blending into the surrounding breast tissue
B. Hardness
C. Excessive mobility within breast tissue
D. Tethering to underlying muscular structures

Sabiston: 552
Schwartz: 533

Comments: Although there are many exceptions to the classic physical findings of breast cancer, the typical breast carcinoma is hard and has fairly distinct borders. Fixation to deeper structures is highly suggestive of malignancy. A smooth, rubbery, mobile mass is more suggestive of fibroadenoma. Fibrocystic disease may present as a disc-like or polynodular thickening with one or more of the borders blending indistinctly into the surrounding breast tissue.

Answer: B, D

23. Which of the following statements is/are true regarding subcutaneous mastectomy?

A. It involves removal of all breast tissue
B. It includes removal of the lower axillary lymph nodes
C. The best reconstruction results are associated with this type of mastectomy
D. It is the treatment of choice for early (less than 1 cm) microinvasive cancers with clinically negative nodes

Sabiston: 557
Schwartz: 542

Comments: Subcutaneous mastectomy is the removal of the breast (most often through a submammary incision) with preservation of the rim of the nipple. Axillary nodes are not removed as part of this operation; in fact, exposure of the axilla to remove the entire tail of the breast is at times difficult. As a result it is estimated that approximately 1 to 2% of breast tissue remains after subcutaneous mastectomy. Because of the preservation of some of the nipple and most of the subcutaneous fat, and because of the more cosmetic incision, it certainly offers the opportunity for reconstruction with the most favorable result. There have, however, been rare reports of cancer developing in the remaining nipple and small amount of remaining breast parenchyma. Its most appropriate use is in clinical settings of recognized high risk of cancer development, when the patient wishes to retain breast contour and the physiognomy of the breast accommodates to such an operation. Despite its virtues as described above, it is not recommended in the therapeutic management of breast carcinoma.

Answer: C

24. Which of the following statements is/are true in regard to cystosarcoma phylloides?

A. It bears a histologic relationship to fibroadenoma
B. Ten percent are malignant
C. As with ductal carcinoma, it has a high incidence of multicentricity within the breast
D. Axillary lymph nodal metastases are uncommon
E. Wide local excision or total (simple) mastectomy will usually suffice for treatment

Sabiston: 569
Schwartz: 539

Comment: Although only approximately 10% of all cystosarcomas are malignant, cystosarcoma is still the most common primary sarcoma of the breast. The benign variant of cystosarcoma is considered by many to be a giant fibroadenoma, and as such usually presents clinically as a solitary, discrete, mobile mass within the breast (usually quite a bit larger than the average fibroadenoma). The diagnosis of malignancy in these lesions is at times difficult, because of the poor correlation between histology and clinical behavior. The malignant cystosarcoma has no significant incidence of multicentricity within the breast (unlike ductal or lobular carcinoma). Furthermore, as with other malignant mesenchymal tumors, its pattern of metastasis is more likely borne to distant sites by blood rather than to the regional lymph nodes via lymphatic spread. In the absence of metastases, wide local excision probably suffices in the management of this lesion, but total mastectomy is also appropriate and may be required because of the size of the tumor.

Answer: A, B, D, E

25. Regarding breast carcinoma in men, the following is/are true:

A. It accounts for approximately 1% of all cases of breast cancer
B. The prognosis is poorer in affected men than it is in affected women
C. Radical mastectomy is utilized for treatment of breast cancer in a higher percentage of cases in men than in women
D. Unlike breast cancer in women, endocrine manipulation plays no significant role in its management
E. Gynecomastia is usually seen in association with male breast cancer

Sabiston: 563

Comment: Breast cancer in men accounts for approximately 1% of all cases of breast cancer in this country. Its clinical presentation and natural history is quite similar to that in women. A mass in the male breast must be differentiated from gynecomastia (which is clearly the more common cause of breast enlargement in men); gynecomastia does not usually occur in association with male breast cancer. Because of the small amount of breast tissue present in men, pectoralis muscle involvement may

be seen more frequently. As a consequence, most of the time it is necessary to perform the classic Halsted radical mastectomy for its proper removal. Stage for stage the results of treatment are quite similar to those in women; men, however, tend to present in later stages of the disease (due in part to lack of awareness that breast cancer can occur in men), and therefore the overall prognosis for male breast cancer is poorer. As with breast cancer in women, that in men may be affected by endocrine manipulation to a varying degree, and significant response rates in cases of advanced disease have been seen following orchiectomy.

Answer: A, B, C

26. Current American Cancer Society recommendations regarding mammography as a screening tool include:

A. An initial screening mammogram should be obtained sometime between ages 35 and 40
B. Following initial screening, mammograms should be obtained between ages 40 and 50 only if there is clinical suspicion of a lesion present
C. Routine screening mammograms should be performed annually after the age of 50
D. Routine screening mammograms should be performed every 3 years after the age of 50

Schwartz: 530

Comment: The principal determinant of recommendations for routine mammography relate to the risk/benefit ratio of tumor induction by unnecessary radiation versus detecting cancers at an earlier, and therefore more curable, stage. Although unnecessary exposure to irradiation should always be avoided, especially in younger persons, the benefits of appropriately prescribed and performed mammography probably outweigh the possible risks of oncogenesis. Weighing all of these factors, the American Cancer Society has recommended an initial screening mammogram sometime between the ages of 35 and 40. Annual mammography should be obtained after the age of 50. Between the time of the first screening mammogram and age 50, mammography should be performed at a variable interval ranging from every year to every 5 years depending on the patient's risk factors, findings on breast examination, and the results of the initial and subsequent mammograms.

Answer: A, C

27. Estrogen/progesterone receptor–positive tumors are associated with which of the following?

A. Better response to hormone manipulation
B. Better response to chemotherapy
C. Better response to surgical therapy
D. Better overall prognosis
E. More well differentiated tumors

Schwartz: 550

Comment: Although estrogen and progesterone receptor analysis is performed in order to predict the response of breast cancers to endocrine manipulation, tumors that are receptor-positive appear to have a generally improved response to all forms of therapy. Also, receptor-positive tumors tend to be well differentiated more often. The hormone receptor status is sufficiently reliable prognostically that some have considered making receptor status an integral part of the staging of breast cancer. Because of the importance of the results of hormone receptor analysis and the wide availability of this assay, it is considered inappropriate not to save tissue for receptor analysis whenever a lump that may be a carcinoma is removed. The only exception would be a tumor that is so small that all of the specimen is required for histologic examination.

Answer: A, B, C, D, E

28. When considering wide local excision (WLE), axillary dissection, and radiotherapy as the definitive treatment for a breast carcinoma, which factor(s) below would bear favorably on that choice?

A. A T1 tumor
B. Central (subareolar) location within the breast
C. An extremely large breast
D. A very small breast
E. A synchronous second primary cancer within the breast

Sabiston: 563

Comment: The choice of WLE (lumpectomy), axillary dissection, and radiotherapy versus modified radical mastectomy for Stage I and Stage II breast cancer is at times a difficult one and depends in part upon the patient's desires. Certain features of the tumor and/or breast itself, however, may play a role in the appropriateness of the therapeutic choice. Small lesions require a smaller resection and therefore usually offer a better cosmetic result. The size of the breast tumor, however, must be considered in relation to the size of the breast itself. Extremely small breasts do not lend themselves particularly well to a WLE, as a significant portion of the breast must be removed in order to achieve clear margins. The very large breast develops sufficient edema during radiotherapy that mastectomy may be a more favorable choice in such circumstances. Very large primary tumors, regardless of breast size, are a relative contraindication to WLE. A synchronous second primary cancer within the breast is considered a contraindication to the wide local excision option. Central or subareolar lesions have a higher likelihood of multiple primary cancers within the breast. Also, WLE for lesions in this location usually necessitate loss of the nipple-areolar complex. For these reasons, the usual choice for a subareolar carcinoma is mastectomy.

Answer: A

CHAPTER 18

Head and Neck

1. Which of the following statements is/are true regarding disorders of the external ear?

A. The so-called "cauliflower" ear as seen in wrestlers and boxers is caused by repeated soft tissue infection of the pinna
B. Full thickness lacerations of the pinna should be managed with sutures placed on both cutaneous surfaces as well as through the disrupted cartilage
C. Infections of the pinna superficial to the perichondrium should not be surgically drained as this may be the cause of perichondritis
D. The preferred method for removing a foreign body from the ear canal is to retrieve it with a blunt hook passed deep to it.

Sabiston: 1301

Comments: The presence of cartilage and its relationship to the perichondrium is an important anatomic consideration to determining management of disorders of the pinna. Hematomas usually occur between the perichondrium and underlying cartilage and should be drained. Untreated, these can organize and calcify, resulting in a "cauliflower" ear. • In full thickness lacerations of the pinna, sutures placed through cartilage are unlikely to help, may lead to a perichondritis, and should be avoided. Such full thickness lacerations should be repaired by reapproximating both skin surfaces and providing appropriate splinting. • Infections superficial to the perichondrium should not be surgically drained for fear of initiating a perichondritis. Infections deep to the perichondrium should be drained, however, because untreated, they may lead to cartilage necrosis. • Foreign bodies in the ear canal are a problem particularly common in children, and when possible they should be removed by passing a blunt instrument deep to them and teasing them out. The use of forceps for this may result in pushing the foreign body further into the ear canal and injuring the tympanic membrane. In an uncooperative child, general anesthesia may be warranted for removing foreign bodies from the ear canal.

Answer: C, D

2. Which of the following statements is/are true regarding neoplasms of the ear?

A. The majority of carcinomas of the pinna are related to excessive exposure to the sun
B. Involvement of cartilage with squamous carcinoma of the pinna is an indication for radiation therapy
C. Chemodectomas are relatively avascular tumors that, in most cases, can be treated by surgical excision only
D. Acoustic neuromas are self-limiting neoplasms that should be excised via a translabyrinthine approach

Sabiston: 1309

Comments: The majority of carcinomas of the pinna are squamous cell and basal cell in type and usually are associated with excessive exposure to the sun. Early lesions can be treated surgically or with irradiation. When there is invasion of cartilage, however, they are best treated by a full thickness V-shaped wedge excision. • Chemodectomas of the middle ear are paragangliomas that may arise in the tympanic plexus (glomus tympanicus) or near the jugular bulb (glomas jugulare). These tumors are extremely vascular and grossly appear as pulsatile, red masses that blanch on compression. Their growth pattern is that of a progressive, slow expansion with or without associated bone erosion. Smaller lesions may be treated by operation only; large lesions, however, are best treated with irradiation. • Acoustic neuromas account for approximately 7% of all intracranial neoplasms and may arise from either the vestibular or the auditory division of the 8th cranial nerve. Initial presentation may involve neural hearing loss or unsteadiness. Over time, these tumors may grow into the cerebellar pontine angle, with compression of the cerebellum and brain stem and involvement of the 5th and 7th cranial nerves. Small acoustic neuromas can be excised through a translabyrinthine route using microsurgical technique; larger tumors require occipital craniotomy.

Answer: A

3. Which of the following statements is/are true regarding nasal trauma?

A. Undisplaced nasal fractures require wire fixation to prevent subsequent displacement during the healing process
B. Septal hematomas are clinically significant conditions that require surgical intervention
C. Cerebrospinal fluid rhinorrhea requires urgent surgical intervention if one is to prevent meningitis
D. Foreign bodies in the nose are best removed by grasping them and pulling gently

Sabiston: 1311

Comments: Nasal fractures are the most common fractures of the facial skeleton and are nearly always associated with tearing of the overlying mucosa, thereby making them open fractures. Clinical examination revealing displacement of the nasal bones or crepitance on light palpation will usually suggest the diagnosis. Nonetheless, facial x-rays should be obtained to confirm the fracture, as well as to look for fractures of other facial bones. Displaced fractures should be reduced in order to prevent permanent deformity. Undisplaced simple fractures, however, require no specific therapy except for external splinting. Septal hematomas develop between the perichondrium and the underlying cartilage of the nasal septum. These hematomas frequently become infected and also may produce avascular necrosis of the underlying cartilage because of separation from the perichondrium. They should, therefore, be incised and drained upon diagnosis. ● Severe nasal injury may be associated with cerebrospinal fluid rhinorrhea. This may be suspected if clear fluid drains from the nose after injury; it is strongly suggested if there is a high glucose content in the fluid; it can be confirmed by instilling fluorescein dye in the subarachnoid space and detecting it in the nasal discharge, or even by a radioactive isotope scan. Initial management is with observation and the giving of antibiotics to prevent meningitis. If the leak persists beyond 2 to 3 weeks, it should be repaired via a frontal craniotomy or transethmoid approach to the roof of the nasal cavity. ● Foreign bodies in the nasal cavity are quite common in children and, like foreign bodies of the auditory canal, are best managed by placing a blunt hook deep to the foreign body and gently teasing it out. Attempting to grasp these foreign bodies with forceps may simply push them further into the nasal cavity.

Answer: B

4. Which of the following statements is/are true regarding epistaxis?

A. In the majority of cases, epistaxis occurs from the anteroinferior part of the nasal septum
B. Antibiotics are rarely required when nasal packing is employed
C. Hypoxemia is a potential complication of nasal packing
D. Ligation of the internal maxillary artery is ineffective in controlling epistaxis and should be avoided

Sabiston: 1313

Comments: Approximately 90% of cases of epistaxis occur from a plexus of vessels in the anteroinferior part of the nasal septum. In the majority of instances, this is easily controlled with simple digital pressure. When this fails and if the bleeding site can be visualized, it can be cauterized chemically or electrically; occasionally, anterior nasal packing is required. In 10% of cases of epistaxis, the source is posterior, near the junction of the inferior meatus and the nasopharynx. This poses a potentially serious problem, as frequently it occurs in patients with arteriosclerosis and hypertension and may be difficult to control; it has an associated mortality of 4 to 5%. The initial attempt at controlling the bleeding should be either with balloon obstruction of the choana or by a combined anterior/posterior gauze packing. When such packing is utilized, antibiotics should be given prophylactically in an effort to prevent sinusitis and otitis media. Air exchange is frequently hindered by the packing and, as many of these patients have associated systemic and cardiopulmonary disease, supplemental oxygen should be administered. Posterior epistaxis that cannot be controlled with packing may be treated by transmaxillary ligation of the internal maxillary artery.

Answer: A, C

5. Which of the following statements is/are true regarding malignant tumors of the nasal cavity and paranasal sinuses?

A. The majority are of minor salivary gland origin
B. Presenting symptoms are uncommon; the majority are diagnosed incidentally during routine physical examination
C. Most tumors of the paranasal sinuses occur in the maxillary antrum
D. Even in an advanced stage, tumors of the maxillary sinus rarely are associated with abnormal physical findings; conventional or computed tomographic x-rays are required to make the diagnosis

Schwartz: 582

Comments: Cancers of the nasal cavity and paranasal sinuses account for approximately 1% of all malignancies, and there is an approximate 3:1 male:female predominance. Roughly 50% of these tumors are epidermoid carcinomas, 20% of minor salivary gland origin, and 10% lymphomas. The remaining 20% comprise sarcomas, melanomas, and other rare tumors. In at least half of cases, patients present with facial pain, nasal obstruction, or persistent nasal discharge. The majority of paranasal sinus cancers are found in the maxillary antrum where, in their advanced state, they may present with swelling or ulceration of the palate, superior buccal gingival sulcus, or cheek, or with ocular signs which may include elevation of the globe, proptosis, or impairment of extraocular movements. The ethmoid sinuses are the next most frequently involved; cancers of the frontal sinus and sphenoid sinus are rare.

Answer: C

6. Which of the following statements is/are true regarding the management of cancer of the maxillary sinus?

A. In contradistinction to lymphomas elsewhere in the body, those of the maxillary sinus are best treated with surgical excision
B. Cancers of the frontal and sphenoidal sinuses are best treated with irradiation

C. Surgery with or without irradiation is the treatment of choice for maxillary carcinoma
D. The surgical management of epidermoid carcinoma of the maxilla should include radical neck dissection if the tumor is greater than 3 cm

Sabiston: 1316
Schwartz: 582

Comments: Most lymphomas (including those of the maxillary antrum) are very radiosensitive and rarely sufficiently localized for operative excision only to be appropriate. Radiation therapy is the treatment of choice for maxillary lymphomas when they are localized; chemotherapy may be indicated in many instances. Epidermoid carcinomas and minor salivary gland tumors of the maxillary antrum and ethmoid sinuses are best treated by surgical excision; the addition of radiation therapy is reserved for particularly large or aggressive tumors. Tumors eroding the floor of the orbit may require orbital exenteration as part of the operative procedure. If the globe is not involved, it should be preserved; a proper maxillectomy can still be performed with excellent cosmetic results through the use of dental maxillary prostheses. Tumors of the frontal and sphenoid sinuses are best managed by radiotherapy because of the inability to achieve an adequate surgical margin without a high probability of injury to the central nervous system. Radical neck dissection in cases of maxillary carcinoma is generally performed only when clinically positive cervical lymph nodes are present.

Answer: B, C

7. Which of the following statements is/are true regarding pharyngeal foreign bodies?

A. Round or oval foreign bodies tend to lodge in the conical pyriform sinus
B. Long, sharp objects tend to lodge in the tonsillar area
C. Because of the protection afforded by the soft palate, foreign bodies reach the nasopharynx only via the nasal cavity
D. Foreign bodies of the pharynx should be retrieved under general anesthesia

Sabiston: 1316

Comments: Foreign bodies of the pharynx are most likely found in one of four locations: the palatine tonsils, pyriform sinuses, valleculae, or nasopharynx. Small round or oval objects (e.g., peanuts) are usually found in the valleculae since in other locations they would probably be easily swallowed. Long, sharp objects such as fish bones are likely to lodge in the palatine tonsils and lingual tonsil. Smaller sharp or irregularly shaped objects are frequently found in the pyriform sinuses of the hypopharynx. Foreign bodies in these locations can usually be removed by direct laryngoscopy with the patient under local anesthesia or light sedation. Occasionally, foreign bodies of any type may be coughed into the nasopharynx. Entrapment of foreign bodies in this location usually requires induction of general anesthesia for their removal.

Answer: B

8. Which of the following statements is/are true regarding nasopharyngeal angiofibromas?

A. They are most often found in adolescent males
B. Epistaxis and nasal obstruction are the most common presenting symptoms
C. Although these lesions are extremely vascular, they can usually be excised with minimal blood loss
D. Surgical excision is the only reasonable therapeutic option

Sabiston: 1317

Comments: Juvenile nasopharyngeal angiofibromas are vascular neoplasms that most often occur in pubescent males. They usually present with nasal obstruction or bleeding. Despite their benign histology, they can grow to very large size with accompanying bone destruction and invasion into the cranial cavity. They are best assessed radiographically with CT scan and angiography. Most of these lesions are treated surgically, but the associated blood loss may be considerable. This may be reduced by preoperative embolization of the internal maxillary artery. Other forms of treatment, including radiation therapy, cryotherapy, and administration of estrogens, have also yielded some favorable results. Radiotherapy is particularly indicated in large lesions invading the cranium.

Answer: A, B

9. Which of the following statements is/are true regarding neoplasms of the nasopharynx?

A. Lymphoma is the most common nasopharyngeal neoplasm among children
B. A viral etiology for squamous carcinoma of the nasopharynx has been suggested
C. There is an unusually high incidence of nasopharyngeal carcinoma among the Chinese
D. Surgery is the treatment of choice for small, well-localized nasopharyngeal carcinomas

Sabiston: 1317

Comments: Malignant neoplasms of the nasopharynx include squamous carcinoma, adenocarcinomas (usually of minor salivary gland origin) sarcoma, lymphoma, and melanoma. Among children, the lymphomas are the most common malignancy in the nasopharynx. In adults, squamous carcinoma and its variant of lymphoepithelioma are the most common types. There is an unusually high incidence of nasopharyngeal carcinoma among the Chinese and it appears at an earlier age than other squamous carcinomas of the upper aerodigestive tract. Elevated titers of anti–Epstein-Barr virus antibodies are seen in almost half of patients with nasopharyngeal carcinoma, suggesting a possible viral etiology. Clinical presentation may include bleeding or nasopharyngeal obstruction as well as the sequelae of invasion of the base of the skull, which would include cranial nerve involvement. Carcinoma of the nasopharynx is best treated with radiation. Difficult access and the inability to obtain any reasonable surgical margin due to the proximity of the nasopharynx to the base of the skull and vertebral column make surgical excision of even the earliest lesions inappropriate. The overall 5-year survival for carcinoma of the nasopharynx is approximately 35%.

Answer: A, B, C

10. Which of the following statements is/are true regarding oropharyngeal abscesses?

A. Peritonsillar, parapharyngeal, and retropharyngeal abscesses occur with approximately equal frequency among children under 10 years of age
B. Aspiration of pus into the lungs is a distinct hazard of drainage of oropharyngeal abscesses
C. Drainage of peritonsillar, parapharyngeal, and retropharyngeal abscesses is best accomplished through the pharyngeal wall
D. As with abscesses in other locations in the body, small drains should be placed into transpharyngeally drained abscesses to promote ongoing evacuation of the abscess cavity

Sabiston: 1318

Comments: Oropharyngeal abscesses have distinct characteristics regarding their epidemiology and management, depending on their location. **Peritonsillar** abscesses are rare in children under the age of 10, even though they represent complications of acute tonsillitis. The patient may appear quite ill and present with trismus and severe odynophagia. An initial trial of antibiotics may be warranted; if there is no response within 24 hours, drainage through the tonsillar bed should be performed. **Retropharyngeal** abscesses tend to occur in infants and younger children and are rare after the age of 10 years. These infections are due to the lymphadenitis associated with pharyngitis. The infant may present in opisthotonus, and the clinical picture is often confused with that of meningitis. Physical examination reveals a boggy, fluctuant texture to the retropharyngeal tissues and inability to palpate the normally palpable vertebral bodies. Antibiotics and surgical drainage through the posterior pharyngeal wall are the treatment of choice. In these two entities, aspiration of pus into the tracheobronchial tree is a distinct hazard and can be prevented by appropriate positioning of the patient prior to drainage. Drains are not required, as these abscess cavities tend to empty themselves during each swallowing motion. **Parapharyngeal** abscesses occur in all age groups and may be secondary to pharyngitis or tonsillitis. Since these abscesses occur more laterally, drainage through the oropharynx is hazardous, because of the proximity to the internal carotid artery and jugular vein. In contradistinction to peritonsillar and retropharyngeal abscesses, parapharyngeal abscesses should be drained through the lateral neck and a drain left in place to permit ongoing evacuation of the cavity.

Answer: B

11. Which of the following statements is/are true regarding carcinoma of the tonsil?

A. Because of the irritation from the passage of food, tonsillar carcinomas tend to present very early
B. Cervical lymph node metastases are rare because of the ability of the abundant peritonsillar lymphatic network to confine regional spread of the tumor

C. The heavy use of tobacco and alcohol has been associated with tonsillar carcinoma
D. Appropriate therapeutic options include surgery and radiation, alone or in combination

Sabiston: 1319

Comments: The most common malignant tumor of the tonsil is squamous carcinoma and, like most squamous carcinomas of the upper aerodigestive tract, there is a distinct male predominance and an association with excessive use of tobacco and alcohol. Tonsillar carcinoma usually remains asymptomatic until it has reached considerable size. This fact, as well as the abundant lymphatics of the tonsillar fossa, are in part responsible for the relatively high frequency of cervical lymph node metastases. Depending on the size of the primary lesion and the presence or absence of cervical lymph node metastases, initial curative therapy may involve surgical excision, or radiation alone or in combination.

Answer: C, D

12. Which of the following statements is/are true regarding laryngeal trauma?

A. Trauma is the most common cause of laryngeal stenosis
B. Iatrogenic laryngeal stenosis is most often in the supraglottic location due to traumatic intubation attempts
C. Since the rigid component of the larynx is cartilage and not bone, fractures of the larynx do not occur
D. Laryngeal trauma with associated difficulty in breathing should be initially managed with urgent tracheostomy rather than endotracheal intubation

Sabiston: 1321

Comments: Because of appropriate vaccination programs and improved antibiotic therapies, trauma has replaced infectious diseases as the most common cause of laryngeal stenosis. A significant proportion of laryngeal injuries are iatrogenic, relating primarily to subglottic injury caused by prolonged intubation with a cuffed endotracheal tube. However, the incidence of complications has been reduced significantly by the use of endotracheal tubes with soft, low-pressure cuffs. These post-traumatic stenoses may be managed by dilatation, laser therapy, or local excision with reconstruction of the stenotic segment. ● Direct blows to the neck may result in fracture of the laryngeal cartilage, or tracheolaryngeal disruption. When such an injury is suspected and the patient is having difficulty breathing, urgent tracheostomy should be performed, as attempts at endotracheal intubation may be unsuccessful and further compound the injury. Once control of the airway is established and other associated injuries have been appropriately managed, assessment of the laryngeal injury should be performed with direct laryngoscopy and tracheoscopy. When the patient's condition is stabilized, surgical reduction and repair of the fracture is carried out.

Answer: A, D

13. Which of the following statements is/are true regarding foreign bodies of the larynx and tracheobronchial tree?

A. The ability to speak is an important differentiating sign in diagnosing the cause of cyanosis and respiratory difficulty occurring while eating
B. Complete occlusion of the larynx with a food bolus should be managed immediately by tracheostomy
C. Radiographs may be of benefit in localizing the site of bronchial obstruction by radiolucent foreign bodies
D. The cessation of coughing 30 minutes after inhalation of a foreign body indicates that the foreign body has been coughed out
E. Infectious complications are the principal long-term sequelae of retained tracheobronchial foreign bodies

Sabiston: 1322

Comments: The so-called "café coronary," in which a patient becomes dyspneic and cyanotic while eating, may be due to myocardial infarction, arrhythmia, or airway obstruction from a food bolus. The inability to exchange air and to speak suggests aspiration as the cause of the difficulty. If the choking person is able to exchange adequate amounts of air, he should be left alone, but observed very closely. If there is complete obstruction to air exchange, initial treatment should include an attempt to dislodge the foreign body with the Heimlich (abdominal thrust) maneuver. Emergency tracheostomy is extremely hazardous and should be employed only as a last-resort, life-saving measure. ● Inhalation of foreign bodies into the tracheobronchial tree, in which air exchange can occur, usually produces severe coughing that may last for up to 30 minutes. By this time, however, the foreign body has settled into one specific location, and because of adaptation the coughing may stop. This may be erroneously interpreted as a sign that the foreign body has been expelled. In most cases of retained foreign body, this relatively asymptomatic latent period is followed by a cough productive of purulent sputum. Infectious complications including bronchiectasis, recurrent pneumonitis, lung abscess, and empyema can follow. ● Even when radiolucent objects have been inhaled, standard chest radiographs may assist in localizing the site of bronchiolar obstruction, as in cases in which a ball-valve type of expiratory obstruction produces a localized pulmonary emphysema. The proper initial management of aspirated foreign bodies is retrieval via tracheobronchial endoscopy.

Answer: A, C, E

14. Which of the following statements is/are true regarding foreign bodies of the esophagus?

A. The majority of esophageal foreign bodies are found just below the cricopharyngeus muscle
B. The risk of esophageal perforation increases the longer the foreign body remains in the esophagus
C. Dysphagia without pain is the clinical hallmark of the presence of a foreign body in the esophagus
D. Retrieval of esophageal foreign bodies through a rigid esophagoscope with the patient under general anesthesia is the treatment of choice

Sabiston: 1323

Comments: Approximately 95% of all esophageal foreign bodies are found immediately below the cricopharyngeus muscle. Large foreign bodies in this area may produce partial airway obstruction due to extrinsic pressure on the membranous trachea. In most instances, the clinical presentation is that of dysphagia and associated suprasternal pain. Perforation may occur immediately or may be delayed; however, the risk of perforation increases with the length of time that the foreign body remains in the esophagus. Perforation is diagnosed by the presence of soft tissue crepitance or the radiographic demonstration of air in soft tissues. Documentation of the presence of a foreign body may be achieved by standard and contrast radiography. Appropriate treatment involves endoscopic retrieval of the foreign body with the patient under general anesthesia.

Answer: A, B, D

15. Which of the following may be appropriate indications for tracheotomy?

A. Inability to handle upper respiratory secretions
B. Inability to handle lower respiratory secretions
C. Respiratory obstruction
D. Endotracheal intubation exceeding 5 days

Sabiston: 1324

Comments: The principal indications for tracheotomy include respiratory obstruction that cannot be properly managed with endotracheal intubation and the inability to evacuate secretions from the upper or lower respiratory tree. Prolonged endotracheal intubation may lead to the complication of subglottic stenosis and require tracheotomy; however, the currently available low-pressure soft cuffs allow safe endotracheal intubation for up to several weeks. Although tracheobronchial toilette is more easily obtained through a tracheotomy tube, the presence of a tracheotomy tube is not without complications. These include the inability of the patient to cough (because of bypass of the glottic closure mechanism), the bypassing of the normal warming and humidification of inspired air in the upper respiratory tract, and the direct exposure of the lower respiratory tract to environmental pathogens.

Answer: A, B, C

16. Match the labeled parts of the drawing of the oropharynx with the anatomic structures listed below.

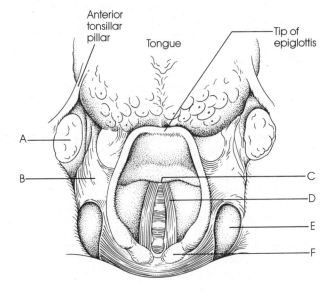

Anterior tonsillar pillar

Tongue

Tip of epiglottis

A. Arytenoid process
B. Vocal cord
C. Pharyngoepiglottic fold
D. Anterior commissure
E. Palatine tonsil
F. Pyriform sinus

Sabiston: 1319

Comments: Anatomically, the larynx may be divided into three regions: the subglottic, glottic, and supraglottic larynx. The **glottic** larynx consists of the true vocal cords only. The **supraglottic larynx** consists of those structures superior to the true vocal cords and includes the laryngeal ventricle, false vocal cords, arytenoids, aryepiglottic folds, and epiglottis. The **subglottic larynx** consists of that mucosa immediately beneath the true vocal cords. The **hypopharynx** is made up of the pyriform sinuses (including both medial and lateral walls), the postcricoid mucosa, and the posterior pharyngeal wall. Knowledge of these anatomic sites is required for proper staging of tumors in this area as well as for the planning of appropriate therapy.

Answer: A–e; B–c; C–d; D–b; E–f; F–a

17. Match the following clinical characteristics of laryngeal/pharyngeal carcinoma with their appropriate anatomic site of origin:

Clinical Characteristics	Anatomic Site
A. Symptoms occur early	a. Supraglottic larynx
B. Regional node metastases common	b. Glottic larynx
C. May be managed with voice preservation	c. Hypopharynx
D. Radiotherapy may be treatment of choice even in symptomatic patients	

Sabiston: 1325

Comments: Glottic carcinomas, in contradistinction to other laryngeal and hypopharyngeal tumors, develop symptoms early because of the relatively small degree of anatomic change required to produce hoarseness. Because of this, glottic carcinomas tend to be diagnosed in their early stages. Additionally, true glottic cancers have limited access to lymphatics, so the likelihood of regional nodal metastases is very low. Although cordectomy may be performed for early glottic lesions, radiotherapy is clearly the treatment of choice because of the lower treatment risk and the better quality of the preserved voice. ● Carcinomas of the supraglottic larynx and hypopharynx usually grow to a considerable size before producing symptoms (hoarseness, dysphagia, dyspnea). Because of this larger tumor size and the greater access to the abundant lymphatics of the supraglottic and hypopharyngeal areas, regional lymph node metastases are relatively common (30–50%) at the time of initial clinical presentation. Symptomatic tumors in these areas can rarely be successfully managed, for these same reasons, by radiotherapy alone. Surgery, with or without radiation therapy, is the preferred treatment. ● Direct involvement of the glottic larynx or paralysis of the vocal cords by supraglottic or hypopharyngeal lesions usually requires total laryngectomy. In selected patients with the glottis free of

tumor and fully mobile, resection can be carried out with preservation of voice function.

Answer: A–b; B–a, c; C–a, b, c; D–b

18. Regarding cleft lip and palate, match the clinical characteristics with the appropriate anatomic defect:

Clinical Characteristics	Anatomic Defect
A. Involves lip and/or alveolus	a. Cleft of primary palate
B. Involves hard and soft palate	b. Cleft of secondary palate
C. Should be closed within the first 3 months of life	
D. Should be closed between 1 and 2 years of age	

Sabiston: 1331

Comments: Vertical paramedian clefts of the lip and palate are considered in two principal categories: clefts of the primary palate (the lip and alveolar ridge) and clefts of the secondary palate (hard and soft palate). These may occur alone or in association with each other, but the most common anomaly is a combined cleft lip and palate. The timing of surgical correction varies with the specific type of defect. Clefts of the lip are best repaired during the first 3 months of life, which enables the infant to achieve more normal patterns of feeding. Repair of a cleft palate is usually delayed until sometime between 1 and 2 years of age, to facilitate the technical closure. Delay beyond age 2, when the child is beginning to develop skills of speech, may result in permanent speech disability. These closures are usually performed utilizing local rotation flaps.

Answer: A–a; B–b; C–a; D–b

19. Which of the following statements accurately pertain(s) to the management of full thickness lacerations of the lip?

A. Layered closure is preferred
B. A frequent cause of wound breakdown is ischemic necrosis secondary to the relatively poor labial blood supply
C. The extent of soft tissue loss in labial lacerations is frequently underestimated
D. Proper apposition of the vermilion border is the principal determinant of cosmetic outcome

Sabiston: 1334

Comments: The proper management of full thickness labial lacerations involves débridement of devitalized tissue and a layered closure of the mucosa, labial musculature, and skin using fine absorbable and nonabsorbable with particular attention paid to the accurate apposition of the vermilion border. Because of the circular and radial orientation of the labial musculature, labial lacerations frequently open widely, leading to the erroneous assumption that there has been significant soft tissue loss. The blood supply of the perioral area is excellent and is rarely of concern in the repair of these wounds. Pathogenic oral anaerobes have occasionally been implicated as the cause of wound breakdown and local infection, and for this reason some clinicians recommend prophylactic penicillin therapy.

Answer: A, D

20. Match the following benign conditions of the lips with their appropriate clinical characteristics:

Characteristics	Condition
A. Pyogenic granuloma	a. May be premalignant
B. Epidermal inclusion cyst	b. No surface epithelial component
C. Keratoacanthoma	c. Large central crater
D. Keratoses	d. Surgical excision frequently indicated
E. Leukoplakia	

Sabiston: 1338

Comments: There are numerous benign conditions of the lips, the diagnosis of which usually is made on clinical grounds alone. **Pyogenic granulomas** are superficial polypoid masses devoid of surface epithelium. They bleed easily with minimal trauma. Infection has been implicated but not proven as the etiology of these lesions. **Epidermal inclusion cysts** result from the occlusion of the pores of sebaceous glands and appear as subcutaneous and intradermal nodules with a small central punctum. **Keratoacanthomas** are benign tumors that arise from hair follicles. The rapid growth and histologic appearance of keratoacanthoma are responsible for the occasional misdiagnosis of this lesion as a squamous carcinoma. Untreated, the surface of the lesion usually breaks down, revealing a central keratin plug which later detaches, leaving a crater-shaped defect. **Keratoses** are scaly and slightly raised lesions which may occur at the vermilion subcutaneous junction and are often associated with a history of excessive exposure to the sun. Untreated, they may develop into squamous cell carcinoma. **Leukoplakia** is a descriptive term applied to white plaque-like lesions that may occur anywhere in the oral cavity or lip; it is frequently associated with previous use of tobacco. Leukoplakia may remain dormant for many years, may spontaneously involute, or may progress to squamous cell carcinoma. In all of these lesions, surgical excision can usually be performed with excellent cosmetic results. In the case of keratoses and leukoplakia, this may involve a "lip shave" procedure with advancement of buccal mucosa for reconstruction.

Answer: A–b, d; B–d; C–c, d; D–a, d; E–a, d

21. Carcinoma of the lip is accurately described by which of the following statements?

A. Carcinomas are approximately equally distributed between the upper and lower lip
B. Carcinoma of the lip has a strong relationship to prior excessive exposure to the sun
C. Over 90% are epidermoid carcinomas
D. Regional nodal metastases usually first appear in the submental and submandibular triangles

Sabiston: 1338

Comments: The vast majority (as many as 99%) of all lip cancers are epidermoid carcinoma. These are found more frequently in patients with a fair complexion and in those who have a history of excessive exposure to the sun. Excessive use of tobacco (particularly pipes) and heavy consumption of alcohol are also considered to be risk factors. Sun exposure as a risk factor may explain why these carcinomas are almost always found on the lower lip. Regional node metastases usually occur late in the course of the disease and tend to be found initially in the submental and submandibular triangles and later along the internal jugular chain. Distant metastases are rare at initial presentation.

Answer: B, C, D

22. Which of the following statements is/are true regarding the principles of management of carcinoma of the lip?

A. The majority of these tumors are adequately treated by V-excision and primary closure
B. When simple V-excision is not possible, radiotherapy is the treatment of choice
C. Prophylactic cervical lymph node dissection should not be employed in the primary management of carcinoma of the lip
D. Mandibular involvement is usually by way of blood-borne metastases

Sabiston: 1339

Comments: Most carcinomas of the lip can be treated with a local V-excision with primary closure. Larger lesions or lesions near the commissure may require more complicated reconstruction, including rotation flaps from the upper lip. In general, operation is preferred over radiotherapy because of the long-term unfavorable sequelae of radiotherapy to this area. Extremely large lesions may properly be treated with radiotherapy alone or in combination with surgery. Prophylactic neck dissection is usually not required in early carcinomas of the lip. However, certain patients with clinically negative neck examinations and a high likelihood of subclinical disease may still benefit from prophylactic neck dissection. The factors that may predict this likelihood include the size of the lesion, an endophytic vs. exophytic morphology, the degree of cellular differentiation, and a history of recurrence of a previously treated tumor. Mandibular involvement from labial carcinomas is usually due to direct extension of the primary tumor.

Answer: A

23. Which of the following anatomic sites are considered to be part of the oral cavity?

A. The floor of the mouth
B. Palatine tonsil
C. Posterior upper gingiva
D. Soft palate
E. Posterior third of tongue

Sabiston: 1339

Comments: When considering neoplasms of the upper aerodigestive tract, it is important to be specific in terms of the site of origin of the tumor, as this may have a bearing on management and prognosis. The **oral cavity** is bounded **anteriorly** by the lips and includes the vestibule of the mouth (including buccal mucosa and buccal gingival sulcus), the buccal, alveolar, and lingual aspects of the gingiva, the floor of the mouth, the anterior two thirds of the tongue, and the hard palate. **Posteriorly** the oral cavity is bounded by the junction between the hard and soft palate and the junction between the anterior two thirds and posterior third of the tongue. The **lateral** borders are described by the anterior tonsillar pillars laterally. The **oropharynx**, which is not considered part of the oral cavity, is bounded by the palatine tonsils, soft palate, posterior third of the tongue, and posterior pharyngeal wall. The more posterior oropharyngeal tumors have a higher likelihood of regional lymph node metastases than those in a more anterior location. Within the oral cavity, there are also general differences in the likelihood of regional nodal disease (e.g., tumors of the gingiva are less likely to have nodal metastases than are tumors of the floor of the mouth).

Answer: A, C

24. Which of the following statements is/are true regarding carcinoma of the oral cavity?

A. Most cancers of the oral cavity are epidermoid carcinomas
B. Male predominance and a history of excessive use of tobacco and of alcohol characterize the epidemiology of most oral cavity carcinomas
C. Minor salivary gland carcinomas are the second most common type of oral cavity cancer
D. Radiotherapy should be avoided in the management of oral cavity cancers because of the debilitating side effects of xerostomia

Sabiston: 1344

Comments: As with all cancers of the upper aerodigestive tract, epidermoid carcinoma accounts for the vast majority of cancers in the oral cavity. Most patients have a history of significant use of tobacco and alcohol. Men have a greater incidence of cancer of the aerodigestive tract, but that difference is narrowing, apparently as a result of increased smoking by women. The second most common cancer in the oral cavity is of minor salivary gland origin. These tumors should be considered in the differential diagnosis of any submucosal lesion in the upper aerodigestive tract. Sarcomas, lymphomas, and melanoma of the oral cavity are extremely rare. There is not a general agreement on the proper therapy for cancers in the oral cavity. Early lesions may be treated by surgical excision or irradiation alone. In order to arrive at a treatment plan, one must weigh the relative risks of anesthesia, and cosmetic and functional deficits caused by surgery, against the problems of xerostomia, dental disease, and poor healing caused by irradiation. Advanced lesions of the oral cavity are frequently treated by surgery and radiotherapy in combination. The use of chemotherapy, alone and in combination with radiotherapy and surgery, is currently under investigation and has yielded excellent short-term results in selected patients.

Answer: A, B, C

25. Cancers of the oropharynx differ from those of the oral cavity in which of the following ways?

A. Oropharyngeal cancers have an equal distribution between males and females
B. Minor salivary gland tumors are the most common malignancies of the oropharynx
C. Lymphoma is more common in the oropharynx
D. The overall prognosis of cancer in the oropharynx is worse

Sabiston: 1345

Comments: Like carcinoma of the oral cavity and other sites in the upper aerodigestive tract, there is a male predominance and the majority of cancers are epidermoid carcinomas. In contrast to the oral cavity, however, there is a much higher incidence of lymphoma (occurring primarily in the lymphoid-rich Waldeyer's ring). Overall, the prognosis of oropharyngeal carcinoma is worse than that found in the oral cavity. This is due to a number of factors, including the greater likelihood of lymph node metastases being present at the time of clinical presentation as well as the larger size that the primary tumor usually achieves before it produces symptoms or is detected clinically.

Answer: C, D

26. Which of the following statements is/are true regarding reconstruction techniques in head and neck cancer surgery?

A. The most significant advance in the rehabilitation of the head and neck cancer patient in recent years has been the development of the technique of esophageal speech following laryngectomy
B. The use of myocutaneous flaps has significantly reduced the total time required for reconstruction of defects in head and neck cancer surgery
C. Free microvascular composite grafts have contributed significantly to the reconstruction of surgical defects particularly those involving mandibulectomy
D. The increasingly complicated extirpative procedures utilized in the last 10 years in head and neck surgery have resulted in a corresponding increase in the need for staged reconstruction techniques

Sabiston: 1346
Schwartz: 596

Comments: Aside from the increased safety of anesthesia and the development of larynx conservation techniques, there have been few major advances in the extirpative portion of the sugical management of head and neck cancer. In contrast, the increasing use in recent years of myocutaneous flaps and the development of free microvascular composite grafts have significantly simplified the reconstruction of large defects. As a consequence, it has facilitated the rehabilitation of these patients. Prior to this development, reconstruction frequently involved the delay and staged transfer of pedicle flaps. It is now common even in complicated cases for the entire reconstruction to be performed at the same time as the extirpative surgery. In addition to reducing the cost and time of the reconstruction, this has also permitted the patient to begin adjuvant radiation therapy or chemotherapy at an earlier time, if indicated. An important additional benefit has been the opportunity for these patients to avoid the prolonged disfigurement and social ostracization they might otherwise suffer. Although much has yet to be learned regarding the use of free composite grafts with microvascular anastomoses, their value in the reconstruction of the patient with head and neck cancer (particularly in cases involving mandibulectomy) appears to be well established.

Answer: B, C

28. Match the following benign conditions involving the tongue with their appropriate description.

Condition	Characteristics
A. Lingual thyroid	a. Failure of fusion
B. Thyroglossal duct cyst	b. Arise from perineural fibroblasts
C. Median rhomboid glossitis	c. Resection may necessitate lifelong medication
D. Granular cell myoblastoma	d. Surgical treatment involves resection of bone

Sabiston: 1346
Schwartz: 571

Comments: The four entities above are among many benign conditions that may involve the tongue. **Lingual thyroid** results from failure of descent of the thyroid gland into the lower anterior neck. This results in the clinical appearance of a reddish-brown mass emanating from the base of the tongue. Resection of a lingual thyroid may be necessitated because of pharyngeal obstruction from the mass. One must be alert, however, to the possibility that this may represent the patient's only thyroid tissue. In such cases, resection would render the patient hypothyroid and necessitate thyroid replacement therapy. **Thyroglossal duct cysts** also represent an anomaly of thyroid embryology in which there is a failure of obliteration of the midline pharyngeal diverticulum during thyroid descent. Clinical presentation is that of a midline cystic mass usually appearing in childhood or adolescence. Proper surgical treatment involves excision of the entire tract, including the midportion of the hyoid bone. **Median rhomboid glossitis** (grooved tongue) results from the failure of fusion of the lateral halves of the tongue. It is a clinically innocuous anomaly and requires no treatment. **Granular cell myoblastoma** is a benign tumor (presumed to arise from perineural fibroblasts) that frequently occurs in the tongue. It may appear clinically similar to carcinoma of the tongue but has no malignant potential and is properly treated by local surgical excision.

Answer: A–c; B–d; C–a; D–b

29. Which of the following statements is/are true regarding carcinoma of the tongue?

A. Most tongue carcinomas occur on the large dorsal surface
B. Lymph node metastases are present in approximately half of all patients presenting with carcinoma of the tongue
C. When tongue carcinomas are sufficiently large to involve the mandible, surgery is no longer an appropriate option and the patient should be treated with radiation therapy

D. Iron deficiency anemia may be associated with carcinoma of the tongue

Sabiston: 1347
Schwartz: 571

Comments: The epidemiology of carcinoma of the oral tongue is similar to that of other oral cavity tumors (male predominance, epidermoid carcinoma prevalence, history of tobacco and alcohol abuse, etc.). There is also an increased incidence of tongue carcinomas in patients with Plummer-Vinson syndrome (cervical dysphasia, iron deficiency anemia, atrophic oral mucosa, brittle spoon-shaped fingernails). Despite its larger surface area, the dorsum of the tongue is rarely the site of epidermoid carcinoma; the majority of these tumors occur on the lateral and ventral surfaces. Since 50% of patients with carcinoma of the tongue present with cervical lymph node metastases, combined treatment of the primary lesion with the ipsilateral cervical lymph nodes should be considered in most cases. Carcinoma of the tongue may frequently present with close approximation to or invasion of the inner table of the mandible. In such circumstances, resection must involve a partial mandibulectomy. Radiation therapy alone is unlikely to be successful in such large lesions, and the majority of them are currently treated with surgery in combination with radiation therapy and/or chemotherapy.

Answer: B, D

30. Which of the following statements is/are true regarding mandibular trauma?

A. Most fractures of the mandible are clinically undetectable and require x-ray for diagnosis
B. Most mandibular fractures are effectively treated with simple intermaxillary wiring or elastic band fixation
C. Teeth lying within the fracture line of the mandible should be removed in order to prevent root abscesses
D. For dislocations of the temporomandibular joint, open reduction and repair of the anterior capsule with the patient under general anesthesia is usually required

Sabiston: 1350
Schwartz: 2140

Comments: The diagnosis of mandibular fracture is usually easily made on careful clinical examination, common signs to look for being point tenderness, malocclusion, instability on bimanual manipulation, and numbness of the lower lip due to inferior alveolar nerve damage. Radiographs should be obtained to confirm the clinical impression as well as to search for associated occult facial bone fractures. Most mandibular fractures are adequately treated by intermaxillary wiring or with archbars and elastic band stabilization. Open reduction of mandibular fractures reduces the period of time required for intermaxillary fixation and is gaining popularity. It was formerly recommended that teeth lying within the fracture line be removed; however, more recently, it has been recognized that many of these teeth are salvageable if the fracture is managed conservatively. Temporomandibular joint dislocations usually occur when the head of the mandibular condyle moves forward through a tear in the anterior joint capsule. This usually can be managed with injection of anesthetic into the joint capsule and downward traction on the posterior molar teeth. Cases of recurrent dislocation may require operative intervention.

Answer: B

31. Match the following type of maxillary fractures with their appropriate anatomic descriptions.

Type of Fracture	Anatomic Description
A. Le Fort I	a. Transverse maxillary fracture
B. Le Fort II	b. Craniofacial dysjunction
C. Le Fort III	c. Pyramidal fractures

Sabiston: 1353
Schwartz: 2140

Comments: In 1900, René Le Fort classified mid-face fractures as described above. In Le Fort I fractures (transverse), fracture segments include the upper teeth, palate, lower portions of the pterygoid processes, and portion of the wall of the maxillary sinus. Le Fort II fractures (pyramidal) also contain the nasal bones and frontal processes of the maxilla. Clinically, the malar eminences are usually not displaced, but there may be significant widening of the inner canthi of the eyes and bridge of the nose. Le Fort III fractures (craniofacial dysjunction) involve separation of the maxillae, nasal bones, and zygomas from their usual cranial attachments. Treatment of these fractures is best carried out with direct operative exposure and wiring of the fracture segments.

Answer: A–a; B–c; C–b

32. Match the following tumors of the jaws with their appropriate characteristics.

Tumor	Characteristics
A. Radicular cyst	a. Usually requires multimodality therapy
B. Ameloblastoma	b. Local excision or curettage is appropriate
C. Osteogenic sarcoma	c. Slow-growing malignancy with "soap-bubble" radiographic appearance
D. Carcinoma	d. May be metastastic from other primary site

Sabiston: 1356
Schwartz: 582

Comments: Although the mandible and maxilla are most often involved in head and neck cancer by virtue of direct extension of contiguous epithelial tumors, a number of benign and malignant primary tumors of the jaws exist. **Radicular cysts** (dental cysts or root cysts) usually are easily diagnosed by their appropriate lucent appearance on x-ray. Local resection or enucleation with curettage of the cyst cavity is usually all that is required for treatment. **Ameloblastoma** (adamantinoma) is a slow-growing, low-grade malignancy which has the capability to metastasize to distant sites. The characteristic x-ray appearance is that of "soap bubbles." Wide excision with appropriate bone reconstruction is the treatment of choice. **Osteogenic sarcoma** may occur in either the man-

dible or maxilla and usually carries a grave prognosis. Wide surgical excision alone may be curative, but recent studies have shown improved results with multimodality therapy including preoperative chemotherapy and possible adjuvant radiotherapy. **Carcinoma** from another site (most often breast, thyroid or prostate) can metastasize to the mandible and present as a primary tumor.

Answer: A–b; B–c; C–a; D–d

33. Which of the following statements is/are true regarding acute suppurative parotitis?

A. This tends to occur in the elderly or debilitated patient
B. Dehydration is a major contributing factor
C. Immediate surgical drainage is mandatory
D. *Staphylococcus aureus* is the organism most likely to be found

Sabiston: 1358
Schwartz: 458

Comments: Acute suppurative parotitis is a severe, life-threatening infection most often seen in dehydrated elderly or debilitated patients. Its pathogenesis is thought to relate to stasis within the salivary ducts due to increased viscosity. *Staphylococcus aureus* is the organism most often found in this severe infection. Initial treatment with appropriate intravenous hydration and antibiotics active against *Staphylococcus* may be successful. If improvement is not seen within 12 hours of initiating this treatment, surgical drainage is warranted.

Answer: A, B, D

34. Which of the following statements is/are true regarding non-neoplastic parotid disease?

A. Lacerated Stensen's duct may be successfully reapproximated over a small catheter stent
B. Recurrent acute sialadenitis is thought to be an ascending infection from the oral cavity
C. Most calculi within the parotid duct are found near the duct orifice
D. Parotidectomy, with its inherent risk of facial nerve injury, is considered too morbid a procedure for use in the treatment of non-neoplastic conditions of the parotid gland

Sabiston: 1357

Comments: Transection of Stensen's duct should be repaired, if possible, with direct sutured approximation over a small catheter stent. Ligation of the duct is at times required but may result in atrophy of the parotid gland, producing contour deformity of the face. Inflammatory conditions of the parotid gland include calculous disease and sialectasis, both of which may result in recurrent sialadenitis. Infection is thought to result from ascending involvement of the parenchyma from the oral cavity by way of the major duct. In the case of calculous disease, improper diet and abnormal salivary pH may predispose to the formation of stones in the major ducts. These stones are usually present near the duct orifice and may be successfully treated by incising the duct and removing the stone transorally. Occasionally, infections continue to occur despite stone extraction, alteration of diet and oral hygiene, stimulation of salivary secretions, adequate hydration, and antibiotics. In such circumstances, parotidectomy may be indicated. Observing the principles of facial nerve identification and dissection reduces the risk of the surgery.

Answer: A, B, C

35. Which of the following questions regarding the anatomy of the major salivary glands is/are correct?

A. The parotid gland is divided into two well-defined lobes (superficial and deep) based on neurovascular supply of the gland and embryologic lobar encapsulation
B. The facial nerve and its branches course superficial to the external parotid fascia, and therefore may be injured during parotid surgery
C. Injury to one or more branches of the facial nerve may occur during operations on the submandibular salivary gland as well as the parotid gland
D. There are approximately 40 to 60 minor salivary glands scattered in the submucosal plane of the oral cavity of most individuals

Sabiston: 1359
Schwartz: 583

Comments: Were it not for the relationship of the parotid gland to the facial nerve, parotid surgery would not be particularly challenging technically. The parotid gland is a unilobar structure embryologically, and is considered clinically to be divided into a superficial and deep lobe as defined by the portions of the gland that lie respectively superficial and deep to the facial nerve, which ramifies through the gland. Superficial lobe tumors usually require identification of the trunk and branches of the facial nerve with dissection of the tumor and superficial lobe off of the underlying nerve. Deep lobe tumors are usually approached by an initial superficial lobectomy followed by removal of the deep lobe from between or underneath the branches of the facial nerve. Injury to the marginal mandibular branch of the facial nerve may also occur in submandibular salivary gland surgery, as this nerve courses deep to the platysma over the external facial vessels, which are in close approximation to the lateral capsule of the gland. The lingual nerve is also at risk during submandibular gland surgery, particularly during the more cephalad dissection and ligation of Wharton's duct. ● Minor salivary glands, formerly and incorrectly considered to be ectopic salivary tissue, are scattered throughout the submucosal plane of the entire upper aerodigestive tract. They are particularly numerous in the oral cavity beneath the palatal, buccal, and labial mucosa. In the normal individual, the number of minor salivary glands is probably counted in the thousands.

Answer: C

36. Match the site of salivary gland tumor with its likelihood of being malignant.

Location of Tumor	Likelihood of Being Malignant
A. Parotid gland	a. 75% malignant
B. Submandibular gland	b. 50% malignant
C. Minor salivary gland	c. 25% malignant

Sabiston: 1359
Schwartz: 585

Comments: The above likelihood of malignancy among the different salivary gland tumors is a rough approximation with variation depending on the series quoted. Although the likelihood of a given tumor being malignant is lowest in the parotid gland, one must remember that since approximately 70% of all salivary gland tumors occur in the parotid gland, the parotid gland accounts for the majority of malignant salivary gland tumors. Although the sublingual gland is considered by many to be a major salivary gland, the likelihood of malignancy in sublingual glands is approximately that seen in minor salivary glands. The clinical approach to tumors of the sublingual gland is likewise similar to that of minor salivary glands.

Answer: A–c; B–b; C–a

37. Match the following histologic types of salivary gland tumor with their appropriate characteristics.

Histologic Type	Characteristics
A. Pleomorphic adenoma	a. High likelihood of perineural involvement
B. Warthin's tumor	b. Most common salivary gland tumor
C. Mucoepidermoid carcinoma	c. Widest range of biologic aggressiveness
D. Adenoid cystic carcinoma	d. May represent malignant change in a previously benign tumor
E. Malignant mixed tumor	e. Marked male predominance

Sabiston: 1359
Schwartz: 585

Comments: Tumors of the major and minor salivary glands represent a broad array of clinical presentation and biologic variability. Among the benign tumors, the **pleomorphic adenoma** (benign mixed tumor) is the most common overall. It is found most often in the parotid gland and is best managed by appropriate lobectomy with dissection of the facial nerve. Attempts to remove this tumor by a more limited "enucleation" has led to a 40 to 50% recurrence rate. The second most common benign tumor is **Warthin's tumor** (papillary cystadenoma lymphomatosum). Ninety-five percent of these tumors are seen in males, and it is the only salivary gland tumor with any significant degree of bilaterality (10%). One can frequently detect a cystic component to it on physical examination. **Mucoepidermoid carcinomas** as a group represent an extremely wide range of biologic aggressiveness. Low-grade mucoepidermoid carcinomas carry a very good prognosis, whereas high-grade mucoepidermoid carcinomas are rarely controlled by surgery alone and carry a poor prognosis. **Adenoid cystic carcinoma** (formerly cylindroma) is characterized by an indolent clinical course in which there may be long disease-free intervals followed by local and/or regional recurrence. A 5- or even 10-year disease-free status is no guarantee against eventual recurrence. These tumors have a propensity to invade and proliferate along perineural spaces, which may account for their high likelihood of local recurrence. **Malignant mixed tumors** are considered by many to be a malignant transformation of a previously benign mixed tumor. This has been suggested by the finding of malignant elements in tumors that otherwise appear to be pleomorphic adenomas. This supports the generally held surgical principle that major salivary gland tumors should be removed, even if they have been present and unchanged for many years.

Answer: A–b; B–e; C–c; D–a; E–d

38. Which of the following statements regarding the technical aspects of parotid surgery is/are correct?

A. The facial nerve is best identified by locating its trunk after it has exited the stylomastoid foramen near the posterior aspect of the parotid gland
B. Complete postoperative paralysis of the muscles supplied by one or more divisions of the facial nerve suggests that there has been disruption of or permanent injury to that division during surgery
C. The auriculotemporal nerve, while not specifically sought during parotid surgery, may be involved in a postoperative morbidity from parotid surgery
D. The sectioning of the facial nerve during parotid surgery results in a permanent degeneration of the nerve distal to the cut, making attempts at nerve reconstruction futile

Sabiston: 1359
Schwartz: 592

Comments: Proper identification and preservation of the facial nerve and its branches is the key to successful parotid surgery. Formerly, it was felt that most parotid malignancies should be treated by radical parotidectomy with deliberate sacrifice of the facial nerve. Currently, it is generally felt that deliberate sacrifice of the nerve or its branches may be required only in instances of direct nerve invasion by tumor. Nerve preservation and adjuvant postoperative radiation therapy have yielded local control rates equivalent to those of the more radical surgery, but without the inherent morbidity of facial nerve sacrifice. • The facial nerve is best protected by identifying its trunk as it exits the stylomastoid foramen at the posterior aspect of the gland. When scarring or tumor prevent dissection in this area, the nerve may be found in a retrograde fashion by dissecting out its more peripheral branches first. • Paresis or even complete paralysis of the muscles supplied by the facial nerve may occur in the absence of obvious nerve injury. This is almost always a temporary phenomenon, and function usually returns within several months. If the facial nerve or one of its major branches is deliberately or inadvertently cut during parotid surgery, immediate nerve repair or interposition nerve graft should be attempted, as there is at least some expectation of partial recovery in such circumstances. When this fails, there are numerous techniques of neuromusculofascial transfers that may be employed in an effort to restore facial symmetry. • Although the auriculotemporal nerve is not specifically sought during parotid surgery, its disruption and subsequent possible cross-reinnervation with branches of the sympathetic supply to the skin may result in postoperative gustatory sweating (Frey's syndrome).

Answer: A, C

39. Which of the following structures are routinely sacrificed in the performance of a classic radical neck dissection?

A. Internal jugular vein
B. Phrenic nerve
C. Spinal accessory nerve
D. Sternocleidomastoid muscle
E. Levator scapulae muscle
F. External carotid artery

Schwartz: 590

Comments: The classic radical neck dissection is an operation designed to remove the lymph node–bearing tissue that accompanies the great vessels within the carotid sheath as well as that found in the submandibular and posterior cervical triangles. This involves removal of the sternocleidomastoid muscle, internal jugular vein, spinal accessory nerve, and submandibular salivary gland and the associated lymph node–bearing fibrofatty tissue. Although branches of the external carotid artery may be sacrificed during this operation, the external, internal, and common carotid arteries are left intact. The cervical branch of the facial nerve is of necessity sacrificed, but the marginal branch is preserved. The sensory branches of the anterior roots of C2, C3, and C4 are sacrificed during the procedure, accounting for the relative absence of significant pain in the postoperative period. The phrenic nerve and its contributing cervical roots are preserved, as are the branches of the brachial plexus and the intrinsic deep musculature of the neck.

Answer: A, C, D

40. Which of the following statements is/are true regarding modifications in the standard approach to neck dissections?

A. Bilateral simultaneous radical neck dissections are well tolerated and should be performed in cases of midline lesions that may have metastasized to either size of the neck
B. The term "modified neck dissection" refers to the dissection of all but the posterior triangle portion of the classic radical neck dissection
C. Modified neck dissection may be used in the treatment of the clinically negative neck in which there is a significant risk of occult nodal metastases
D. The dissection and preservation of the spinal accessory nerve significantly reduces the morbidity of neck dissection in most patients

Schwartz: 591

Comments: Occasionally, clinical, bilateral cervical nodal disease necessitates bilateral radical neck dissection. Such an operation significantly increases the morbidity of the surgery in terms of marked facial and pharyngeal edema (usually requiring tracheostomy) as well as occasional changes in mental status due to increases in central nervous system venous pressures. Staging the neck dissections to allow some collaterals to develop and preservation of one of the internal jugular veins, if technically feasible, may reduce these postoperative risks. Prophylactic or elective bilateral simultaneous neck dissections should be avoided. • Modified radical neck dissection means different things to different people, but in general the term refers to a full dissection of the lymph node–bearing areas dealt with in the classic radical neck dissection, but with preservation of one or more of the sternocleidomastoid muscle, internal jugular vein, or spinal accessory nerve. This has gained acceptance in dissection of the clinically negative neck that is being explored because of the possibility of occult nodal disease. It is also valuable in the management of the clinically positive neck in patients with metastatic well-differentiated thyroid cancer. The shoulder droop, discomfort, and weakness that accompany loss of the spinal accessory is a major source of morbidity following neck dissection. In patients who are candidates for modified neck dissection, preservation of this nerve significantly reduces the likelihood of this aspect of postoperative morbidity.

Answer: C, D

41. Which of the following statements is/are true regarding the diagnosis and management of a solitary lump in the neck?

A. A 1-month period of observation and antibiotic therapy should be carried out in all patients because of the possibility of the lump being an inflammatory lymph node
B. The first step in management is an incisional or excisional biopsy to establish the diagnosis in order to avoid other unnecessary testing
C. One must consider primary tumors in the chest and abdomen to be potential sources of cervical lymph node metastases
D. Radical neck dissection should not be performed for a metastatic cervical disease if the primary tumor has not been found

Schwartz: 587

Comments: Solitary lumps in the neck may represent inflammatory lymph nodes, metastatic carcinoma from sites in the upper aerodigestive tract, metastases from sites other than the upper aerodigestive tract (lung, breast, gastrointestinal tract, kidney, etc.), lymphoma, or rare primary tumors (e.g., carotid body tumor). The age of the patient, clinical presentation, and physical characteristics of the mass will frequently give some indication as to the nature of the pathology. The first step in the management should be a thorough examination of the head and neck area, including indirect laryngoscopy and nasopharyngoscopy. If no primary pathology is found in the upper aerodigestive tract and the mass is felt clinically to be inflammatory in nature, it is reasonable to observe it over a brief period of time (2–4 weeks) with or without antibiotics. If the mass persists or enlarges during this time, one is obligated to consider the diagnosis

of neoplasm. Needle aspiration biopsy should be considered as an early diagnostic test insofar as it is safe, is fairly accurate when positive, and has not been shown to result in implantation of tumor cells along the needle tract. One is cautioned, however, not to accept a negative needle aspiration result if the clinical index of suspicion of malignancy is high. Incisional or excisional biopsy of the mass may be required to establish the diagnosis. A finding of squamous carcinoma suggests a primary site in the upper aerodigestive tract or lung; the location of the mass within the neck will give some guidance as to the possible site of primary tumor. In cases of metastatic squamous cell carcinoma and no obvious primary site on clinical examination, direct laryngoscopy under anesthesia with multiple random biopsies of the likely sites of occult primary tumors (e.g., nasopharynx, tonsillar fossa, base of tongue, pyriform sinus) may be warranted. When no primary tumor is found despite these efforts, it is generally believed that the cervical metastatic disease should be treated for cure by radical neck dissection, radiation therapy, or a combination of the two. Approximately one third of the patients so managed will survive 5 years free of disease despite the fact that the primary tumor may never be found. A finding of adenocarcinoma suggests gastrointestinal tract, breast, or lung as likely primary sites. One must remember, however, that salivary gland malignancies can metastasize to regional nodes.

Answer: C

42. Which of the following persons may have a role to play in the management of the head and neck cancer patient?

A. Reconstructive surgeon
B. Oral surgeon
C. Prosthetist
D. Speech therapist
E. Family members
F. Psychiatrist/psychologist

Schwartz: 597

Comments: The overall care of the head and neck cancer patient does not end with the surgical, radiotherapeutic, or chemotherapeutic effort. Rehabilitation following treatment is a major aspect contributing to success in the care of these patients. The significant cosmetic and functional (speech, swallowing, etc.) deficits created in the treatment of advanced head and neck cancer necessitate a coordinated effort among many disciplines to restore appearance and function to as a great a degree as possible as well as to assist in the psychologic rehabilitation of the patient.

Answer: A, B, C, D, E, F

CHAPTER 19

Thyroid

1. Which of the following statements regarding the vascular relationships of the thyroid gland is/are correct?

A. The average blood supply of 5 ml/gm/min to the thyroid gland makes it one of the most vascularized organs in the body
B. The inferior thyroid artery is the only named arterial branch of the common carotid artery
C. The thyroidea ima arteries are paired bilateral arteries supplying the lower poles of the gland
D. The inferior thyroid veins parallel the inferior thyroid arteries in their anatomic course
E. The superior thyroid vein is the only thyroid vein that drains directly into the internal jugular vein

Sabiston: 580
Schwartz: 1546

Comment: There are few tissues (e.g., carotid body) with a blood supply (per gram of tissue) greater than that of the thyroid gland. This blood supply comes from paired superior thyroid arteries arising from the external carotid, paired inferior thyroid arteries arising from the thyrocervical trunk, and an inconstant midline thyroidea ima artery usually arising from the aortic arch. Venous drainage of the thyroid is via the superior and middle thyroid veins, which drain directly into the internal jugular vein, and the inferior thyroid veins, which drain directly into the innominate vein. The rich blood supply of the thyroid gland may explain in part the ease and relative frequency with which central necrosis in a thyroid nodule results in hemorrhage into it, accounting for a sudden increase in its size.

Answer: A

2. Which of the following statements is/are true regarding the association of the thyroid gland to nearby nerves?

A. Both the superior and inferior thyroid arteries bear a fairly constant relationship to the laryngeal nerves
B. The superior laryngeal nerve is both sensory and motor to the larynx
C. The laryngeal nerves do not directly innervate the

thyroid gland and therefore are of significance only because of their proximity to the gland
D. The "recurrent" nature of the recurrent laryngeal nerves is one of the few anatomic relationships in which anomalies or variations have not been reported
E. Injury to one or both recurrent laryngeal nerves results in airway compromise that frequently requires tracheostomy

Sabiston: 580
Schwartz: 1546

Comment: The innervation of the thyroid gland is via both sympathetic fibers from the cervical ganglion and parasympathetic fibers from the vagus reaching the gland through the laryngeal nerves. The importance of the laryngeal nerves relates to their proximity to the gland and risk of injury during thyroidectomy. The superior laryngeal nerve is both sensory and motor to the larynx; it is the external branch (motor to the cricothyroid muscle) that is at risk during thyroid surgery because of its close relationship to the superior thyroid vessels. Injury to this branch results in a bowing of the vocal cord during phonation. The recurrent laryngeal nerve is so named because of its oblique ascent to the cricothyroid membrane, having coursed around the subclavian artery on the right and the aorta near the ductus arteriosus on the left. In their usual course the nerves bear a fairly constant relationship to branches of the inferior thyroid arteries as they near the larynx. Occasionally, on the right side, a nonrecurrent nerve exists, usually in association with vascular anomalies of the aortic arch. In such circumstances, the nerve approaches the cricothyroid membrane obliquely from above and may be inadvertently divided if not recognized. The recurrent laryngeal nerve provides motor function to most of the intrinsic laryngeal muscles, and its unilateral injury results in paralysis of the vocal cord which changes the quality of the voice but rarely compromises the airway significantly. Bilateral recurrent laryngeal nerve injury, on the other hand, may severely compromise air flow, necessitating tracheostomy.

Answer: A, B

3. Which of the following thyroid anomalies may relate to variations in embryologic development?

A. Lingual thyroid
B. Thyroglossal duct cyst
C. Persistent pyramidal lobe
D. Mediastinal thyroid
E. Lateral aberrant thyroid rest

Sabiston: 581, 1346
Schwartz: 1546

Comment: Embryologically the thyroid gland results from a joining of the median anlage, which arises from the pharyngeal floor in the area of the foramen cecum, with lateral components from the ultimobranchial bodies of the fourth and fifth branchial pouches. Abnormalities in descent of the thyroid tissue from the pharyngeal floor may result in a lingual thyroid or persistence of solid or cystic structures along the course of the midline descent, resulting respectively in persistent pyramidal lobe or a thyroglossal duct cyst. The initial embryologic descent of the thyroid may proceed into an abnormally caudad position, resulting in a mediastinal or substernal thyroid, although the majority of intrathoracic goiters represent inferior extension of acquired thyroid pathology from a normally located gland. The existence of benign lateral aberrant thyroid rests has been questioned by those who feel that such structures represent metastases of well differentiated thyroid cancers. In cases in which papillary features or severely atypical follicular features are found, this is probably the case. In some instances, however, a failure of the lateral thyroid elements to be incorporated into the thyroid capsule may, indeed, result in embryologic thyroid rests in the lateral neck.

Answer: A, B, C, D, E

4. Regarding lingual thyroid, which one or more of the following statements is/are correct?

A. They are usually associated with a smaller than average thyroid gland in the normal anatomic position
B. They may cause obstructive symptoms in the pharynx
C. Diagnosis depends upon tissue confirmation from biopsy
D. There is a 40% risk of malignancy when the thyroid is in an aberrant location
E. Surgical excision is generally recommended because of the risk of pharyngeal obstruction and malignancy

Sabiston: 581
Schwartz: 1547

Comment: On rare occasions, when the normal descent of the thyroid is arrested, a lingual thyroid may result; in 70% of cases this may be the only thyroid tissue present. Lingual thyroids normally are asymptomatic but may enlarge to produce dysphagia, dyspnea, and other sequelae of pharyngeal obstruction. Grossly lingual thyroid may be confused with other submucosal lesions of the base of the tongue, including lymphoma and minor salivary gland tumors; a technetium or iodine scan, however, will be positive in that area if thyroid tissue is present. The risk of malignancy is relatively low (approximately 3%). When symptoms are present or the suspicion of malig-

nancy is high, treatment may be either by radioiodine or surgical excision. A thyroid scan should be performed to see if this is the only thyroid tissue present. In such a case, autotransplantation can be performed or, if the tissue is excised, permanent thyroid replacement will be necessary following treatment.

Answer: B

5. Thyroid hormones are involved in the regulation of which one or more of the following metabolic processes?

A. Oxygen consumption
B. Protein synthesis
C. Glycogenolysis
D. Lipid metabolism
E. Oxidative phosphorylation

Schwartz: 1549

Comment: See Question 6.

6. Which of the following statements is/are true regarding thyroid hormone synthesis and physiology?

A. The iodine utilized in thyroid hormone synthesis is derived primarily from dietary sources
B. The role of TSH in thyroid physiology is limited to regulation of the release of thyroid hormone into the plasma
C. Enough T4 is stored in the normal thyroid to provide a euthyroid state for 2 months despite absence of iodine uptake
D. The regulation of thyroid function involves pituitary but not hypothalamic input

Sabiston: 581
Schwartz: 1548

Comment: Thyroid hormones play an active regulatory role in many aspects of energy substrate metabolism. These include increased oxygen consumption and calorigenesis, stimulation of protein synthesis, regulation of most aspects of carbohydrate metabolism, and metabolism of cholesterol and phospholipids. Furthermore, they play an important role in many other physiologic processes, including other endocrine, thermoregulatory, and cardiodynamic events. Thyroid hormone synthesis begins with the active transport of iodine from dietary sources into the thyroid gland. Successive iodinization of amino acids results in the eventual production of T3 and T4, which may be stored in sufficient quantities in the thyroid gland to provide a euthyroid state despite 2 months of iodine deprivation or synthesis inhibition. When the active T3 and T4 hormones are released into the plasma they become bound to thyroxin-binding globulin (TBG) for transport. Peripherally, the greater portion of T4 is converted to T3, which may in fact be the only active hormone intracellularly. Most of the aspects of iodine uptake and organification as well as thyroid hormone release are regulated by TSH, which is elaborated from the anterior pituitary. Hypothalamic input in the form of thyrotropin-releasing hormone (TRH) and even cortical influences also have a role in thyroid regulation. Of course, proper thyroid function is dependent upon the availability of adequate dietary iodine.

Answer: Question 5: A, B, C, D, E
Question 6: A, C

7. Match the following thyroid tests with their ability to assess either thyroid function or thyroid nodules:

a. Technetium scan
b. Iodine uptake and scan
c. Ultrasound
d. T4 assay
e. Needle aspiration cytology
f. Thyroid autoantibodies

a. Useful in assessing metabolic thyroid function
b. Useful in assessing the nature of thyroid nodules
c. Both
d. Neither

Sabiston: 583
Schwartz: 1551

Comment: With the exception of inflammatory or infectious thyroid disease, most thyroid pathology can be considered as either an abnormality of metabolic thyroid function or the presence of a potentially neoplastic nodule. **Scanning** techniques (both technetium and iodine) are used primarily to determine the presence of nodules within the thyroid gland. However, the amount of radioactivity detected during the scan is a measure of the uptake of the nuclide and, thus, indirectly indicates the metabolic activity of the gland. With iodine scanning, this can be quantitated and is an excellent measure of thyroid activity. **Ultrasound** of the thyroid is useful in determining the number of thyroid nodules and their cystic vs. solid nature, but does not contribute to assessment of thyroid function. **Thyroid hormone** (T3 or T4) and TSH assays of peripheral blood are useful in determining the presence of hyper- or hypofunction of the gland, as well as the status of the thyroid/pituitary feedback mechanism. **Needle aspiration** of the thyroid gland is used primarily in the evaluation and/or treatment of thyroid nodules. If cystic, the lesion can be entirely treated by aspiration, whereas if the lesion is solid, cytology can be performed to assess the likelihood of underlying malignancy. Assay of thyroid **autoantibodies** does not in and of itself directly assess thyroid nodules or thyroid function. These autoantibodies may be seen in Graves' disease (hyperfunction) or Hashimoto's disease (hyper- or hypofunction), both of which may or may not be associated with discrete thyroid nodules.

Answer: A–c; B–c; C–b; D–a; E–b; F–d

8. Which of the following statements is/are true regarding thyroid function tests?

A. Estrogens increase the amount of thyroxin-binding globulin (TBG) and, therefore, may falsely suggest hyperthyroidism
B. Administration of exogenous thyroid may lead to an increase in the radioactive iodine uptake (RAIU)
C. Both barium enema and intravenous pyelography may affect RAIU
D. Failure of exogenous T3 to suppress TSH secretion may be seen in Graves' disease, toxic adenoma, and functioning carcinoma

Sabiston: 583
Schwartz: 1551

Comment: Because of the difficulty in measuring free T4, most assays of plasma T4 measure total T4, which re-flects the free element as well as that which is bound to TBG. Estrogen administration or pregnancy usually results in elevated TBG values, which may be reflected as an elevated total T4 even though the patient is not hyperthyroid and has a normal free T4. Androgens have the opposite effect. Assessment of the amount of radioactive iodine taken up by the thyroid gland is another useful determination of thyroid function. Administration of exogenous thyroid hormone or dietary or intravenous iodine will usually result in a reduction of RAIU even though the patient is not clinically hypothyroid. Contrast studies that do not involve iodine use obviously do not affect the iodine uptake assay. Assessment of the thyroid/pituitary feedback loop can be achieved with TSH suppression tests in which T3 is administered and the amount of TSH production is evaluated. Normally plasma TSH levels should fall to 50% of control values when T3 is administered for 7 to 10 days. In conditions with autonomous function of the thyroid (as may be seen in Graves' disease, toxic adenomas, functioning carcinomas, and chronic lymphocytic thyroiditis), TSH may already be suppressed and further depression cannot be obtained by administration of exogenous thyroid hormone.

Answer: A, D

9. Which of the following statements is/are true regarding thyroid scanning?

A. The dose of radiation delivered to the thyroid is the same regardless of whether I-131, I-123, or Tc-99m is used
B. Thyroid scanning is of use in assessing the thyroid gland when it is in the normal position but does not evaluate ectopic thyroid tissue
C. Thyroid imaging is highly accurate even in detecting lesions as small as 1 cm
D. Metastases from well differentiated thyroid carcinoma are unlikely to be detected by T-131 imaging if significant normal thyroid tissue is present

Sabiston: 181
Schwartz: 1553

Comment: Thyroid scanning involves the uptake of a radionuclide by the thyroid gland with subsequent emission of radioactivity which is detected and displayed by the scanner. Its greatest utility is in demonstrating "cold" or nonfunctioning nodules. Its accuracy in detecting nodules less than 1.5 cm in size may be reduced depending on the technique of the scan and where in the thyroid gland the nodule is located. I-131 was the standard agent for many years but has for the most part been replaced by technetium or I-123, which emit considerably less radiation. I-131 remains useful for the detection of retrosternal masses or for total body scanning to search for metastatic disease. Other ectopic sites of thyroid tissue (e.g., lingual thyroid) are also detectable with thyroid scanning. The capacity of normal thyroid tissue to take up iodine is so great that the ability of thyroid imaging to detect metastatic disease is significantly hindered by the presence of normal functioning thyroid tissue. For this reason, the use of iodine scanning for metastatic disease depends upon prior surgical or radio-therapeutic ablation of the gland.

Answer: D

10. With which of the following thyroid abnormalities may thyrotoxicosis be associated?

A. Diffuse painless enlargement
B. Diffuse painful or tender enlargement
C. Multinodular goiter
D. Solitary solid nodule

Sabiston: 585
Schwartz: 1554

Comment: See Question 11.

11. Match the following causes of thyrotoxicosis with their appropriate description(s): (more than one match possible)

A. Graves' disease
B. Toxic multinodular goiter
C. Toxic adenoma

a. Autonomous function independent of TSH, LATS, TSI
b. Diffuse gland involvement with increased vascularity and lymphoid aggregate
c. Extrathyroidal manifestations
d. Cervical compression symptoms may be present

Sabiston: 585
Schwartz: 1554

Comment: Overactivity of the thyroid gland may be manifested only by elevation of the amount of circulating thyroid hormone or may be made clinically evident by a number of signs and symptoms, many of which mimic catecholamine excess (e.g., hypertension, tachycardia, flushing, sweating). Overproduction of thyroid hormone may occur in the setting of a diffuse enlargement of the gland (diffuse toxic goiter or Graves' disease) or it may occur in the setting of a single "hot" nodule or in a multinodular gland. Additionally, some forms of thyroiditis, particularly Hashimoto's thyroiditis, may be associated with hyperthyroidism. In cases of the toxic adenoma or toxic multinodular goiter, the hyperfunctioning nodules are thought to simply represent adenomas which are autonomously functioning. In contradistinction, Graves' disease is thought to be an autoimmune phenomenon in which TSH receptors within the thyroid gland are stimulated by binding with immunoglobulins (LATS—long-acting thyroid stimulator, and TSI—thyroid-stimulating immunoglobulins). Among the entities producing hyperthyroidism, Graves' disease is unique in its association with extrathyroidal manifestations (exophthalmos, pretibial myxedema) which may bear no relationship to the presence or severity of thyroid overactivity. Any enlargement of the thyroid gland (diffuse or nodular) may produce tracheal or pharyngoesophageal compression symptoms.

Answer: Question 10: A, B, C, D
Question 11: A–b, c, d; B–a, d; C–a, d

12. Match the following clinical situations with their most appropriate initial treatment:

A. A 25-year-old with Graves' disease and a markedly enlarged gland with compressive symptoms
B. An 8-year-old with Graves' disease
C. A 38-year-old with a toxic adenoma
D. A 35-year-old with a toxic multinodular goiter who forms very large unsightly keloids

a. Surgery
b. Radioiodine
c. Antithyroid drugs

Sabiston: 586
Schwartz: 1558

Comment: The treatment of Graves' disease is controversial and may be effectively carried out with either a subtotal thyroidectomy, radioiodine therapy, or antithyroid drugs; all of these forms of treatment have their particular advantages and disadvantages. **Antithyroid drugs,** which exert their effect by interfering with iodine binding, require long-term treatment—up to 2 years—and may be associated with drug fever, rash, and agranulocytosis, which is occasionally fatal. Furthermore, recurrence of hyperthyroidism after cessation of the drugs may occur in as many as 70% of patients. **Radioiodine** may take several weeks to months to exert its effect and is associated with the almost certain occurrence of future hypothyroidism. **Subtotal thyroidectomy** confers the risk of anesthesia and surgery, the latter including trauma to the recurrent laryngeal nerve or permanent hypoparathyroidism. However, it has the advantage of an immediate response and reduction of compression symptoms. Hypothyroidism after subtotal thyroidectomy is also very common. Any of these three forms of treatment may be appropriate as the initial treatment for a particular patient with Graves' disease, with specific circumstances occasionally influencing the therapeutic choice. For example, radioiodine is generally avoided in children because of the possible deleterious effects of radiation in that age group. If there are relative contraindications to surgery, then antithyroid drugs would be the treatment of choice in such a setting. Those with extremely large glands with compressive symptoms would be most readily treated by subtotal thyroidectomy. Toxic multinodular goiters are probably most effectively treated by surgical excision. Radioiodine is an acceptable alternative but may be less effective than it is in Graves' disease because of the inhomogeneous uptake of the nuclide by the multinodular gland. Toxic adenomas are best treated by surgery involving lobectomy on the involved side. This provides an immediate effective treatment, frequently with preservation of enough thyroid tissue that there is no need for thyroid replacement therapy.

Answer: A–a; B–c; C–a; D–b

13. Which of the following is/are true regarding the use of radioiodine to treat hyperthyroidism?

A. If hypothyroidism is to occur following radioiodine, it will do so within 2 years of treatment
B. There is a marked increased risk of future thyroid cancers following radioiodine therapy

C. The risk of leukemia following radioiodine therapy is approximately 10%
D. Mutational abnormalities are seen in 15% of infants following maternal treatment during pregnancy with radioiodine
E. Radioiodine may pass through the placenta and lactating breast to produce hypothyroidism in the fetus and infant

Sabiston: 587
Schwartz: 1558

Comment: Radioiodine is an effective form of treatment of hyperthryoidism, particularly that due to Graves' disease; however, it has several undesirable sequelae which must be considered: **Hypothyroidism** develops in nearly 100% of patients after treatment, although this may take as long as 10 years to become manifest. The **carcinogenic** effects of radioiodine have long been a theoretical consideration, mitigating against its use; however, clinical experience has not supported this contention. In the case of thyroid carcinoma, there is an increase in the incidence of thyroid nodules following radioiodine treatment; however, the risk of subsequent thyroid carcinoma does not appear to be appreciably increased. This is in contradistinction to the increased risk of thyroid carcinoma following low-dose external beam irradiation for conditions such as thymic enlargement in infancy, lymphadenopathy, and acne. Similarly, the risk of leukemia does not appear to be appreciably increased by radioiodine therapy. The radionuclide can pass through the placenta and the lactating breast; however, its propensity to produce **genetic abnormalities** in this way appears to be low, with its principal effect being the induction of hypothyroidism in the infant.

Answer: E

14. Which one or more of the following may precipitate a thyroid storm?

A. Surgery on the thyroid gland
B. Appendectomy
C. Pregnancy
D. Lobar pneumonia
E. Compound fracture of tibia
F. Diabetic acidosis

Sabiston: 592
Schwartz: 1575

Comment: See Question 15.

15. Which of the following are appropriate elements in the management of thyroid storm?

A. Oxygen administration
B. Large amounts of intravenous glucose
C. Hypothermia blanket
D. Propranolol
E. Sodium or potassium iodide
F. Emergency radioiodine therapy

Sabiston: 592
Schwartz: 1575

Comment: Thyroid storm results when there is excessive release of thyroid hormone from a toxic gland. The clinical manifestations are those of hyperthermia, tachycardia, irritability, sweating, anxiety, and hypertension, which can eventually lead to prostration, hypotension, and death. This may be precipitated by any number of metabolically stressful situations, including surgery on the thyroid gland or for non-thyroid conditions, pregnancy, infection, trauma, or other metabolic stresses such as diabetic acidosis. Formerly, surgery was the most common inciting event. However, with the more current prophylactic measures available, it now is a rare cause of thyroid storm. More often, it is precipitated by trauma, infection, or toxemia of pregnancy in patients whose underlying thyrotoxic state had not previously been recognized. The fundamentals of treating thyroid storm center on providing those factors needed to support the increased metabolic rate (oxygen, glucose, fluid), counteracting the peripheral adrenergic manifestations of the syndrome (propranolol, hypothermia) and preventing iodinization and release of thyroid hormone (large doses of sodium or potassium iodide). Radioiodine therapy does not have a role in the treatment of thyroid storm, and in fact may itself precipitate thyroid storm.

Answer: Question 14: A, B, C, D, E, F
Question 15: A, B, C, D, E

16. A 50-year-old woman presents with a 2-year history of mild, diffuse, tender thyroid enlargement with a 10-pound weight gain and fatigue. Of the following, which is the most likely diagnosis?

A. Riedel's thyroiditis
B. Hashimoto's thyroiditis
C. Subacute thyroiditis
D. Suppurative thyroiditis
E. Papillary thyroid carcinoma

Sabiston: 593
Schwartz: 1562

Comment: Hashimoto's disease is the most common form of chronic thyroiditis. It most often occurs in middle-aged women and commonly presents as a mild to moderate diffuse thyroid enlargement which may be tender. Although evidence of hyperthyroidism may be present in patients with Hashimoto's disease, most patients either are euthyroid or show evidence of mild to moderate hypothyroidism. The disease is thought to involve an autoimmune process, and one of the confirming diagnostic findings is the presence of antithyroid antibodies. Frequently, no treatment is needed; however, thyroid replacement therapy is used if the patient is hypothyroid. The incidence of thyroid carcinoma in Hashimoto's disease may be slightly greater than that in the general population, but not enough so to warrant prophylactic thyroidectomy. Operation generally is reserved for symptoms of compression or to remove nodules within the diseased gland that potentially may be malignant.

Answer: B

17. Match the following forms of thyroiditis with their proper clinical description:

A. Acute suppurative
B. Subacute (de Quervain's)
C. Hashimoto's
D. Riedel's struma

a. May be associated with retroperitoneal fibrosis
b. Acutely ill patients; bacterial origin
c. Most common form of thyroiditis
d. Probable viral origin

Sabiston: 593
Schwartz: 1561

Comment: As discussed at Question 16, **Hashimoto's disease** is the most common form of thyroiditis encountered. Of the other three recognized forms of thyroiditis, each has a distinctive clinical picture. **Acute suppurative thyroiditis** is extremely rare. It is manifested by the sudden onset of severe pain associated with fever, chills, and dysphagia. It almost always follows an acute upper respiratory infection and is of bacterial origin. Treatment is with antibiotics and occasionally drainage. **Subacute thyroiditis** is of debatable origin (many consider it to be of viral etiology) and, as with suppurative thyroiditis, frequently follows an upper respiratory infection. Although of fairly abrupt onset, its clinical course is less fulminant than that of suppurative thyroiditis and is characterized by a moderately swollen and tender thyroid gland with repeated exacerbations and remissions over several months. Recovery is frequently spontaneous, but may be facilitated by a course of salicylate or occasionally corticosteroid therapy. **Riedel's struma** is a rare chronic inflammatory condition of the thyroid gland characterized by increasing dense fibrosis throughout the gland and the periglandular tissues, frequently resulting in hypothyroidism and symptoms of tracheal and esophageal compression. Occasionally it has been associated with other fibrotic reactions, including retroperitoneal fibrosis and sclerosing mediastinitis. When unilateral it is difficult to distinguish from carcinoma. Treatment usually includes thyroid hormone therapy, and operation may be necessary for relief of tracheoesophageal obstruction.

Answers: A–b; B–d; C–c; D–a

18. Which one or more of the following statements regarding goiter is/are correct?

A. The term "goiter" can refer to any enlargement of the thyroid gland
B. The term "familial goiter" falsely implies that a genetic defect may play a role in the etiology.
C. The most identifiable cause of endemic goiter is iodine deficiency
D. Operation is indicated for patients with extremely large iodine deficiency goiters because of the increased risk of cancer in the larger glands

Schwartz: 1564

Comment: The term "goiter" refers broadly to any abnormal enlargement of the thyroid gland, either diffuse or nodular. In the majority of instances it is unrelated to hyper- or hypothyroidism. Occasionally there may be a familial tendency toward diffuse thyroid enlargement, and in some circumstances this may be due to an inherited enzymatic defect resulting in impaired iodine metabolism. These patients are usually hypothyroid. More commonly, however, diffuse thyroid enlargement is due to environmental effects. These may include the ingestion of goitrogenic foods or drugs (e.g., para-aminosalicylic acid) or more commonly, dietary iodine deficiency. In many countries, there are so-called goiter belts due to environmental iodine deficiencies occurring in specific geographic locations. In the United States, these regions included mountainous areas, the upper Northwest, and the Great Lakes region. This is of primarily historical in-

terest today, as the use of iodinized table salt has become nearly routine. Sporadic cases of iodine deficiency goiter still occur and may be treated with iodine administration. Diffuse goiters may cause problems by virtue of their cosmetic effect, or compression symptoms. They occasionally can be made smaller with iodine or thyroid hormone administration, but may require operation for correction of these problems. The risk of cancer is not increased in these glands and is not an indication for operation.

Answer: A, C

19. Which of the following are considered risk factors for the development of thyroid carcinoma?

A. A family history of medullary carcinoma of the thyroid
B. A family history of papillary carcinoma of the thyroid
C. History of abnormally low iodine ingestion during childhood
D. Exposure to low-dose radiotherapy (less than 2,000 rads)
E. Exposure to high-dose radiotherapy (greater than 2,000 rads)
F. Previous exposure to radioiodine therapy for hyperthyroidism

Sabiston: 602
Schwartz: 1566

Comments: A family history of thyroid neoplasms, benign or malignant, of follicular cell origin does not appear to increase the risk of thyroid cancer significantly. However, a history of medullary carcinoma of the thyroid (parafollicular cell origin) does increase one's risk of developing the same type of thyroid cancer. It has long been recognized that exposure of the thyroid gland to low-dose radiation therapy increases the subsequent risk of thyroid cancer. More recently, it has been determined that this risk is also increased in patients exposed to higher doses (for example, those receiving upper mantle radiation therapy for Hodgkin's disease—up to 5,000 rads). Therapeutic radioiodine administration as is used in the treatment of hyperthyroidism has not been associated with an increased subsequent risk of thyroid cancer; and it is presumed that this is due to the nearly total destruction of the follicular cells by the iodine therapy.

Answer: A, D, E

20. Which of the following thyroid adenomas is most strongly associated with thyroid carcinoma?

A. Colloid adenoma
B. Embryonal adenoma
C. Fetal adenoma
D. Hürthle cell adenoma

Sabiston: 598

Comments: The clinical significance of thyroid adenomas relates to the need to differentiate them from thyroid carcinoma. This frequently requires partial thyroidectomy for tissue diagnosis; and once histologic diagnosis is known, no further treatment is necessary (some clinicians believe that thyroid suppression should be used to reduce the risk of development of future adenomas). The colloid, embryonal, and fetal adenoma are all considered subcategories of follicular adenoma and are differentiated from each other by the relative amount of colloid present and the architectural arrangement of the epithelial cells. Cytologically, these cells all appear to be quite similar to the normal thyroid follicular cell. These follicular adenomas are entirely benign (although one must recognize that the histologic differentiation of follicular adenoma from follicular carcinoma may occasionally be difficult) and do not increase the risk of carcinoma. In contradistinction, the Hürthle cell adenoma, so named because of the characteristic Hürthle cell (variable enlargement, hyperchromatic nuclei, and granular cytoplasm), is considered by many pathologists to be in fact a low-grade follicular carcinoma. For that reason, the noncommital term of "Hürthle cell tumor" has been used to describe these tumors. As a consequence of this possible identity as a low-grade carcinoma, some feel that a more aggressive surgical approach (total thyroidectomy) is indicated in the management of these tumors.

Answer: D

21. Select which one from each pair of features of thyroid nodules is associated with the greater likelihood of malignancy.

A. Solid vs. cystic
B. Solitary vs. multiple
C. "Hot" vs. "cold"
D. Rapid enlargement overnight vs. slow enlargement over many months
E. Hard vs. soft
F. Male vs. female
G. Child vs. adult

Sabiston: 600
Schwartz: 1567

Comments: The management of thyroid nodules, particularly the decision as to whether surgical intervention is required, depends upon one's clinical index of suspicion that the nodule may be malignant. Numerous factors in the history, physical examination, and laboratory examination of the patient raise or lower one's index of suspicion. Epidemiologically, thyroid cancers are more common in adults than in children and in women than in men. However, that is due to the fact that thyroid nodules themselves are more common in those populations. The likelihood that a given nodule may be malignant, however, is greater in males than in females and in children as compared with adults. Most thyroid cancers are manifested by a slow, indolent growth, that which is described as sudden enlargement overnight, is usually due to hemorrhage into a previously undetected nodule; and although this underlying nodule may be a carcinoma, it usually is a follicular adenoma. A history of recent voice change or difficulty swallowing, particularly when the lesion is small, should raise one's index of suspicion of malignancy as well. On physical examination, soft or fleshy lesions suggest benign disease, whereas hardness of texture is more associated with malignancy. Examination of the vocal cord function by indirect laryngoscopy should be performed to search for ipsilateral paresis or paralysis, which suggests that the thyroid nodule may be invading or compressing the recurrent laryngeal nerve. Noninvasive laboratory workup usually consists of a radionuclide scan and/or ultrasound of the thyroid. Radionuclide scan gives information regarding the metabolic activity of the nodule as well as the number of nodules present, whereas ultrasound gives information relating to the number of nodules and the solid vs. cystic nature of them. Uninodularity, decreased or absent function ("cold"), and solid characteristics all increase the likelihood of malignancy as compared with their respective counterparts. Taking all comers, a solitary, solid, cold nodule in the thyroid gland carries approximately a 20% risk of malignancy, whereas cystic structure, multinodularity, and normal or hyperfunctioning status carry risks in the range of 5% or less.

Answer: A–solid; B–solitary; C–cold; D–slow; E–hard; F–male; G–child

22. Which one or more of the following statements is/are true regarding the technique of needle aspiration biopsy of the thyroid?

A. It is generally contraindicated owing to the extremely vascular nature of the thyroid gland
B. False positives are rare
C. False negatives are rare
D. There is a 3% risk of cancer cells implanting along the needle tract
E. Benign versus malignant follicular neoplasms are fairly easily differentiated

Sabiston: 601
Schwartz: 1567

Comment: In recent years needle biopsy of the thyroid gland has gained popularity. Needle core biopsy was initially the technique employed but was associated with a significant risk of hematoma. This technique has more recently been supplanted by fine needle aspiration cytology (18- to 25-gauge needles). In the absence of coagulopathy, hemorrhagic complications are extremely rare with this technique. The theoretical complication of implantation of cancer cells along the needle tract has been proposed but not observed. Because of the possibility of a sampling error in any needle aspiration technique, one must look upon negative results with caution. False positive results, however, are extremely rare when the specimen is examined by an experienced cytologist. The area of greatest difficulty in interpretation is that dealing with follicular neoplasms, in which differentiation of benignity from malignancy depends more upon gross and histologic tumor architecture than upon cytology. In cases in which the clinical index of suspicion of malignancy is high, a negative needle aspiration result should probably be ignored.

Answer: B

23. Match each of the following types of thyroid cancer with the appropriate descriptive phrase:

Thyroid Cancer	Descriptive Phrase
A. Papillary carcinoma	a. Most likely to respond to radioiodine
B. Follicular carcinoma	b. Almost uniformly fatal
C. Medullary carcinoma	c. Propensity to local and regional recurrence
D. Anaplastic carcinoma	d. Usually requires radiation therapy and/or chemotherapy
E. Lymphoma	e. Familial tendency

Sabiston: 602
Schwartz: 1568

Comment: Cancers of the thyroid gland encompass a wide range of biological aggressiveness, depending on the histologic type. At the favorable extreme are the papillary carcinomas with their propensity to local or regional recurrences as opposed to systemic metastases. Follicular carcinomas also carry a generally favorable prognosis, but are characterized by a propensity for blood-borne distant metastases. Fortunately, many of these tumors respond to radioiodine therapy. Medullary carcinomas may occur sporadically or in a familial pattern, occasionally as part of the MEN-2 syndrome (medullary carcinoma of the thyroid, pheochromocytoma, parathyroid hyperplasia). These tumors carry an intermediate prognosis, depending on the presence or absence of nodal involvement and distant metastatic disease. Lymphomas of the thyroid gland also carry an intermediate prognosis, depending on the stage at presentation. Rarely, patients with thyroid lymphoma may be cured by surgery alone; but in the vast majority of cases, the disease is considered to be part of a more widespread process and regional radiation therapy and/or chemotherapy are indicated. Anaplastic thyroid carcinoma is an extremely rapidly growing and nearly uniformly fatal disease which presents characteristically with massive involvement in the neck associated with tracheoesophageal obstruction. Palliative surgery, radiotherapy, or chemotherapy may result in occasional short-lived responses.

Answer: A–c; B–a; C–e; D–b; E–d

24. Which one or more of the following statements is/are true regarding papillary thyroid carcinoma?

A. It is the second most common form of thyroid cancer
B. The presence of resectable lymph node metastases does not appear to worsen prognosis
C. The 30% mortality seen in this disease is due primarily to distant metastases
D. It is the type of thyroid cancer most often associated with prior radiation exposure
E. There is a high likelihood of clinical or occult multicentric disease

Sabiston: 603
Schwartz: 1568

Comment: Papillary thyroid carcinoma is the most common form of thyroid cancer and carries the best prognosis. It manifests itself primarily by local and regional involvement, with distant metastases present in less than 1% of patients at initial presentation. It accounts for the vast majority of thyroid cancer seen after prior exposure to radiation therapy. There is a high likelihood (up to 80%) of occult multicentric disease when the gland is examined carefully enough pathologically. These data, as well as autopsy data showing a much higher incidence of occult disease than clinical disease, raise the question as to the biologic importance of these occult papillary cancers. Unlike with most other epithelial cancers, the presence of regional lymph node metastases in the younger population (less than 40 years old) does not appear to adversely affect prognosis as long as the disease is resectable. The overall mortality from papillary thyroid cancer ranges from 1 to 10% and is usually due to aggres-

sive local regional behavior with tracheoesophageal and mediastinal involvement or from dedifferentiation to a more anaplastic tumor over time.

Answer: B, D, E

25. A 29-year-old man presents with a 2-cm firm mass in the right thyroid lobe that is positive for papillary carcinoma on needle aspiration cytology and a 1.5-cm ipsilateral lower deep jugular lymph node metastasis. Which of the following would be inappropriate treatment plans?

A. Thyroid lobectomy with external beam radiotherapy to the involved neck
B. Total thyroidectomy and ipsilateral radical neck dissection
C. Thyroid lobectomy followed by radioiodine therapy
D. Total thyroidectomy with ipsilateral modified radical neck dissection
E. Total thyroidectomy and bilateral modified radical neck dissection
F. Excision of thyroid lobe and isthmus with ipsilateral modified radical neck dissection
G. Enucleation of the primary tumor from the thyroid gland and external beam radiotherapy to the involved neck
H. Excision of thyroid lobe and isthmus and paratracheal node dissection

Sabiston: 604
Schwartz: 1569

Comment: Papillary thyroid cancer is primarily a surgically treated disease, with radiation therapy reserved for unresectable disease. Management of the primary tumor is somewhat controversial in terms of the extensiveness of the thyroidectomy required. Enucleation of the tumor without anatomic dissection of the involved lobe is generally discouraged because of the risk of hemorrhage and inadvertent injury to the recurrent laryngeal nerve and parathyroid glands. Excision of the involved thyroid lobe and isthmus is an acceptable approach for small papillary carcinomas that are contained within that lobe. Those preferring this approach do so because of the risk of hypoparathyroidism and nerve injury incurred when the clinically uninvolved contralateral lobe is resected. Others believe that a more extensive resection to include the near total or total removal of the contralateral lobe is warranted. The rationale for this more aggressive approach is based on the recognized incidence of multicentric disease (albeit with an unclear clinical significance) and the facilitation of possible postoperative radioiodine therapy by surgical ablation of the remaining thyroid parenchyma. ● The management of cervical lymph node metastases has become considerably more conservative in recent decades; it is now generally accepted that a modified radical neck dissection (sparing the sternocleidomastoid muscle, internal jugular vein, and spinal accessory nerve) is appropriate for the management of clinically evident cervical node metastases. Some feel that even less radical surgery with the removal of only the grossly positive nodes (the so-called berry-picking procedure) may also be appropriate. Prophylactic dissection of the clinically uninvolved neck (ipsilateral or contralateral) is discouraged for management of papillary thyroid carcinoma, as it has not been shown to be beneficial. For patients with a clinically uninvolved neck from a proven papillary carcinoma, prophylactic paratracheal lymph node dissection may be appropriate, as it can easily be performed without extending the incision and without functional or cosmetic compromise. Further, it removes the station I lymph nodes that are most likely to be involved by papillary carcinoma. • Radioiodine therapy may be beneficial in the management of papillary thyroid carcinoma, although pure papillary carcinomas do not take up radioiodine as frequently as follicular carcinomas. Nonetheless, many clinicians would manage the patient with lateral cervical metastases described above with postoperative residual thyroid ablation with radioiodine and subsequent iodine scanning for clinically occult metastases. Others would delay such treatment until clinical evidence of disease occurred. • External beam radiation therapy has little utility in the management of papillary carcinoma except in instances in which disease is unresectable and unresponsive to radioiodine.

Answer: A, B, C, E, G, H

26. Which of the following statements is/are correct regarding follicular thyroid carcinoma?

A. The diagnosis is based more on the individual cytologic characteristics than on the overall tumor growth characteristics
B. The presence of a discrete capsule around the tumor essentially rules out malignancy
C. Distant metastases are more common than regional nodal metastases
D. The incidence of multicentricity is approximately the same as with papillary thyroid carcinomas

Sabiston: 606
Schwartz: 1570

Comment: Like papillary carcinoma, follicular carcinoma of the thyroid is considered a well differentiated form of thyroid cancer. Frequently characteristics of both papillary and follicular tumors are found within the same neoplasm. The pure follicular carcinoma is difficult to diagnose on cytologic characteristics alone, as the cell appears quite similar to its benign counterpart found in follicular adenomas. The diagnosis is more reliably obtained by the identification of vascular or capsular invasion by the tumor. Such invasive characteristics may be present, even though the capsule appears to be quite discrete and intact grossly. Unlike papillary carcinomas of the thyroid, follicular carcinomas spread primarily hematogenously and their metastatic potential is more likely distant than regional. The favored sites of distant metastases are bone, lung, and liver. Multicentricity within the thyroid gland does not appear to be nearly as common with follicular carcinomas as it is with papillary carcinomas.

Answer: C

27. A 45-year-old woman with a firm 3-cm nodule of the left thyroid lobe undergoes left thyroid lobectomy and is found by frozen section to have a follicular carcinoma with capsular invasion. Which of the following additional treatment modalities may be appropriate in this situation?

A. Performance of a near total or total thyroidectomy
B. Radical neck dissection on the involved side

C. Exogenous thyroid administration to suppress TSH
D. Radioiodine scan to detect pulmonary metastases with appropriate surgical resection if found
E. Ablation of residual thyroid tissue and any demonstrated metastases with radioiodine

Sabiston: 606
Schwartz: 1570

Comment: As is the case with papillary thyroid carcinoma, the extent of thyroid resection in follicular thyroid carcinoma is controversial. Some favor removing only the involved lobe because of the reduced morbidity and relying on subsequent radioiodine ablation of the remaining thyroid tissue if necessary. Others favor total thyroidectomy, as this facilitates the detection of metastases by radioiodine postoperatively. The relatively low likelihood of multicentric follicular carcinoma does not alone warrant the performance of a total thyroidectomy. Regional lymph node metastases from pure follicular thyroid carcinomas are relatively uncommon and certainly make prophylactic neck dissection inappropriate. When involved cervical lymph nodes are found, they are best managed by a modified neck dissection with preservation of the sternocleidomastoid muscle, internal jugular vein, and spinal accessory nerve. Resection of the grossly apparent regional lymph nodes alone may be appropriate. Radioiodine scanning for the presence of metastases is useful in follicular thyroid carcinoma, but its accuracy increases when the residual normal thyroid tissue has been ablated, either by surgery or a prior dose of radioiodine. When metastases are found by radioiodine scanning, these are best treated by ablative doses of radioiodine. Resection of isolated metastases may occasionally be appropriate if they do not have an affinity for iodine. The growth of well differentiated thyroid carcinomas may to some extent be under the influence of TSH. For that reason, patients should receive exogenous thyroid hormone in doses that keep the serum TSH at a low level. Many cases of regression of known metastatic follicular carcinoma with exogenous thyroid therapy alone have been reported.

Answer: A, C, E

28. Which one or more of the following statements regarding medullary thyroid carcinoma is/are correct?

A. It is derived from a dedifferentiated variant of the same cell that produces papillary/follicular carcinomas
B. Its pattern of metastatic spread is almost exclusively to distant sites
C. The serum calcitonin level is useful in diagnosis and management
D. The prognosis is approximately as favorable as that of papillary carcinoma

Sabiston: 612
Schwartz: 1571

Comment: Medullary carcinoma accounts for approximately 10% of all thyroid carcinomas. Its cell of origin is the C-cell or parafollicular cell, which is believed to be of neural crest origin and bears no embryologic association with the epithelial cell origin of papillary and follicular tumors. This cell is responsible for production of calcitonin, which is involved in calcium homeostasis. Marked elevations of serum calcitonin levels are diagnostic for C-cell hyperplasia (considered to be a premalignant condition) and frank medullary carcinoma; and changes in the serum calcitonin level may be useful in reflecting the success of treatment and the presence of recurrent disease. Medullary thyroid carcinoma has the propensity to spread to both regional lymph nodes and distant metastatic sites, and its prognosis depends on the presence or absence of regional and distant metastases. The overall 5-year survival is approximately 50%, which is considerably less than that of the well differentiated thyroid carcinomas.

Answer: C

29. Match the following characteristics of medullary thyroid carcinoma with their appropriate associations with either the sporadic or the familial form.

A. More likely to be multi-   a. Sporadic
    centric   b. Familial
B. Occurs at an earlier age
C. Better prognosis
D. More likely associated
    with marked hyperten-
    sion
E. More likely associated
    with hypercalcemia

Schwartz: 1571

Comment: Medullary carcinoma of the thyroid may occur as a sporadic case (approximately 75%) or as a familial form (approximately 25%) inherited as an autosomal dominant. There is no clear-cut sex predilection; and although these tumors may be found in virtually all age groups, there is a propensity for the familial form to occur at a much earlier age (median age—early 20's). The familial form is also characterized by an extremely high likelihood of multicentricity within the gland. The familial form frequently occurs as part of the multiple endocrine neoplasia Type II syndrome, which is associated with hyperparathyroidism and pheochromocytoma. Owing in part to the associated endocrine abnormalities and in part to the more virulent biologic behavior, medullary carcinoma of the thyroid in the familial form carries a considerably worse prognosis than the sporadic form.

Answer: A–b; B–b; C–a; D–b; E–b

30. Which of the following statements is/are correct regarding the management of a patient with medullary thyroid carcinoma?

A. The patient should be screened for hyperparathyroidism and pheochromocytoma only if hypercalcemia and hypertension, respectively, exist
B. If the familial form is present, total thyroidectomy is indicated
C. If cervical lymph node metastases are present without distant disease, radical neck dissection should be performed even though the likelihood of long-term survival is less than 10%
D. If pheochromocytoma is found, the adrenal surgery should precede the thyroid surgery
E. If hyperparathyroidism is found, this may be surgically managed at the time of thyroidectomy by removing the two largest parathyroid glands

Sabiston: 612
Schwartz: 1571

Comment: The incidence of familial medullary thyroid carcinoma is probably underestimated, as the disease may have been unrecognized or unreported in other family members. One must be alert to the possibility of multiple endocrine neoplasia, therefore, in all patients with medullary thyroid carcinoma with or without a family history of same. Therefore, it is reasonable to screen for hyperparathyroidism (PTH and calcium levels) and pheochromocytoma (urinary catecholamines and VMA) in all patients with medullary thyroid carcinoma. If evidence of pheochromocytoma exists, this problem must be dealt with first, as there is a significant risk of catastrophic blood pressure fluctuations during surgery in the presence of pheochromocytoma. If hyperparathyroidism is found, this is almost always due to four-gland hyperplasia and is best treated by excision of three and one-half glands or, more popularly, total parathyroidectomy with implantation of a small amount of parathyroid tissue in the forearm musculature. The parathyroid surgery should be carried out at the same time as the thyroid surgery. Although sporadic cases of medullary carcinoma can be managed by excision of the involved thyroid lobe and isthmus, total thyroidectomy is considered to be the treatment of choice, and especially so in the familial form. Medullary thyroid carcinoma tends to spread first to the regional lymph nodes and then to distant sites, and therefore thyroidectomy with radical neck dissection in the presence of clinically evident cervical lymph nodes is appropriate therapy and is associated with 10-year survivals approaching 50%.

Answer: B, D

CHAPTER 20

Parathyroid

1. Which of the following statements regarding the embryology of the parathyroid glands is/are correct?

A. The upper parathyroids arise from the third branchial pouch

B. The lower parathyroids arise from the fourth branchial pouch

C. The upper parathyroids are embryologically associated with the thyroid gland

D. The lower parathyroids are embryologically associated with the thymus gland

E. In the adult, the lower parathyroid glands are found over a wider anatomic range than are the upper parathyroids

Sabiston: 620
Schwartz: 1578

Comments: The upper parathyroid glands arise from the fourth branchial pouch in association with the lateral thyroid complex. Paradoxically, the lower parathyroid glands rise from a higher branchial pouch (the third) in association with the thymus. They achieve their characteristically lower position in the adult because of the more caudal descent of the thymus gland into the mediastinum. Because of the longer range of descent that these elements of the third branchial pouch undergo, the lower parathyroids are found over a wider anatomic range (from the pharynx to the pericardium) than are the upper parathyroids, which bear a fairly constant relationship to the posterolateral aspect of the thyroid gland.

Answer: C, D, E

2. Which of the following statements about parathyroid anatomy is/are correct?

A. The superior parathyroids usually receive their blood supply from the superior thyroid artery

B. The inferior parathyroids usually receive their blood supply from the inferior thyroid artery

C. A parathyroid weighing 25 to 30 mg should be considered to be hypoplastic

D. Variations from the usual four parathyroid glands are found in at least 30% of cases

Sabiston: 620
Schwartz: 1579

Comments: Normal parathyroid glands in adults are flat, ovoid structures measuring approximately 3×6 mm and weighing approximately 25 to 30 mg each. Both the superior and inferior parathyroids derive their blood supply from the inferior thyroid artery in the majority of cases. Occasionally the superior parathyroids may be supplied by branches of the superior thyroid artery. Eighty to 90% of patients have four parathyroid glands. The other 10 to 20% of patients may have supernumerary glands (usually totaling five or six), which may be due to fragmentation of the original four glands during embryologic descent. The presence of fewer than the usual four glands has been reported; however, this must be viewed with caution as inability to find a gland does not prove its absence.

Answer: B

3. Which of the following statements about the physiology of parathyroid hormone (PTH) is/are correct?

A. Normally, PTH secretion is inversely related to the serum calcium level

B. PTH secretion is under partial control of the pituitary via parathyroid stimulating hormone (PSH)

C. PTH has a direct action on bone, causing calcium release via active transport mechanisms

D. PTH has an indirect effect on the renal reabsorption of phosphate, which is controlled primarily by the action of vitamin D

E. PTH has a direct effect on the gut, promoting intestinal absorption of dietary calcium

Sabiston: 621
Schwartz: 1586

Comments: Parathyroid hormone, the principal mediator of calcium homeostasis, is secreted from the parathyroid gland in response to fluctuations in serum calcium concentration. This is a direct feedback system in which the secretion of PTH is inversely related to the serum calcium level. There is no pituitary control over PTH secretion. PTH has direct effects on the bone and kidney and an indirect effect on the gut, all of which result in an increased serum calcium concentration. In the bone, PTH stimulates calcium release via active transport mechanisms as well as lysosomal enzyme systems. In the kidney, PTH causes a decrease in calcium clearance, as well as an increased excretion of renal phosphate via inhibition of tubular reabsorption. Intestinal absorption of dietary calcium appears to be primarily under the control of metabolites of the vitamin D complex, the formation of which is facilitated by PTH.

Answer: A, C

4. Which of the following statements regarding vitamin D physiology is/are correct?

A. The major nondietary source of Vitamin D is hepatic synthesis
B. Hydroxylation of vitamin D_3 results in a loss of metabolic activity
C. Vitamin D increases intestinal absorption of dietary calcium
D. Vitamin D has a direct effect on bone, resulting in calcium and phosphorus mobilization

Sabiston: 622
Schwartz: 1583

Comments: The natural form of vitamin D (vitamin D_3 or cholecalciferol) is produced primarily by ultraviolet activation of 7-dehydrocholesterol in the skin. Vitamin D_3 undergoes an initial hydroxylation in the liver and a second hydroxylation in the kidney under PTH control to its most active form. This dihydroxy vitamin D_3 is the form of the vitamin complex that is responsible for its primary physiologic functions, namely, facilitation of intestinal absorption of dietary calcium and mobilization of calcium and phosphorus from bone.

Answer: C, D

5. Which of the following statements regarding calcitonin is/are correct?

A. It is manufactured by follicular cells that originate at the base of the tongue
B. It induces urinary excretion of phosphate
C. It inhibits bone resorption
D. It is of greater physiologic importance in humans than in other mammals

Sabiston: 622
Schwartz: 1584

Comments: Calcitonin is a hormone secreted by the parafollicular (C) cells of the thyroid. These cells are probably of neural crest origin and migrate to join the lateral thyroid lobes of branchial pouch origin during embryologic development. The principal effect of calcitonin is to lower serum calcium levels, primarily by inducing urinary excretion of phosphate and inhibiting bone resorption of calcium and phosphorus. These physiologic effects appear to be much more important in the calcium homeostasis of phylogenetically lower mammals than they are in humans, as exemplified by the relatively normal calcium metabolism that is found in patients who have undergone total thyroidectomy.

Answer: B, C

6. Match the laboratory or physiologic findings in the left-hand column with the appropriate categorization of hyperparathyroidism in the right-hand column:

A. High-normal to high serum calcium; high serum PTH
B. Low-normal to low serum calcium; high serum PTH
C. Compensatory hyperfunction
D. Autonomous hyperfunction
E. Underlying renal disease
F. Underlying malabsorption syndrome

a. Primary hyperparathyroidism
b. Secondary hyperparathyroidism
c. Tertiary hyperparathyroidism

Sabiston: 622
Schwartz: 1587, 1617

Comments: Hyperparathyroidism refers to the production of abnormally large amounts of parathyroid hormone. This may be associated with high, normal, or low serum calcium levels depending on the underlying mechanism. In primary hyperparathyroidism, one or more parathyroid glands are autonomously functioning without the normal negative feedback response to the serum calcium level. This usually results in elevations of both serum calcium and PTH levels. Secondary hyperparathyroidism is considered a compensatory response by the parathyroid glands to hypocalcemia. Most often the hypocalcemia is secondary to underlying renal disease (causing hyperphosphatemia and a reduction of 1,25[OH]$_2$ vitamin D_3) and intestinal malabsorption syndromes. In secondary hyperparathyroidism, the PTH level is elevated; however, because of abnormal calcium losses, the serum calcium level rarely rises above the low-normal range. Tertiary hyperparathyroidism generally refers to cases of secondary hyperparathyroidism in which long-standing stimulation of the parathyroid glands by hypocalcemia results in the autonomous hyperfunction of those glands. In such cases, the parathyroid hormone level remains high and the serum calcium level becomes high-normal to elevated.

Answer: A–a, c; B–b; C–b; D–a, c; E–b, c; F–b

7. Which of the following entities may be responsible for hypercalcemia?

A. Vitamin D intoxication
B. Milk-alkali syndrome
C. Multiple basal cell carcinomas
D. Multiple myeloma
E. Metastatic carcinoma
F. Hyperthyroidism
G. Hypothyroidism

Sabiston: 629
Schwartz: 1607

Comments: All of the above entities except for multiple basal cell carcinomas and hypothyroidism may result in hypercalcemia. **Vitamin D intoxication** causes increased intestinal absorption of calcium and calcium resorption from the bone. The **milk-alkali syndrome** is seen in patients taking large amounts of milk and antacids for peptic ulcer disease, resulting in increased calcium available for intestinal absorption and decreased renal excretion of calcium. **Multiple myeloma** may cause hypercalcemia because of the bone destruction associated with that disease. **Metastatic carcinoma** may also produce hypercalcemia. Initially this was thought to be due solely to bone destruction from osseous metastases; however, many cancers produce a PTH-like substance that may also result in hypercalcemia. **Hyperthyroidism** may cause hypercalcemia by virtue of the increased bone turnover from the hypermetabolic state.

Answer: A, B, D, E, F

8. Which of the following is the least common presenting condition in patients found to be hypercalcemic?

A. Completely asymptomatic
B. Arthralgia
C. Muscle weakness
D. Confusion
E. Constipation

Sabiston: 623
Schwartz: 1593

Comments: See Question 9.

9. Which of the following disease states is/are associated with hyperparathyroidism?

A. Hypertension
B. Peptic ulcer disease
C. Diabetes mellitus
D. Pancreatitis

Sabiston: 623
Schwartz: 1593

Comments: Because of the importance of calcium in bone structure, neuromuscular activity, and membrane stabilization, the symptoms of hypercalcemia may vary widely in nature (from asymptomatic to multi–organ system complaints) and severity (from asymptomatic to coma and death). With the increasing application of polychemistry serum testing, asymptomatic hypercalcemia is being diagnosed with greater frequency and, in fact, probably represents the most common clinical presentation of the hypercalcemic patient. The most common complaints seen at initial presentation include muscle weakness, arthralgia, constipation, and polyuria. Many other presenting symptoms may also be seen, including bone pain, myalgia, abdominal pain, and mental status changes; however, these are less common initial symptoms. Hyperparathyroidism may also be associated with other disease states. It has been shown to have a variable association with hypertension, usually in more severe cases of hyperparathyroidism. The mechanism for this association is thought to be related to underlying renal disease. Hyperparathyroidism has also been associated with an increased incidence of peptic ulcer disease (possibly related to increased gastrin production stimulated by PTH excess) and pancreatitis (possibly due to calcium deposition and an increased incidence of cholelithiasis).

Answer: Question 8: D
Question 9: A, B, D

10. Which of the following bone and cartilage abnormalities is/are characteristic of hyperparathyroidism?

A. Subperiosteal bone resorption
B. Sclerosis of the calvarium
C. Calcium deposition in articular cartilage
D. Multiple bone cysts
E. Increased bone density

Sabiston: 624
Schwartz: 1594

Comments: One of the principal actions of PTH is the stimulation of calcium resorption from bone. As expected, this produces characteristic radiographic findings of demineralization. Radiographically, this is most readily demonstrated on x-ray films of the hands in which subperiosteal resorption is seen (most easily along the radial aspect of the middle phalanx of the second and third digits). This is considered pathognomonic of hyperparathyroidism and may further be associated with tufting of the distal phalanges. The calvarium is also commonly involved with radiographic evidence of demineralization. This is seen as a mottled granular appearance with obliteration of the normal vascular grooves. Osteoclastomas or "brown tumors" appearing as bone cysts with sharp margins near the cortex are also characteristic of hyperparathyroidism. Excess calcium may be abnormally deposited in many tissues in hyperparathyroidism, including articular cartilages and menisci.

Answer: A, C, D

11. Which of the following laboratory determinations is/are characteristic of primary hyperparathyroidism?

A. A borderline elevated serum calcium with borderline elevated PTH
B. Low serum phosphate
C. Chloride/phosphate ratio greater than 33
D. Elevated alkaline phosphatase

Sabiston: 626
Schwartz: 1596

Comments: The effects of excess PTH on bone (increased calcium resorption) and on the kidneys (increased phosphorus and bicarbonate excretion and chloride retention) account for the characteristic biochemical laboratory findings in primary hyperparathyroidism: elevated serum calcium, elevated serum PTH level, elevated serum chloride, elevated serum alkaline phosphatase, and decreased serum phosphate. It is important to remember, however, that the relationships between two or more of these determinations may be more diagnostic than the absolute value of any one alone. For example, it is possible to have both serum calcium and PTH levels within the normal range; however, if they are both within the high-normal range, this is highly suggestive of primary hyperparathyroidism, insofar as the normal inverse relationship between the two would suggest that a high-normal calcium would cause a reduction in PTH production. Similarly, the serum chloride level may be in the high-normal range and the serum phosphate level in the low-normal range, and yet if their ratio exceeds 33, this is highly suggestive of underlying primary hyperparathyroidism. Since the calcium, phosphate, chloride, and alkaline phosphatase levels are all measurable by standard polychemistry screening tests, the diagnosis of primary hyperparathyroidism is usually easily suggested by these simple tests. Confirmation, however, generally requires the simultaneous determination of serum PTH and calcium levels.

Answer: A, B, C, D

12. Which of the following statements regarding renal diseases associated with hyperparathyroidism is/are correct?

A. The term nephrolithiasis refers to minute calcifications within the renal parenchyma
B. Nephrocalcinosis is more common than nephrolithiasis in hyperparathyroidism
C. Permanent renal damage is more likely to occur with nephrocalcinosis than with nephrolithiasis
D. Nephrolithiasis is more easily treated than nephrocalcinosis

Sabiston: 623
Schwartz: 1596

Comments: The excess serum calcium seen in primary hyperparathyroidism may induce renal damage in two principal ways. Nephrolithiasis is the formation of stones within the collecting system of the kidneys. These may cause mechanical irritation, infection, or obstruction of the collecting system, and if chronic and severe may lead to decreased renal function. Fortunately, nephrolithiasis is reasonably easily treated by the surgical removal of the stones or by awaiting their spontaneous passage. The propensity to form these stones is reversed when the offending parathyroid gland(s) is/are removed. Nephrocalcinosis is a process of renal parenchymal calcification leading fairly predictably to decreased renal function, which is irreversible even after correction of the underlying hyperparathyroid state. Of the two forms of renal damage, nephrolithiasis is more commonly seen (30%) than is nephrocalcinosis (5 to 10%).

Answer: C, D

13. The incidence of primary hyperparathyroidism is correctly described by which one or more of the following statements?

A. There has been an overall increased incidence in recent years
B. It is most often due to a single adenoma (in approximately 80% of cases)
C. The incidence of four-gland hyperplasia is decreasing
D. Approximately 10% of cases are seen in children under 10 years of age
E. The incidence may be increased in patients with a history of exposure to low-dose radiotherapy

Sabiston: 622
Schwartz: 1587

Comments: The reported incidence of primary hyperparathyroidism has increased in recent years, probably owing in great part to the increased application of polychemistry screening profiles, which have detected increasing numbers of asymptomatic hypercalcemic patients. The incidence of primary hyperparathyroidism increases with age; the disease is extremely rare in

individuals under 10 years of age. A history of prior low-dose ionizing radiation to the head and neck area appears to increase one's risk of developing primary hyperparathyroidism, and this would be analogous to the increased incidence of well-differentiated thyroid cancer and salivary gland tumors in similarly exposed patients. For those with primary hyperparathyroidism, the cause in approximately 80% of cases is a single adenomatous gland. However, the incidence of four-gland hyperplasia as the cause of primary hyperparathyroidism has been increasing. This may be due in part to increased recognition of hyperplasia on the part of pathologists.

Answer: A, B, E

14. Which of the following statements regarding the pathology of primary hyperparathyroidism is/are correct?

A. The presence of hyperplastic tissue surrounded by a rim of normal-appearing parathyroid tissue essentially confirms the diagnosis of adenoma
B. Chief cell hyperplasia is the most common form of parathyroid hyperplasia
C. Clear cell hyperplasia of the parathyroid gland is incapable of producing primary hyperparathyroidism
D. When more than one gland is pathologically enlarged, the diagnosis of hyperplasia must be made

Sabiston: 634
Schwartz: 1587

Comments: The differentiation of adenoma from hyperplasia as the cause of primary hyperparathyroidism is at times difficult. The classic gross finding of a single enlarged gland with three normal or small remaining glands associated with the histologic finding of hyperplastic tissue surrounded by a rim of normal-appearing parathyroid tissue in the large gland is diagnostic of an adenoma. Such adenomas may be found in more than one gland at exploration, in which case the diagnosis of multiple adenomas rather than hyperplasia should be made. This is uncommon, however, probably accounting for fewer than 5% of cases. When more than one gland is abnormally enlarged, the more likely diagnosis is hyperplasia. Chief cell hyperplasia is the most common subtype of parathyroid hyperplasia. Clear cell hyperplasia as a cause of primary hyperparathyroidism was more commonly diagnosed in the past. The frozen section evaluation of parathyroid glands during exploration to differentiate hyperplasia from adenoma may at times be difficult. Unless the characteristic rim of normal tissue is seen, the hyperplastic nature of both adenomas and true hyperplasia is quite similar. Frequently the intraoperative decision as to whether one is dealing with an adenoma or a hyperplasia problem depends upon the gross characteristics of the glands identified at exploration.

Answer: A, B

15. Which of the following statements is/are correct regarding parathyroid carcinoma?

A. It accounts for less than 5% of all cases of primary hyperparathyroidism
B. Only 5 to 10% of patients with parathyroid carcinoma manifest hypercalcemia

C. The cytologic criteria differentiating parathyroid carcinoma from adenoma are fairly well established
D. Among patients with parathyroid carcinoma, more deaths are due to the effects of hypercalcemia than to the tumor bulk or metastases
E. Surgical resection should not be undertaken unless there is a reasonable expectation to remove all known disease

Sabiston: 627
Schwartz: 1590

Comments: Parathyroid carcinoma as a cause of hyperparathyroidism is rare, accounting for only 1 to 3% of cases. Like many other neuroendocrine tumors, carcinoma of the parathyroid does not prevent the gland from carrying out its endocrine function (namely PTH production); however, regulation of PTH production is usually impaired, and as many as 85% of patients with parathyroid carcinoma will present with hypercalcemia. Of note is that the hypercalcemia is usually quite severe, frequently manifesting serum calcium concentrations in excess of 14 mg/dl. Again, as with several other neuroendocrine tumors, the cytologic criteria for malignancy are poorly defined, and it may be quite difficult at times to differentiate a parathyroid carcinoma from adenoma based on histology alone. Evidence of local invasion or regional or distant metastases may be needed to confirm the diagnosis of carcinoma. Obviously, the greatest likelihood of cure exists when all known disease can be surgically resected with or without adjuvant radiation therapy. However, surgical "debulking" of known disease can be beneficial in reducing the PTH levels and thereby palliating the symptoms of severe hypercalcemia.

Answer: A, D

16. A patient previously diagnosed as having primary hyperparathyroidism presents with rapidly developing muscular weakness, nausea, vomiting, and confusion, and the diagnosis of hyperparathyroid crisis is made. Which one or more of the following statements is/are correct?

A. One can expect the serum calcium level to be in the range of 16 to 20 mg/dl
B. Fluid restriction is an appropriate first step in management
C. Vigorous hydration with intravenous saline should be started immediately
D. Intravenous furosemide is likely to be helpful in management
E. Intravenous mithramycin is contraindicated because of its toxic effect
F. Immediate parathyroid exploration should be carried out to prevent coma and death
G. Surgical intervention has little chance of success in such severe cases of hyperparathyroidism

Sabiston: 628
Schwartz: 1610

Comments: For reasons that are unclear, patients with mild to moderate hypercalcemia from primary hyperparathyroidism may suddenly develop a hyperparathyroid crisis in which the serum calcium rises to levels frequently greater than 16 mg/dl. This should be considered

a medical emergency, the initial management of which is designed to lower the serum calcium level acutely. This is best accomplished by vigorous saline diuresis via intravenous infusion and diuretic therapy. When such therapy is ineffective or contraindicated because of other medical conditions, intravenous mithramycin can effectively lower the serum calcium within 24 hours of administration and should probably be employed despite its side effects and potential renal and hepatic toxicity. Parathyroid exploration with resection of the offending gland(s) represents the definitive treatment of this entity, but should be delayed until the serum calcium is brought down to a safer level.

Answer: A, C, D

17. A patient requires parathyroid exploration for primary hyperparathyroidism. During the exploration an abnormally large parathyroid gland is found posterior to the lower pole of the right thyroid lobe. Which of the following choices is the appropriate course to take at this point?

A. Excise the enlarged gland without identification of the other parathyroid glands
B. Excise the enlarged gland, then identify the three remaining glands, and if they appear normal, perform biopsies of all three to confirm normal histology
C. Identify the remaining glands, and if they appear normal in size, excise the large one and perform a biopsy of one of the remaining ones
D. Identify the remaining glands and excise the large one and two of the three remaining ones

Sabiston: 631
Schwartz: 1613

Comments: See Question 18.

18. On further exploration of the patient described in Question 17, the three remaining glands are encountered and all appear to be abnormally enlarged similar to the first gland found. Which one or more of the following options would be appropriate at this point?

A. Resect all four glands
B. Resect the two largest glands only
C. Resect three glands and a portion of the fourth
D. Resect all four glands and implant a portion of one in the forearm musculature
E. Resect the largest gland and one half of each of the three remaining glands

Sabiston: 633
Schwartz: 1613

Comments: The differentiation between an adenoma and four-gland hyperplasia as the cause of hyperparathyroidism is frequently more easily made by the gross findings at operation than by the histologic findings. When a large gland is found during exploration, the surgeon needs to identify at least one additional normal-sized gland in order to feel confident that one is dealing with an adenoma. Ideally, all three remaining glands should be found; if they are normal in size, the surgeon is fairly secure in removing only the enlarged gland. A shave biopsy of one of the three normal-appearing glands is useful in confirming its normal histology. A biopsy of all three remaining glands carries the risk of injuring or devascularizing all three, rendering the patient permanently hypoparathyroid. If one large and one normal-sized gland are found, but the other two glands are not easily identified, many surgeons would not pursue a more intense search for the remaining glands on the grounds that the risk of injuring those glands and rendering the patient hypoparathyroid may outweigh the very small possibility of the patient harboring multiple adenomas. If more than one enlarged gland is found, it is likely that four-gland hyperplasia is the cause of the hyperparathyroidism. In such an instance, it is more important that all four glands be identified. If indeed, all four are enlarged, the generally accepted options for management include either resecting three glands and a portion of the fourth (leaving approximately 40 to 60 mg of a single gland in place), or resecting all four glands and implanting a morcellated portion of one of the glands into a readily accessible muscle. Implantation into the forearm musculature permits re-exploration of that area should hyperparathyroidism persist without the inherent dangers of a cervical re-exploration. The obvious goal in managing four-gland hyperplasia is to leave enough parathyroid tissue to prevent permanent hypoparathyroidism.

Answer: Question 17: C
Question 18: C, D

19. During exploration for primary hyperparathyroidism, two normal-appearing glands on the left and one normal-appearing gland on the right are found after exploring the paratracheal areas bilaterally. The fourth gland is not found after a thorough search of its expected anatomic location. The most appropriate course of action would be:

A. Terminate the operation with no further dissection
B. Extend the exploration through the existing cervical incision to include the parathymic and paraesophageal areas of the upper mediastinum, the carotid sheath, and the para- and retroesophageal areas down to the vertebral bodies and terminate the operation if the fourth gland is not found
C. Resect the three glands found, leaving the fourth to maintain normal PTH levels
D. Extend the incision into the right neck laterally to explore the entire neck, including the posterior triangle
E. Close the cervical incision and perform a median sternotomy to explore the mediastinum for an ectopic parathyroid

Sabiston: 631
Schwartz: 1613

Comments: One of the more frustrating aspects of parathyroid surgery is the inability to find one of the parathyroid glands that is suspected to be the cause of the hyperparathyroidism. In the above clinical situation, three normal-appearing glands were found, raising the likelihood that an adenoma of the fourth gland exists in an ectopic location. Understanding the embryology of parathyroid descent enables one to select those areas in which the gland is most likely to be found. This includes the central compartment of the neck from carotid to ca-

rotid, posteriorly to the vertebral body, superiorly to the level of the pharynx and carotid bulb, and inferiorly into the mediastinum. All of these areas, including the upper portion of the mediastinum, can be explored through the existing cervical collar incision, and this exploration should be carried out at the time of the initial operation. If the adenoma is not found after this more extensive search, it is likely that the adenoma is in the mediastinum in an area not accessible through the collar incision. A small possibility exists that the adenoma is truly subcapsular within the ipsilateral thyroid lobe, and some would perform a thyroid lobectomy on the side of the missing gland. Extending the cervical exploration to include the posterior triangle will not be fruitful, as the parathyroid gland would not be found in that location. Although sternotomy may be required to identify the missing gland, most surgeons would delay this procedure until after the performance of sophisticated localization studies. Prior to closing, normal histology (i.e., nonhyperplastic tissue) should be confirmed by biopsy of one or two of the three normal-appearing glands that were found. It would be inappropriate to resect all three glands, as the patient would then be rendered hypoparathyroid once the adenoma is found and resected.

Answer: B

20. Which of the following parathyroid localization studies would be inappropriate to obtain before an initial parathyroid exploration?

A. Sonography
B. Technetium-thallium scan
C. CT scan
D. Angiography
E. Selective venous sampling for PTH

Sabiston: 630
Schwartz: 1600

Comments: Preoperative localization of one or more enlarged parathyroid glands may greatly facilitate parathyroid exploration and in selected circumstances reduce the morbidity of the surgery by allowing the surgeon to avoid unnecessary dissection near clinically normal glands. However, one must weigh the risk versus the benefit of the localization studies employed before obtaining them. All of the studies listed above are useful in localizing abnormally enlarged or hyperfunctioning parathyroids. Sonography and CT scan are noninvasive techniques that will demonstrate abnormally enlarged glands in a significant percentage of cases. Sonography seems to be a little more accurate (approximately 70% accuracy) and is less expensive than CT scanning and therefore is preferred as the initial localization procedure by many. Technetium-thallium scanning is a radionuclide subtraction technique in which the thyroid (which takes up both technetium and thallium) is "erased" from the scan image of the parathyroid glands (which take up thallium, not technetium), leaving an image of any enlarged parathyroid glands. This technique is also relatively noninvasive and has an accuracy in the 70% range. Any of these three studies may be appropriate in the preoperative evaluation of a patient with hyperparathyroidism. Angiography, which may localize parathyroid glands by creating a vascular blush with the contrast material, may be useful; however, it is potentially hazardous, carrying the risk of reaction to the contrast material and myelitis with hemi- or quadriplegia. Selective venous sampling from the brachiocephalic venous circulation may be useful in detecting the source of abnormally high production of PTH, but, like angiography, is a moderately invasive procedure. These two latter procedures are generally reserved for use in patients undergoing a second cervical exploration or a sternotomy to locate a gland not found at initial exploration.

Answer: D, E

21. A patient presents with hypercalcemia, severe recurrent peptic ulcer disease, and acromegaly. Of the following, the most likely diagnosis is:

A. MEN-I
B. MEN-IIA
C. MEN-IIB
D. MEN-III
E. Pituitary adenocarcinoma

Sabiston: 627
Schwartz: 1604

Comments: See Question 23.

22. A patient presents with hypercalcemia, markedly elevated and labile blood pressure, and a thyroid mass. Of the following, the most likely diagnosis is:

A. MEN-I
B. MEN-IIA
C. MEN-IIB
D. MEN-III

Sabiston: 627
Schwartz: 1604

Comments: See Question 23.

23. Following the proper documentation of the diagnosis, the correct management of the patient described in Question 22 would be:

A. Urgent parathyroid exploration to reduce serum calcium followed by subsequent resection of the pheochromocytoma, followed in turn by resection of the thyroid tumor
B. Immediate resection of the pheochromocytoma followed in several weeks by thyroid/parathyroid exploration
C. Pharmacologic management of the blood pressure followed by resection of the pheochromocytoma and then by thyroid/parathyroid exploration
D. Pharmacologic management of the blood pressure followed by simultaneous resection of the pheochromocytoma and thyroid and parathyroid abnormalities during the same operation

Sabiston: 615
Schwartz: 1528

Comments: Most cases of primary hyperparathyroidism occur in a sporadic distribution in the general population. There is a small subset of patients, however, who

manifest a familial tendency to develop hyperparathyroidism. This may occur alone as the only endocrine abnormality or may occur in association with other endocrine abnormalities (multiple endocrine neoplasia or MEN syndromes). The MEN-I syndrome in its fully expressed state consists of pituitary adenomas (usually producing acromegaly), parathyroid hyperplasia, and neoplasms of the pancreatic islet cells (e.g., gastrinoma, insulinoma). The MEN-II syndrome consists of medullary carcinoma of the thyroid variably associated with parathyroid hyperplasia and pheochromocytoma. In the fully expressed form of the subtype MEN-IIA, all three of these entities exist. MEN-IIB syndrome consists of medullary carcinoma of the thyroid and pheochromocytoma in association with ganglioneuromatous soft tissue nodules and a marfanoid habitus, but no hyperparathyroidism. There is no MEN-III syndrome. The management of patients with MEN-I depends on the severity of symptomatology associated with the individual components. Resection of the pituitary adenoma, parathyroidectomy, and pharmacologic or surgical management of the pancreatic tumor may all be appropriate and need not be performed in any set sequence. In the case of fully expressed MEN-IIA syndrome, however, the labile and severe hypertension associated with pheochromocytoma represents a significant risk to the patient's life, especially when under the stress of surgery. For this reason, the pheochromocytoma should be treated first, and this is best accomplished by an initial pharmacologic management of the hypertension with alpha and beta blockade followed by appropriate surgical exploration, depending on the location and number of tumors present. Following recovery from this surgery, the medullary carcinoma of the thyroid and the parathyroid hyperplasia should be treated simultaneously at a subsequent operation.

Answer: Question 21: A
Question 22: B
Question 23: C

24. The most common cause of hypoparathyroidism is:

A. Prior thyroid surgery
B. Prior parathyroid surgery
C. Prior viral infection involving the parathyroid glands
D. Genetic disorder of PTH metabolism
E. "Innocent bystander effect" from radioiodine therapy of the thyroid

Sabiston: 636
Schwartz: 1620

Comment: The most common cause of hypoparathyroidism is surgical trauma to the parathyroid glands during thyroid or parathyroid exploration. Because of the much greater frequency of thyroid operations than parathyroid operations, prior thyroid surgery represents the most common cause of hypoparathyroidism. There is a genetic disorder (pseudohypoparathyroidism) in which there is a normal to elevated serum PTH level but an abnormal end-organ response of the kidney to circulating PTH, resulting in hyperphosphatemia and hypocalcemia. Postoperative hypocalcemia is usually temporary, and if viable parathyroid tissue does remain, the PTH levels and serum calcium will return to normal. These patients may need to be supported temporarily with exogenous calcium and vitamin D; however, if they remain asymptomatic, it is usually wise to avoid calcium administration based on the low serum level alone, as this low level serves as the stimulus for the compensatory growth and function of the remaining parathyroid tissue. If the patient develops clinical signs of hypocalcemia (e.g., carpopedal spasm, tetany, Chvostek's sign, Trousseau's sign, electrocardiographic changes) or if the hypoparathyroidism appears to be permanent, then treatment with exogenous calcium (up to 2 gm of elemental calcium/day) and vitamin D_3 (up to 100,000 units/day) will be needed.

Answer: A

CHAPTER 21

Pituitary

1. Match the following synonymous terms:

A. Infundibular process
B. Pars distalis
C. Infundibulum
D. Infundibular stem

a. Median eminence
b. Anterior pituitary
c. Posterior pituitary
d. Pituitary stalk

Sabiston: 643
Schwartz: 1476

Comment: To some degree there is a lack of standardization of the nomenclature pertaining to pituitary anatomy. The most widely accepted terminology is attributed to Wislocki. Using this terminology, the pituitary is considered to be composed of the neurohypophysis and the adenohypophysis. The **neurohypophysis** is composed of the infundibulum (median eminence), the infundibular stem (pituitary stalk), and the infundibular process (posterior lobe, posterior pituitary, or pars nervosa). The **adenohypophysis** consists of the pars tuberalis (wrapping around the infundibular stem) and the pars distalis (anterior lobe or anterior pituitary). The conceptualization of the pituitary gland as two separate but closely related entities—the neurohypophysis, or posterior pituitary, and the adenohypophysis, or anterior pituitary—is important in considering the numerous aspects of clinical pituitary pathology.

Answer: A–c; B–b; C–a; D–d

2. Which of the following statements regarding the anatomy of the pituitary gland is/are correct?

A. As with other portions of the central nervous system, there is an anatomic and physiologic blood-brain barrier present within the neurohypophysis
B. The adenohypophysis does not have its own direct arterial blood supply
C. The neurohypophysis contains both neuronal cell bodies and axons
D. The adenohypophysis contains axons only
E. No nerves terminate within the adenohypophysis

Sabiston: 639
Schwartz: 1477

Comment: The special neuroendocrine function of the pituitary gland and its interrelationship with the hypothalamus are facilitated by several distinct anatomic features. For example, the hormonal mediators released within the neurohypophysis gain access to the vascular system through fenestrated epithelium, and thus the neurohypophysis does not have a "blood-brain barrier" like the barrier that characterizes most of the rest of the central nervous system. The vascular anatomy of the adenohypophysis is unusual in that it does not derive its blood supply from a direct arterial source, but rather from a system of portal vessels which pass first through the capillary bed of the neurohypophysis. Since no nerves directly terminate within the adenohypophysis, it is dependent upon this portal capillary system for receiving the hormones that influence its function. The neurohypophysis, on the other hand, is regulated in part by hormonal influences from the periphery (and possibly feedback directly from the adenohypophysis) as well as by direct neural input from the hypothalamus. This is by means of axons, the cell bodies of which lie within the hypothalamus. The neurohypophysis itself contains no cell bodies. Such an anatomic arrangement allows for the complicated interplay of neural and endocrine factors between the hypothalamus, neurohypophysis, adenohypophysis, and peripheral endocrine function.

Answer: B, E

3. Match the secretions with the portion of the pituitary from which they originate:

A. Growth hormone
B. Oxytocin
C. Thyrotropin-releasing factor
D. ACTH
E. Cortisol
F. Vasopressin
G. Prolactin

a. Adenohypophysis
b. Neurohypophysis
c. Both
d. Neither

Sabiston: 641
Schwartz: 1478

Comment: Hormones secreted by the anterior pituitary (e.g., growth hormone, ACTH, TSH, LH, FSH, prolactin) are controlled in part by direct feedback inhibition from the periphery, as well as by releasing factors from the hypothalamus and neurohypophysis (e.g., thyrotropin, corticotropin, gonadotropin, or growth hormone releasing factor). In addition to these releasing factors, the neurohypophysis also produces two hormones (oxytocin and vasopressin) that have their primary effect peripherally.

Answer: A–a; B–b; C–b; D–a; E–d; F–b; G–a

4. Which of the following statements is/are true regarding pituitary releasing factors?

A. Releasing factors are formed in the hypothalamus and proceed directly to the adenohypophysis, bypassing the neurohypophysis
B. Releasing factors are derivatives of steroids similar to those seen in the adrenal cortex
C. Release of thyroid stimulating hormone (TSH) is under partial control of thyrotropin releasing hormone and partial control of peripheral T3 and T4 levels
D. The concept of feedback inhibition of pituitary function is outdated

Sabiston: 641
Schwartz: 1479

Comment: The concept of feedback inhibition is fundamental to the understanding of the hypothalamic–pituitary–peripheral endocrine axis. In its most simplified form, the hypothalamus, sensing and reacting to peripheral blood hormone levels, synthesizes releasing factors (small peptides) which are released as neurosecretory granules from the axons within the neurohypophysis. These are then transported through the portal vascular system to the adenohypophysis to influence adenohypophyseal hormone output. These hormones in turn influence endocrine function of the peripheral end organ that alters blood levels, completing the cycle. The adenohypophysis may be directly sensitive to blood levels of circulating hormones, as in the case of TSH production, which may be altered not only by thyrotropin releasing hormone but also by peripheral T3 and T4 levels.

Answer: C

5. Which of the following statements is/are true regarding the neurohypophysis?

A. Releasing factors, as well as vasopressin and oxytocin, come from similar hypothalamic neurons
B. Oxytocin has few physiologic effects in males but has a marked inhibitory effect on the contraction of the gravid uterus
C. Marked water retention with hyponatremia may result from neurohypophyseal dysfunction
D. Marked dehydration and hypernatremia may result from neurohypophyseal dysfunction
E. Most metastases to the pituitary are found in the neurohypophysis

Sabiston: 643
Schwartz: 1478

Comment: The dual physiologic function of the neurohypophysis (i.e., production of releasing factors affecting the adenohypophysis and production of hormones with direct peripheral effects) is reflected anatomically in the cells of origin within the hypothalamus. From the parvicellular neurons of the hypothalamus come the neurosecretory peptides that function as releasing factors for adenohypophyseal function. From the magnocellular neurons of the supraoptic and paraventricular nuclei in the hypothalamus project neurons that contain larger neurosecretory peptides (vasopressin and oxytocin) coupled to a carrier protein (neurophysin) that, when uncoupled and released, exert their direct hormonal effects peripherally. Oxytocin has few physiologic effects in the male, but exerts a marked stimulatory effect on the contraction of the gravid uterus, and is used pharmacologically to facilitate labor. Vasopressin has numerous systemic effects, the most prominent of which is its antidiuretic effect on the distal nephron. When vasopressin is secreted in inappropriately high amounts (inappropriate ADH), large amounts of water are retained, leading to overhydration and hyponatremia. When inappropriately small amounts of vasopressin are released (diabetes insipidus), inappropriately high volumes of dilute urine are excreted, resulting in dehydration and hypernatremia.

Answer: C, D, E

6. Which of the following statements about growth hormone is/are correct?

A. Growth hormone is a peptide that affects the growth of somatic structures such as bone and muscle, but does not affect the growth of visceral organs or physiologic homeostasis
B. Growth hormone secretion is stimulated by a hypothalamic releasing factor, but, to date, no hypothalamic inhibitory factor has been identified
C. Under normal circumstances, the largest surge of growth hormone in the peripheral blood occurs in the evening
D. Growth hormone secretion may be stimulated by exercise, stress, or hypoglycemia

Sabiston: 646
Schwartz: 1480

Comment: Growth hormone is a large peptide secreted from the lateral aspect of the adenohypophysis. Its secretion is regulated by both releasing factors and inhibitory factors (somatostatin) from the hypothalamus. Furthermore, its release is stimulated either directly or indirectly by exercise, physiologic stress, and hypoglycemia. In addition to its positive effect on the growth of somatic structures, it also stimulates the growth of visceral organs. Furthermore, it has numerous anabolic effects, including the elevation of blood glucose and free fatty acid levels and the incorporation of amino acids into protein. Growth hormone is released into the peripheral blood as a result of secretory surges occurring six to eight times daily, the largest one being in the early morning hours. During adolescence, the total amount of growth hormone secreted daily increases owing to an increase in the number of surges.

Answer: D

7. Which of the following statements regarding prolactin secretion and physiology is/are correct?

A. Prolactin is secreted from the neurohypophysis in response to suckling
B. Nonpregnant females and males have similar blood levels of prolactin
C. Prolactin has physiologic effects on the breast, ovary, and testis
D. The principal hypothalamic effect on prolactin secretion is inhibitory
E. Prolactin secretion may be stimulated by pregnancy, stress, exercise, and breast stimulation

Sabiston: 646
Schwartz: 1480

Comment: Prolactin is a peptide secreted from eosinophilic cells of the adenohypophysis in response to numerous peripheral factors, including pregnancy, stress, exercise, and direct breast stimulation. Hypothalamic control of prolactin secretion is primarily inhibitory via prolactin inhibiting factor (PIF), which some evidence suggests may be dopamine. In the nonstimulated state, men and women have similar blood levels of prolactin. Its most significant physiologic effect is mammotropic, stimulating duct development and lactation. It also has gonadal effects, however, and is thought to modulate to some degree ovarian progesterone synthesis and testicular testosterone synthesis.

Answer: B, C, D, E

8. Which of the following statements is/are true regarding thyroid stimulating hormone (TSH)?

A. TSH is released under the influence of the hypothalamus by means of thyrotropin releasing hormone (TRH)
B. TSH is released under the direct influence of circulating thyroid hormones
C. As with other adenohypophyseal hormones, TSH has numerous effects in addition to its stimulatory effect on the thyroid gland
D. TSH levels can be pharmacologically manipulated so as to possibly affect the growth of thyroid neoplasms

Sabiston: 645
Schwartz: 1480

Comment: Unlike prolactin and growth hormone, which have numerous metabolic effects, TSH appears to exert influence only on the thyroid gland, stimulating growth of the gland and secretion of thyroid hormones. Circulating thyroid hormones in turn exert a very well defined feedback inhibition on TSH-producing cells in the adenohypophysis, possibly by inhibiting the effect of hypothalamically derived TRH. The growth of thyroid neoplasms, like the normal thyroid gland, may be stimulated by high TSH levels. For this reason, pharmacologic reduction of TSH levels through the administration of exogenous thyroid hormone may result in the shrinkage of both benign and malignant thyroid tumors.

Answer: A, B, D

9. Which of the following statements is/are true regarding ACTH?

A. ACTH release is presumed to be under partial hypothalamic control

B. ACTH release may be affected by direct feedback inhibition of circulating cortisol levels on the adenohypophysis
C. ACTH levels are fairly constant during any given 24-hour period but may rise abruptly in response to stress
D. There is a circadian rhythm to ACTH release which usually cannot be overcome by peripheral stimulatory influences

Sabiston: 645
Schwartz: 1481

Comment: Adrenocorticotropic hormone (ACTH) is secreted by the adenohypophysis under the influence of both hypothalamic control via corticotropin releasing factor (CRF—presumed to be present but not yet identified) and the negative feedback control of circulating cortisol levels. Although there are several surges of ACTH release during a given 24-hour period, the largest one occurs characteristically at night and in the early morning hours, accounting for the typical diurnal variation of blood cortisol levels. These central and negative feedback regulatory mechanisms are easily overridden during periods of stress such as acute illness, fever, hypoglycemia, and emotional upset. An abrupt increase in ACTH secretion in response to these factors can lead to as high as a tenfold increase in cortisol production within a very short period of time.

Answer: A, B

10. Match the following physiologic effects with the respective gonadotropic hormone:

A. Promotes spermatogenesis   a. FSH
B. Stimulates testicular testosterone production   b. LH
C. Facilitates development of corpus luteum   c. Both
D. Promotes ovarian follicle maturation   d. Neither
E. Production stimulated by gonadotropin releasing hormone (GnRH)

Sabiston: 643
Schwartz: 1481

Comment: Sexual and reproductive physiology involves a complex interaction of hypothalamic, pituitary, gonadal, adrenal, and circulating hormonal factors. The pituitary's role in this complex scheme involves the production of FSH (follicle stimulating hormone) and LH (luteinizing hormone). These two hormones are produced by the same basophilic adenohypophyseal cell under the influence of a single gonadotropic releasing hormone from the hypothalamus. This hypothalamic pituitary interaction is modulated by feedback from adrenal and gonadal hormone production. The principal gonadal effects of these two hormones are outlined above.

Answer: A–a; B–b; C–b; D–a; E–c

11. Pituitary endorphins are characterized by which one or more of the following statements?

A. These are opiate-like peptides
B. They share a common amino acid sequence with other adenohypophyseal hormones
C. They are also found in the brain and gut
D. Despite their biochemical identification, physiologic or behavioral effects of these substances have not yet been demonstrated

Sabiston: 645
Schwartz: 1481

Comment: During the past 10 years, much has been learned about the presence of pituitary endorphins, which are opiate-like peptides that represent fragments of a larger prohormone called pro-opiocortin. MSH (melanocyte stimulating hormone) and ACTH possess amino acid sequences that are identical to portions of the pro-opiocortin and β-lipotropin structures. These endorphins, which are also found throughout the brain and gut, are capable of exerting potent analgesic effects and may be key factors in an individual's behavioral and physiologic response to pain.

Answer: A, B, C

12. Amenorrhea and progressive hypothyroidism occurring after recovery from shock due to placental hemorrhage may be known as (one or more may apply):

A. Sheehan's syndrome
B. Postpartum pituitary ischemia
C. Thyrogenital syndrome
D. A form of pituitary apoplexy

Sabiston: 656
Schwartz: 1482

Comment: During pregnancy, the pituitary may increase in size as much as 50% with a proportionate increase in blood flow requirements. If a state of hypoperfusion should occur during late pregnancy or delivery, the pituitary may become ischemic and subsequently necrotic, resulting in panhypopituitarism. The most obvious clinical manifestations of this would be amenorrhea and hypothyroidism. Once the diagnosis is made, treatment involves appropriate hormonal replacement therapy.

Answer: A, B, D

13. Chromophobe adenomas are characterized by which one or more of the following statements?

A. They are the most common type of pituitary tumor
B. Almost all of them are nonsecreting tumors
C. They may produce binasal hemianopsia
D. Large tumors may compress the adjacent pituitary, leading to what is usually a predictable sequential loss of the various pituitary functions

Sabiston: 656
Schwartz: 1482

Comment: Pituitary tumors were originally designated as acidophilic, basophilic, or chromophobic as a result of their affinity for different dyes. From this standpoint alone, chromophobe adenomas do represent the most common form of pituitary tumor. With the development of immunohistochemical staining techniques, however, as many as 40% of chromophobe adenomas are found to secrete prolactin, FSH, or TSH, although clinical manifestations of hypersecretion of these hormones is usually absent. As a consequence, these tumors may achieve a relatively large size, with their initial clinical presentation being that of a mass effect. Cephalad extension produces visual loss, characteristically a bitemporal hemianopsia. Lateral enlargement may result in compression of the third, fourth, first portion of fifth, and sixth cranial nerves. Progressive enlargement of the tumor may also compress the surrounding pituitary tissue, leading to loss of pituitary function. Of note is that the functional losses tend to be in a fairly predictable sequence: growth hormone first, gonadotropic secretion next, thyrotropic secretion third, and ACTH secretion last.

Answer: A, D

14. True statements regarding growth hormone hypersecretion include:

A. Acromegaly may occur in both adults and children
B. Growth hormone–secreting adenomas may be eosinophilic or chromophobic
C. Growth hormone–secreting tumors may produce symptoms that are not related to growth hormone excess
D. Acromegalics frequently die of cardiac complications
E. Surgery has been supplanted by radiation therapy as the treatment of choice for excessive growth hormone secretion

Sabiston: 652
Schwartz: 1483

Comment: Excessive production of growth hormone by pituitary adenomas (usually chromophobic, but occasionally eosinophilic) produces morphologic changes which differ according to the age and skeletal maturity of the patient. In children (before epiphyseal closure) there is generalized overgrowth of most of the somatic structures, resulting in gigantism. In adults (after epiphyseal closure) the somatic enlargement is most evident in the face, hands, and feet and is termed acromegaly. In patients with acromegaly, enlargement of the heart with subsequent valvular dysfunction and cardiomyopathy may also occur and is a common cause of death. Although the characteristic physical appearance of patients with growth hormone excess dominates the clinical presentation, the adenoma itself may occasionally grow to such a size as to produce symptoms due to an expanding pituitary mass (e.g., visual disturbances, headache, pituitary hypofunction). Surgical excision of the adenoma remains the treatment of choice in most circumstances; however, radiation therapy is finding increasing applicability in this area.

Answer: B, C, D

15. Which one or more of the following statements is/are true regarding ACTH excess of pituitary origin?

A. Cushing's syndrome and Cushing's disease are synonymous terms
B. ACTH-producing pituitary adenomas are the most common cause of excess adrenal cortisol production
C. The majority of cases of hypothalamic/pituitary causes of excess ACTH production are due to pituitary microadenomas

D. The sella is enlarged in the majority of patients with ACTH-producing pituitary adenomas

E. Bilateral adrenalectomy is preferable to hypophysectomy for the management of Cushing's disease

Sabiston: 655
Schwartz: 1484, 1495

Comment: Cushing's syndrome refers to the clinical sequelae of excess adrenal cortisol production. This may be due to an adrenal carcinoma, adrenal adenoma, nodular dysplasia of the adrenal, or diffuse adrenal hyperplasia in response to excess CRF production from the hypothalamus, ectopic ACTH production, or excess ACTH production from a pituitary adenoma. When Cushing's syndrome is due to a pituitary adenoma, this is known as Cushing's disease, which in fact is a relatively uncommon cause of the syndrome itself. Of the hypothalamic/pituitary causes of Cushing's syndrome, it was formerly felt that the pituitary accounted for only 10 to 20% of cases. However, current pathologic studies have demonstrated that up to 80% of these patients harbor a pituitary microadenoma that produces ACTH. In the majority of these cases, the adenoma is too small to cause any changes in the radiographic appearance of the sella. When appropriate studies have revealed a pituitary adenoma to be the cause of bilateral adrenal hyperplasia, the preferred method of treatment is transsphenoidal excision of the adenoma rather than bilateral adrenalectomy. (Please refer to Chapter 22 regarding the adrenal gland for further questions on Cushing's syndrome.)

Answer: C

16. Which of the following statements is/are true regarding prolactinomas?

A. Excess prolactin secretion is the most common clinically detectable disorder of pituitary function

B. They may produce amenorrhea and galactorrhea in females

C. They may produce priapism and breast enlargement in males

D. They may be successfully managed with bromocriptine

Sabiston: 651
Schwartz: 1484

Comment: Excess prolactin secretion is indeed the most common clinically observed disorder of pituitary function. In females excess prolactin production may result in amenorrhea and galactorrhea, while in males it causes breast enlargement and impotence. All of these symptoms are reversible if the serum prolactin level can be reduced. This is most quickly accomplished by surgical excision of the adenoma. In some centers, however, the preferred treatment for prolactinomas is bromocriptine, which is an ergot derivative effective in inhibiting prolactin production and reducing tumor bulk.

Answer: A, B, D

17. Which of the following statements correctly describe(s) craniopharyngiomas?

A. They contain squamous epithelium

B. They may occur cephalad or caudad to the diaphragma sellae

C. They may cause dwarfism

D. They will recur unless radiotherapy is added to surgical excision

Sabiston: 656
Schwartz: 1485

Comment: Craniopharyngiomas are squamous cell tumors of the pituitary that arise as remnants of the embryologic Rathke's pouch. They may present in childhood or adulthood, and their clinical presentation depends in part on their size and location, which may be above or below the diaphragma sellae. Those that develop within the sella turcica usually result in hypofunction of the adenohypophysis and therefore may be a cause of dwarfism. Those arising above the sella may produce headache, visual loss, and other neurologic sequelae commonly associated with expanding lesions in the area of the hypothalamus. When craniopharyngiomas are well encapsulated, they may frequently be totally excised with excellent long-term results. Poorly encapsulated or very large tumors may need to be treated by partial excision or cyst drainage combined with radiation therapy.

Answer: A, B, C

18. Match the following surgical approaches to the pituitary with one or more appropriate characteristics:

A. Transcranial
B. Transfrontal
C. Transsphenoidal

a. Current approach of choice for pituitary microadenomas
b. Treatment of choice prior to the antibiotic era
c. Unilateral anosmia
d. Allows assessment of associated intracranial anatomic variations

Sabiston: 651
Schwartz: 1485

Comment: Prior to the antibiotic era, transsinus (frontal or sphenoid) approaches to the pituitary gland were considered hazardous because of the risk of bacterial contamination of the central nervous system. The transcranial technique was therefore preferred. This technique, like the transfrontal technique, approaches the pituitary from above the diaphragma sellae and therefore permits assessment of associated intracranial anatomic variations. Disadvantages to these approaches include the need to retract the frontal lobe physically and, in the case of the transfrontal approach, the resultant postoperative unilateral anosmia. The transsphenoidal approach involves an incision in the buccal gingival sulcus with a transnasal/transsphenoidal entry into the infradiaphragmatic sellae. It is more cosmetically appealing, causes less morbidity, and is considered to be the treatment of choice for surgical excision of pituitary tumors confined to the sella.

Answer: A–b, d; B–c, d; C–a

19. Current or former indications for hypophysectomy include which of the following disease states?

A. Breast carcinoma
B. Prostate carcinoma
C. Diabetic neuropathy
D. Diabetic retinopathy

Sabiston: 657
Schwartz: 1487

Comment: The clinical course of metastatic breast carcinoma and prostate carcinoma may be favorably influenced by a reduction in the level or end organ effectiveness of circulating estrogens or androgens, respectively. Because of the pituitary influence on the adrenal and gonadal production of these hormones, some patients who have responded clinically to oophorectomy or orchiectomy have also shown a clinical response to hypophysectomy. In the case of breast cancer, this treatment modality has largely been supplanted by the use of tamoxifen (an antiestrogen), aminoglutethimide (for blockade of adrenal and peripheral estrogen production), and other pharmacologic endocrine manipulations. In the case of prostate cancer, this approach has rarely been employed because of its short duration of response and the availability of other chemotherapeutic and supportive measures. Quite serendipitously, it was observed that diabetic retinopathy occasionally improved in patients who had undergone postpartum necrosis of the pituitary. As a result, hypophysectomy in the past was used in the treatment of rapidly progressive diabetic retinopathy. This technique has largely been replaced by the use of laser photocoagulation and vitrectomy.

Answer: A, B, D

CHAPTER 22

Adrenal

1. Which of the following statements is/are true regarding adrenal gland embryology?

A. The adrenal cortex is derived from endodermal tissue
B. The adrenal medulla is derived from ectodermal tissue
C. The adrenal medulla bears a close embryologic relationship to the sympathetic ganglia
D. The adrenal glands are extremely small during mid-fetal life but gradually enlarge through the first postpartum year
E. Extra-adrenal cortical tissue is found more commonly than is extra-adrenal medullary tissue

Sabiston: 657
Schwartz: 1489

Comments: The adrenal gland is composed of a cortex and a medulla, which have different embryologic origins and widely differing physiologic functions. The cortex is derived from primitive mesoderm between the fourth and sixth weeks of fetal development. The medulla is derived from ectodermal cells of the neural crest during the seventh week of fetal development. Migration of these ectodermal cells from the neural crest to the periaortic area is responsible for the eventual development of the sympathetic ganglia as well as the adrenal medulla. In lower vertebrates the cortical and medullary tissues remain separate, whereas in humans the cortex envelops the medulla to form a single gland structurally. This gland is actually larger than the kidney during the midportion of fetal development, but gradually decreases in size through the end of the first postpartum year. During the course of fetal development, both adrenal cortical and adrenal medullary rests may persist along the paths of cellular migration. Extra-adrenal medullary (chromaffin) tissue is found more commonly and over a much wider anatomic range than is extra-adrenal cortical tissue and is responsible for the occurrence of extra-adrenal pheochromocytoma. Extra-adrenal cortical tissue tends to be found adjacent to the adrenal glands and is responsible for the persistence of Cushing's syndrome following bilateral adrenalectomy.

Answer: B, C

2. Match the following anatomic findings with the appropriate adrenal gland:

Anatomic Findings	Adrenal Gland
A. Contiguous with the upper pole of the kidney	a. Right
B. Contiguous with the "bare" area of the liver	b. Left
C. Fairly constant arterial supply directly from the aorta	c. Both
D. Variable arterial supply from the aorta, phrenic artery, and renal artery	d. Neither
E. Single vein draining directly to the inferior vena cava	

Sabiston: 658
Schwartz: 1489

Comments: The triangular adrenal glands lie in close association to the upper pole of the kidneys, occasionally extending medially and as inferiorly as the renal hilus. On the right side the gland also is closely associated with the liver, which may have a bearing on the difficulty of resecting large right adrenal tumors. The arterial supply of the adrenal gland is usually from a variable combination of three possible sources: a branch from the inferior phrenic artery, a vessel directly from the aorta, and a branch of the renal artery. In contrast, the venous drainage of the adrenal gland is fairly constant in that it is via a single vein. On the left it drains into the renal vein. On the right it drains directly into the inferior vena cava via a short, and occasionally wide, adrenal vein, which increases the difficulty of performing a safe right adrenal dissection.

Answer: A–c; B–a; C–d; D–c; E–a

3. Match the hormones in the left-hand column with the appropriate part of the adrenal gland where they are primarily manufactured:

Hormone	Part of Adrenal Gland
A. Cortisol	a. Zona glomerulosa
B. Aldosterone	b. Zona fasciculata
C. Sex steroids	c. Zona reticularis
D. Epinephrine	d. Adrenal medulla
E. Norepinephrine	

Sabiston: 658
Schwartz: 1489

Comments: Adrenal cortical hormones are manufactured as a result of hydroxylation and oxidation on certain sites of the cholesterol molecule. These processes occur in different areas of the adrenal cortex as a consequence of the presence or absence of specific enzymes in those areas. Anatomically, the adrenal cortex consists of three zones arranged concentrically from the capsule inward to the medulla: zona glomerulosa, zona fasciculata, and zona reticularis. All three of these zones contain 11- and 21-hydroxylating enzymes; the zona glomerulosa alone contains 18-oxidase; the zona fasciculata and zona reticularis alone contain 17-hydroxylating enzyme. As a consequence, aldosterone is produced exclusively by the zona glomerulosa, while cortisol is produced in both the zona fasciculata and zona reticularis. The sex steroids are thought to be produced primarily by the zona reticularis, but debate persists as to whether these androgens and estrogens may also be manufactured by cells within the zona fasciculata. Norepinephrine and epinephrine are produced in the adrenal medulla. Of note is that the conversion from norepinephrine to epinephrine is in part under the influence of glucocorticoids, which are obviously present in very high concentration in the venous blood draining from the cortex through the medulla.

Answer: A–b, c; B–a; C–c; D–d; E–d

4. Which one or more of the following may be associated with cortisol excess?

A. Gluconeogenesis
B. Redistribution of body fat
C. Somatic muscular development
D. Immunosuppression
E. Impaired wound healing

Sabiston: 659
Schwartz: 1497

Comments: Glucocorticoid excess, either endogenously as is seen in Cushing's syndrome or exogenously from steroid administration, produces far-reaching multisystem effects. Cortisol exerts influence over carbohydrate metabolism, promoting gluconeogenesis and glycogen deposition in the liver. This is frequently achieved owing to a redistribution of metabolites away from skeletal muscle and a breakdown of skeletal muscle protein to provide substrate, all of which may result in muscle wasting. For reasons that are unclear, cortisol excess also results in a centripedal redistribution of body fat, causing truncal obesity and the "buffalo hump" appearance of the patient with Cushing's syndrome. The catabolic actions of glucocorticoids also may result in inhibition of normal lymphocyte, macrophage, other hematopoietic cell, and fibroblast function. This in turn may lead to impairment of both the afferent and efferent limbs of the immune response as well as impaired wound healing.

Many other disturbances, including mental aberrations, gastrointestinal bleeding, and fluid and electrolyte disorders, are seen in states of glucocorticoid excess.

Answer: A, B, D, E

5. Which of the following statements is/are correct regarding aldosterone physiology?

A. Aldosterone is one of several potent mineralocorticoids found in humans
B. Aldosterone secretion is primarily influenced by serum levels of ACTH, sodium, and potassium
C. The classic serum electrolyte findings of hyperaldosteronism include hypernatremia and hypokalemia
D. Primary hyperaldosteronism implies an aberrancy in the normal feedback inhibition loop of aldosterone physiology
E. Documentation of an elevated serum aldosterone level implies the presence of a primary adrenal abnormality

Sabiston: 661
Schwartz: 1492

Comment: In humans, aldosterone is the only clinically important mineralocorticoid present. It is secreted by the zona glomerulosa of the adrenal cortex under the influence of the renin-angiotensin system, serum sodium and potassium concentrations, and plasma ACTH levels. Of these, the plasma ACTH influence appears to be the weakest, being seen only when pathologic states of ACTH excess are present or when pharmacologic doses of ACTH are given. The major regulator of aldosterone secretion is the renin-angiotensin system, in which changes in serum sodium or blood pressure stimulate renin secretion from the juxtaglomerular cells of the kidney. This precipitates a series of enzymatic conversions from angiotensinogen through angiotensin I to angiotensin II, which functions as both a potent vasoconstrictor and a stimulant of aldosterone secretion. Aldosterone acts primarily on the renal tubule, resulting in sodium and chloride retention in exchange for potassium and hydrogen. In pathologic states, this results in the classic findings of hypernatremia and hypokalemia. Hyperaldosteronism may be a "primary" event in which autonomous production of aldosterone (e.g., an aldosterone-producing adenoma) functions outside the influence of the normal negative feedback loop. "Secondary" hyperaldosteronism is a normal physiologic compensatory mechanism in which elevated serum aldosterone levels are found in response to hyponatremia, hypovolemia, or hypotension.

Answer: C, D

6. Which of the following statements is/are true regarding androgen and estrogen physiology?

A. Adrenocortical production of androgens and estrogens slightly exceeds gonadal production during most of childhood and early adult life
B. During fetal development, male physiognomy will occur "by default" unless estrogens are present in sufficient quantity to direct feminization
C. Virilization of a prepubertal female is not known to occur if at birth the genitalia are appropriate for age and sex

D. Virilizing tumors in adult males are very difficult to detect on clinical grounds alone

E. Estrogen-producing tumors are clinically silent in adult females

Sabiston: 661
Schwartz: 1488

Comments: Both the adrenal cortex and the gonads are responsible for androgen and estrogen production, with the largest quantity of these steroids produced by the gonads under normal circumstances. During fetal development, the "dominant" sexual development pattern will be female unless androgens are present in sufficient quantity to direct masculinization. Abnormally high androgen and/or estrogen production by the adrenal may occur during fetal development, childhood, or adulthood as a result of adrenocortical hyperplasia, adrenal enzymatic defects, or adrenal neoplasms. The clinical syndrome produced depends upon the age of the patient and the degree of hormone excess. Probably the most difficult syndrome to detect clinically would be virilization in an adult male. Estrogen-producing tumors in adult females may also be difficult to detect but frequently are manifested by abnormal breast enlargement and menstrual abnormalities. In prepubertal patients, estrogen excess will produce precocious breast development and menstruation in females and gynecomastia in males, whereas androgen excess will produce clitoral or phallic enlargement, increased muscle mass, and precocious development of axillary and pubic hair.

Answer: D

7. Which one of the following is the most common cause of Cushing's syndrome?

A. Adrenocortical adenoma
B. Adrenocortical carcinoma
C. Adrenocortical hyperplasia
D. Adrenal response to ectopic ACTH production

Sabiston: 662
Schwartz: 1495

Comments: It is important to differentiate Cushing's syndrome from Cushing's disease. Cushing's syndrome refers to the sequelae of excess cortisol secretion. This may result from autonomous adrenocortical function as may be seen in the presence of an adrenal adenoma or carcinoma, or it may result from diffuse bilateral adrenocortical hyperplasia in response to elevated levels of circulating ACTH. Excess ACTH production most often is due to pituitary adenomas, but may result from ectopic sources such as tumors of the lung, pancreas, and thymus. In 1932, Harvey Cushing published his classic article describing eight patients with Cushing's syndrome, six of which were noted to have pituitary adenomas. After the cause-effect relationship of the pituitary pathology to the cortisol excess was established years later, it became customary to refer to patients with cortisol excess as a consequence of pituitary ACTH production as having "Cushing's disease." Considering all causes of Cushing's syndrome, bilateral adrenocortical hyperplasia is the most common cause (approximately 70% followed in turn by adrenal adenoma, adrenal carcinoma, and ectopic ACTH production.

Answer: C

8. Which of the following is/are not expected to occur in patients with Cushing's syndrome?

A. Obesity
B. Hirsutism
C. Ankylosing spondylitis
D. Hypertension
E. Pathologic fractures
F. Alopecia

Sabiston: 663
Schwartz: 1497

Comments: Most of the signs and symptoms of Cushing's syndrome are due to excess cortisol secretion and may be produced in normal patients by exogenous corticosteroid administration. The most common findings seen clinically are truncal obesity, hirsutism, hypertension, facial plethora, muscular weakness, moon facies, and acne or other rashes. In women, menstrual abnormalities are also extremely common. Other problems, seen less commonly or in advanced cases, include pathologic fractures, major mental aberrations, neuropathies, virilism, and exophthalmos, among many others. Ankylosing spondylitis and alopecia are not considered to be sequelae of cortisol excess.

Answer: C, F

9. A 30-year-old man presents with progressive truncal obesity, hypertension, and purple striae on the abdomen. Which one or more of the following tests would be appropriate to confirm your clinical impression?

A. Iodocholesterol adrenal scan
B. Urinary free cortisol level
C. Morning and afternoon plasma cortisol levels
D. CT scan of the abdomen
E. X-ray of the sella turcica

Sabiston: 663
Schwartz: 1497

Comments: The initial laboratory evaluation of a patient suspected of having Cushing's syndrome involves the documentation of excess cortisol production. This may be done by looking for excess urinary free cortisol excretion or by detecting abnormally high plasma cortisol levels with disruption of the normal diurnal variation of these levels (which are high in the morning and low in the evening). The other tests listed above may be useful in detecting bilateral adrenal enlargement, adrenal neoplasms, or pituitary neoplasms as the cause of the Cushing's syndrome but are not appropriate as initial screening tests.

Answer: B, C

10. Which of the following laboratory findings would be expected in a patient with hypercortisolism due to a pituitary adenoma (Cushing's disease)?

A. Elevated urinary free cortisol level
B. Elevated plasma ACTH level
C. Persistence of elevated urinary 17-hydroxycorticosteroids after high-dose dexamethasone administration

D. Further increase in urinary 17-hydroxycorticosteroids after metyrapone administration

Sabiston: 663
Schwartz: 1497

Comments: See Question 12.

11. Which of the following laboratory findings would be expected in a patient with hypercortisolism due to an adrenal adenoma or carcinoma?

A. Elevated urinary free cortisol level
B. Depressed plasma ACTH level
C. Decrease in urinary 17-hydroxycorticosteroids after both low-dose and high-dose dexamethasone administration
D. No change in urinary 17-hydroxycorticosteroid levels after metyrapone administration

Sabiston: 663
Schwartz: 1497

Comments: See Question 12.

12. Which of the following laboratory findings would be expected in a patient with hypercortisolism due to an ectopic source of ACTH production?

A. Elevated urinary free cortisol levels
B. Elevated plasma ACTH level
C. Persistence of elevated 17-hydroxycorticosteroid levels after both low-dose and high-dose dexamethasone administration
D. No change in urinary 17-hydroxycorticosteroid levels after metyrapone administration

Sabiston: 663
Schwartz: 1497

Comments: Elevated urinary free cortisol levels would be expected in all patients with hypercortisolism. It is important, however, to differentiate the causes of hypercortisolism, as the management of patients with that problem varies widely depending on the etiology. Plasma ACTH levels would obviously be elevated in patients with Cushing's syndrome due to pituitary or ectopic sources of excess ACTH production. These levels would be expected to be suppressed when hypercortisolism is due to autonomous production of cortisol by an adrenal adenoma or carcinoma. The dexamethasone suppression test (low-dose and high-dose) and the metyrapone test have been useful in differentiating cases of adrenal hyperplasia due to pituitary sources of ACTH from those due to ectopic sources of ACTH. In the dexamethasone suppression test, urinary 17-hydroxycorticosteroids are measured over a 2-day control period, then following administration of 2 mg per day of dexamethasone in divided doses over a 2-day period, and finally following administration of 8 mg per day of dexamethasone in divided doses over a 2-day period. Dexamethasone is a potent synthetic corticosteroid which in the normal individual will suppress urinary 17-hydroxycorticosteroid levels after both low-dose and high-dose administration. In patients with adrenal hyperplasia due to a pituitary source of ACTH production, low-dose dexamethasone will not affect the pituitary secretion of ACTH, and therefore urinary 17-hydroxycorticosteroid levels remain the same.

However, high doses of dexamethasone are able to suppress the ACTH production from the pituitary, resulting in a decrease in urinary 17-hydroxycorticosteroids. Hypercortisolism due to autonomous adrenal hyperfunction (adenoma or carcinoma) is already associated with low plasma ACTH levels, and it is obvious that further suppression of these levels with dexamethasone administration (low-dose or high-dose) would not affect the urinary 17-hydroxycorticosteroid levels. In cases of ectopic ACTH production, neither low-dose nor high-dose dexamethasone administration is able to suppress the ACTH production, and therefore urinary 17-hydroxycorticosteroid levels remain unchanged. The metyrapone test is based on the ability of this agent to inhibit the function of 11-beta-hydroxylase and therefore prevent the conversion of 11-deoxycortisol to cortisol in the adrenal cortex. As a result, in the normal individual, metyrapone administration results in an increase in ACTH secretion, resulting in increased adrenal production of biologically inactive cortisol precursors which are detected in the urine as increased quantities of 17-hydroxycorticosteroids. In patients with hypercortisolism due to increased pituitary ACTH secretion, metyrapone administration results in a further stimulation of the already hyperfunctioning pituitary gland, leading to further increase in urinary 17-hydroxycorticosteroid levels. In patients with hypercortisolism from autonomous adrenal function or ectopic ACTH production, the pituitary gland has been chronically suppressed by high plasma levels of cortisol and therefore is insensitive to the stimulatory effect of metyrapone administration. Hence, the urinary 17-hydroxycorticosteroid levels remain unchanged.

Answer: Question 10: A, B, D
Question 11: A, B, D
Question 12: A, B, C, D

13. A 29-year-old man presents with truncal obesity, hypertension, and muscular weakness and is found to have increased serum cortisol levels, an elevated plasma ACTH level, and suppression of urinary 17-hydroxycorticosteroids after high-dose, but not low-dose, dexamethasone administration. A CT brain scan reveals a small mass in the pituitary confined to the sella. The treatment of choice for this individual is:

A. Pituitary irradiation
B. Transsphenoidal hypophysectomy
C. Bilateral adrenalectomy
D. Aminoglutethimide administration

Sabiston: 668
Schwartz: 1484, 1501

Comments: See Question 15.

14. An adult patient presents with clinical and laboratory evidence of Cushing's syndrome and is found to have a depressed plasma ACTH level and a well-defined 3-cm left adrenal mass. The preferred treatment is:

A. Bilateral adrenalectomy
B. Left adrenalectomy
C. *o,p'*-DDD administration
D. Left adrenal irradiation

Sabiston: 667
Schwartz: 1501

Comments: See Question 15.

15. A 45-year-old man presents with Cushing's syndrome and a 7-cm right adrenal mass invading the perinephric fat compatible with an adrenal carcinoma. There is no other evidence of disease after thorough evaluation. The preferred treatment is:

A. External beam radiation therapy to the right adrenal area
B. *o,p'*-DDD administration
C. Right radical adrenalectomy
D. Interarterial adriamycin via the right adrenal artery

Sabiston: 667
Schwartz: 1500

Comment: The management of the patient with Cushing's syndrome depends upon the specific etiology involved. In Cushing's disease, wherein the primary pathology relates to excess pituitary production of ACTH, most feel that initial therapy should be directed at the pituitary. In cases where there is a small pituitary adenoma present within a normal-sized sella, transsphenoidal hypophysectomy is the treatment of choice. In cases in which the pituitary pathology becomes extrasellar, pituitary irradiation may be preferred but offers long-term control in only approximately 30% of patients. When a surgical or radiotherapeutic approach to the pituitary fails to control the disease, bilateral adrenalectomy is warranted and will be curative except in rare instances in which there is extra-adrenal cortical tissue. Pharmacologic management of patients with Cushing's disease has been tried with drugs such as aminoglutethimide, which blocks the production and secretion of adrenocortical steroids. This treatment may be of value in patients who are not good operative candidates, but certainly would not be considered an appropriate initial treatment. Hypercortisolism due to ectopic ACTH production is best approached by attempting to control the tumor that is producing the ACTH. If this cannot be achieved, bilateral adrenalectomy may be appropriate, depending on the overall status of the patient and the likelihood of long-term survival from the primary tumor. Cushing's syndrome due to adrenal adenomas or carcinomas is best approached by surgical resection of the involved gland. In cases of adenoma, total adrenalectomy of the involved side is preferable to a partial adrenalectomy. Adrenocortical carcinoma, which appears localized, is best managed by aggressive surgical resection, even if this may require en bloc resection of contiguous involved resectable tissues. Radiation therapy may be beneficial in situations in which all gross disease cannot be removed or when margins are quite close. However, data supporting the use of adjuvant postoperative radiation therapy are sparse. In cases of metastatic adrenocortical carcinoma producing Cushing's syndrome, resection of metastases may be palliative in terms of reducing cortisol levels. The administration of *o,p'*-DDD (related to the insecticide DDT) may produce regression of metastatic disease in up to 60% of patients.

Answer: Question 13: B
Question 14: B
Question 15: C

16. Which one of the following findings is most consistent with the diagnosis of primary hyperaldosteronism?

A. Sodium 145 mEq/l, potassium 4.8 mEq/l, blood pressure 148/96, retinal hemorrhages, expanded blood volume
B. Sodium 132 mEq/l, potassium 5.4 mEq/l, blood pressure 160/110, retinal hemorrhages, expanded blood volume
C. Sodium 149 mEq/l, potassium 2.9 mEq/l, blood pressure 190/140, normal retina, contracted blood volume
D. Sodium 149 mEq/l, potassium 2.9 mEq/l, blood pressure 150/98, normal retina, expanded blood volume

Sabiston: 671
Schwartz: 1508

Comments: See Question 18.

17. Which one of the following is the most common cause of primary hyperaldosteronism?

A. Bilateral adrenal cortical hyperplasia
B. Adrenocortical carcinoma
C. Solitary adrenal adenoma
D. Pituitary neoplasm
E. Ovarian or testicular neoplasm

Sabiston: 672
Schwartz: 1508

Comments: See Question 18.

18. Which of the following treatment modalities would be appropriate as the initial treatment for the two most common causes of primary hyperaldosteronism?

A. Spironolactone therapy
B. Aminoglutethimide therapy
C. Unilateral adrenalectomy
D. Bilateral adrenalectomy
E. Transsphenoidal hypophysectomy

Sabiston: 673
Schwartz: 1514

Comments: Primary hyperaldosteronism is a condition in which there is autonomous excess secretion of aldosterone from the adrenal cortex. In 80 to 90% of cases this is due to a solitary adrenal adenoma. Most of the remaining cases are due to bilateral adrenocortical hyperplasia, the exact cause of which is unknown. Pituitary adenomas as the cause of this aldosterone-producing bilateral hyperplasia have not been found. Occasionally adrenocortical carcinoma may be associated with excess aldosterone secretion, and there have been a few reports of ectopic production of aldosterone from ovarian neoplasms. The clinical and laboratory findings that are characteristic of primary hyperaldosteronism are all explainable on the basis of aldosterone's physiologic effect on the distal convoluted tubule, causing sodium retention in exchange for potassium excretion. This leads to hypernatremia, hypokalemia, expanded blood volume, and a mild sustained hypertension without associated retinopathy. Alkalosis, polydipsia, nocturnal polyuria, proteinuria, and paresthesias are also commonly seen. Appropriate treatment in cases of primary hyperaldosteronism caused by an adrenal adenoma is unilateral adrenalectomy. When bilateral adrenocortical hyperplasia is the cause, initial management with spironolactone thereapy is appropriate. If the clinical and laboratory findings are refractory to this therapy, bilateral adrenalectomy may be required.

Answer: Question 16: D
Question 17: C
Question 18: A, C

19. Match each of the following clinical forms of the adrenogenital syndrome (congenital adrenal hyperplasia) with its associated enzymatic defect:

Adrenogenital Syndrome	Enzymatic Defect
A. Most common clinical form, virilization with or without salt losing	a. 3-beta-hydroxydehydrogenase deficiency
B. Virilization and hypertension	b. 11-beta-hydroxylase deficiency
C. Mild degrees of pseudo-hermaphroditism and severe salt losing	c. 17-hydroxylase deficiency
D. Sexual infantilism and hypertension	d. 21-hydroxylase deficiency

Sabiston: 674
Schwartz: 1503

Comments: Numerous enzymes are required for the appropriate conversion of cholesterol to the various adrenal corticosteroids required for normal physiology. Insufficient amounts of one or more of these enzymes may result in excesses or deficits in glucocorticoids, mineralocorticoids, and the sex steroids, leading in turn to various combinations of electrolyte abnormalities, sexual maldevelopment, and hypertension. The most common enzymatic defect, accounting for approximately 95% of patients with the various adrenogenital syndromes, is 21-hydroxylase deficiency, which causes excess formation of androstenedione and a variable deficit in aldosterone production. The defect may be partial, in which one sees virilization in females and precocious sexual development in males, or it may be complete, in which the above sexual changes are also associated with a salt-losing syndrome. 11-Beta-hydroxylase deficiency leads to an accumulation of adrenal androgens and the mineralocorticoid desoxycorticosterone, resulting in the clinical findings of virilization and hypertension. 3-Beta-hydroxydehydrogenase deficiency leads to a marked deficit of cortisol and aldosterone production, with a severe and usually fatal salt-losing syndrome associated with mild degrees of pseudohermaphroditism. 17-Hydroxylase deficiency results in deficits of androgens, estrogens, and cortisol, leading to sexual infantilism and hypertension.

Answer: A–d; B–b; C–a; D–c

20. Which of the following statements regarding adrenal tumors that produce sex steroids is/are correct?

A. Virilizing adrenal tumors are more common in females than in males
B. Most feminizing adrenal tumors occur in adult males
C. Gynecomastia in young males (ages 13 to 15) is highly suggestive of an underlying feminizing tumor
D. Urinary 17-ketosteroid levels are elevated in the presence of virilizing, but not feminizing, adrenal tumors

E. Pharmacologic therapy is preferred over surgical resection as the initial therapy of these tumors

Sabiston: 676
Schwartz: 1505

Comments: Adrenal tumors producing primarily virilization or feminization are extremely rare. Virilizing tumors are seen twice as commonly in females as in males and are frequently seen during childhood. They are manifested by heterosexual or isosexual precocious puberty, depending on the sex of the patient. Feminizing adrenal tumors are most often seen in adult males during the second through fourth decades of life and are manifested clinically by gynecomastia and testicular atrophy. One must remember, however, that mild degrees of bilateral or unilateral gynecomastia may be seen as a normal physiologic pubertal change in up to 90% of young males. With both feminizing and virilizing adrenal tumors, there may be marked elevation in the urinary 17-ketosteroid levels. Resection of the gland harboring the tumor should be undertaken when possible. In cases of metastatic or unresectable disease, aminoglutethimide or o,p'-DDD may be useful in palliating symptoms.

Answer: A, B

21. A 35-year-old man with a history of pulmonary tuberculosis presents with weight loss, anorexia, dehydration, hyponatremia, and hyperkalemia. Of the following, the most likely diagnosis is:

A. Recurrent pulmonary tuberculosis
B. Pulmonary scar cancer with metastases
C. MEN-II syndrome
D. Addison's disease
E. Drug-induced nephropathy

Sabiston: 676
Schwartz: 1515

Comments: See Question 23.

22. The most common noniatrogenic cause of adrenal insufficiency is:

A. Tuberculosis
B. Autoimmune disease
C. Intra-adrenal hemorrhage
D. Metastases to the adrenal gland
E. Adrenal trauma

Sabiston: 676
Schwartz: 1515

Comments: See Question 23.

23. The proper treatment of chronic adrenal insufficiency includes which one or more of the following?

A. ACTH administration
B. Allogeneic adrenal transplantation
C. Administration of sheep adrenal extract
D. Cortisone acetate therapy
E. Fludrocortisone therapy

Sabiston: 677

Comments: The signs and symptoms of adrenocortical insufficiency (first described by Addison in 1855) are due to the sequelae of glucocorticoid and mineralocorticoid deficiencies. These include anorexia, nausea, vomiting, weight loss, lethargy, hypoglycemia, hypovolemia, hyponatremia, and hyperkalemia. Tuberculous involvement of the adrenal glands used to be the most common etiology and even today accounts for up to 17% of cases. The most common cause recognized today is an autoimmune destruction of the adrenal cortex involving antiadrenal antibodies, lymphocytic infiltration of the cortex, and progressive fibrosis. All of the other causes listed in the question do occur but with much less frequency. The treatment of adrenocortical insufficiency is glucocorticoid and mineralocorticoid replacement therapy. Cortisone acetate administered twice daily provides the glucocorticoid needs of the patient under baseline conditions. Fludrocortisone also has glucocorticoid activity but, more importantly, has potent mineralocorticoid activity which must be provided to the patient with a chronic adrenal insufficiency. This medication is administered two to three times per week.

Answer: Question 21: D
Question 22: B
Question 23: D, E

24. A 46-year-old woman who has been on long-term prednisone therapy for rheumatoid arthritis requires an abdominal hysterectomy for bleeding fibroid tumors. Which one or more of the following complications might this patient be expected to encounter with greater than average frequency?

A. Poor wound healing
B. Pancreatitis
C. Duodenal ulcer
D. Gastric ulcer
E. Adrenocortical insufficiency

Schwartz: 1517

Comments: All of the above responses are seen with greater frequency in patients on chronic corticosteroid therapy when compared with the average population. Poor wound healing, pancreatitis, duodenal ulcer, and gastric ulcer are due to the steroid treatment itself. In the case of poor wound healing, exogenous corticosteroids are known to blunt the inflammatory response and inhibit normal fibroblast function, resulting in poor wound healing. The etiology of steroid-induced pancreatitis is unclear. Both gastric and duodenal ulcers are seen with greater frequency in patients on corticosteroid therapy and, at least in the case of gastric ulcer, this is thought to be due to an alteration in the protective mucosal barrier with subsequent increased back-diffusion of hydrogen ions into the mucosa. Gastric and duodenal perforation as a complication of these ulcers is also seen with greater frequency. Adrenocortical insufficiency is also seen in patients on chronic corticosteroid therapy because of the inhibition by exogenous steroids of the normal adrenal response to stress. Both pituitary ACTH and endogenous adrenal steroid production are suppressed by exogenous steroid administration and therefore cannot respond to physiologic or surgical stress in a normal physiologic manner. To protect the patient against this

complication of exogenous steroid use, a "steroid prep" should be administered prior to surgery. One of the acceptable regimens includes cortisone acetate 100 mg intramuscularly 8 hours and 2 hours prior to operation, with 100 mg of hydrocortisone intravenously administered during the operative procedure. Cortisone, 300 mg per day, will usually protect the patient even in cases of maximum stress. This is then tapered to the patient's baseline steroid requirements over a time course that is dictated by the preoperative steroid dose, length of preoperative steroid treatment, and degree of stress induced by the operative procedure and postoperative course.

Answer: A, B, C, D, E

25. The pathway of catecholamine synthesis does not include which one or more of the following?

A. L-Tyrosine
B. Cholesterol
C. Dopamine beta-hydroxylase
D. 17-alpha-hydroxylase
E. Phenylethanolamine *N*-methyl transferase

Sabiston: 678
Schwartz: 1517

Comments: The corticosteroids of the adrenal cortex are derived from enzymatically mediated alterations in the cholesterol molecule. Catecholamine synthesis that occurs in the adrenal medulla begins with the amino acid L-tyrosine derived either from the diet or by endogenous conversion of phenylalanine. L-Tyrosine is hydroxylated (tyrosine hydroxylase) to L-dihydroxyphenylethylamine (DOPA), which undergoes decarboxylation (aromatic L-amino acid decarboxylase) to form dopamine. L-Norepinephrine is then formed by hydroxylation of dopamine (dopamine beta-hydroxylase). Finally, L-norepinephrine may be converted to L-epinephrine via phenylethanolamine *N*-methyl transferase. The metabolites of catecholamine degradation include normetanephrine, metanephrine, vanillylmandelic acid (VMA), and methoxy-hydroxy phenyl glycol (MHPG). These breakdown products are measurable in the urine and of great use in the diagnosis of states of catecholamine excess as is seen in pheochromocytoma.

Answer: B, D

26. Which one or more of the following would be an unexpected finding in a patient with known pheochromocytoma?

A. Paroxysmal hypertension
B. Persistent hypertension
C. Excessive sweating
D. Absence of sweating
E. Palpitations

Sabiston: 681
Schwartz: 1520

Comments: The clinical signs and symptoms seen in a patient with pheochromocytoma are due to the excessive secretion of catecholamines. One would expect, therefore, to see the typical physiologic response to catecholamine excess in these patients: hypertension, tachycardia, palpitations, excessive sweating, anxiety, tremulousness, and nausea and vomiting, among many others. The catecholamine secretion from these tumors may be episodic, in which case one sees paroxysmal hypertensive episodes, or it may be a sustained secretion, in which case one sees persistent hypertension.

Answer: D

27. With which one or more of the following syndromes may pheochromocytoma be associated?

A. MEN I
B. MEN IIa
C. MEN IIb
D. von Recklinghausen's disease
E. von Willebrand's disease

Sabiston: 681
Schwartz: 1528

Comment: Although the majority of cases of pheochromocytoma occur in isolated form, one must be alert to the association of pheochromocytoma with several other neuroendocrine and neuroectodermal abnormalities. Pheochromocytoma is one of the tumors found in the MEN IIa (pheochromocytoma, medullary carcinoma of the thyroid, and parathyroid hyperplasia) and MEN IIb (pheochromocytoma, medullary carcinoma of the thyroid, and multiple mucosal neuromas) syndromes. It is also seen in several other neurocutaneous syndromes, including von Recklinghausen's disease (neurofibromatosis), Bourneville's disease (tuberous sclerosis), and Sturge-Weber disease (meningofacial angiomatosis). Because of the danger of a catastrophic hypertensive crisis occurring in patients with undiagnosed pheochromocytoma, it is generally felt that patients presenting with other manifestations of these syndromes should be screened for the presence of pheochromocytoma.

Answer: B, C, D

28. Which one or more of the following statements regarding pheochromocytoma is/are correct?

A. There are only rare anecdotal reports of pheochromocytoma occurring outside the adrenal medulla
B. Pheochromocytoma is found bilaterally in 50% of cases
C. Malignant pheochromoctyomas occur in approximately 50% of cases
D. Approximately 10% of pheochromocytomas occur in patients less than 20 years of age

Sabiston: 682
Schwartz: 1531

Comment: Pheochromocytomas may occur in locations other than the adrenal medulla, they may be bilateral, they may be malignant, and they may occur in patients less than 20 years of age. When one considers all patients afflicted with pheochromocytoma, each of the above clinical situations occurs in approximately 10 to 20% of cases. It is important to realize, however, that within subsets of patients with pheochromocytoma the likelihood of one or more of the above presentations may increase. For example, in familial cases of pheochromocytoma there is a significantly increased risk of bilateral

tumors, extra-adrenal tumors, and malignancy occurring. Also, in familial cases, the tumors tend to appear at an earlier age. In all cases of pheochromocytoma, one must be alert to the possibility of the tumor being present in an extra-adrenal location. These may occur at any site where chromaffin tissue is located but most often are found in paraganglia of the periaortic area and specifically in vestigial structures located in the area of the inferior mesenteric artery and aortic bifurcation (organ of Zuckerkandl). Pheochromocytomas have also been reported in the urinary bladder and outside the abdomen (carotid body and glomus jugulare). Among the adrenal pheochromocytomas, there is a definite right-sided predominance for reasons that are unclear.

Answer: D

29. Of the following studies used to localize pheochromocytomas, which two are least likely to be ordered routinely?

A. Radionuclide adrenal imaging
B. CT scan with and without infusion
C. Adrenal venography
D. Selective adrenal arteriography
E. Ultrasonography

Sabiston: 686
Schwartz: 1525

Comments: The evaluation of a patient with clinical evidence of pheochromocytoma begins with the biochemical confirmation of catecholamine excess (most easily obtained by measuring urinary VMA and catecholamine levels). Once the diagnosis has been established, it is important to localize the pheochromocytoma prior to exploration. This is particularly important because of the significant incidence of bilateral and extra-adrenal tumors. Ultrasonography is the least expensive and invasive and is able to identify adrenal or other retroperitoneal masses when they are larger than 2 to 3 cm, but is relatively insensitive to the presence of tumors smaller than that. Computed tomography can identify adrenal masses as small as 1 cm and, being noninvasive, is probably the first localization study performed in the majority of cases. Radionuclide scanning with iodocholesterol has been useful in some cases of pheochromocytoma and is relatively noninvasive but lacks adequate sensitivity. Recent reports regarding the use of I-131 MIBG scanning appear to be promising. Selective arteriography and venography may be very useful in demonstrating adrenal masses, but in the case of pheochromocytomas may precipitate a severe and occasionally lethal hypertensive crisis due to the sudden increase in intraglandular vascular pressure during the study. For that reason, those studies are not usually obtained unless all other less invasive studies have failed to localize the tumor.

Answer: C, D

30. Of the following, which one or more would be appropriate to administer in the preoperative preparation of a patient with pheochromocytoma?

A. An alpha antagonist
B. A beta antagonist
C. A beta agonist

D. Fluid and/or blood
E. A diuretic

Sabiston: 685
Schwartz: 1532

Comments: The principal physiologic mechanism at work in cases of pheochromocytoma relates to excessive alpha and (frequently) beta catecholamine stimulation. This leads to an increase in peripheral vascular resistance, hypertension, tachycardia, and a contracted blood volume. At operation, when the pheochromocytoma is removed, there is an abrupt cessation of this stimulation which may lead to catastrophic hypotension and hypovolemia. To protect against this possibility, patients should be prepared preoperatively with alpha and beta blockade. Alpha blockade may be achieved by administration of phentolamine or the more preferred phenoxybenzamine. Beta blockade is indicated when patients present with significant tachycardia and may be achieved by propranolol administration. It is important to achieve alpha blockade prior to administration of propranolol, since beta blockade alone in a patient with pheochromocytoma may lead to bradycardia, increasing hypertension, and congestive heart failure. Since vasodilation occurs as a result of effective alpha-adrenergic blockade, there is frequently the need to administer fluid and/or blood to provide an effective circulating blood volume prior to operation. Diuretics would, of course, be contraindicated in such a situation, as diuresis would lead to further contraction of the blood volume.

Answer: A, B, D

31. In which of the following situations would resection of an adrenal gland be indicated?

A. A clinically silent, solid adrenal mass 4 cm in diameter recently discovered
B. A clinically silent, cystic adrenal mass 7 cm in diameter
C. A functioning solid adrenal mass 2 cm in diameter
D. A clinically silent, solid adrenal mass 5 cm in diameter that has increased in size from 3 cm over the past 12 months

Sabiston: 689

Comments: The increasing use of computed tomography in recent years has led to the discovery of many clinically silent adrenal masses. Retrospective study of numerous patients with adrenal masses has resulted in the general view that silent masses less than 6 cm in size are unlikely to be malignant and therefore, can safely be observed with repeat CT scans at appropriate intervals (every 6 to 12 months). If an increase in size is detected, resection should be performed. Clinically silent adrenal masses larger than 6 cm in size, whether cystic or solid, should probably be resected, as the incidence of malignancy in these lesions is sufficient to warrant the risk of the surgery. It is generally felt that hormonally active or clinically functioning tumors should be resected regardless of their size.

Answer: B, C, D

32. Which of the following statements regarding the surgical approach to adrenal lesions is/are correct?

A. The anterior (transabdominal) approach is generally safer than the posterior approach and results in faster recovery
B. Abdominal pheochromocytomas are most often approached anteriorly
C. Bilateral adrenal adenomas should be approached anteriorly because of the increased morbidity associated with bilateral posterior incisions
D. A large unilateral adrenocortical carcinoma is best approached posteriorly in order to avoid contamination of the peritoneal cavity

Sabiston: 689

Comments: It is generally agreed that recovery from a posterior or flank approach to an adrenal mass is faster and less complicated than a transabdominal approach. This is due in part to the intestinal ileus associated with the anterior approach and the greater likelihood of postoperative adhesive bowel obstruction. Respiratory complications also seem to be less with a posterior approach. Even bilateral posterior approaches are considered by many to be preferable to an anterior approach when bilateral adenomas are present. Many feel that pheochromocytomas should be approached anteriorly because of their significant association with multicentric, contralateral, or extra-adrenal tumors. Increasing accuracy in the localization of pheochromocytoma preoperatively, however, has led to the relatively low likelihood of encountering unsuspected extra-adrenal or multicentric pheochromocytomas at exploration and raises the issue as to whether the posterior approach may in fact be more advantageous for unilateral pheochromocytoma. Adrenocortical carcinomas, especially when large, should be approached anteriorly in order to fully assess the extent of disease and to provide a wider operative field for the tumor removal, which frequently involves excision of contiguous structures.

Answer: B

CHAPTER 23

Gastrointestinal Dysfunction:
Physiologic Principles

1. Which of the following accurately describe(s) the act of deglutition?

A. The mylohyoid muscle is important in speech, but not in swallowing
B. Elevation of the soft palate closes off the nasopharynx
C. The respiratory tract is normally completely sealed off by approximation of the vocal cords and posterior displacement of the epiglottis
D. Relaxation of the cricopharyngeal muscle permits the food bolus to enter the esophagus

Schwartz: 1027

Comments: Deglutition is a complicated orchestration of neuromuscular events which are classically considered in three stages. In the **oral** stage the food bolus is moved into the pharynx by action of the oral tongue and mylohyoid muscle. In the **pharyngeal** stage, the bolus is transported through the pharynx by involuntary contractions of the pharyngeal muscles. During this stage reflux into the nasopharynx is prevented by elevation of the soft palate; aspiration into the trachea is prevented by apposition of the vocal cords, posterior displacement of the epiglottis, and reflex inhibition of respiration. The food bolus enters the cervical esophagus through the relaxed cricopharyngeus muscle, and the third stage proceeds with **esophageal** peristalsis.

Answer: B, C, D

2. Which of the following statements is/are true regarding dysphagia?

A. Esophageal motility disorders causing dysphagia are always of the hypomotility type
B. The reason painful lesions of the mouth or tongue do not cause dysphagia is that they are not involved in the involuntary swallowing mechanism of the pharynx and esophagus
C. Dysphagia may be a common manifestation of emotional disorders

D. In cases of mechanical obstruction causing dysphagia, the patient can usually pinpoint the site of obstruction

Sabiston: 705
Schwartz: 1027

Comments: The term dysphagia refers to difficulty in swallowing, which may be due either to a disturbance of muscular action or to a physical obstruction. This is in contradistinction to odynophagia, which is simply painful swallowing. Since swallowing involves oral, pharyngeal, and esophageal stages, painful lesions or disorders in any of these areas may cause not only odynophagia but dysphagia as well. Abnormalities not necessarily intrinsic to the deglutition mechanism may also be responsible for dysphagia, and include neuromuscular disturbances (e.g., poliomyelitis, myasthenia gravis), acute thyroiditis, and emotional disorders (e.g., anxiety states, conversion hysteria, anorexia nervosa). Esophageal dysphagia may be caused by both hypermotility and hypomotility states. In cases of obstruction due to tumor or stricture, the patient is frequently able to localize the site of obstruction.

Answer: C, D

3. Which of the following statements is/are true regarding nausea and vomiting?

A. Reversed peristalsis of the stomach plays a significant role in the mechanism of vomiting
B. The chemoreceptor trigger zone is important in the mechanism of vomiting due to drugs, uremia, and radiation sickness
C. Afferent pathways to the vomiting center emanate almost exclusively from the stomach and duodenum, the exception being the terminal common duct
D. The act of vomiting involves muscular activity limited to the gastrointestinal muscular systems

Schwartz: 1029

Comments: The pathophysiology of nausea and vomiting is multifactorial and incompletely understood. There is general agreement that vomiting is controlled through two medullary centers: a sensory chemoreceptor trigger zone and an integrated center that coordinates the physical act of vomiting. The chemoreceptor trigger zone is important in initiating emesis associated with drugs, uremia, infections, and radiation sickness. Other afferent impulses causing vomiting may involve the autonomic nervous system and may emanate from virtually all sites within the body. Mechanical obstruction, autonomic disorders of the alimentary tract, severe somatic and visceral pain, sepsis, shock, metabolic derangements, and emotional disturbances are among the many causes of nausea and vomiting. The physical act of vomiting is a complicated and coordinated motor function involving the respiratory, somatic, and gastrointestinal muscular systems. Appropriately timed contraction or relaxation of abdominal musculature, intrinsic gastric musculature, the diaphragm, and pharyngeal and laryngeal muscles result in the forceful expulsion of gastrointestinal contents through the mouth with protection of the airway. Reversed peristalsis in the stomach does not contribute significantly to the mechanism of vomiting.

Answer: B

4. Match the items in the two columns (multiple combinations possible).

Vomiting Characteristic	Associated Cause
A. No antecedent nausea	a. Chronic gastric outlet obstruction
B. Projectile	b. Central nervous system lesion
C. Immediately following eating	c. Hypertrophic pyloric stenosis
D. Large amounts of partially digested food at 12- to 48-hour intervals	d. Toxic etiology

Sabiston: 1269
Schwartz: 1030

Comments: Recognition of the pattern of vomiting can often assist in diagnosing the underlying cause. Although none of the associations listed above are present in every instance, taken together with other aspects of the patient's history and physical findings, they may be valuable in suggesting the cause of vomiting.

Answer: A–b; B–b, c; C–c; D–a

5. Which of the following accurately characterizes the metabolic consequences of protracted vomiting?

A. Hypovolemia
B. Hypokalemia
C. Hypochloremia
D. Alkalosis
E. Compensatory alkaline urine

Sabiston: 72, 830
Schwartz: 1030

Comments: Protracted vomiting results in significant loss of fluid, hydrogen, chloride, and sodium in the vomitus. This results in a hypovolemic, hypokalemic, hypochloremic alkalosis. Volume depletion stimulates adrenocortical and renal mechanisms to conserve sodium at the ex-

pense of hydrogen and potassium. This results in a worsening of the hypokalemia and the excretion of a paradoxically acid urine with subsequent worsening of the systemic alkalosis. The proper initial management to offset these changes includes the administration of appropriate amounts of fluid, sodium, and chloride. In severe disturbances administration of hydrochloric acid may be indicated.

Answer: A, B, C, D

6. Which of the following pathophysiologic mechanisms may result in diarrhea?

A. Excessive intestinal secretion
B. The presence of poorly absorbable substances within the gastrointestinal tract
C. Malabsorption of ions
D. Altered bowel motility

Sabiston: 953
Schwartz: 1032

Comments: Diarrhea is usually produced by one or more of the four pathophysiologic mechanisms described above. The first mechanism is considered to be **secretory** diarrhea, the most important aspect of which is excessive active ion secretion by the small intestine. This may be a response to such underlying factors as bacterial toxins and gastrointestinal hormones. Secretory diarrhea is characterized by voluminous isotonic diarrhea, which usually persists even during fasting. The second mechanism, **osmotic** diarrhea, results from the presence of poorly absorbable solutes within the intestine. This may be due to the type of food ingested or the inability of pancreatic or mucosal enzyme systems to properly digest and absorb the solutes present. Osmotic diarrhea usually abates when the patient fasts. The third mechanism, **malabsorption** of a normal ion, is a rare cause of diarrhea. Congenital chloridorrhea, in which there is a defective transport mechanism for the absorption of chloride across the bowel mucosa, is an example. **Altered motility** may be seen with diseases such as diabetic enteropathy and scleroderma.

Answer: A, B, C, D

7. Which of the following statements is/are true regarding the clinical manifestations of intestinal obstruction?

A. Severe cramping pain follows the associated hyperperistalsis by several minutes
B. Abdominal distension is not considered an early sign of obstruction
C. In long-standing bowel obstruction, the vomitus frequently becomes dark and malodorous, representing regurgitated feces
D. Vomiting is a feature of all forms of bowel obstruction

Sabiston: 907
Schwartz: 1037

Comments: The cramping pain associated with bowel obstruction is a direct result of the hyperperistalsis proximal to the obstruction, and therefore, occurs simultaneously with it. Abdominal distension occurs as the bowel proximal to the obstruction distends with air and fluid. As this may take hours or days to develop, abdominal distension is not a very early sign of obstruction. In cases of high intestinal obstruction, where the contents of the obstructed gastrointestinal tract may be expelled by vomiting, abdominal distension may not be a feature at all. The vomitus from a patient who has been obstructed over a longer period of time may be dark and malodorous and even feculent. This is due to bacterial overgrowth within the stagnant intestinal contents and does not represent regurgitated feces. In cases of colonic obstruction with a competent ileocecal valve, there can be massive distension and severe pain, even perforation of the colon, without vomiting being present.

Answer: B

8. Which of the following statements is/are true regarding the physical findings of a patient with a mechanical bowel obstruction?

A. Fever and tachycardia are usually present within the first 12 hours of the obstruction
B. Dehydration is rarely present before vomiting develops, since, up to that point, fluid has not actually been lost from the body
C. Even in the absence of peritonitis, palpation during attacks of pain may reveal tenderness and cause guarding
D. Except for instances in which blockage is incomplete, auscultatory findings are sufficiently nonspecific that they do not assist in the evaluation of the patient with a bowel obstruction

Sabiston: 907
Schwartz: 1038

Comments: The physical examination of a patient presumed to have a suspected bowel obstruction is of value not only in diagnosing the obstruction but also in determining the presence of complications of obstruction such as strangulation. In a simple mechanical obstruction there may be few, if any, physical findings within the first 24 hours. Fever and tachycardia would be rare in the absence of peritonitis or significant dehydration. Even before vomiting develops, large amounts of fluid can be sequestered within the lumen and wall of the bowel, resulting in significant intravascular volume depletion and subsequent oliguria. Although tenderness to palpation may be absent between episodes of pain, it may be quite severe during colicky episodes, sufficiently so to even falsely suggest the presence of peritonitis. The typical bursts or rushes of loud, high-pitched bowel sounds are characteristics of mechanical obstruction. Paralytic ileus is usually characterized by a fairly quiet abdomen, but a few bowel sounds may remain. Complete silence may suggest the presence of gangrenous bowel. Evidence of systemic sepsis or toxemia is a grave sign, also suggesting the presence of gangrenous bowel.

Answer: C

9. Which of the following statements is/are true regarding the laboratory findings associated with intestinal obstruction?

A. Significant electrolyte abnormalities are unusual in the early stages of intestinal obstruction

B. The acid-base disturbances associated with intestinal obstruction vary according to the duration and location of the obstruction
C. The white blood cell count is sufficiently variable as to be of minimal help in differentiating between different types of obstruction
D. Serum amylase level may be of benefit in suggesting the presence of ischemic bowel

Sabiston: 909
Schwartz: 1038

Comments: Although the diagnosis of bowel obstruction is generally a clinical and radiographic one, some laboratory findings may be of benefit in the evaluation of patients with bowel obstruction. Although serum amylase levels may be elevated because of primary pancreatic pathology or abnormal renal amylase clearance, their presence in cases of bowel obstruction should alert the clinician to the possibility of ischemic bowel. Mild leukocytosis is commonly seen in uncomplicated mechanical obstruction; moderate elevations of the white cell count strongly suggest the presence of strangulation; marked leukocytosis suggests primary mesenteric vascular occlusion. Acid-base abnormalities may be severe in longstanding bowel obstruction, but there is no one characteristic picture. Metabolic acidosis may be seen as a result of dehydration, ketosis, and loss of alkaline secretions; metabolic alkalosis may be seen in high jejunal obstructions because of loss of the acidic gastric contents through vomiting. Even respiratory acidosis may be seen when the abdominal distension is so severe that diaphragmatic excursion is hindered. Although significant dehydration does occur and may result in an associated rise in the hematocrit, the plasma concentrations of sodium, potassium, and chloride rarely are affected.

Answer: A, B, D

10. Which of the following statements accurately characterize(s) normal gastrointestinal transit of food?

A. Following a meal, the stomach usually empties within 3 to 4 hours
B. Digested food reaching the cecum in less than 4 hours suggests abnormally increased small bowel motility
C. Most of the large intestinal water absorption occurs in the right colon
D. Man differs from lower quadripeds in that defecation is entirely under voluntary control

Schwartz: 1030

Comments: Although there is a relatively wide range of "normal" transit times through the gastrointestinal tract, ingested food usually leaves the stomach within 3 to 4 hours. It passes through the small intestine at an average rate of 1 inch per minute, with a total passage of a meal into the cecum requiring between 2 and 9 hours. The chyme entering the cecum and right colon is semiliquid, and it is at this segment of the colon that most of the water reabsorption occurs. Beyond the hepatic flexure the primarily solid stool is propelled by mass peristaltic waves down to the rectum. Defecation is a complicated physiologic act depending on afferent and efferent fibers of both the somatic and autonomic nervous systems.

Answer: A, C

11. Match the following terms with their associated type of abdominal pain:

A. Diffuse, poorly localized
B. Hollow viscus wall tension
C. Parietal peritoneum
D. Convergence-projection hypothesis
E. Associated sweating, nausea, tachycardia

a. Visceral pain
b. Somatic pain
c. Referred pain

Sabiston: 790
Schwartz: 1022

Comments: Appreciation of the mechanisms of abdominal pain is important in understanding the pathophysiology of intra-abdominal disease processes. **Visceral** or **splanchnic** pain is caused by stimulation of visceral afferent fibers, which are part of the autonomic nervous system. Visceral afferent nerve endings are located in the visceral peritoneum and wall of hollow viscera and in the capsules of solid viscera. They are sensitive to increasing wall tension or stretching, and because of their relatively sparse numbers result in sensation of pain that is diffuse and poorly localized. **Somatic** pain arising from the abdomen is mediated by segmental spinal nerves whose endings are in the abdominal wall (including the parietal peritoneum), root of the mesentery, and respiratory diaphragm. Somatic pain tends to be more localized. **Referred** pain relates to the perception of pain in an area that is separate from the actual site of pathology. It is explained according to the convergence-projection hypothesis, which suggests that pain fibers from multiple visceral and skin sites converge on a single tract for projection to the thalamus or brain cortex. The pain may be interpreted as having come from one of the converging afferent fibers that may not be involved in the pathologic process. Both visceral and somatic pain, when severe enough, can cause associated autonomic responses, including, among others, sweating, nausea, vomiting, tachycardia, and hypotension.

Answer: A–a; B–a; C–b; D–c; E–a, b

12. Neurosurgical intervention is required occasionally for the management of intractable abdominal pain. Match the following statements with their associated form(s) of neurosurgical intervention:

Statement	Neurosurgical Procedure
A. Alleviates visceral pain	a. Splanchnicectomy and celiac ganglionectomy
B. Alleviates somatic pain	b. Posterior rhizotomy
C. Subsequent painful paresthesias	c. Anterolateral chordotomy
D. Altered reaction to pain	d. Prefrontal lobotomy

Sabiston: 1414
Schwartz: 1023

Comments: In cases of intractable pain, prolonged opiate use may become ineffective, necessitating neurosurgical intervention. Splanchnicectomy and celiac ganglionectomy are useful in controlling abdominal pain of visceral afferent origin, but will not alleviate somatic pain. Posterior rhizotomy and interruption of the spinothalamic tract (anterolateral chordotomy) occur at a point at which the visceral and somatic afferent fibers have joined and, therefore, are effective in controlling both forms of pain. Unfortunately, pain and temperature sensation are also lost as a result of these procedures and introduce the risk of subsequent injury to the anesthetized area. The anesthetic areas created by rhizotomy and chordotomy are frequently replaced (after approximately 1 year) by painful paresthesias. This may be a consideration in choosing this form of neurosurgical intervention for patients with a long life expectancy. Prefrontal lobotomy does not alter the degree of pain but rather the patient's reaction to pain, and results in the flattening of affect globally.

Answer: A–a, b, c; B–b, c; C–b, c; D–d

13. Which of the following statements is/are true regarding some characteristics of pain?

A. Sensitivity to pain remains approximately the same throughout the life of an individual
B. Repeated painful stimuli result in an accommodation to the stimuli and a subsequent raising of the threshold
C. Underlying metabolic disorders can alter an individual's response to pain
D. Pain produces some degree of sympathetic response in virtually all cases

Schwartz: 1024

Comments: The perception of pain is a subjective reaction to noxious stimuli requiring the highest levels of integration of the central nervous system. This perception of pain and the physical responses to it vary with a number of factors. Sensitivity to pain tends to increase from infancy to adult life and then gradually decreases in the elderly. This explains, in part, the somewhat atypical presentation of peritonitis that may occur in the very young and very old. Repeated painful stimuli result in a hypersensitivity (facilitated pain) in which the threshold for pain perception is lowered. The pain threshold may also be affected by underlying metabolic conditions such as hyperthyroidism and hyperadrenalism, which are associated with a lowered threshold, and by hypothyroidism, which is associated with a higher threshold. Pain frequently results in sympathetic nervous system responses. Severe deep pain, however, may be accompanied by bradycardia and hypotension.

Answer: C

14. In the clinical evaluation of abdominal pain, which of the following characteristics of the pain is/are important to elicit?

A. Character
B. Severity
C. Location
D. Timing
E. Aggravating and alleviating factors

Sabiston: 790
Schwartz: 1025

Comments: In clinical practice, as we come to rely more and more on laboratory and radiographic investigation to diagnose the cause of abdominal pain, our ability to interpret its clinical features has tended to suffer. Obviously, all of the features listed above are important in determining the cause of abdominal pain. In teaching centers, where patients frequently must repeat their history for several observers, one must be alert to the possibility that some aspects of the patient's pain may have been "suggested" to the patient by earlier examiners. When possible, questioning a patient about abdominal pain should be open-ended and the terms used to describe the pain and its associated characteristics should be of the patient's choosing. Also, one should take one's own history of abdominal pain and not rely on that given to him by earlier examiners, as it is not uncommon for new and potentially helpful aspects of the pain to be elicited on repeated questioning. One should learn how the specific characteristics of abdominal pain, listed above, relate to specific underlying disease processes. As a general rule, however, abdominal pain persisting for over 6 hours or associated with clinical signs of peritoneal irritation should raise the possibility of an underlying surgically correctible cause. The decreased response to abdominal pain in the elderly makes evaluation of their pain more difficult.

Answer: A, B, C, D, E

15. Which of the following extra-abdominal processes may cause abdominal pain?

A. Pneumonia
B. Myocardial ischemia
C. Sickle cell anemia
D. Spinal cord tumors
E. Uremia
F. Porphyria
G. Insect bites

Sabiston: 808
Schwartz: 1025

Comments: The causes of abdominal pain are myriad. Processes within the abdomen tend to produce pain in the same general anatomic location as the process itself. Therefore, the possible causes of localized abdominal pain should always include consideration of inflammatory or neoplastic conditions of the organs present within that general area of the abdomen. One's sophistication in diagnosing the cause of abdominal pain increases as one considers the numerous extra-abdominal processes that may be causally related. These include numerous abnormalities in the cardiopulmonary, hematologic, neurologic, orthopedic, metabolic, and toxic categories.

Answer: A, B, C, D, E, F, G

16. Which of the following statements is/are true regarding anorexia?

A. Anorexia is mediated through spinal reflexes
B. Anorexia may be associated with extra-abdominal endocrinopathies
C. Anorexia is a potential side effect of many drugs
D. The presence of anorexia is of significant help in differentiating between various forms of intra-abdominal pathology

Sabiston: 792
Schwartz: 1028

Comments: Anorexia refers to the absence of the desire to eat. It is thought to be mediated through a satiety center in the hypothalamus. It is a nonspecific symptom that can be found in association with most forms of inflammatory and neoplastic abdominal pathology. It is similarly associated with many extra-abdominal and systemic abnormalities, including endocrine disorders such as adrenal insufficiency and hyperparathyroidism. Most drugs are capable of causing anorexia through either toxic or idiosyncratic reactions. Anorexia is a sufficiently common complaint that it is not often helpful in making a specific diagnosis. Its absence, however, may be valuable in excluding certain pathologic processes. For example, appendicitis rarely occurs in the absence of some degree of anorexia.

Answer: B, C

17. Constipation may be associated with which of the following?

A. Psychogenic factors
B. High-fiber diet
C. Marked ascites
D. Spinal cord tumor
E. Anal fissure

Schwartz: 1031

Comments: Constipation is considered to be an abnormal retention of feces or delay in fecal discharge. It has numerous causes. Improper toilet training during childhood can cause psychogenic constipation. Diets consisting of highly refined foods and minimal fiber are also associated with constipation. Expulsion of fecal matter depends upon involuntary bowel contraction as well as voluntary somatic contraction, principally of the abdominal and diaphragmatic muscles. Weakness of the abdominal muscles, as can be seen in pregnancy and marked ascites, as well as atony of the intrinsic intestinal muscle as seen in some electrolyte imbalances, can cause constipation. Neurogenic abnormalities (e.g., multiple sclerosis, spinal cord tumors) may affect the autonomic intestinal function, leading to constipation. One must also consider that constipation may be a side effect of numerous drugs. Painful anorectal conditions also may be the cause of constipation; it may be an unsuspected cause in children. Of course, a new onset of constipation must always cause the clinician to consider mechanical obstruction to the gastrointestinal tract as, for example, by tumors, strictures, and impactions.

Answer: A, C, D, E

18. Which of the following are potential consequences of prolonged diarrhea?

A. Acidosis
B. Elevated hematocrit
C. Hyperkalemia
D. Hyponatremia

Sabiston: 69
Schwartz: 1033

Comments: Diarrhea usually contains concentrations of sodium and chloride that are lower than those found in plasma and concentrations of potassium and bicarbonate that are higher than those found in plasma. The relative losses of these electrolytes, together with the fluid loss and associated dehydration, lead to the predictable findings of acidosis, hypokalemia, and elevated hematocrit (as a result of dehydration) seen in prolonged diarrhea. Serum sodium concentrations are usually not significantly affected.

Answer: A, B

19. Match each of the following clinical situations with the cause of intestinal obstruction most likely to be involved:

Clinical Situation	Cause of Obstruction
A. A 5-year-old boy with small bowel obstruction	a. Neoplasm
B. A 68-year-old man with colonic obstruction; no previous surgery	b. Adhesive bands
	c. Incarcerated hernia
C. A 40-year-old woman with small bowel obstruction 3 years after abdominal hysterectomy for fibroids	d. Volvulus
	e. Diverticulitis

Sabiston: 905
Schwartz: 1034

Comments: Grouping all ages together, adhesive bands followed by incarcerated hernia, followed in turn by neoplasm, are the most common causes of intestinal obstruction. This order may vary, however, in specific age groups. For example, hernia is a much more common cause of obstruction in childhood, and colorectal carcinoma is a much more common cause in the elderly. In a given patient, the historical features and physical findings associated with the obstruction, together with the presence or absence of a history of previous abdominal surgery, will assist greatly in determining the cause of obstruction.

Answer: A–c; B–a; C–b

20. Which of the following statements is/are true regarding the abdominal distension seen in intestinal obstruction?

A. The gaseous distension of the intestine is due primarily to bacterial production of gas
B. Intraluminal sequestration of fluid is the only significant way in which intra-abdominal fluid contributes to distension
C. Free peritoneal fluid implies a perforation of the intestine and suggests the presence of severe concomitant peritonitis
D. In distal small bowel obstruction, repetitive vomiting of large volumes of fluid does not prevent the development of significant abdominal distension

Sabiston: 906
Schwartz: 1035

Comments: The abdominal distension seen in intestinal obstruction is due to the accumulation of both gas and fluid. Although gas can be produced by intestinal bacteria, it is swallowed air that accounts for the major portion of intraluminal gas seen in both normal and pathologic states. The fluid component of abdominal distension is primarily due to both the sequestration of fluid within the lumen of the bowel and that within the wall of the bowel. The edematous bowel can exude fluid into the peritoneal cavity without perforation being present. Thus, the finding of free peritoneal fluid in cases of intestinal obstruction does not imply that perforation or peritonitis is present. In the absence of other pathologic states (e.g., portal hypertension), the free peritoneal fluid seen in intestinal obstruction does not contribute significantly to the abdominal distension. Vomiting is effective in emptying the stomach and even the duodenum of its gaseous and fluid contents and is responsible for the occasional appearance of a nondistended abdomen in the setting of high intestinal obstruction. In low intestinal obstruction, the abdominal distension is due primarily to intraluminal fluid and gas that cannot be evacuated by vomiting.

Answer: D

21. Match the following types of intestinal obstruction with their appropriate characteristics:

Type of Clinical Characteristics	Obstruction
A. May lead to perforation	a. Closed loop; small bowel
B. Most rapid clinical progression	b. Simple mechanical; ileum
C. Law of Laplace predicts location of perforation	c. Colon; competent ileocecal valve
D. May have minimal distension	d. Colon; incompetent ileocecal valve

Sabiston: 906
Schwartz: 1036

Comments: When an obstructed segment of bowel loses its blood supply, this is referred to as strangulation and is the most hazardous consequence of intestinal obstruction. Strangulation may occur either because of a twist of the mesentery leading to obstruction of its vessels or because of a pressure phenomenon within the lumen of the obstructed bowel leading to occlusion of the venules, then the capillaries, and finally the arterioles. Untreated, strangulation will eventually lead to perforation; this is a potential complication of any bowel obstruction. A closed-loop obstruction occurs when both the afferent and efferent limbs of the involved bowel are obstructed. This leads to rapid distension of the loop and a clinical progression to strangulation that is faster than in other forms of obstruction. Because of this, strangulation and perforation can occur in closed-loop small bowel obstruction in the presence of minimal abdominal distension. Colonic obstruction may also be a form of closed loop obstruction when the ileocecal valve is competent. In such cases, there usually will be massive colonic and abdominal distension that may lead to perforation. In colon obstruction the site of perforation is usually the cecum, as dictated by Laplace's law, which states that wall tension is directly related to intraluminal pressure and diameter. When the ileocecal valve is incompetent and the small bowel also can distend, the clinical course may be slower, but with more abdominal distension, and the patient is less likely to go on to colonic perforation.

Answer: A–a, b, c, d; B–a; C–c, d; D–a

22. Match the following radiographic findings with the appropriate form of bowel obstruction:

Radiographic Findings	Type of Obstruction
A. Moderate gaseous dilatation of the entire small and large bowel	a. Colonic obstruction with competent ileocecal valve
B. Gaseous distension of the small bowel with no gas in the colon	b. Ileus
C. Gaseous distension of the small bowel with small amount of gas in colon	c. Complete small bowel obstruction
D. Distended colon from cecum to descending colon with no small bowel gas	d. Partial small bowel obstruction

Sabiston: 908
Schwartz: 1038

Comments: The origin of the term *ileus* suggests that it should mean intestinal obstruction from any cause. By common usage, however, ileus has come to mean failure of progression of bowel contents due to disordered motility. The characteristic radiographic findings of ileus include moderate gaseous distension of both the small and large bowel. If the large bowel is not distended all the way to the rectum, one must also consider a left-sided colonic obstruction with an incompetent ileocecal valve. A colonic obstruction with a competent ileocecal valve will cause distension of the colon alone. An incomplete small bowel obstruction will cause significant distension proximal to the obstruction but with some gas present distal to the obstruction because of its incomplete nature. When an incomplete obstruction goes on to completion, it takes some time for the gas beyond the obstruction to be expelled, and therefore early complete small bowel obstructions may be confused radiographically with partial small bowel obstructions. When fully established, however, the characteristic appearance of distended small bowel with absent colonic gas is seen.

Answer: A–b; B–c; C–c, d; D–a

23. Which of the following statements is/are appropriate principles of management of intestinal obstruction?

A. Closed-loop obstructions represent a surgical emergency
B. In a partial small bowel obstruction, there is no advantage to a delay in surgical intervention
C. The use of "long" intestinal tubes is sufficiently cumbersome and time-consuming that it has no significant role in the modern management of intestinal obstruction
D. Most strangulated obstructions progress sufficiently quickly that fluid and electrolyte abnormalities rarely coexist

Sabiston: 909
Schwartz: 1040

Comments: All forms of intestinal obstruction should be considered as surgical problems, the urgency for correction being dictated by the likelihood of associated strangulation. In cases of colonic obstruction (particularly with a competent ileocecal valve) or closed loop obstruction of the small bowel, or when the diagnosis is bowel strangulation, the situation should be considered a surgical emergency and the patient prepared as rapidly as possible for abdominal exploration. Dehydration and electrolyte abnormalities may be significant in all forms of obstruction, and the time one has to correct these abnormalities depends upon the presence or absence of the factors listed above. In instances of partial small bowel obstruction without evidence of strangulation, it is appropriate first to correct fluid and electrolyte abnormalities before considering operation. In such instances, decompression of the proximal bowel with a long intestinal tube may result in relief of the obstruction and obviate the need for an operation. If not, this maneuver may be of benefit in reducing abdominal distension and relieving the intraluminal pressure, which may subsequently reduce the bowel wall edema. This may in turn lead to a safer exploration; as there will be less likelihood of spillage of intestinal contents, and more secure anastomoses if they are required.

Answer: A

24. Which of the following statements is/are true regarding adynamic ileus?

A. Ileus may be considered as due to muscular inhibition, muscular spasticity, or vascular occlusion
B. Except for the stomach, all segments of the gastrointestinal tract recover from adynamic ileus at approximately the same rate
C. Pseudo-obstruction of the colon is easily differentiated from mechanical colonic obstruction with plain films of the abdomen
D. In most instances, the management of ileus is nonoperative and is directed at the underlying predisposing abnormality

Sabiston: 906, 913
Schwartz: 1044

Comments: The most common form of ileus seen in surgical practice is adynamic ileus, which is due to the inhibition of intestinal neuromuscular function, usually in response to manipulation at the time of operation or from localized inflammation or infection. In uncomplicated cases, the recovery of intestinal motility from adynamic ileus occurs at rates that are specific for the area of the gastrointestinal tract involved (small bowel—8 hours; stomach—48 hours; colon—3 to 5 days). Spastic ileus refers to uncoordinated hyperactivity of the intestine and is seen in toxic and metabolic states. Specific therapy here is directed at the underlying pathology. Ileus of vascular occlusion results from the inability of ischemic muscle to contract properly. In chronic states, this may be improved by revascularization. A specific form of adynamic colonic ileus (Ogilvie's syndrome) is a form of colonic pseudo-obstruction; on plain films it appears similar to a mechanical obstruction of the left colon, and contrast study or colonoscopy may be required to differentiate between the two. One must always consider underlying electrolyte abnormalities and drugs as contributing to adynamic ileus. The therapy in general is expectant relative to etiology but includes nasogastric and rectal decompression and correction of underlying fluid and electrolyte abnormalities.

Answer: A, D

Sabiston: 828
Schwartz: 1048

25. Which of the following statements is/are true regarding gastrointestinal bleeding?

A. The definition of hematemesis is limited to the vomiting of fresh blood from a source proximal to the ligament of Treitz
B. Approximately 500 ml of gastrointestinal blood loss is required to produce melena
C. The presence of occult blood in the stool may persist for up to 3 weeks following an acute episode of gastrointestinal bleeding
D. The hematocrit level is a reliable measure of one's blood volume during the first 6 hours following an acute gastrointestinal bleed
E. The degree of azotemia seen in gastrointestinal bleeding relates in part to the site of bleeding and the status of bacterial colonization of the gut

Schwartz: 1045

Comments: Hematemesis may occur as a result of any significant bleeding occurring at a site from the pharynx to the ligament of Treitz. The blood vomited may be fresh and red, indicating fairly rapid or recent bleeding, or it may be dark and "coffee ground" in character owing to the acid effect on the blood that may occur at slower rates of bleeding. Melena refers to the passage of tarry stool and may be seen with as little as 50 ml of blood in the intestinal tract. Melena may persist for as long as 5 days after a significant gastrointestinal bleed, and occult blood may be detected for up to 3 weeks. Since it takes several hours for extracellular fluid shifts to occur in the setting of acute blood loss, the hematocrit is an unreliable indicator of the degree of hemorrhage in the early clinical period. Tachycardia and orthostatic blood pressure changes are more reliable indicators of significant blood loss. Azotemia may be seen in many forms of gastrointestinal hemorrhage, although this is most commonly seen in bleeding from esophageal varices because of the frequently associated liver disease. The production of urea from intraluminal blood requires bacterial action and therefore may vary with changes in the bacterial colonization of the gut (e.g., as occurs with the use of broad-spectrum antibiotics). Other factors, such as the site of bleeding within the gastrointestinal tract and co-existing renal impairment or hypotension, may also affect the degree of azotemia.

Answer: A, C, E

26. Match the following techniques of assessment of upper gastrointestinal hemorrhage with one or more appropriate characteristics:

Assessment Technique	Characteristics
A. Upper gastrointestinal contrast study	a. Single most important assessment technique
B. Endoscopy	b. May hinder subsequent assessment
C. Arteriography	c. May be utilized for therapy as well as diagnosis
	d. Most hazardous

Comments: The three techniques listed above are the most common ones used in the assessment of upper gastrointestinal bleeding. Despite its relative safety, **upper gastrointestinal contrast study** should not be employed as an initial technique in cases of active bleeding. It fails to adequately determine the presence of erosive gastritis, for example. Also, the retained barium handicaps any subsequent arteriography. Instead, it is more appropriately utilized in the chronically bleeding patients when one is looking for a tumor or a discrete ulcer. **Endoscopy** has become the favored technique for evaluating these patients; it has the advantage of being able to directly visualize such causes as ulcers, erosive gastritis, esophageal varices, Mallory-Weiss tears, or tumors. Also, it can be used therapeutically in the sclerosis of esophageal varices and the electrocoagulation and laser photocoagulation of bleeding sites. Its effectiveness is determined in great part by the prior ability to clear the stomach of retained blood and clots. **Arteriography,** although the most invasive and hazardous of these three techniques, may pinpoint the site of bleeding in selected patients; for this to be possible, bleeding must be at a rate of approximately 5 ml/minute. Following the diagnostic phase of the study, the arteriographic catheter may be left in place and used for therapeutic administration of vasopressin or embolic materials. Radionuclide imaging utilizing technetium-labeled erythrocytes is also a useful study, providing diagnostic information similar to that obtained by arteriography.

Answer: A–b; B–a, c; C–c, d

27. Which of the following statements is/are true regarding lower gastrointestinal tract bleeding?

A. Bleeding from the proximal jejunum usually presents as both hematemesis and melena
B. Recognition of the right colon as the site of colonic bleeding has increased in recent years
C. Diverticulitis and tumor are the most common causes of massive rectal bleeding in the adult
D. The presence of inflamed hemorrhoids in the presence of rectal bleeding should preclude further investigation of the rectum and colon

Schwartz: 1050

Comments: Bleeding from sites distal to the ligament of Treitz usually is manifested by the passage of bloody stools, which may vary from bright red to tarry depending on the site and rate of bleeding. Hematemesis is rarely associated with even high jejunal bleeding. Causes of bleeding from the distal small bowel include Meckel's diverticulum, intestinal duplication, inflammatory bowel disease, neoplasms, and vascular ectasia. In the colon the causes include diverticular disease, vascular ectasia, and neoplasm. Increasingly, vascular ectasia (particularly in the right colon) has been recognized as the cause of lower gastrointestinal bleeding; indeed, in some patient populations it may be the most common cause. The rate of bleeding may give some clue as to its source; the bleeding episodes from vascular ectasia and diverticulosis are more likely to be moderate to massive; those from diverticulitis or colorectal cancer tend to be mild. Hemorrhoids and the benign anorectal conditions that may present with bleeding are sufficiently common that their presence should not preclude evaluation of the remainder of the rectum and colon to search for other causes of rectal bleeding.

Answer: B

28. Match the following disease states that produce jaundice with their appropriate pathophysiology:

Disease	Pathophysiology
A. Gilbert's disease	a. Bilirubin production exceeds excretory capacity
B. Hemolysis	b. Extrahepatic biliary obstruction
C. Physiologic neonatal jaundice	c. Deficient hepatocyte secretion
D. Crigler-Najjar syndrome	d. Deficient hepatocyte uptake
E. Dubin-Johnson syndrome	e. Deficient conjugation
F. Suppurative cholangitis	

Schwartz: 1051

Comments: It is useful to consider patients with jaundice in terms of the possible pathophysiologic mechanisms: excess bilirubin production, deficient hepatocyte uptake, deficient conjugation, deficient hepatocyte secretion, and deficient bilirubin excretion. These have been classically grouped as prehepatic, hepatic, and posthepatic causes. One of the first tests to be performed in the evaluation of the jaundiced patient is a fractionated bilirubin assessment to determine the relative proportion of conjugated and unconjugated bilirubin. A predominance of unconjugated bilirubin suggests prehepatic causes (hemolysis) or hepatic deficiencies of uptake or conjugation of bilirubin. Predominance of conjugated bilirubin suggests defects in hepatocyte secretion into the bile ducts, or biliary excretion into the gastrointestinal tract. Combined conjugated and unconjugated hyperbilirubinemia usually suggests complex pathophysiology in which there has been acquired liver damage, or in which prehepatic or posthepatic causes have become associated with hepatocyte damage. Gilbert's disease is a relatively common abnormality of hepatic uptake of bilirubin and usually presents as a mild hyperbilirubinemia without other associated abnormalities. The Crigler-Najjar syndrome represents an inability to conjugate bilirubin within the hepatocyte due to a deficiency of glucuronal transferase. The physiologic jaundice of the newborn also represents a deficiency in conjugation; however, this is due to a self-correcting immaturity of bilirubin glucuronide synthesis. The Dubin-Johnson syndrome is caused by a deficiency in liver cell secretion and therefore presents as an intrahepatic form of obstructive jaundice. Clearly, the most significant category of jaundice as relates to surgical practice is that of extrahepatic biliary obstruction. This is usually caused by gallstones, stricture, or neoplasm. Clinically, the patient may present with a spectrum of findings ranging from asymptomatic jaundice to the sepsis and moribund state of the patient with acute suppurative cholangitis. The latter is among the most urgent general surgical situations one may encounter.

Answer: A–d; B–a; C–e; D–e; E–c; F–b

29. Match the following diagnostic procedures utilized in the evaluation of jaundice with one or more appropriate characteristics.

Diagnostic Test	Characteristics
A. Computerized tomography (CT)	a. Overall the most cost-effective initial procedure
B. Percutaneous transhepatic cholangiography (PTC)	b. May be of help in obtaining tissue diagnosis
C. Endoscopic retrograde cholangiopancreatography (ERCP)	c. Greater utility in assessing periampullary causes of obstruction
D. Upper gastrointestinal contrast study	d. May be utilized in biliary decompression
E. Ultrasonography	e. Helps determine resectability
	f. Rarely indicated

Schwartz: 1058

Comments: Proper evaluation of a patient with obstructive jaundice involves assessment of the intra- and extrahepatic biliary tree and the periampullary area of the duodenum, and all of the tests listed above may have a role to play in this assessment. Of these, upper gastrointestinal contrast study is the least helpful and would be of benefit only in showing an intraduodenal mass or extrinsic involvement of the duodenum with a periduodenal tumor. Ultrasonography as the initial method of investigation is probably the most cost-effective in that it can confirm the presence of biliary dilatation and assess the pancreas, liver, and retroperitoneal nodal areas for the presence of mass lesions or involvement which may preclude curative resection. Furthermore, under ultrasound control, needle aspiration biopsy may be performed of mass lesions. Computerized tomography is also useful in demonstrating biliary dilatation and in searching for mass lesions in the periampullary area and liver. It may further help in assessing resectability by defining the relationship of the peripancreatic vessels (particularly the superior mesenteric vessels) to the tumor mass. As with ultrasonography, CT scans may also be utilized for directing percutaneous needle biopsies. PTC is useful in visualizing the site of biliary obstruction. During this procedure, transbiliary brush biopsies for cytology may be obtained and drainage catheters may be placed to decompress the biliary tree. ERCP is also useful in determining the site of obstruction, and when this site is suspected to be distal in the biliary tree, offers the added advantage of visual inspection of the ampulla as the possible source of neoplastic obstruction. During ERCP, biopsies for histology and cytology may be performed and therapeutic intervention in the form of catheter drainage or endoscopic papillotomy may be carried out.

Answer: A–b, e; B–b, d; C–b, c, d; D–f; E–a, b, e

Esophagus

1. Which of the following statements is/are true regarding the anatomy of the esophagus?

A. The esophagus lacks a serosal layer
B. The upper esophagus is composed of striated muscle, while the lower esophagus is composed of smooth muscle
C. The narrowest point of the esophagus occurs where it traverses the diaphragm
D. The blood supply is segmental and derived from cervical, thoracic, and abdominal sources
E. The phrenoesophageal membrane is a continuation of the transversalis fascia of the abdomen

Sabiston: 698
Schwartz: 1063

Comments: Proper surgical management of diseases of the esophagus is predicated upon a thorough understanding of esophageal anatomy. The esophagus is a muscular tube with an inner circular and an outer longitudinal layer. The absence of a serosal covering may contribute to the risk of leakage following esophageal anastomosis or repair of transmural esophageal defects. In its course from the pharynx to the stomach, the esophagus is positioned to the left or to the right of the midline at various levels, thus influencing surgical accessibility. The cervical and lower thoracic portions of the esophagus are best approached from the left, whereas the subcarinal portion is more accessible from the right side. ● The normal esophagus is not of uniform diameter, but rather has predictable areas of narrowing at the levels of the cricopharyngeus, the aortic arch, and the diaphragm; of these, the upper cervical narrowing is generally the most marked. ● The arterial blood supply and venous drainage of the esophagus are segmental from numerous sources. Lymphatic drainage may extend longitudinally in the wall of the esophagus before continuing on to regional lymph nodes; this is an important consideration when performing esophagectomy for malignant disease. ● The esophagogastric junction is a complex area, both anatomically and physiologically. Supportive structures in this area include the diaphragmatic crura and the phrenoesophageal ligament. This is a continuation of the endoabdominal fascia and circumferentially attaches the esophagus to the muscular diaphragm. The anatomy of the phrenoesophageal membrane is an important factor in the pathophysiology of gastroesophageal reflux.

Answer: A, B, D, E

2. Which of the following is/are true regarding normal esophageal motility?

A. The negative intraluminal pressure of the thoracic esophagus is the main stimulus to transportation of a food bolus
B. Primary, secondary, and tertiary peristaltic waves are voluntarily initiated by swallowing
C. The esophagus contains two high-pressure zones corresponding to the upper and lower esophageal sphincters
D. Normal post-deglutition contraction of both the upper and lower esophageal sphincters results in pressures greater than pre-deglutition resting pressure

Sabiston: 701
Schwartz: 1066

Comments: Manometric studies have defined normal esophageal motility and characterized anomalies in various pathologic states. Typically, studies are performed using multiple perfused catheter systems and pull-through techniques. Within the esophagus, two high-pressure zones can be identified: one corresponding to the upper esophageal sphincter at the level of the cricopharyngeal muscle, and another representing the lower esophageal sphincter near the gastroesophageal junction. The normal act of deglutition involves coordination of both voluntary and involuntary movements. After swallowing, the upper esophageal sphincter relaxes, allowing a food bolus to enter the esophagus. A primary peristaltic wave progressively moves the food to the stomach, which is entered following coordinated relaxation of the lower esophageal sphincter. Following relaxation, a post-deglutition contraction of the sphincters occurs prior to resumption of a resting pressure. If the esophagus is not cleared of material by the primary peristaltic wave, secondary peristaltic waves are initiated in the smooth muscle of the lower two thirds of the esophagus. Tertiary waves are not peristaltic. Numerous hormonal, neural, pharmacologic, chemical, and mechanical factors can affect esophageal motility, although the precise mechanisms of control are incompletely defined.

Answer: C, D

3. Which of the following is the most important mechanism for maintaining competence of the gastroesophageal junction?

A. Intact vagus nerve
B. Diaphragmatic crural "pinch"
C. Angle of esophageal entry into the stomach
D. Orientation of muscle fibers of the lower esophageal sphincter
E. Intra-abdominal segment of esophagus

Sabiston: 703, 754
Schwartz: 1067, 1074

Comments: The anatomic arrangement of the gastroesophageal (GE) junction and the physical means by which competence of the GE junction is maintained have long been studied but are still not completely understood. It is clear that in man, unlike other animals, there is not a distinct, intrinsic muscular sphincter and that several anatomic considerations affect competence of the GE junction. It is generally agreed, however, that the presence of a segment of esophagus exposed to intra-abdominal pressure is the most important. Both the laws of physics pertaining to wall tension and pressure in hollow tubes of different diameters and many years of clinical experience with various antireflux operations support this concept. A critical anatomic factor in the maintenance of an intra-abdominal segment of esophagus appears to be the insertion of the phrenoesophageal membrane onto the esophagus at a point several centimeters above the manometrically determined gastroesophageal junction.

Answer: E

4. Which of the following statements is/are true regarding the relationship between sliding hiatal hernia and gastroesophageal reflux?

A. Reflux occurs in all patients regardless of the presence or absence of hiatal hernia
B. Symptomatic GE reflux does not occur without a hiatal hernia
C. Most patients with hiatal hernia have symptomatic GE reflux
D. Most patients with symptomatic GE reflux have hiatal hernia

Sabiston: 758
Schwartz: 1074, 1078

Comments: Limited acid reflux into the esophagus is a normal physiologic event. Clinically significant reflux and its attendant complications occur when the high-pressure zone at the lower end of the esophagus is of inadequate degree and/or length. This is not necessarily related to the presence of a sliding hiatal hernia in which the stomach and transversalis (endoabdominal) fascia protrude through the esophageal hiatus. Most patients

with significant reflux, however, can be demonstrated to have a sliding hiatal hernia. The cause of the reflux is not the hernia per se; in fact, most patients with sliding hiatal hernias do not have significant or symptomatic reflux.

Answer: A, D

5. Which of the following is the most sensitive test for the detection of GE reflux?

A. Barium swallow
B. Esophagoscopy
C. 24-hour pH monitoring
D. Acid perfusion (Bernstein) test

Sabiston: 705, 760
Schwartz: 1066

Comments: The overlap between the symptoms of gastroesophageal reflux and those of other upper abdominal or mediastinal problems makes accurate documentation of pathologic reflux important prior to embarking upon definitive therapy. Numerous tests have been used to identify abnormal reflux. Acid reflux tests, which are performed by placing a pH electrode above the manometrically determined gastroesophageal junction and measuring changes during various maneuvers (standard acid reflux test) or during normal daily activities (24-hour pH monitoring) are considered the most accurate. During 24-hour pH monitoring, a log is kept to document symptomatic episodes and the patient's activities, and these are correlated with both the frequency and the duration of reflux as recorded from the pH electrode. Tests in which 0.1 normal hydrochloric acid is instilled into the esophagus in an attempt to reproduce symptoms and acid-clearing tests in which there is measurement of the ability of the esophagus to remove instilled acid are both less accurate. Reflux can be demonstrated radiographically in many patients regardless of clinical significance. Endoscopy is useful in assessing anatomic damage produced by reflux such as esophagitis, ulceration, or stricture, but does not convey accurate physiologic information.

Answer: C

6. For each of the factors in the left-hand column, select its appropriate effect upon distal esophageal sphincter pressure.

A. Atropine
B. Bethanacol
C. Metoclopramide
D. Nicotine
E. Gastric acidification

a. Increased lower esophageal sphincter pressure
b. Decreased lower esophageal sphincter pressure
c. No significant effect

Sabiston: 704
Schwartz: 1068

Comments: Control of the distal high-pressure zone in the esophagus that acts as a physiologic sphincter is complex and is affected by neural, hormonal, chemical, and mechanical factors. Therapeutic administration of agents that increase sphincter pressure and avoidance of factors that reduce sphincter pressure are important in the medical management of patients with symptomatic reflux. The basal tone of the sphincter appears to be an intrinsic muscular property independent of autonomic innervation; relaxation or contraction of the sphincter zone, however, is modulated by neurohormonal stimulation. Cholinergic agents (and anticholinesterases) and alpha-adrenergic agents increase sphincter tone, while anticholinergic agents, alpha-adrenergic antagonists, and beta-adrenergic agonists decrease sphincter pressure. Nicotine, alcohol, chocolate, and fatty meals all tend to have detrimental effects upon sphincter tone (i.e., they cause a decrease in sphincter tone and thereby increase the likelihood of reflux). Hormonal influences include the stimulatory effects of gastrin and inhibitory influences of secretin and cholecystokinin; it is not clear, however, what effect these hormones have in physiologic doses. Gastric alkalinization and distension tend to increase lower esophageal sphincter pressure, while gastric acidification decreases sphincter tone.

Answer: A–b; B–a; C–a; D–b; E–b

7. Recognized complications of gastroesophageal reflux include which one or more of the following?

A. Anemia
B. Aspiration
C. Barrett's esophagus
D. Motility disturbance
E. Lower esophageal ring (Schatzki)

Sabiston: 758, 764
Schwartz: 1075

Comments: Significant reflux of acid gastric contents into the esophagus can produce mucosal inflammation, ulceration, chronic blood loss, and eventual stricture or shortening from scar contracture. Pulmonary aspiration of refluxed material can lead to recurrent pneumonia, bronchiectasis, and lung abscess. The chronic destructive influences of reflux can produce metaplasia of the normal squamous esophageal epithelium, resulting in esophageal lining by columnar epithelium, known as Barrett's esophagus. A constricting mucosal ring of the lower esophagus can also follow as a minor complication of reflux. Motility disorders, including spasm and disordered peristalsis, can result from chronic reflux or stenosis. In general, indications for operative intervention include symptoms or complications intractable to medical management. Medical management consists of mechanical measures, such as avoidance of recumbency (particularly after meals), weight loss, and avoidance of constricting garments, as well as pharmacologic measures that might include antacids, H_2-blockers, and metoclopramide. Fortunately, medical management is sufficient for the majority of patients with symptomatic GE reflux; even the complication of esophageal stenosis can often be effectively treated by esophageal dilatation.

Answer: A, B, C, D, E

8. Which of the following statements is/are true regarding Barrett's esophagus?

A. It may be congenital in origin
B. The columnar lining may be discontinuous with the gastric epithelium
C. It is associated with an increased risk of epidermoid cancer of the esophagus

D. Antireflux operation is indicated at time of diagnosis
E. Esophageal resection is indicated at time of diagnosis

Sabiston: 764
Schwartz: 1076

Comments: See Question 9.

9. Which one or more of the following describe the effect of antireflux operations on Barrett's esophagus?

A. Regression of esophagitis
B. Prevention of further columnar metaplasia
C. Regression of columnar esophageal lining
D. Prevention of malignancy

Sabiston: 764
Schwartz: 1076

Comments: Barrett's esophagus is a columnar metaplasia of the normal squamous epithelial lining of the esophagus. The condition is usually acquired as the result of chronic irritation from gastroesophageal reflux, but it may occasionally be congenital. Both continuous and discontinuous patterns of involvement occur. Complications include esophageal stenosis, ulceration in the columnar epithelium (Barrett's ulcer), and an increased risk of dysplasia and subsequent development of adenocarcinoma of the esophagus. The exact risk of malignant transformation is unknown. The indications for antireflux operations in Barrett's esophagus not complicated by malignancy are no different from the indications in any patient with GE reflux—that is, complications and intractibility. Antireflux operations are effective in relieving esophagitis and in preventing further metaplastic epithelial change, but they do not cause the columnar lining already present to regress, nor have they been shown to prevent the risk of cancer. Any patient with a Barrett esophagus, whether symptomatic or not, requires careful follow-up with serial endoscopic examination and biopsy. If severe dysplasia is demonstrated, esophageal resection is indicated.

Answer: Question 8: A, B
Question 9: A, B

10. Which one or more of the following principles are common to the Belsey, Nissen, and Hill antireflux operations?

A. Narrowing of the esophageal hiatus
B. Gastric plication around the distal esophagus
C. Restoration of normal gastroesophageal anatomy
D. Restoration of an intra-abdominal segment of esophagus
E. Vagotomy

Sabiston: 761
Schwartz: 1079

Comments: See Question 11.

11. Match the characteristic in the left-hand column with the appropriate operation(s) in the right-hand column.

A. Thoracic approach only   a. Belsey
B. Abdominal approach only   b. Nissen
                                  c. Hill
C. Median arcuate ligament

Sabiston: 761
Schwartz: 1079

Comments: Simple reconstitution of normal gastroesophageal anatomy is not an effective antireflux operation. Several well-conceived and standardized operations have now been devised as effective antireflux procedures. These operations include the Nissen fundoplication, the Belsey Mark IV operation, and the Hill posterior gastropexy with calibration of the cardia. Common to all of these procedures are restoration of an intra-abdominal segment of esophagus, a variable degree of gastric plication around the distal esophagus, and a narrowing of the esophageal hiatus. Illustrations in the referenced surgical texts should be referred to for a simple anatomic understanding of these operations. The **Belsey** operation, performed through the chest only, involves two layers of plicating sutures placed between the gastric fundus and the lower esophagus with subsequent creation of approximately a 280-degree anterior gastric wrap and posterior approximation of the crura. In the **Nissen** fundoplication, which can be performed either via an abdominal or thoracic approach, a 360-degree circumferential wrap of the gastric fundus around the distal esophagus is created. In the **Hill** operation, performed only through the abdomen, a posterior approximation of the crura is followed by anchoring of both the anterior and posterior aspects of the gastroesophageal junction to the median arcuate ligament adjacent to the aorta, thus creating a gastric wrap of approximately 180 degrees. Calibration of the plication by intraoperative manometric measurements is considered critical to success of the Hill procedure. All of these operations can be effective in the prevention of GE reflux; whether one operation is clearly superior to another is controversial. Each has a place in the management of GE reflux, depending upon individual patient characteristics, technical considerations, and the surgeon's experience.

Answer: Question 10: A, B, D
Question 11: A–a, B–c, C–c

12. Which of the following is/are true regarding paraesophageal hiatal hernias?

A. Symptomatic GE reflux is the most common complication
B. Often there is an associated sliding hiatal hernia
C. Large asymptomatic hernias require repair
D. Surgical treatment usually involves an antireflux procedure

Sabiston: 757
Schwartz: 1081

Comments: The anatomic defect in a paraesophageal (type II) hiatal hernia involves a defect in the phrenoesophageal membrane with herniation of the stomach in a peritoneal-lined pouch adjacent to the esophagus. The gastroesophageal junction may remain located in its normal position, but often there is an associated sliding hiatal hernia as well. Occult gastrointestinal bleeding from gastritis or ulceration in the herniated portion of the stomach and gastric volvulus are the most common complications. Acute gastric volvulus is a surgical emergency; it may present with a classic triad of pain, nausea with inability to vomit, and inability to pass a nasogastric tube. There is a significant risk of serious complications with paraesophageal hernias, even when asymptomatic; for this reason repair is generally indicated when the condition is diagnosed. Although a pure paraesophageal hernia is not associated with GE reflux and theoretically should not require an antireflux procedure for its correction, a significant incidence of postoperative reflux has been observed following simple reduction. This has been attributed to attenuation of tissues and the consequences of the dissection required for the reduction of large paraesophageal hernias. An antireflux procedure therefore is performed by many surgeons when the paraesophageal hernia is reduced, even if there is not an associated sliding component.

Answer: B, C, D

13. A 45-year-old man complains of dysphagia and regurgitation. The esophagogram shows a narrow distal esophagus. Manometric studies demonstrate absence of peristaltic waves and a lower esophageal sphincter that does not relax with swallowing. The main defect in this condition is located in the:

A. Cervical esophagus
B. Upper esophageal sphincter
C. Body of the esophagus
D. Lower esophageal sphincter

Sabiston: 708
Schwartz: 1068

Comments: See Question 16.

14. Appropriate treatment for the patient described in Question 13 may include which one or more of the following?

A. Nitrates
B. Balloon dilatation
C. Cervical esophagomyotomy
D. Thoracic esophagomyotomy
E. Esophagectomy

Sabiston: 708
Schwartz: 1068

Comments: See Question 16.

15. A 40-year-old woman complains of chest pain and dysphagia. Esophagogram is normal. Manometric studies demonstrate simultaneous high-amplitude contractions with normal relaxation of the lower esophageal sphincter. The most likely diagnosis is:

A. Cricopharyngeal dysfunction
B. Diffuse esophageal spasm
C. "Vigorous" achalasia
D. Scleroderma
E. Psychogenic dysphagia

Sabiston: 717
Schwartz: 1072

Comments: See Question 16.

16. Appropriate initial treatment of the patient described in Question 15 should include which one or more of the following?

A. Antispasmodics
B. Balloon dilatation
C. Cervical esophagomyotomy
D. Thoracic esophagomyotomy
E. Esophagectomy

Sabiston: 717
Schwartz: 1072

Comments: Esophageal motility disorders may be primary or they may occur secondarily as the result of mechanical obstruction or of various neuromuscular disorders. Exclusion of mechanical problems such as tumor or stricture and accurate characterization of the type of motility disorder are mandatory prior to definitive therapy. Motility disorders can often be differentiated based upon the findings of esophagoscopy, esophagography, manometric studies, and acid reflux tests. • In achalasia, the absence or degeneration of intramural ganglion cells in the body of the esophagus eliminates normal esophageal peristalsis and produces a characteristic failure of the lower esophageal sphincter to relax with deglutition. An esophagogram may demonstrate esophageal dilatation and a typical "bird's beak" narrowing of the distal esophagus. Clinically, patients experience dysphagia, regurgitation, and weight loss. Although the problem may occur at any age, it is most commonly diagnosed in those between 30 and 50 years of age and is somewhat more frequent in males. Therapy is focused on destruction of the muscular apparatus of the hypertonic lower esophageal sphincter. This can be effectively accomplished in about 85% of patients either by forceful dilatation with hydrostatic or pneumatic balloons or by surgical myotomy of the lower thoracic esophagus. Operative treatment may be somewhat more effective and has a lower risk of perforation. The extent to which the myotomy should be carried down onto the stomach and the necessity for concomitant performance of an antireflux procedure are controversial features about the surgical management of achalasia. • Diffuse esophageal spasm presents with chest pain and dysphagia. The etiology is unclear, although in many patients it is associated with emotional factors and functional GI disorders. Manometric studies demonstrate aperistaltic, high-amplitude contractions, although peristalsis may be observed in the upper, striated portion of the esophagus. Unlike achalasia, the lower esophageal sphincter usually has a normal relaxation response. Manometric findings may be intermittent, obscuring the diagnosis. The esophagogram is frequently normal, although the classic "corkscrew" esophagus may occasionally be demonstrated. Surgical treatment of diffuse esophageal spasm is less satisfactory than that of achalasia. For this reason, medical management with antispasmodics, dietary modulation, and psychiatric counseling constitute the initial therapeutic management. When surgical therapy is necessary, an extended thoracic esophagomyotomy is indicated. Esophagectomy may occasionally be indicated for patients with advanced esophageal dilatation due to motility disorders of any type. • Variants of these two classic problems may be seen, and precise diagnosis is sometimes difficult. One example is so-called vigorous achalasia in which patients may present with symptoms of dysphagia, regurgitation, and chest pain and have manometric findings suggestive of diffuse spasm as well as abnormal relaxation of the lower esophageal sphincter. A

note of caution remains: In any patient with a suspected esophageal motility disorder, organic obstruction and, in particular, carcinoma must carefully be excluded.

Answer: Question 13: C
Question 14: B, D
Question 15: B
Question 16: A

17. Cricopharyngeal myotomy may be an appropriate treatment for which one or more of the following conditions?

A. Sideropenic dysphagia
B. Cricopharyngeal dysfunction
C. Scleroderma
D. Zenker's diverticulum

Sabiston: 705, 726, 728
Schwartz: 1087, 1103

Comments: The symptom of cervical dysphagia may be a manifestation of a neurologic, muscular, or mechanical disorder affecting the pharyngoesophageal region. Conditions that result from abnormal contraction of the cricopharyngeal muscle, such as a pharyngoesophageal diverticulum (Zenker's) and cricopharyngeal dysfunction, may be effectively treated by surgical division of the muscle. The etiology of a Zenker's diverticulum has been related to premature contraction of the cricopharyngeus during swallowing; hypertonic contraction of the inferior constrictor mechanism may be seen in patients with so-called cricopharyngeal spasm or dysfunction. Cervical dysphagia occurs in patients with sideropenic dysphagia (Plummer-Vinson, Paterson-Kelly syndromes), in which the mechanism is usually an upper esophageal web related to a nutritional deficiency. Treatment consists of esophageal dilatation and nutritional supplementation. Esophageal motility problems can occur in scleroderma and in other collagen vascular diseases. The primary disturbance is not specific to the cricopharyngeal region, however, and generally involves motility disturbance of the distal esophagus and incompetence of the gastroesophageal junction.

Answer: B, D

18. Which of the following statements is/are true regarding a Zenker's diverticulum?

A. Severity of symptoms is primarily determined by the size of the diverticulum
B. Diagnosis is best established endoscopically
C. Cricopharyngeal myotomy alone without diverticulectomy may be adequate treatment
D. Complete surgical excision generally requires thoracotomy

Sabiston: 726
Schwartz: 1087

Comments: A pharyngoesophageal diverticulum may result when premature contraction of the cricopharyngeus produces a posterior mucosal protrusion between the horizontal fibers of the cricopharyngeus and the more superior oblique fibers of the thyropharyngeus. Characteristic symptoms include cervical dysphagia and regurgitation; respiratory symptoms may occur as the result of aspiration. The severity of symptoms is primarily related to the degree of cricopharyngeal dysfunction and not simply to the size of the diverticulum. The diagnosis is established by esophagography. The operative approach is one of an incision in the left neck. Cricopharyngeal myotomy alone is adequate treatment for small lesions; larger diverticula should be excised as well.

Answer: C

19. Match the characteristic in the left-hand column with the appropriate type(s) of esophageal diverticulum(a) in the right-hand column:

Characteristic	Diverticulum
A. Acquired	a. Zenker's
B. Muscular wall	b. Traction
C. Esophagobronchial fistula	c. Epiphrenic
D. Treatment usually non-operative	d. None of the above

Sabiston: 727
Schwartz: 1089

Comments: At any level of the alimentary tract diverticula can occur; they can be considered as "true" diverticula, meaning that they contain a complete wall of mucosa, submucosa, and muscle, or as "false" diverticula, which lack a muscular layer. Diverticula can further be categorized as acquired or congenital. In the esophagus most herniations are acquired defects. The pharyngoesophageal and epiphrenic outpouchings lack a muscular layer (false diverticula) and result from functional or mechanical obstruction. Traction diverticula are generally located in the mid-esophagus; they represent a small area of distortion that involves the entire wall of the esophagus (true diverticulum) caused by inflammation in adjacent mediastinal lymph nodes, which is usually due to granulomatous disease. Traction and epiphrenic diverticula usually are inconsequential; operation is occasionally necessary for a large epiphrenic diverticulum or for a traction diverticulum complicated by perforation or esophagorespiratory fistula.

Answer: A–a, b, c; B–b; C–b; D–b, c

20. Which of the following is the most common benign tumor of the esophagus?

A. Congenital cyst
B. Leiomyoma
C. Fibrovascular polyp
D. Hemangioma
E. Lymphangioma

Sabiston: 736
Schwartz: 1092

Comments: Benign esophageal tumors are far less common than malignant neoplasms. Oftentimes they are completely asymptomatic, although large lesions may cause obstruction. **Leiomyomas** are the most common benign esophageal lesions; they are extramucosal lesions that produce a characteristic smooth defect with intact mucosa on radiographic studies. Treatment consists of simple enucleation. **Esophageal cysts** are the second most common type of benign tumor; these also are extra-

mucosal lesions treated by enucleation. **Benign esophageal polyps** represent unusual mucosal lesions that most commonly are encountered in the cervical esophagus. They can be treated endoscopically or by resection via a cervical esophagotomy. Other types of benign esophageal neoplasms are rare.

Answer: B

21. Which one or more of the following is/are associated with an increased risk of epidermoid carcinoma of the esophagus?

A. Achalasia
B. Barrett's esophagus
C. Caustic stricture
D. Ectopic gastric mucosa
E. Upper esophageal web

Sabiston: 738
Schwartz: 1092

Comments: Most malignant esophageal neoplasms are epidermoid carcinomas; adenocarcinoma may occur in the distal esophagus at the columnar epithelial junction or in other columnar-lined areas of the esophagus, as observed with Barrett's esophagus or ectopic gastric mucosa. Adenocarcinoma in the distal esophagus may also be seen as an extension of a primary gastric neoplasm. There are notable worldwide variations in the incidence of epidermoid cancer of the esophagus, with high rates in certain areas of China, Japan, Iran, South Africa, and Russia. In the United States, esophageal cancer is much more common in men than in women and occurs approximately four times more frequently in black men than in white men. The numerous carcinogenic etiologies that have been implicated include alcohol, tobacco, nutritional deficits, and chronic inflammation. Patients with achalasia, corrosive esophageal stricture, and sideropenic dysphagia are well recognized to be at increased risk of developing esophageal epidermoid cancer.

Answer: A, C, E

22. Select one or more of the following. When diagnosed, esophageal cancers are most often:

A. Multicentric
B. Metastatic to lung
C. Metastatic to liver
D. Metastatic to lymph nodes
E. Radiosensitive

Sabiston: 738
Schwartz: 1093

Comments: Esophageal cancer is a disease with a dismal outlook. The extensive submucosal lymphatic network of the esophagus predisposes to early involvement of mediastinal, supraclavicular, and abdominal lymph nodes. Hematogenous spread to lung and liver may occur. Furthermore, these tumors tend to be locally invasive, with involvement of adjacent mediastinal structures such as the tracheobronchial tree, recurrent laryngeal nerve, aorta, pericardium, and diaphragm. When all of these factors are combined, it is not surprising that the vast majority of esophageal cancers are unresectable for cure at the time of diagnosis. Epidermoid cancers are radio-sensitive, but the extent of involvement at the time of diagnosis usually precludes cure by this local-regional modality of therapy. Chemotherapy, often combined with radiation, may play an important role in treatment of advanced esophageal cancer, and evaluation of various treatment protocols is ongoing. In China and Japan, where esophageal cancer is more prevalent, aggressive screening programs have led to detection of earlier lesions, and improved cure rates are being reported. Nonetheless, in the West, treatment of esophageal cancer remains predominantly palliative, with 5-year survival rates of 10% or less.

Answer: D, E

23. Select one or more of the following. Esophagectomy for esophageal cancer is:

A. Indicated only if potentially curative
B. Indicated for palliation, only if endoscopic intubation is unsuccessful
C. The preferred method of providing palliation when there is a tracheoesophageal fistula
D. Preferable to operative bypass for palliation of an obstructing lesion

Sabiston: 739
Schwartz: 1094

Comments: Although operation for esophageal cancer is most often noncurative, many consider esophagectomy the best method of providing palliation. Reconstruction is generally performed by pulling up the stomach; if necessary, it can be used to replace the entire length of the esophagus. Colon interposition can be used when the stomach is not available. The mortality rate for esophagectomy is 2 to 5 per cent. Endoscopic intubation of unresectable obstructing esophageal cancers would seem an attractive technique, but has not been uniformly acceptable owing to complications of tube obstruction or dislodgment, or esophageal perforation. Placement of an esophageal tube, however, may be the preferred method of palliation for the difficult problem of malignant tracheoesophageal fistula. Use of the stomach or colon for retrosternal bypass of the obstructed esophagus has a high attendant morbidity and has not proved superior to esophagectomy for palliation.

Answer: D

24. Advantages of esophagectomy performed without thoracotomy for esophageal cancer may include which one or more of the following?

A. Prolonged disease-free survival
B. Decreased incidence of anastomotic leak
C. Decreased incidence of gastroesophageal reflux
D. Decreased blood loss
E. Elimination of need for pleural drainage

Sabiston: 745

Comments: Standard approaches to the thoracic esophagus include a left thoracoabdominal incision or a combined abdominal incision and separate right thoracotomy. Esophagectomy can also be accomplished without thoracotomy using abdominal and cervical incisions. This approach, which has more recently been popularized, involves a transhiatal blunt or "blind" resection of the thoracic esophagus from the abdomen with subsequent pull-up of the stomach and an esophagogastric anastomosis in the neck. Such an approach violates the dictum of traditional cancer surgery that calls for en bloc resection of the affected organ and regional lymph nodes in planes away from the tumor. Nonetheless, proponents of blunt esophagectomy argue that the avoidance of thoracotomy minimizes morbidity of the operation, that leakage from the cervical anastomosis is far less catastrophic than an intrathoracic leak, that postoperative gastroesophageal reflux is less common than with an intrathoracic anastomosis, and that the technique has not detrimentally affected survival. Blunt esophagectomy is not without complication, however; pneumothorax is common, and serious injury to the trachea, recurrent laryngeal nerve, or aorta can occur. Randomized prospective clinical trials comparing the blunt technique to standard radical esophagectomy have not been reported.

Answer: C

25. A 4-year-old child is brought to the emergency room 15 minutes after ingesting drain cleaner. The patient is hoarse and stridorous. Initial treatment should include which one or more of the following?

A. Syrup of ipecac
B. Gastric lavage
C. Fiberoptic endoscopy
D. Steroids
E. Antibiotics

Sabiston: 768
Schwartz: 1102

Comments: See question 27.

26. Which of the following statements is/are true regarding the role of endoscopy in the acute therapy of one who has ingested a corrosive substance?

A. It should be performed within 12 to 24 hours if the patient is stable
B. It is contraindicated prior to esophagography because of the risk of perforation
C. It is contraindicated if obvious oropharyngeal burns are present
D. It is contraindicated if perforation is suspected
E. The full extent of the injury must be visualized to determine appropriate therapy

Sabiston: 768
Schwartz: 1103

Comments: See Question 27.

27. Which of the following is the most appropriate in the initial management of a patient with confirmed esophageal corrosive injury?

A. Prompt institution of serial esophageal dilatation
B. Parenteral hyperalimentation and prohibition of oral intake for 2 to 3 weeks
C. Steroids for 3 weeks
D. Esophagectomy with gastrostomy, cervical esophagostomy, and delayed reconstruction
E. Esophagectomy with immediate reconstruction

Sabiston: 769
Schwartz: 1103

Comments: When caustic alkaline burns of the esophagus are suspected, the ingested agent should be promptly identified and an early assessment of the extent of injury made. Superficial burns usually heal without complication, whereas full-thickness injury must be aggressively treated to avoid late formation of stricture. Early endoscopy is important to verify the presence or absence of esophageal injury and to assess its severity. It is critical that the endoscope not be advanced any farther than the proximal extent of injury if a burn is identified, in order to avoid perforation. The distal extent of injury can be assessed radiographically. Esophagoscopy is contraindicated in patients with evidence of perforation or potential airway obstruction. The child presented in Question 25 has findings of laryngeal or epiglottic edema, and preservation of the airway must be the priority of treatment. Endoscopy is therefore deferred, and tracheostomy may be required. Induced emesis and lavage are also contraindicated, as they may aggravate the injury. When an esophageal burn is confirmed or when the presence or absence of esophageal injury cannot be verified because of airway considerations, treatment consists of the administration of steroids and antibiotics. This regimen reduces the late formation of stricture and is felt to be more effective and safe than early esophageal dilatation. Steroids may be better avoided in patients with suspected perforation or acid ingestion; in these patients the site of injury is more frequently the stomach rather than the esophagus, and the addition of steroid therapy may increase the risk of hemorrhage. In most cases, oral intake is allowed after several days when the edema of the initial injury has subsided and the patient can swallow effectively. Oral intake, in fact, provides a natural method of esophageal dilatation and may help to prevent stricture formation. The presence or absence of oropharyngeal burns in a patient with suspected corrosive ingestion is not a reliable indicator of esophageal injury.

Answer: Question 25: D, E
Question 26: A, D
Question 27: C

28. Which of the following is/are true regarding the late sequelae of ingestion of corrosive substances?

A. Stricture is best treated by injection of steroids endoscopically
B. Acid ingestion is more commonly complicated by gastric outlet obstruction than by esophageal stricture
C. The late development of esophageal cancer is more common with strictures following acid ingestion than alkali ingestion
D. Cancer following corrosive injury has a better prognosis than esophageal cancer in general

Sabiston: 770
Schwartz: 1103

Comments: Late complications of corrosive burns of the esophagus include stricture, gastroesophageal reflux, and malignancy. The standard treatment for stricture is esophageal dilatation, often performed retrogradely through a gastrostomy. There is limited experience with treatment of localized strictures by the direct injection of steroids. Refractory strictures may require esophagectomy or a bypass operation. For patients who develop severe GE reflux as the result of scarring and gastroesophageal incompetence, dilatation of the stricture may be detrimental. This situation also requires more definitive surgical treatment. • In contradistinction to alkaline ingestion, acid ingestion more commonly produces gastric injury. This is because the squamous epithelium of the esophagus is somewhat resistant to acid injury and also because the pylorospasm that accompanies acid ingestion prolongs contact time with the stomach. • Malignant degeneration is a well-recognized complication of corrosive esophageal stricture and should be suspected in any patient with a long-standing stricture who then has a change in symptoms. The prognosis of these cancers, however, has been more favorable than in patients without chronic stricture, and resection may provide cure.

Answer: B, D

29. Following diagnostic esophagoscopy, a patient complains of odynophagia and chest pain. Which of the following is the most appropriate next step in management?

A. Analgesics and observation
B. Repeat endoscopy
C. X-ray with Gastrografin swallow
D. X-ray with barium swallow

Sabiston: 735, 751
Schwartz: 1099

Comments: Chest pain, fever, tachycardia, subcutaneous emphysema, dysphagia, and dyspnea are all typical symptoms of esophageal perforation. Perforation may result from iatrogenic (endoscopy, periesophageal operations) or external trauma, primary esophageal disease, or postemetic ("spontaneous") esophageal hypertension. The mortality of esophageal perforation is clearly related to the time interval between perforation and definitive treatment. Whenever perforation is suspected, a contrast study should be performed with water-soluble contrast material. If a perforation is not demonstrated, an immediate barium swallow study should be performed. Barium is more accurate in delineating an esophageal leak, but potentially more dangerous. Contrast studies are important not only for verification of esophageal rupture but for documenting the level of injury, which has important implications for treatment. Although endoscopy can be used in cases of suspected esophageal perforation, and may allow foreign body retrieval, it is associated with the potential hazard of extending the perforation and is usually not required.

Answer: C

30. For each clinical situation described in the left-hand column, choose the most appropriate treatment in the right-hand column:

Clinical Situation

A. Septic patient with 48-hour-old perforation of the thoracic esophagus and pneumohydrothorax
B. Stable patient with fever, subcutaneous emphysema, and cervical perforation 2 hours after endoscopy
C. Patient with epidermolysis bullosa, minimal chest pain, and low-grade fever 2 days following endoscopy. Esophagogram shows thoracic perforation with limited mediastinal involvement
D. Patient with 6-hour-old stab wound, fever 102° F, left pleural effusion, and thoracic esophageal perforation

Most Appropriate Treatment

a. Antibiotics, nothing orally, parenteral nutrition
b. Emergency esophagectomy
c. Pleural drainage, esophageal exclusion, gastrostomy, cervical esophagostomy
d. Primary transthoracic esophageal repair
e. Transcervical esophageal repair and drainage

Sabiston: 735, 751
Schwartz: 1100

Comments: Treatment of esophageal perforation depends upon the site and extent of injury, the etiology, the presence or absence of underlying esophageal disease, the patient's general status, and, importantly, the time interval between perforation and diagnosis. Cervical perforations can usually be handled with transcervical drainage; repair is desirable if technically possible. Patients with recently recognized perforations of the thoracic esophagus can be successfully managed by primary esophageal repair, the principles of which include layered closure of the esophagus, buttressing of the repair, and thoracic drainage. The gastric fundus or pleural or pericardial flaps can be useful for buttressing the sutured closure and are important in decreasing postoperative leakage. For late perforations in septic patients, the mortality is high. These patients require aggressive control of the septic focus; attempts at primary repair are doomed to failure. Techniques of esophageal exclusion may be useful in this setting; some also favor esophagectomy. In patients with esophageal perforations and underlying esophageal disease such as obstructing distal lesions, surgical management of the perforation should include definitive treatment of the underlying pathology. This may require esophagectomy, for example, in patients with perforation proximal to an esophageal carcinoma. There is a subset of patients who may be managed conservatively without operation. This includes patients with late-recognized perforations who are clinically stable and improving and whose perforation is radiographically limited without pleural extension and preferably with evidence of spontaneous drainage of the periesophageal cavity back into the esophagus.

Answer: A–c; B–e; C–a; D–d

CHAPTER **25**

Stomach and Duodenum

1. Concerning the blood supply of the stomach, which of the following statements is/are true?

A. The right gastric artery arises from the common hepatic artery and constitutes the major vascular supply to the antrum
B. The left gastric artery often originates anomalously from the superior mesenteric artery
C. The gastroepiploic arcade arises from both the gastroduodenal and splenic arteries
D. Ligation of the splenic artery results in necrosis of the greater curvature of the stomach

Sabiston: 810
Schwartz: 1113

Comments: The arterial blood supply of the stomach is derived primarily from branches of the celiac axis. The **left gastric artery** usually arises directly from the celiac trunk. The **right gastric artery,** from the common hepatic artery, supplies a portion of the duodenum and the pyloric region. The **gastroepiploic arcade** along the greater curvature arises from both the gastroduodenal artery and the splenic artery. The **splenic artery** also contributes the short gastric vessels, but because the stomach has an abundant collateral blood supply, necrosis is infrequent following ligation of the splenic artery. The left hepatic artery may arise anomalously from the left gastric artery.

Answer: C

2. When the stomach is mobilized for esophageal replacement, the arterial supply is primarily based upon the:

A. Left gastric artery
B. Right gastric artery
C. Left gastroepiploic artery
D. Right gastroepiploic artery
E. Superior mesenteric artery

Sabiston: 743
Schwartz: 1095

Comments: The left gastric artery and short gastric vessels are routinely divided when the stomach is mobilized for esophageal replacement. The main blood supply, then, is derived from the right gastroepiploic artery, so the gastroduodenal artery must be preserved during dissection. The right gastric artery and the superior mesenteric artery may also contribute.

Answer: D

3. Match the items in the two columns related to gastric innervation.

A. Anterior vagus
B. Posterior vagus
C. Hepatic vagal branch
D. Celiac vagal branch
E. Criminal nerve of Grassi
F. Nerve of Laterjet
G. "Crow's foot"
H. Sympathetic innervation

a. Right vagus nerve
b. Left vagus nerve
c. Both
d. Neither

Sabiston: 811
Schwartz: 1114

Comments: The left thoracic vagus continues as the anterior vagus, which gives off a hepatic branch and continues along the lesser curvature as the anterior nerve of Laterjet, terminating in the "crow's foot" at the pyloroantral region. The thoracic right vagus becomes the posterior vagal trunk, which gives off a celiac branch and continues as the posterior nerve of Laterjet, terminating as does the anterior nerve. Selective vagotomy divides the nerves of Laterjet below the hepatic and celiac branches; highly selective vagotomy divides individual branches of the nerve of Laterjet, preserving the "crow's foot." Sympathetic innervation of the stomach is via the splanchnic nerves.

Answer: A–b; B–a; C–b; D–a; E–a; F–c; G–c; H–d

4. Match the cell types with their secretory function.

177

Cell Type	Secretory Function
A. Parietal cell (fundus)	a. Intrinsic factor
B. Chief cell (fundus)	b. Gastrin
C. Neck cell	c. Pepsinogen
D. G-cell (antrum)	d. Hydrochloric acid
E. Surface epithelial cell	e. Mucus
	f. Bicarbonate

Sabiston: 811
Schwartz: 1116

Comments: The various areas of the stomach have different secretory functions; this is an important consideration in the surgical management of peptic ulcer disease. Subtotal gastrectomy removes a large portion of the acid-secreting, parietal cell mass; antrectomy removes the main source of acid-stimulating gastrin; the effectiveness of highly selective vagotomy depends upon denervation of the parietal cell mass. Following resections involving the fundus, periodic injections of vitamin B_{12} may be required to prevent a deficiency caused by the lack of intrinsic factor.

Answer: A–a, d; B–c; C–e; D–b; E–e, f

5. Gastric acid secretion is:

A. Stimulated by vagally released acetylcholine
B. Inhibited by secretin
C. Stimulated by gastrin released from the duodenal mucosa
D. Stimulated by gastrin released from the fundal mucosa
E. Inhibited by calcium

Sabiston: 815
Schwartz: 1118

Comments: There are cephalic, gastric, and intestinal phases of gastric acid secretion. Vagal stimulation directly releases acid from parietal cells in addition to releasing gastrin from the antrum and sensitizing the parietal cells to the gastrin released. Although the antrum is the predominant source of gastrin, some secretion from the duodenal mucosa also occurs. Calcium stimulates acid secretion. Duodenal acidification releases secretin, which inhibits gastric acid secretion.

Answer: A, B, C

6. Which of the following enhance(s) the secretion of gastrin?

A. Antral acidification
B. Duodenal acidification
C. Antral distension
D. Sympathetic neural stimulation
E. Antral carbohydrates and fat content

Sabiston: 815
Schwartz: 1119

Comments: Vagal stimulation, antral distension, and antral protein stimulate gastrin release. A feedback mechanism exists so that the secretion of gastrin and subsequent acid release are inhibited as gastric pH decreases. Gastrin release decreases with a pH below 5 and essentially ceases when the pH is 1.5.

Answer: C

7. Effects of gastrin include:

A. Stimulation of gastric acid secretion
B. Stimulation of pepsin secretion
C. Stimulation of gastric mucosal blood flow
D. Stimulation of pancreatic enzyme secretion
E. Trophic influence on gastric mucosa

Sabiston: 816

Comments: Gastrin, in addition to its numerous effects on gastrointestinal secretory function, is thought to be an important trophic factor for the gastric mucosa.

Answer: A, B, C, D, E

8. Concerning digestive function of the stomach:

A. The antrum functions as an efficient one-way valve for distal propagation of particulate matter
B. Gastric secretion of lipase aids early fat digestion
C. Proteolytic activity of pepsin is pH-dependent
D. Activity of salivary amylase is enhanced by gastric acidification
E. The antral mucosa contains both chief cells and parietal cells

Schwartz: 1117

Comments: The stomach has both a mechanical and a chemical role in digestion. Food particles are reduced in size by the grinding action of the antrum, which returns material to the proximal stomach for further processing. Enzymatic breakdown of proteins, carbohydrates, and fat occurs in the stomach. Salivary amylase is inactivated at low pH, whereas the conversion of pepsinogen to its active form requires a low intragastric pH.

Answer: B, C

9. Gastric emptying patterns:

A. May be delayed by truncal vagotomy
B. Can be quantitatively assessed by radionuclide scans
C. Are best assessed by the saline load test
D. Are similar for solids and for liquids
E. Are usually accelerated in diabetes owing to an osmotic phenomenon

Schwartz: 1120

Comments: Gastric emptying is influenced by meal composition and by neural and hormonal factors. Although truncal vagotomy may produce delayed emptying, its effects are variable. Radioisotope scans, which provide an objective assessment of gastric emptying, have, in fact, a relatively poor correlation with clinical impressions. One advantage of highly selective vagotomy over truncal vagotomy is the preservation of more normal emptying patterns. Alterations have been observed following this type of vagotomy, but the clinical effects are usually minimal. Emptying of liquids is exponential and depends on fundal tone. Emptying of solids is linear after an initial lag period and depends on antral peristalsis. Diabetes may be associated with delayed gastric emptying.

Answer: A, B

10. The most common pathophysiologic mechanism of duodenal ulcer is primarily related to:

A. Gastric acid hypersecretion
B. Fasting hypergastrinemia
C. Deficient duodenal buffers
D. Rapid gastric emptying
E. Hyperpepsinogenemia

Sabiston: 820
Schwartz: 1124

Comments: Duodenal ulcer is a heterogenous disorder. Forty percent of patients are hypersecretors of gastric acid owing to an increase in the parietal cell mass. While fasting gastrin levels are not generally elevated, some patients with duodenal ulcer have postprandial hypergastrinemia. Subgroups have also been identified with a familial elevation in serum pepsinogen I levels or rapid gastric emptying, which delivers an early acid load to the duodenum. Defects in the release of secretin or other duodenal buffers have been postulated to play a role, but this has not been demonstrated.

Answer: A

11. Hemorrhage complicating duodenal ulcer:

A. Usually is massive, resulting from erosion of the gastroduodenal artery
B. Is a more frequent complication of duodenal ulcer than is either obstruction or perforation
C. Can be controlled by endoscopic techniques with decreased mortality and a decreased need for operation
D. Usually requires gastric resection for its control
E. Can be controlled by ligation, which should be accompanied by a definitive acid-reducing procedure

Sabiston: 828
Schwartz: 1125

Comments: Hemorrhage, the most common complication of duodenal ulcer, usually presents with melena or minor bleeding, although massive bleeding may occur from an eroded gastroduodenal artery. Endoscopic coagulation techniques are sometimes effective in controlling hemorrhage, but it remains controversial whether or not they decrease mortality rates or the need for subsequent operation. When operation is necessary, bleeding is controlled by suture ligation. A definitive anti-ulcer operation should then be performed, because of the high risk of recurrent hemorrhage.

Answer: B, E

12. Which one or more of the following describe(s) the classic metabolic abnormality associated with gastric outlet destruction?

A. Hypochloremic, hypokalemic, metabolic alkalosis
B. Hyperchloremic, hypernatremic, metabolic acidosis
C. Potassium loss, primarily renal
D. Alkaline urine
E. Usually treated with administration of HCl

Sabiston: 830
Schwartz: 1125

Comments: Prolonged loss of gastric fluid produces a hypochloremic, hypokalemic metabolic alkalosis. As volume is depleted, renal compensatory mechanisms conserve sodium at the expense of potassium and eventually hydrogen ion so that a paradoxical aciduria develops. The abnormality can generally be corrected by appropriate administration of volume expanders, potassium, and chloride. Occasionally, administration of hydrochloric acid may be indicated.

Answer: A, C

13. Perforated duodenal ulcer:

A. Can be excluded if pneumoperitoneum is not demonstrated
B. Can be treated nonoperatively
C. Requires a definitive ulcer operation at the time of closure
D. Most commonly occurs with posterior ulcers
E. Is a contraindication to parietal cell vagotomy because of the risk of mediastinal contamination

Sabiston: 829
Schwartz: 1125

Comments: Perforation is usually a complication of anterior duodenal ulcers. Approximately 20% of patients will not demonstrate pneumoperitoneum. In the United States, nonoperative management has generally been reserved for *forme fruste* type perforations or for critically ill patients who are unable to withstand operations. Following simple closure of a perforated duodenal ulcer, approximately one third of patients will have recurrent symptoms that can be managed medically and an additional one third will require a subsequent operation. It has been suggested that chronicity of symptoms prior to perforation or operative findings of chronic ulcer disease correlate with a higher risk of future problems. Some surgeons advocate a routine anti-ulcer operation in any patient with perforation who is clinically stable. The risk of mediastinal contamination in the setting of perforated ulcer was a theoretical objection to the performance of parietal cell vagotomy but has not proved to be clinically significant.

Answer: B

14. Regarding the surgical treatment of intractable duodenal ulcer:

A. Partial gastrectomy (three fourths) has the lowest recurrence rate but the highest mortality
B. Parietal cell vagotomy without drainage has the lowest mortality but the highest recurrence rate
C. Truncal vagotomy and drainage has a recurrence rate similar to that of truncal vagotomy and antrectomy
D. Truncal vagotomy and antrectomy has lower recurrence rates than parietal cell vagotomy, but undesirable postoperative sequelae are more common
E. Selective vagotomy produces diarrhea less often than does truncal vagotomy

Sabiston: 830, 837
Schwartz: 1128

Comments: The goal of surgical therapy for duodenal ulcer is to reduce acid in a manner that is safe and has few side effects. Acid can be reduced by eliminating vagal stimulation and by removing the antral source of gastrin or the parietal cell mass. Traditionally, partial gastrectomy has the highest mortality. Truncal vagotomy and antrectomy has the lowest recurrence rate. Parietal cell vagotomy has the lowest mortality, the lowest incidence of side effects, and the highest recurrence rate. Procedures that involve gastric resection, pyloroplasty, or truncal vagotomy may be complicated by diarrhea, "dumping," or bile reflux. Selective vagotomy, which preserves the hepatic and celiac vagal branches, has been associated with a lower rate of diarrhea than truncal vagotomy.

Answer: B, D, E

15. Which of the following may produce elevated basal serum gastrin levels?

A. Retained antrum
B. Vagotomy
C. H2 receptor antagonist
D. Renal failure
E. Gastric outlet obstruction
F. G-cell hyperplasia
G. Duodenal ulcer

Sabiston: 817

Comments: Marked elevations of serum gastrin are seen with gastrinoma; lesser elevations may occur in a variety of clinical settings. Vagotomy of any type may be associated with hypergastrinemia due to a loss of vagal inhibition of gastrin release. Duodenal ulcer may be associated with postprandial hypergastrinemia, but is not characterized by elevations of basal serum gastrin.

Answer: A, B, C, D, E, F

16. Which of the following is/are true regarding the diagnosis of Zollinger-Ellison syndrome?

A. Serum gastrin levels must be greater than 1,000 pg/ml
B. Gastrin levels are decreased by the infusion of secretin
C. Gastrin levels are increased by the infusion of calcium
D. BAO/MAO ratio greater than 0.6
E. MAO 10 to 15 mEq/hr

Sabiston: 833
Schwartz: 1125

Comments: Zollinger-Ellison syndrome is characterized by elevated serum gastrin levels and an elevated basal acid output (BAO) that is at least 60% of the maximal acid output (MAO). Normally, the BAO is 2 to 3 mEq/hr and the MAO is in the range of 10 to 15 mEq/hr. In Zollinger-Ellison syndrome, the BAO may be 50 mEq/hr. Although marked elevations of serum gastrin are often seen, the elevations may be only mild. Provocative testing with infusion of secretin or calcium produces an increase in gastrin in patients with Zollinger-Ellison syndrome.

Answer: C, D

17. Appropriate management of patients with Zollinger-Ellison syndrome may include:

A. Enucleation of a duodenal gastrinoma
B. High doses of an H2 receptor antagonist
C. Total palliative pancreatectomy
D. Total gastrectomy
E. Subtotal gastrectomy and vagotomy

Sabiston: 834
Schwartz: 1129

Comments: Pancreatic gastrinomas are often multiple, usually are malignant and metastatic, and therefore are not resectable for cure. Surgical therapy involves tumor removal if possible, but in most instances it is limited to focusing on the end organ. Tumor resection has been successful for the occasional duodenal gastrinoma. High-dose H2 receptor antagonists have been used to control the ulcer diathesis, but patients may become refractory to treatment or experience side effects, and the efficacy of drug therapy must repeatedly be assessed by acid-secretion studies. Total gastrectomy has been the standard surgical treatment for nonresectable disease; a newer approach includes parietal cell vagotomy combined with H2 receptor antagonists. Subtotal gastrectomy is contraindicated because of the high risk of recurrent ulceration.

Answer: A, B, D

18. Regarding the medical treatment of duodenal ulcer:

A. Anticholinergics are best reserved for nighttime administration because of their side effects
B. Minimal relapse has been observed after an adequate 6-week course of cimetidine
C. Antacids alone provide symptomatic relief but have not been demonstrated to promote healing
D. Diets have not been demonstrated to promote healing
E. Omeprazole binds to necrotic tissue at the ulcer base to prevent back-diffusion of hydrogen ion

Sabiston: 827
Schwartz: 1126

Comments: Much of the traditional medical therapy for duodenal ulcer is unfounded. Controlled clinical studies have not demonstrated any type of diet or feeding schedule to affect ulcer healing or recurrence, although aspirin and cigarettes should be avoided. Antacids and H_2 receptor antagonists are equally effective, and both have been demonstrated to promote ulcer healing as compared with placebo. There is a high rate of relapse following cessation of any medical therapy; there is no medical treatment that alters the natural history of the disease; the possible exception to this may be nocturnal administration of H_2 antagonists. Omeprazole is a specific inhibitor of hydrogen-potassium ATPase. Sucralfate binds to ulcers preventing diffusion of hydrogen ion and pepsin and also works to absorb pepsin and bile. Currently available anticholinergics have not been convincingly effective in the treatment of duodenal ulcer, but may sometimes be a useful adjunct to other therapy.

Answer: A, D

19. Regarding "stress" bleeding from acute erosive gastritis, which of the following statements is/are true?

A. Prophylactic treatment with cimetidine or with antacids is equally effective
B. It has been decreasing in incidence
C. The site of hemorrhage most often is in the antrum
D. There is minimal rebleeding after treatment by oversewing of bleeding sites, vagotomy, and pyloroplasty
E. Effective surgical treatment requires total gastrectomy

Sabiston: 832, 836
Schwartz: 1129

Comments: Stress bleeding in critically ill patients is best prevented by the use of antacids whose dosage is monitored by titration of the gastric pH. H2 receptor antagonists alone are not as effective as antacids alone, but their use conjointly may decrease the volume of buffer required. Bleeding most often occurs in the fundus. If operation is required, vagotomy and pyloroplasty may have a fairly high rate of rebleeding, but often are performed to avoid the morbidity of gastric resection in these critically ill patients.

Answer: B

20. As compared with duodenal ulcer, isolated gastric ulcer:

A. Occurs at a relatively younger age
B. Has a female preponderance
C. Is less responsive to vagotomy or H2 receptor antagonists
D. Is often associated with massive hemorrhage

Sabiston: 830
Schwartz: 1131

Comments: Chronic gastric ulcer occurs more commonly in older patients and in women than does duodenal ulcer. The female/male ratio is 2:1. When complicated by obstruction, perforation, or bleeding (which usually is not massive) the prognosis is often thought to be worse than for the corresponding complications of duodenal ulcer. Although H2 receptor antagonists and vagotomy may be effective therapy for gastric ulcer, they are not as useful as for duodenal ulcer or for combined disease involving both the stomach and duodenum.

Answer: B, C

21. The following procedure(s) may be appropriate treatment for gastric ulcer not associated with duodenal ulcer:

A. Subtotal gastrectomy
B. Antrectomy and excision of ulcer
C. Parietal cell vagotomy and excision of ulcer
D. Truncal vagotomy, drainage, and biopsy of ulcer
E. Total gastrectomy for high proximal lesions

Sabiston: 832
Schwartz: 1132

Comments: The standard surgical treatment of isolated gastric ulcer is subtotal gastrectomy including resection of the ulcer. Vagotomy has not proved superior to resec-

tion and has been associated with an increased rate of recurrence in controlled trials. It is, however, appropriate in situations where one wishes to avoid the morbidity of resection. Evaluation of parietal cell vagotomy for the treatment of gastric ulcer has been limited. Controlled trials have indicated higher recurrence rates, but these have not been statistically significant. High gastric ulcers may pose technical problems; excision is preferred, but the ulcer may be left provided that malignancy can be excluded.

Answer: A, B, C, D

22. Concerning the Mallory-Weiss syndrome, which of the following statements is/are true?

A. It involves a longitudinal mucosal tear near the gastroesophageal junction
B. Profuse hemorrhage is the most common manifestation
C. It can generally be managed medically
D. An antisecretory operation is a useful adjunct for patients requiring surgical treatment
E. It is often associated with the drinking of alcohol

Sabiston: 846
Schwartz: 1136

Comments: Retching may produce a tear of the mucosa and submucosa near the gastroesophageal junction, usually on the gastric side; there is profuse hemorrhage about 10% of the time. Once the condition is identified, the bleeding can often be managed medically. An acid-reducing operation is not required; should operation be necessary, bleeding can be controlled simply by oversewing the site of the tear. If the tear extends into the esophagus, a fundoplication may also be performed.

Answer: A, C, E

23. Ménétrier's disease:

A. Is characterized by enlarged gastric rugal folds in the antrum
B. Often is associated with polyendocrine adenomatosis
C. May have an increased incidence of gastric cancer
D. Usually requires surgical treatment
E. May be associated with massive protein loss

Sabiston: 857
Schwartz: 1135

Comments: This disorder is characterized by hypertrophic gastric folds involving the proximal stomach. A protein-losing gastropathy may develop which, if severe, may necessitate gastrectomy. There may be a higher incidence of gastric cancer, so these patients should be followed closely.

Answer: C, E

24. Regarding gastric volvulus:

A. The symptoms consist of severe nausea with inability to vomit
B. It is associated with congenital anomalies of gastric fixation

C. It frequently is relieved simply by passage of a naso-gastric tube
D. It constitutes a surgical emergency
E. Is associated with an increased incidence of sigmoid volvulus

Schwartz: 1136

Comments: Two types of gastric volvulus may occur depending upon the axis of rotation. Organoaxial volvulus, the more common type, involves rotation around the axis of a line connecting the cardia and pylorus. In mesenterioaxial volvulus that axis is approximately at a right angle to the cardiopyloric line. Combined types have also been described. Patients generally have severe pain and nausea but are unable to vomit, and a nasogastric tube cannot be passed. Strangulation can follow, so gastric volvulus requires prompt reduction. Because of the risk of volvulus, patients with paraesophageal hiatal hernia should have it repaired.

Answer: A, D

25. The differential diagnosis of hypertrophic gastric folds seen on upper GI series includes:

A. Ménétrier's disease
B. Pernicious anemia
C. Pseudolymphoma
D. Eosinophilic gastroenteritis
E. Adenocarcinoma

Schwartz: 1135

Comments: Numerous disorders may be associated with hypertrophic gastric folds. Pernicious anemia, however, is associated with atrophic gastritis and achlorhydria. In Ménétrier's disease, the proximal stomach is involved, whereas the antrum is involved with eosinophilic gastroenteritis.

Answer: A, C, D, E

26. Regarding the surgical treatment of morbid obesity:

A. Most patients undergoing jejunoileal bypass develop hepatic failure
B. As compared with procedures involving gastric stapling alone, gastric bypass with gastroenterostomy has a lower morbidity
C. Wound infection is the most common major complication of gastric bypass operations
D. Controlled clinical trials suggest that vertical banded gastroplasty is the preferred method of gastric partitioning
E. Both gastric partitioning and gastric bypass operations eventually provide for loss of all excess weight in most patients

Sabiston: 928
Schwartz: 1137

Comments: Jejunoileal bypass operations for morbid obesity were associated with numerous complications, including hepatic disease in 5 to 10% of patients and oxalate calculi in 30 to 50%; these procedures have been abandoned. Numerous operative techniques have been used to reduce gastric capacity and to provide a small

outlet from the gastric pouch. Gastric bypass has been associated with significant rates of morbidity and reoperation; wound infection has been the most common complication. Some feel that the technique of vertical banded gastroplasty is preferred, but controlled trials have not been reported. In most patients, all gastric size-reducing operations produce a roughly equivalent weight loss of 50% of excess weight.

Answer: C

27. Atrophic gastritis is associated with:

A. Pernicious anemia due to chronic gastrointestinal blood loss
B. Achlorhydria or hypochlorhydria
C. Circulating parietal cell antibodies
D. Histologic "intestinalization" of gastric mucosa
E. An increased incidence of adenomatous polyps and gastric cancer

Schwartz: 1137

Comments: Atrophic gastritis is associated with a loss of parietal cells with subsequent achlorhydria and vitamin B_{12} deficiency due to the absence of intrinsic factor required for absorption of vitamin B_{12}. Antibodies to parietal cell have been demonstrated. Patients with atrophic gastritis have a higher risk of developing gastric cancer.

Answer: B, C, D, E

28. Pathogenetic factors in benign gastric ulcer may include:

A. Bile reflux
B. Acid hypersecretion
C. Deficient mucosal barrier
D. Mucosal irritating drugs

Sabiston: 820
Schwartz: 1131

Comments: Numerous factors have been thought important in the development of benign gastric ulcer. Although patients with gastric ulcer are not usually hypersecretors of acid as are patients with duodenal ulcer, some acid must be present. The major pathogenetic factor in gastric ulcer is the back diffusion of hydrogen ion through a deficient mucosal barrier, which may result from a variety of causes. It has been demonstrated that most ulcers occur within 2 cm of the junctional mucosa between the acid-secreting and non–acid-secreting stomach and that most ulcers occur on the acid-secreting side.

Answer: A, B, C, D

29. Concerning the epidemiology of gastric neoplasia:

A. The highest incidence is in Japan and Iceland
B. The death rate from it in the United States is declining
C. There is an increased incidence in patients with blood group O
D. There is an increased incidence following resection for duodenal ulcer
E. There is an associated increased risk with long-term H2 blocker therapy

Sabiston: 882
Schwartz: 1133

Comments: Epidemiologically, gastric adenocarcinoma occurs most frequently in geographic areas where the diet is high in smoked fish. Death rates from gastric cancer in the United States have declined over the last decades to a current rate of approximately 8 per 100,000. The incidence is increased in patients with pernicious anemia and in those with blood group A, suggesting the role of genetic factors. The incidence is higher in patients who have had resection or gastroenterostomy for duodenal ulcer, implicating the role of bile-reflux gastritis. It has been speculated that long-term H2 blocked therapy may lead to an increased risk because of the chronic hypochlorhydria produced and the subsequent increase in nitrosamines from bacterial overgrowth; this, however, has not been proved.

Answer: A, B, D

30. Radiation may play a therapeutic role in which of the following gastric conditions?

A. Adenocarcinoma
B. Leiomyosarcoma
C. Lymphoma
D. Ménétrier's disease
E. Eosinophilic antritis

Sabiston: 861
Schwartz: 1134

Comments: Although the treatment of gastric adenocarcinoma is primarily surgical, radiotherapy may be utilized in instances of recurrent or unresectable tumors. Radiation therapy alone or in combination with operation may produce remission or cure of gastric lymphoma; when the process is limited to the stomach, such therapy gives 5-year survival rates of 85%. Leiomyosarcomas are not responsive to radiation or to chemotherapy. Radiation has no role in the treatment of benign gastric conditions.

Answer: A, C

31. Regarding gastric adenocarcinoma:

A. Death with advanced lesions usually results from obstruction and aspiration
B. Curative gastric resection produces a 5-year survival rate of 50%
C. Cure rates approach 80 to 90% for lesions confined to the mucosa

D. Cancer-free survival is significantly increased by adjuvant chemotherapy and radiotherapy
E. Anticipated survival is worse than that of gastric lymphoma, but better than with the rarer leiomyosarcoma

Sabiston: 891
Schwartz: 1134

Comments: Except for early mucosal lesions, the cure rate of gastric adenocarcinoma is poor. Overall 5-year survival after resection for cure is about 10%. Liver and lung metastases are common. Death is usually the result of cachexia. There is no clear benefit to chemotherapy or radiotherapy following surgical resection for cure. Both lymphoma and leiomyosarcoma have an anticipated long-term survival.

Answer: C

32. Concerning the surgical treatment of gastric malignancy:

A. Because of its multifocal nature, the preferred method of palliation for adenocarcinoma is total gastrectomy
B. Gastric lymphoma may be treated by radiation alone
C. Radical subtotal gastrectomy is appropriate for gastric adenocarcinoma without distant metastases
D. Palliative gastric resection usually ameliorates symptoms for only 2 to 3 months

Sabiston: 861, 889
Schwartz: 1134

Comments: Except for the most advanced cases, gastric adenocarcinoma should be treated by resection, even though in most instances it will be palliative. Generally it is best to avoid total gastrectomy for palliative purposes, although occasionally it may be appropriate. When resection is performed with curative intent, radical subtotal or total gastrectomy including resection of the omentum, spleen, and celiac lymph nodal drainage is appropriate. Palliative resection should be done for immediate need or if the anticipated relief of symptoms will exceed 6 months. Good results with gastric lymphoma have been obtained with radiotherapy alone or in combination with resection.

Answer: B, C

CHAPTER 26

Small Intestine

1. During an operation for presumed appendicitis, the appendix is found to be normal; however, the terminal ileum is markedly thickened and feels rubbery to firm, its serosa is covered with a gray-white exudate, and several loops of apparently normal small intestine are adherent to it. The most likely diagnosis is:

A. Crohn's disease of the terminal ileum
B. Perforated Meckel's diverticulum
C. Ulcerative colitis
D. Ileocecal tuberculosis
E. Acute ileitis

Sabiston: 922
Schwartz: 1148

Comments: **Crohn's disease** can present acutely and, when it involves the terminal ileum, may clinically very closely resemble appendicitis. Segments of bowel involved with Crohn's disease have a characteristic gross appearance; in addition to the features described, the mesenteric fat is seen to "creep" over the serosa. The mesentery is thickened, dull, and rubbery, and may contain lymph nodes as large as 3 to 4 cm in diameter. Not infrequently, partial obstruction of the involved segment can produce dilatation of the proximal bowel. **Acute ileitis** (or regional enteritis) may mimic appendicitis and grossly appear as inflammation of the terminal ileum; the findings, however, do not resemble advanced Crohn's disease. **Meckel's diverticulitis** can mimic appendicitis, but presents as a process located approximately 50 cm proximal to the ileocecal valve and without the bowel wall changes seen with Crohn's disease. **Tuberculosis of the terminal ileum,** rare in the United States, can produce scarring and stenosis of the distal ileum and enlargement of the mesenteric lymph nodes. Demonstration of caseation and acid-fast bacilli on biopsy of a mesenteric granuloma confirms the diagnosis. **Ulcerative colitis** is usually confined to the large bowel, and any associated pain can usually be distinguished from that of appendicitis.

Answer: A

2. True statements regarding Crohn's disease include:

A. It is the most common primary disease of the small intestine requiring operation
B. Black males and males of Mediterranean descent are most commonly affected
C. The disease involves both the terminal ileum and the right colon in 90% of cases
D. The disease may involve any portion of the gastrointestinal tract from esophagus to rectum

Schwartz: 1147

Comments: Although uncommon in comparison with other gastrointestinal diseases, Crohn's disease is the most common primary disease of the small intestine requiring operation. The incidence is highest in the United States, England, and Scandinavia. The disease is three times more common in Jews than in non-Jews, more common in whites than nonwhites, and slightly more common in males. It occurs in all age groups but is most frequently diagnosed in young adults. The distribution of involvement is such that 35% of patients have disease limited to the small intestine, 20% to the colon, and about 50% have both small and large intestine involvement. This usually is in continuity, although diseased segments may be separated by normal bowel (so-called skip areas). Isolated involvement of the esophagus, stomach, or duodenum does occur, but this is rare.

Answer: A, D

3. True statements regarding the microscopic appearance of Crohn's disease include:

A. The disease is confined to the mucosa
B. The disease is confined to the mucosa and submucosa
C. Granulomas demonstrating caseation without acid-fast bacilli confirm the diagnosis
D. Submucosal fibrosis occurs secondary to bacterial invasion
E. Marked lymphangiectasia is a prominent microscopic feature

Sabiston: 918
Schwartz: 1148

Comments: Several microscopic features characterize, but are nonspecific for, Crohn's disease. These features progress from an early to a late phase of involvement and can be described as a granulomatous fibrotic inflammation progressing through all layers of the bowel wall. **Early phase:** Edema of the entire bowel wall accompanied by lymphangiectasis and hyperemia, associated with an increased proportion of goblet cells in an otherwise normal mucosa. **Intermediate phase:** Thickening due to fibrosis of the submucosal and subserosal areas of the bowel. Focal mucosal ulcers become numerous, and in 60% of patients "sarcoid-like" granulomas appear, particularly in the submucosa, subserosa, and regional lymph nodes. These granulomas contain epithelioid giant cells, do not caseate, and do not contain acid-fast bacilli. Lymphangiectasis remains visible throughout the intermediate and late phases. **Late phase:** There is dense fibrosis exceeding that expected from the simple healing of an inflammatory insult, producing a fixed stenosis and partial obstruction of the lumen. The mucosa is denuded over wide areas with occasional islands of intact mucosal cells. Glands deep in the mucosa resemble those of the pyloric region and are termed "aberrant pyloric glands" or Brunner's gland metaplasia. The ulcers can be deep and progression through the bowel wall may occur, sometimes terminating as fistula tracts.

Answer: E

4. True statements regarding the etiology of Crohn's disease include:

A. The primary pathologic mechanism is a progressive, obstructive lymphangitis
B. Crohn's disease is a form of sarcoidosis limited to the gastrointestinal tract
C. A mouse-footpad virus has been identified as the etiologic agent
D. The disease is the result of a local hypersensitivity reaction
E. The disease is primarily a psychosomatic illness
F. The actual etiology is unknown

Sabiston: 918
Schwartz: 1149

Comments: Despite extensive investigation, the actual etiology of Crohn's disease is unknown. The possibility of a transmissible agent has emerged as a result of work demonstrating the development of granulomatous lesions in the mouse footpad following injection of intestinal homogenates obtained from patients with Crohn's disease. These results, however, have been difficult to reproduce, and their precise meaning requires further investigation. Although the granulomas of sarcoidosis and Crohn's disease are similar, the Kveim test, positive in 80% of patients with active sarcoidosis, is almost always negative in Crohn's disease. It is generally felt that the immunologic alterations seen in patients with Crohn's disease reflect a response to the disease rather than its cause.

Answer: F

5. True statements regarding the clinical manifestations of Crohn's disease include:

A. The majority of patients present acutely with pain, nausea, and diarrhea
B. Bloody diarrhea is an infrequent symptom
C. The bloody diarrhea almost always produces anemia
D. Steatorrhea results from pancreatic involvement
E. Fever and signs of systemic toxicity are common

Sabiston: 919
Schwartz: 1150

Comments: While 10% of patients with Crohn's disease present acutely and with a picture mimicking appendicitis, in most the onset is insidious with intermittent pain or discomfort being the most frequent and sometimes the only symptom. Pain is often precipitated by dietary indiscretion. With advanced disease, the pain may become associated with signs and symptoms of partial obstruction. Constant localized pain, especially if associated with a palpable mass, suggests the presence of an abscess or bowel fistula. Diarrhea is the next most frequent symptom and, unlike that in chronic ulcerative colitis, rarely contains mucus, pus, or blood. The diarrhea is the result of several factors. The involved segment of small bowel has a decreased capacity to absorb intestinal contents. Also, the obstruction produced by this involved segment alters the absorptive capacity of the proximal bowel. Decreased absorption of bile salts in the terminal ileum leads to bile salt–induced damage of the absorptive cells of the colonic mucosa. One third of patients will present with fever and 50% of patients present with weight loss, weakness, and easy fatigability. Persistent occult loss of blood frequently produces anemia, which may be aggravated by a vitamin B_{12} deficiency. Hypoproteinemia occurs because of increased loss of protein from the inflamed bowel mucosa. Deficiencies in vitamins and minerals are the result of their decreased ingestion, altered metabolism, and decreased absorption.

Answer: B

6. True statements regarding the complications of Crohn's disease include:

A. When present, obstruction is usually partial rather than complete
B. Perforation of the bowel wall occurs in 15 to 20% of patients
C. Free perforations into the peritoneal cavity are as common as confined perforations
D. Fistulization rarely occurs in patients who have not had an operation
E. Perianal disease rarely occurs in patients with Crohn's disease confined to the small bowel
F. Crohn's disease of the small bowel is not associated with an increased risk of malignancy

Sabiston: 926
Schwartz: 1150

Comments: Complete obstruction is uncommon in Crohn's disease. In contrast, partial obstruction is common; when it is high grade, an elective operation may be necessary. Perforation occurs in 15 to 20% of patients, usually resulting in formation of an abscess or an internal fistula to the bowel, bladder, or vagina. Free perforations into the peritoneal cavity are rare. When they do occur, they usually are on the antimesenteric border of the distal ileum, proximal to a stenotic lesion. Enterocutaneous fistulas rarely occur in patients not previously operated upon. However, they are common after operation. Up to 50% of patients with Crohn's disease of the small bowel develop perirectal abscesses or fistulas, usually without evidence of communication with the diseased small bowel. Frank hemorrhage is rare, but can occur if an ulcer erodes into a large blood vessel. There is an increased risk of developing cancer in patients with Crohn's ·disease compared with the general population, but with respect to the colon, it does not approach the level seen in patients with chronic ulcerative colitis. The risk, however, is not considered high enough to warrant prophylactic resection. Most cases of small bowel cancer associated with Crohn's disease have occurred in patients with long-standing disease and have appeared in a previously bypassed segment of bowel.

Answer: A, B

7. During exploration for a presumed diagnosis of appendicitis, the cecum and appendix appear normal, and the terminal 50 cm of ileum is inflamed, beefy red, and slightly edematous. It is soft to touch and there is no proximal ileal distension. The most appropriate operative choice is:

A. Appendectomy
B. Resection of involved ileum and appendix
C. Placement of irrigation catheters, appendectomy
D. Closure without appendectomy or ileal resection
E. Bypass ileo-ascending colostomy

Sabiston: 925
Schwartz: 1148, 1152

Comments: When acute regional enteritis (of the terminal ileum) is encountered during exploration for presumed appendicitis, the appropriateness of appendectomy is somewhat controversial. The incidence of enterocutaneous fistula after operation in patients with Crohn's disease is high, but the fistulas usually arise from the diseased ileum, not the appendiceal stump. Further, 90% of patients in whom acute regional enteritis is found at operation do not progress to chronic Crohn's disease; their symptoms resolve without sequelae. Therefore, if the stump of the appendix is not involved, most surgeons favor the performance of an appendectomy. This reduces the difficulty of the differential diagnosis if right lower abdominal pain should develop at a later date. In acute regional enteritis that is encountered as in this clinical setting without evidence of obstruction or fistula formation, the ileum should not be resected.

Answer: A

8. True statements regarding the radiographic findings of Crohn's disease of the small intestine include:

A. Barium enema with reflux into the terminal ileum is adequate to define the extent of disease
B. The string sign of Kantor is produced by luminal narrowing
C. When present, fistulas are almost always seen on small bowel follow-through studies
D. Barium should be avoided, since it can convert partial thickness to full thickness bowel wall involvement
E. Mass effects extrinsic to the bowel wall may indicate the presence of abscesses

Sabiston: 922
Schwartz: 1150

Comments: An upper GI series of x-rays with small bowel follow-through, as well as a barium enema with reflux into the terminal ileum, should be obtained when evaluating patients suspected of having Crohn's disease. Luminal narrowing due to acute edema or chronic fibrosis produces the string sign of Kantor seen on barium examination. Thickening of the bowel wall and mesentery increases the space between adjacent loops of bowel and may give the impression of extraluminal abscess formation. Fistulas may be seen, but often are obscured by adjacent loops of bowel. The mucosal pattern may be markedly distorted, but it is more difficult to evaluate than the mucosal changes seen with Crohn's colitis. "Skip areas" of normal bowel between involved segments may also be detected and help to differentiate Crohn's disease from ulcerative colitis.

Answer: B, E

9. True statements regarding medical management of Crohn's disease include:

A. Nonabsorbable antibiotics (sulfasalazine) sometimes improve symptoms and should be tried
B. Steroids relieve symptoms and can induce remission, but do not alter the natural course of Crohn's disease
C. Azathioprine is no more effective than placebo in relief of symptoms or induction of remission
D. 6-Mercaptopurine is more effective than placebo in decreasing symptoms, healing fistulas, and reducing steroid dosage
E. Elemental diets and total parenteral nutrition do not affect the natural course of Crohn's disease
F. Prednisone is more effective for small bowel involvement, while sulfasalazine is most effective for colonic involvement

Sabiston: 924
Schwartz: 1151

Comments: There is no curative therapy for Crohn's disease. Although certain therapeutic agents are effective in controlling symptoms, none have been shown to influence the natural course of the disease. The goal of medical management, therefore, is to control symptoms and to provide nutritional support. Failure of medical therapy that necessitates operation usually results from progression of the disease at the established site, rather than from longitudinal extension along uninvolved bowel. The majority of patients with Crohn's disease will ultimately require an operation. Yet because the rate of recurrence after operation is high, medical management is preferred until a complication makes an operation mandatory. Occasionally, a patient with a high-grade incomplete obstruction or with an internal fistula will respond to aggressive nonoperative management; these complications, therefore, should not be considered as absolute indications for operation.

Answer: A, B, C, D, E, F

10. True statements regarding operation for Crohn's disease include:

A. Operation is curative
B. Perirectal disease may respond to small bowel resection
C. The most common indication for operation is obstruction
D. The recurrence rate after operation is 15%

Sabiston: 925
Schwartz: 1151

Comments: Up to 90% of all patients with Crohn's disease will ultimately need an operation. The most common indications for operation, in decreasing order of frequency, are obstruction, persistent symptomatic abdominal mass, abscess, fistula, perirectal disease that fails to respond to local therapy, and intractability of symptoms despite adequate medical management. Less common indications are free perforation, hemorrhage, and the blind-loop syndrome. Whichever operation the surgeon chooses to perform, the byword is preservation of intestinal length whenever possible. As a consequence, most surgeons practice conservative resection of grossly diseased bowel. Neither the use of frozen section to assess the proximal margin of resection nor resection of involved mesenteric lymph nodes improves long-term cure rates. Simple bypass and bypass with exclusion are no longer used routinely. The bypassed segment often continues to be a source of active disease that is prone to the development of bacterial overgrowth, obstruction, perforation, and possibly malignant degeneration. A bypass procedure is reserved for use in elderly, poor-risk patients, in patients with extensive disease associated with multiple areas of stenosis, in patients with obstructive gastroduodenal disease, and in patients having undergone previous extensive small bowel resection. Recurrence of symptoms after operation occurs in up to 50% of patients, and the yearly rate for reoperation remains constant at approximately 15%.

Answer: B, C

11. Select the correct statements regarding tuberculous enteritis from among the following:

A. Primary infection usually results from ingestion of milk contaminated with the bovine strain of *Mycobacterium tuberculosis*
B. Secondary infection results from the ingestion of bacilli contained in contaminated sputum
C. The ileocecal region is the site of involvement in 85% of cases
D. Primary infection frequently mimics the chronic form of Crohn's disease
E. Secondary infection frequently produces radiographic findings indistinguishable from carcinoma of the colon

Sabiston: 918, 923
Schwartz: 1152

Comments: **Primary tuberculosis** is rare in the United States, but is still common in underdeveloped countries. Usually it produces minimal symptoms; occasionally, however, it can cause a hypertrophic reaction in the ileocecal area that produces stricture and stenosis of the distal ileum and cecum. Radiographic findings are frequently indistinguishable from those of carcinoma of the

colon. In some cases, exploration and biopsy may be advisable, but resection is not performed unless high-grade obstruction is present. Treatment with isoniazid, para-aminosalicylic acid, and streptomycin usually suffices. **Ulcerative tuberculosis** is a form that develops secondary to pulmonary disease. While symptoms are variable, when they are present, they most often consist of pain and diarrhea. The diagnosis is made by barium enema examination; confirmation is by documenting response to antitubercular therapy. The antitubercular chemotherapy effectively allows healing of the lesion, and operation is contraindicated except for the complications of perforation, obstruction, or hemorrhage.

Answer: A, B, C

12. True statements regarding typhoid enteritis include:

A. The diagnosis can be made by culturing *Salmonella typhosa* from the blood or stool
B. Chloramphenicol is the drug of choice for treatment
C. Bleeding requiring operative intervention occurs in 10 to 20% of patients
D. Steroids should be used in patients who are toxic and who fail to respond after several days of antibiotic therapy

Schwartz: 1153

Comments: Typhoid enteritis is a systemic infection caused by *Salmonella typhosa* and is accompanied by fever, headache, cough, maculopapular rash, abdominal pain, and leukopenia. There is hyperplasia and ulceration of Peyer's patches, mesenteric lymphadenopathy, and splenomegaly. Chloramphenicol no longer is the drug of choice because of the emergence of resistant strains of bacteria and the risk of marrow toxicity. Currently, trimethoprim and sulfamethoxazole are preferred. Patients who remain toxic after 1 week of therapy often benefit from a short course of prednisone. Bleeding occurs in 10 to 20% of patients and usually is treated simply with transfusion. Perforation through ulcerated Peyer's patches occurs in 2% of patients, most often being free, solitary, and in the terminal ileum. Operative closure and appropriate peritoneal toilette is required; occasionally, the perforations are multiple, requiring intestinal resection with primary anastomosis.

Answer: A, C, D

13. True statements regarding benign tumors of the small bowel include:

A. Most are found in the ileum
B. Often they produce no symptoms and are difficult to diagnose by either clinical or radiologic examination
C. The most common clinical manifestations are bleeding and obstruction
D. They obstruct the bowel either by encroachment on the lumen or by causing intussusception

Sabiston: 868
Schwartz: 1154

Comments: The types and relative frequency of benign neoplasms of the small intestine vary in different series, but common lesions include leiomyoma, lipoma, adenoma, and hemangioma. Fifteen percent occur in the duodenum, 25% in the jejunum, and about 60% in the ileum, usually the distal third. Often they are asymptomatic, and when symptoms are present they are vague and nonspecific. Bleeding and obstruction are the two most common symptoms, the bleeding usually being occult and intermittent and even leading to iron-deficiency anemia. Leiomyoma and hemangioma are the lesions that most often bleed. The differential diagnosis of small bowel bleeding should include hereditary hemorrhagic telangiectasis (Osler-Rendu-Weber syndrome). Intussusception in adults usually is due to an organic cause; 50% of cases are due to benign small bowel neoplasms. When small bowel neoplasms are suspected, barium small bowel follow-through is indicated and is diagnostic most of the time. When identified, small bowel tumors should be excised because of the risk of complications and the possibility of their being malignant.

Answer: A, B, C, D

14. A 26-year-old man presents in the emergency room with the complaint of recurrent colicky, mid-abdominal pain. On physical exam he has a palpable abdominal mass and several areas of increased pigmentation on his lips, palms, and soles. He states his father had a colon polyp removed several years ago. Your diagnosis is:

A. Familial polyposis with malignant degeneration
B. Gardner's syndrome with intussusception
C. Peutz-Jeghers syndrome with intussusception
D. Symptomatic Crohn's disease

Sabiston: 870
Schwartz: 1155

Comments: Peutz-Jeghers syndrome is a familial disease (autosomal dominant transmission) characterized by intestinal polyposis and mucocutaneous hyperpigmentation. The polyps are hamartomas that most frequently are in the jejunum and ileum, but also can be found in the stomach, duodenum, colon, and rectum. It is felt that their malignant potential is extremely low. Peutz-Jeghers syndrome can produce abdominal symptoms due to intussusception or hemorrhage, up to one third of patients presenting with abdominal pain and a palpable mass. An operation is indicated for obstruction or for bleeding; it should be limited to conservative resection of the involved portion of the bowel rather than an attempt to resect all polyps detected during exploration.

Answer: C

15. True statements regarding malignant small bowel tumors include:

A. They account for 2% of all gastrointestinal malignancies
B. Carcinoid is the most common malignancy of the small intestine
C. Five-year survival is highest with adenocarcinoma, followed by lymphoma, and still lower for leiomyosarcoma
D. Wide resection with regional lymphadenectomy is the preferred operation.

Schwartz: 1155

Comments: Malignant tumors of the small bowel account for 2% of all gastrointestinal malignancies. The most frequent type is adenocarcinoma, followed by carcinoid, lymphoma, and sarcoma, principally leiomyosarcoma. While adenocarcinoma occurs with equal frequency in the duodenum, jejunum, and ileum, the others tend to occur most often in the ileum. Their clinical manifestations may include any combination of diarrhea, obstruction, and/or chronic blood loss with anemia. The preferred therapy is wide resection with regional lymphadenectomy. For each entity, survival is dependent on a number of factors and is variable, but in general leiomyosarcomas and lymphomas have the highest survival (about 40%) and adenocarcinoma the lowest (about 20%). Postoperative chemotherapy and radiation therapy can be useful in treating a patient with lymphoma, but are not useful adjuncts for adenocarcinoma or sarcoma. Histiocytic lymphoma may develop in patients with long-standing celiac sprue and has a worse prognosis than conventional small bowel lymphomas. Another lymphoma variant, the Mediterranean-type lymphoma (associated with monoclonal alpha heavy chains and a dense plasma cell tumor infiltration) also carries a bad prognosis.

Answer: A, D

16. True statements regarding carcinoid tumors include:

A. The cell of origin is the Kupffer cell
B. The rectum is the most common site of origin
C. There is a tendency towards multicentricity
D. Prognosis is related to tumor size, location, and histologic pattern

Sabiston: 949
Schwartz: 1155

Comments: The origin of carcinoid tumors is the Kultschitzky cell, thought to arise from the neural crest. Carcinoids can occur anywhere in the gastrointestinal tract, the most frequent site being the appendix and next the ileum and rectum. Extraintestinal sites include the bronchus and ovary. Small bowel carcinoid tumors tend to be multicentric (30% of cases); a second noncarcinoid neoplasm is present in up to 30% of patients. The prognosis is a function of the size of the tumor and its site of origin. Ileal carcinoids tend to metastasize more commonly than those originating in the appendix. Only 2% of tumors less than 1 cm in diameter metastasize, while for tumors progressively larger than 2 cm, metastases are present in up to 80% of patients. Recent information suggests that the histologic pattern as well may affect prognosis.

Answer: C, D

17. True statements regarding carcinoid tumors and their surgical management include:

A. They produce a characteristic luminal deformity seen on barium examination
B. They are often easily palpable
C. Often their metastases are much larger than the primary tumor
D. The usefulness of surgical therapy is dependent on excision of the primary tumor

Schwartz: 1155

Comments: The usual submucosal location of carcinoid tumors often makes them difficult to find on x-ray examination or with cursory palpation during an exploratory laparotomy. The tumors are sometimes associated with a surrounding fibrosis that can produce luminal narrowing. Mesenteric lymph node metastases can be quite large, and they too may be accompanied by an extensive desmoplastic reaction that results in fixation and kinking of the bowel. Tumors less than 1 cm in diameter and without demonstrable metastases can be treated by excision or segmental resection. Those greater than 1 cm or with regional metastases should be excised widely; this would include right hemicolectomy for lesion of the distal ileum and appendix. In patients with widespread disease, removal of all resectable tumor can provide significant palliation if the carcinoid syndrome is present.

Answer: C

18. True statements regarding the clinical manifestations of the carcinoid syndrome include:

A. Episodic manifestations include cutaneous flushing, hyperperistalsis and diarrhea, and asthma
B. Cardiac manifestations occur early and affect primarily the mitral and aortic valves
C. Cutaneous phenomena are the most characteristic and frequently recognized manifestations
D. Diarrhea is a significant complaint in fewer than 30% of patients
E. Asthmatic attacks occur in the majority of patients

Sabiston: 950
Schwartz: 1158

Comments: Episodic manifestations of the carcinoid syndrome include flushing, diarrhea, and asthma. The cutaneous phenomena are the most characteristic and consist of episodes of flushing of the face, neck, arms, and upper trunk, occasionally accompanied by vasomotor collapse. Diarrhea is significant in over 80% of patients and usually is sudden in onset, watery, and accompanied by cramping pain and borborygmi. Asthmatic attacks occur in 25% of patients. Manifestations of long-standing involvement include the development of facial hyperemia with telangiectasias of the cheeks, nose, and forehead, development of the cutaneous lesions of pellagra, and valvular heart disease. The valves most commonly involved are the tricuspid and pulmonic, although the mitral and aortic valves are sometimes affected. Peripheral edema is present in about 70% of patients and can occur in the absence of valvular disease.

Answer: A, C

19. True statements regarding the carcinoid syndrome include:

A. Carcinoid tumors producing serotonin divert up to 60% of dietary tryptophan
B. The most useful diagnostic test for suspected carcinoid syndrome is the determination of serum serotonin levels
C. Patients with normal sertonin levels do not develop carcinoid syndrome
D. 5-HIAA is the active form of serotonin

Sabiston: 950
Schwartz: 1156

Comments: Functioning carcinoid tumors divert up to 60% of dietary tryptophan into the production of serotonin, thus contributing to the development of pellagra and protein deficiency. Serotonin is metabolized in the liver to 5-HIAA, which then is excreted into the urine. For this reason, the most useful diagnostic test in patients suspected of having the carcinoid syndrome is the determination for 5-HIAA in a 24-hour collection of urine. 5-HIAA is inactive, and tumors drained by the portal system may produce large amounts of serotonin yet not provide evidence of the carcinoid syndrome. Serotonin release into the systemic circulation occurs most commonly from liver metastases or from tumors outside the portal area. While it is generally believed that patients with the carcinoid syndrome have tumors that produce serotonin, the role of serotonin in the mediation of the syndrome is not clear. Not all patients with elevated production of serotonin have the syndrome; some patients with the syndrome have normal levels of 5-HIAA in the urine, and injection of pure serotonin does not create all the manifestations of the disease. It is likely that carcinoid tumors have the capacity to produce a number of biologically active peptides, which accounts for the variability of the syndrome and discrepancies between serotonin levels and the clinical presentation.

Answer: A

20. True statements regarding the treatment of carcinoid syndrome include:

A. Exploration is indicated in nearly all patients with the malignant carcinoid syndrome
B. The antiserotonin agents methysergide, cyproheptadine, and p-chlorophenylalanine may be helpful in controlling bowel symptoms
C. Phenothiazines and alpha-adrenergic blockers may ameliorate flushing attacks
D. Occasionally, corticosteroid therapy can decrease the symptoms of the carcinoid syndrome
E. In some patients with the carcinoid syndrome and unresectable tumor, a combination of streptozotocin and 5-fluorouracil (5-FU) can provide palliation through their antineoplastic effect

Schwartz: 1155

Comments: As previously stated, in patients with the carcinoid syndrome and noncurable spread, exploration may be worthwhile, since in many patients even subtotal tumor excision can provide relief of symptoms for prolonged periods of time. A number of pharmacologic agents can be used to ameliorate the symptoms; a combination of streptozotocin and 5-FU has provided palliation of the syndrome in some patients.

Answer: A, B, C, D, E

21. True statements regarding Meckel's diverticulum include:

A. They occur in 50% of the population, in one form or another
B. They are true diverticula

C. Some can be visualized on Tc-99m pertechnetate scans
D. Most complications occur in the elderly
E. Diverticulitis is the most common complication

Sabiston: 946
Schwartz: 1159

Comments: Meckel's diverticulum is the most frequently encountered diverticulum of the small intestine, occurring in 2 to 4% of the general population. It is a true diverticulum, arising from the antimesenteric border of the ileum, 50 to 75 cm from the ileocecal valve. Often there is a persistent band of tissue extending from the tip of the diverticulum to the umbilicus. Sometimes the diverticulum contains ectopic gastric mucosa capable of producing peptic ulceration and bleeding of adjacent ileal mucosa. This ectopic gastric mucosa can be visualized by scans using Tc-99m pertechnetate. Clinical problems most often present in the pediatric age group. The most frequent complications are bleeding, intussusception, and obstruction, the latter usually due to volvulus or kinking around the persistent band. The least common manifestation is diverticulitis; this often presents clinically as appendicitis. Therapy consists of diverticulectomy for uncomplicated diverticulitis and segmental ileal resection for bleeding or for complicated diverticulitis. Prophylactic diverticulectomy generally is not performed when a diverticulum is found incidentally, unless there is evidence of ectopic gastric mucosa or the neck of the diverticulum is very narrow.

Answer: B, C

22. True statements regarding duodenal, jejunal, and ileal diverticula include:

A. Duodenal diverticula are true diverticula
B. Duodenal diverticula are often multiple, while jejunal diverticula are often solitary
C. Asymptomatic duodenal diverticula should be resected to avoid potentially serious complications
D. Asymptomatic jejunal diverticula do not require therapy

Schwartz: 1159

Comments: Diverticula of the duodenum, jejunum, and ileum are false (pulsion) diverticula containing only mucosa, submucosa, and serosa. Duodenal diverticula usually are solitary and project medially toward the head of the pancreas. While most are asymptomatic, 10% present with nonspecific epigastric symptoms; bleeding and perforation can occur. In instances of perforation, drainage of the local site and the performance of a gastrojejunostomy is the operation most often applicable; occasionally, biliary decompression is necessary. In instances of bleeding without inflammation, diverticulectomy is indicated, either from a dorsal approach utilizing the Kocher maneuver or via a duodenotomy. Jejunal and ileal diverticula are often multiple and project from the mesenteric border of the bowel into the leaves of the mesentery. This type of diverticulum is more common in the jejunum than in the ileum. The usual treatment for symptomatic diverticula in these areas is segmental resection. Asymptomatic diverticula of the duodenum, jejunum, or ileum do not require therapy.

Answer: D

23. A 56-year-old woman has a history of pelvic radiation therapy 5 years ago for cervical cancer. Now, 5 days after she underwent a right hemicolectomy for a villous adenoma of the cecum, her surgical wound is red and tender. You open her wound and the initial drainage is obviously purulent; she becomes afebrile. However, the drainage persists as a continuous brown, liquid discharge. Your differential diagnosis should include:

A. Simple wound infection
B. Clostridial infection
C. Anastomotic leak with enterocutaneous fistula
D. Dehiscence

Schwartz: 1160

Comments: Most fistulas are iatrogenic and are due to an anastomotic leak, inadvertent injury to the bowel during the operation, laceration of the bowel during abdominal closure, or retained foreign bodies. Fewer than 2% of fistulas are the result of diseased bowel, and when this is so, the most common contributing factors are preoperative radiotherapy, intestinal obstruction, or inflammatory bowel disease. Although small bowel fistulas occasionally lead to generalized peritonitis, most commonly they produce a walled-off abscess that presents as an infection of the operative incision. While the initial drainage may be purulent, if the infection is due to an anastomotic leak of the small bowel, the drainage will become enteric within 1 to 2 days.

Answer: C

24. For the patient described in Question 23, appropriate initial management might include:

A. Packing of the subcutaneous tissue with wet to dry dressings
B. Packing of the subcutaneous tissue with dry, absorbent dressings
C. Placement of a rubber sump catheter attached to suction
D. Protection of the skin around the fistula with Stomahesive karaya powder, aluminum paste, or zinc oxide and collection of the draining fluid in an attached plastic bag
E. Insertion of a nasogastric tube and administration of appropriate intravenous fluids

Schwartz: 1161

Comments: The initial management of a small bowel fistula should include the administration of appropriate intravenous fluids, proximal decompression with nasogastric suction, control and quantification of the fistula output, and protection of the surrounding skin. Fistulas are classified according to their location and to the volume of their output. Proximal fistulas tend to have a higher output and lead to more severe electrolyte and fluid imbalance. Nasogastric suction can be helpful in diminishing the output of proximal intestinal fistulas, while the output of those more distal in the gut may not be influenced by this maneuver. Sump catheters can provide a means of controlling and quantifying high-output fistulas, especially early in their formation. Once the fistula tract is established, suction catheters should be replaced with a stoma appliance fixed to the edges of the fistula. Enteric contents are highly erosive, and the skin surrounding the fistula opening should be carefully protected. Most well established fistulas do not produce sepsis, but in patients with persistent fever, administration of antibiotics systemically and a careful search for an undrained abdominal abscess are indicated.

Answer: C, D, E

25. After the first several days, the diagnostic work-up of the patient described in Question 23 to localize the fistula may include:

A. Upper GI series with small bowel follow-through
B. Colon fluoroscopic examination with contrast material
C. Instillation of contrast material via a catheter into the fistula
D. CT scan of the abdomen

Schwartz: 1161

Comments: Localizing the position of the fistula can be achieved using a combination of the tests listed above. In addition, instillation of contrast material through the fistula opening helps define the extent of the associated abscess cavity if one is present.

Answer: A, B, C, D

26. Diagnostic work-up of the woman described in Question 23 reveals that she has a distal ileal fistula in communication with an associated small cavity. Appropriate therapeutic interventions include:

A. Prompt exploration and interruption of the fistula tract
B. Prompt exploration and bypass of the fistula
C. Prompt exploration, with resection of the portion of ileum involved in the fistula and primary reanastomosis
D. A 4- to 6-week trial of intravenous hyperalimentation
E. A 4- to 6-week trial of low-residue or elemental enteral alimentation

Schwartz: 1161

Comments: Knowing the location of the fistula has important prognostic as well as therapeutic implications. The overall mortality rate for small bowel fistulas is 20%, being higher for jejunal fistulas and lower for those of the ileum. With proper supportive care such as intravenous or enteral alimentation and in the absence of distal obstruction, up to 40% of small bowel fistulas close spontaneously. Enteral alimentation has the advantage of avoiding the possible hepatic and septic complications of prolonged total parenteral nutrition. Even if there is a slight increase in fistula output after the start of enteral nutrition, the fistula still may close. Fistulas of the proximal jejunum may require the transnasal insertion of a long tube through the stomach and duodenum and just beyond the fistula before starting enteral alimentation. The preferred operation for correcting a persistent fistula is resection of the fistula in continuity with the segment of involved bowel, followed by a primary anastomosis.

Alternative therapies include complete or partial exclusion with primary anastomosis. After resolution of inflammation, the isolated loop of bowel should be excised. Simple bypass of the fistula without exclusion should be avoided.

Answer: D, E

27. Which of the following statements about the blind-loop syndrome is/are correct?

A. It is manifested by abdominal pain, diarrhea, malabsorption, and vitamin deficiency
B. Bacteria successfully compete for vitamin B_{12}, which may lead to megaloblastic anemia
C. Bacterial deconjugation of bile salts can lead to steatorrhea
D. In the blind-loop syndrome, addition of intrinsic factor in the Schilling test causes urinary B_{12} excretion to return to normal
E. The addition of tetracycline in the Schilling test causes urinary B_{12} excretion to return to normal

Sabiston: 959
Schwartz: 1161

Comments: The blind-loop syndrome is caused by stasis of intestinal contents with subsequent bacterial overgrowth. This stasis can be caused by a number of abnormalities including stricture, stenosis, fistula, diverticula, or the formation of a blind pouch. The syndrome presents with steatorrhea, diarrhea, anemia, weight loss, abdominal pain, multiple vitamin deficiencies, joint pains, and occasionally neurologic disorders. The steatorrhea is the result of bile salt deconjugation that takes place in the stagnant fluid in the blind loop of bowel. Megaloblastic anemia probably is due to successful competition by the bacteria for vitamin B_{12}. The Schilling test reveals a type of urinary excretion of B_{12} much as that seen in pernicious anemia, except that it is not corrected with the addition of intrinsic factor but is corrected with the use of oral tetracycline. Although the administration of tetracycline and parenteral B_{12} can correct megaloblastic anemia, surgical correction of the cause of the bowel stasis is curative.

Answer: A, B, C, E

28. Select the correct statement(s) in regard to the short-bowel syndrome.

A. Serious nutritional deficits are produced with resection of the entire jejunum
B. Abnormal absorption of fat, vitamin B_{12}, and electrolytes and water are the three major nutritional derangements
C. Resection of up to 70% of the bowel can be tolerated if the terminal ileum and ileocecal valve are preserved
D. Relative gastric hyposecretion with increased intestinal pH, in conjunction with interruption of the enterohepatic bile salt circulation are the causes of steatorrhea

Schwartz: 1163

Comments: The entire jejunum can be resected without adverse nutritional sequelae. The entire ileum can be resected without harm as long as vitamin B_{12} is replaced postoperatively. Up to 70% of the small bowel can safely be resected if the terminal ileum and ileocecal valve are left intact; if they are resected, however, loss of 50 to 60% of the small bowel can lead to severely compromised nutrition. The deficiencies created by extensive resection of the small bowel are vitamin B_{12} malabsorption, altered fat absorption, and fluid and electrolyte problems. Vitamin B_{12} malabsorption leads to B_{12} deficiency and megaloblastic anemia. Altered fat absorption produces steatorrhea as a result of several factors: (a) Massive small bowel resection leads to gastric hypersecretion; decreased bowel pH stimulates the intestine, thus shortening transit time and interfering with absorption of ingested fat. (b) Interruption of bile salt resorption interferes with micelle formation. (c) The unabsorbed fats are irritating to the colonic mucosa, thus increasing the diarrhea and steatorrhea associated with the syndrome. Fluid and electrolyte problems are a function of the shortened transit time and the diarrhea that results from loss of small bowel absorptive area.

Answer: B, C

29. True statements regarding the treatment of short-bowel syndrome include:

A. Initial therapy consists of control of diarrhea, restriction of oral intake, and intravenous administration of nutrients, fluid, and electrolytes
B. Diarrhea is best controlled by administration of medium-chain triglycerides
C. The taking of oral bile salts is of central importance in controlling steatorrhea
D. Vagotomy and pyloroplasty, and reversal of a segment of bowel are the two most important operations in the early management of short-bowel syndrome

Sabiston: 136
Schwartz: 1164

Comments: Treatment of the short-bowel syndrome centers on control of diarrhea and parenteral maintenance of nutrition. With time (2 to 3 years), the mucosa of as little as 30 to 45 cm of small bowel may undergo enough hypertrophy to allow withdrawal of intravenous alimentation and the start of carefully modified oral feedings. Diarrhea can be controlled with agents such as Lomotil or codeine, which slow intestinal motility. Oral calcium carbonate is also useful and acts by neutralizing hydrochloric acid and free fatty acids. When oral intake is resumed, dietary fat is restricted to 30 to 50 grams daily. Some patients benefit from the use of medium-chain triglycerides. In some patients oral bile salts are tolerated and aid in the formation of micelles, while in others they cause increased diarrhea. Similarly, cholestyramine is useful in some patients, but poorly tolerated by others. There is no standard approach to the resumption of oral intake, and the treatment must be highly individualized. While some patients ultimately do well with a modified oral diet, others remain dependent on permanent parenteral nutrition. There are no operative procedures that reliably correct this problem, so operative treatment should be considered only in patients who cannot maintain their body weight to within 30% of normal without intravenous supplementation. Operations that may be useful include reversal of a segment of intestine, creation of a recirculating loop of small bowel, creation of an artificial sphincter, and vagotomy and pyloroplasty. Allotransplantation of small bowel in humans has not been successful as of this date.

Answer: A

CHAPTER 27

Appendix

1. Concerning the function of the appendix:

A. It is a vestigial organ with no known function
B. It is a component of the secretory immune system
C. Its immunologic function protects against the development of colon cancer
D. The infantile appendix is the sole source of maturation for thymus-independent lymphocytes
E. None of the above

Sabiston: 980
Schwartz: 1245

Comments: Although the appendix is dispensable, it functions as an immunologic organ, producing immunoglobulins. Lymphoid tissue appears in the appendix during infancy and involutes during adulthood. It has been postulated that the appendix, the tonsils, and Peyer's patches of the intestine are sites where the processing of thymus-independent lymphocytes occurs in the human.

Answer: B

2. The anatomy of the appendix is such that:

A. In the adult, its base is located at the posteromedial aspect of the cecum below the ileocecal valve
B. The position of the tip in acute appendicitis is a function of the source of infection
C. The teniae coli form the outer longitudinal muscle layer
D. The position of the tip is relatively constant and is approximately under McBurney's point
E. None of the above

Sabiston: 967
Schwartz: 1245

Comments: The relation of the base of the appendix to the cecum is relatively constant; the position of the tip, however, is quite variable. Since the teniae coli converge at the base of the appendix, they can be useful landmarks in finding the appendix at the time of appendectomy, if easy visualization of it is difficult.

Answer: A, C

3. Concerning pathogenesis of acute appendicitis:

A. Fecaliths are identified in most patients with uncomplicated appendicitis
B. When examined carefully, a congenital narrowing at the appendiceal-cecal junction can frequently be identified
C. Fecaliths are more often found with gangrenous appendicitis than with simple appendicitis
D. Luminal obstruction is the most important factor in the development of appendicitis

Sabiston: 968
Schwartz: 1246

Comments: Appendicitis is initiated by obstruction of the lumen, which commonly is caused by a fecalith, or by lymphoid hypertrophy; less commonly, inspissated barium, vegetable or fruit seeds, or parasites are the cause. Fecaliths have been identified in approximately 40% of patients with acute simple appendicitis compared with 90% in patients with gangrenous appendicitis with rupture.

Answer: C, D

4. Which of the following statements is/are true about the natural history of acute appendicitis?

A. Rupture occurs most frequently in adolescent females because of the difficulty in establishing the diagnosis and consequent delay in operation
B. Perforation rates correlate with the severity of the initial illness
C. Acute appendicitis does not resolve spontaneously
D. Early antibiotic treatment decreases the incidence of perforation
E. None of the above

Sabiston: 969, 972
Schwartz: 1246

Comments: Although some episodes of appendicitis apparently resolve spontaneously and recurrent appendicitis is a recognized entity, the natural history of acute appendicitis is generally one of persistent obstruction leading to gangrene and perforation. Perforation occurs more commonly in patients at either end of the age spectrum, but clinical manifestations of the disease do not otherwise correlate with the risk of appendiceal rupture. Prompt appendectomy therefore is indicated when the diagnosis is made, since it is the only certain way of preventing perforation and its attendant morbidity.

Answer: E

5. In acute appendicitis:

A. Anorexia is usually present
B. Vomiting usually precedes pain
C. Pain often begins in the periumbilical area
D. Obstipation or diarrhea may occur
E. All of the above

Sabiston: 969
Schwartz: 1247

Comments: Classically, abdominal pain, which begins in the periumbilical region and subsequently localizes to the right lower quadrant, is the hallmark of acute appendicitis. Anorexia is a fairly constant symptom, and the diagnosis should be questioned if it is not present. Vomiting occurs in most patients and typically follows the onset of pain; the sequence has diagnostic significance. Variable patterns of bowel function may be seen and are usually not of diagnostic significance, although repeated diarrhea accompanied by vomiting is suggestive of gastroenteritis.

Answer: A, C, D

6. The most reliable physical findings in acute appendicitis is:

A. Cutaneous hyperesthesia
B. Localized right lower quadrant tenderness
C. Psoas sign
D. Tenderness on rectal examination
E. All of the above are equally reliable

Sabiston: 970
Schwartz: 1247

Comments: In typical acute appendicitis, tenderness is maximal near McBurney's point, although the precise location of maximal tenderness will vary with position of the appendix, being more lateral for a retrocecal appendix, and more medial or suprapublic for a retroileal or pelvic location. Rovsing's sign, the psoas sign, and the obturator sign are indications of local peritoneal or retroperitoneal irritation. Rectal examination is most useful when an abscess or phlegmon is present. Cutaneous hyperesthesia is an inconstant finding, but sometimes a helpful early sign.

Answer: B

7. Radiologic findings consistent with acute appendicitis include:

A. Distended loop of small bowel in the right lower quadrant
B. Partial filling of the appendix on barium enema

C. Gas-filled appendix
D. Mass effect on the cecum on barium enema
E. All of the above

Sabiston: 972
Schwartz: 1248

Comments: The diagnosis of acute appendicitis usually is based on the history and clinical findings, particularly when substantiated by laboratory findings of leukocytosis and normal urinalysis. Radiologic studies are, therefore, useful in terms of the differential diagnosis. A radio-opaque fecalith may be present on plain abdominal x-rays. Barium enema is sometimes helpful when the diagnosis is unclear; appendicitis can be excluded only when the appendix is completely filled.

Answer: E

8. Appendicitis in young children:

A. Is more often self-limited than in adolescents because of the relatively larger diameter of the appendiceal lumen
B. Has a high rate of rupture because of commonly delayed diagnosis and more rapid progression of disease
C. When ruptured, results in a localized periappendiceal abscess more often than in adults
D. Is often associated with higher fever and more vomiting than in adults
E. Is more serious, owing in part to the incomplete development of the omentum

Sabiston: 972
Schwartz: 1251

Comments: Acute appendicitis in infants and young children is a serious disease with a high rate of rupture. Symptoms are often atypical or difficult to elicit, resulting in a delay in diagnosis. In addition, the actual progression of the disease is thought to be more rapid than in older children or adults. When perforation does occur, diffuse peritonitis and distant intra-abdominal abscesses are more common, since the omentum is less developed and is less capable of confining the inflammatory process.

Answer: B, D, E

9. In evaluation of the female patient with right lower quadrant pain, which of the following should be included in the differential diagnosis?

A. Ruptured ectopic pregnancy
B. Twisted ovarian cyst or tumor
C. Diverticulitis of sigmoid colon
D. Epiploic appendicitis

Sabiston: 974
Schwartz: 1249

Comments: The differential diagnosis of appendicitis is basically that of the acute abdomen. Often it is impossible to differentiate these and other inflammatory processes from acute appendicitis. An extensive diagnostic workup is usually not warranted. The surgeon must be prepared to treat other pathologic entities should they be found on exploration for appendicitis.

Answer: A, B, C, D

10. A 16-year-old girl presents at the midpoint of her menstrual cycle with right lower quadrant abdominal pain and tenderness, fever to 39° C, mild diarrhea, and two episodes of vomiting. The white blood count is 12,500. The differential diagnosis includes:

A. Acute appendicitis
B. Ruptured graafian follicle
C. Acute gastroenteritis
D. Pelvic inflammatory disease
E. Crohn's disease

Comment: See Question 11.

11. An appropriate course of action for the patient described in Question 10 might include:

A. Laparotomy through a midline incision
B. Laparoscopy
C. Appendectomy via McBurney incision
D. Observation and antibiotics

Sabiston: 972, 974
Schwartz: 1250

Comments: The etiology of right lower quadrant abdominal pain includes numerous gastrointestinal, genitourinary, and infectious etiologies, which are best differentiated on the basis of the history, the clinical examination, and the laboratory findings. Occasionally, plain abdominal films, x-ray contrast studies of the colon, and ultrasonography are of use; the correct diagnosis will sometimes depend upon laparotomy. A false negative rate of 15% is commonly considered acceptable. Other etiologies most frequently observed include acute mesenteric lymphadenitis, acute pelvic inflammatory disease, torsion of an ovarian cyst, ruptured graafian follicle, acute gastroenteritis, and even no organic pathology.

Answer: Question 10: A, B, C, D, E
Question 11: A, B, C, D

12. Regarding acute appendicitis in the elderly:

A. Symptoms and physical findings may be minimal
B. It is associated with a high rate of perforation
C. Perforation is associated with a 50% mortality rate
D. Perforation often results in diffuse peritonitis
E. All of the above

Sabiston: 973
Schwartz: 1251, 1254

Comments: As in infants, acute appendicitis in the elderly may not present with typical signs and symptoms. Symptoms and clinical findings may be quite minimal or absent; leukocytosis may not be present. A 60 to 90% rate of rupture has been described because of the delay in ascertaining the correct diagnosis. The mortality rate of ruptured appendicitis in the elderly is about 15%. As in infants who have an as yet underdeveloped short omentum, the atrophic omentum in the elderly is less capable of walling off the inflammatory process. As a con-

sequence, rupture may result in diffuse peritonitis or distant intra-abdominal abscess.

Answer: A, B, D

13. Nonoperative therapy of appendicitis may be appropriate for which of the following?

A. A pregnant woman during the first trimester
B. A 35-year-old patient with subsiding symptoms and a right lower quadrant mass
C. An elderly patient with concomitant cardiac disease
D. A 20-year-old woman with Crohn's disease
E. None of the above

Sabiston: 978
Schwartz: 1252

Comments: When the diagnosis of appendicitis is a strong consideration but not certain, in most instances operation should be undertaken because delay has the risk of rupture and the accompanying increased morbidity and mortality. Operation should not be delayed during pregnancy, because there is risk to both the mother and to the fetus; nor should it be delayed in elderly patients, because they carry an increased risk of appendiceal rupture and death. The optimal timing of operation for ruptured appendicitis with established periappendiceal abscess has been controversial; most surgeons favor prompt operation as opposed to nonoperative treatment and delayed appendectomy. Initial nonoperative therapy followed by interval appendectomy may be considered, however, in a patient whose symptoms are clearly subsiding when a discrete right lower quadrant mass is palpable.

Answer: B

14. Appendicitis during pregancy:

A. May present with right upper quadrant or right flank pain
B. Should initially be treated by antibiotics in an attempt to avoid operation
C. Occurs more frequently than in nonpregnant women
D. When perforated, is associated with a fetal mortality of 80% and a maternal mortality of 10%
E. All of the above

Sabiston: 973
Schwartz: 1251

Comments: The gravid uterus pushes the appendix (and cecum) to a more lateral and cephalad position, so that the typical location of somatic pain is altered. The occurrence of abdominal pain, nausea, and leukocytosis during a normal pregnancy may also make the diagnosis more difficult. When the diagnosis is strongly considered, however, prompt operation is indicated. Fetal mortality is approximately 10% overall and rises to 35% with rupture. Maternal mortality is less than 0.5%.

Answer: A

15. A 20-year-old woman is operated on through a McBurney incision for presumed appendicitis; the appendix is normal. Appropriate treatment at this point should include:

A. Exploration and treatment of any associated pathology, as indicated, without appendectomy
B. Exploration and, if no pathology is found, closure without appendectomy
C. Exploration and diverticulectomy if a Meckel's diverticulum is present and normal by inspection and palpation
D. Exploration and ileal resection if the terminal ileum appears acutely inflamed
E. None of the above

Sabiston: 977
Schwartz: 1253

Comments: If appendicitis is not found at the time of operation, a careful exploration for other pathology must be carried out. Appendectomy is performed except in some cases of Crohn's disease. The pelvic organs, gallbladder, colon, and gastroduodenal areas should be inspected to the extent possible. Mesenteric lymph nodes are assessed and the small intestine is inspected in a retrograde manner for evidence of inflammatory bowel disease or a Meckel's diverticulum. Resection of a Meckel's diverticulum is indicated if diverticulitis is present. If acute regional enteritis is discovered, appendectomy alone is indicated.

Answer: E

16. Appropriate management of ruptured appendicitis includes:

A. Drainage and prompt appendectomy for periappendiceal abscess
B. Drainage and interval appendectomy for periappendiceal abscess if the appendix cannot be safely removed
C. Appendectomy, peritoneal lavage, and drainage for diffuse peritonitis
D. Antibiotics and nonoperative therapy when an abscess forms
E. All of the above

Sabiston: 978
Schwartz: 1252

Comments: Ruptured appendicitis may produce a localized periappendiceal abscess, diffuse peritonitis, or abscesses at other abdominal sites, notably in the pelvis, in the right subhepatic region, or between loops of bowel. When a localized abscess is encountered, it should be drained. The appendix should be removed, if possible, but if dissection is hazardous, interval appendectomy is an appropriate alternative. It is not possible to accomplish a generalized drainage of the peritoneal cavity for nonlocalized inflammation.

Answer: A, B

17. Which of the following statements is/are true concerning carcinoid tumors of the appendix:

A. The appendix is the most common location of gastrointestinal carcinoid tumors
B. Carcinoids may present as acute appendicitis since they most often occur at the base
C. Appendiceal carcinoids often are malignant and produce carcinoid syndrome

D. Nearly one third are multiple
E. All of the above

Sabiston: 976
Schwartz: 1155, 1254

Comments: In order of decreasing frequency, the appendix, ileum, and rectum are the most common locations for gastrointestinal carcinoids. Carcinoids of the small bowel are multiple in 30% of cases, whereas appendiceal carcinoids are usually solitary. The classic carcinoid syndrome, seen in patients with liver metastases, most commonly has the primary lesion in the ileum and rarely in the appendix.

Answer: A

18. If an incidental appendiceal carcinoid tumor is recognized 1 day after simple appendectomy, which of the following statements is/are true?

A. If mesoappendiceal lymph nodes are negative and resection margins clear, no further surgical treatment is necessary
B. Right hemicolectomy is routinely indicated regardless of nodal status
C. Right hemicolectomy is indicated if tumor is present at the surgical margins or if nodal involvement is present
D. If mesoappendiceal lymph nodal metastases are present, then surgical cure is unlikely and chemotherapy should be initiated
E. None of the above

Sabiston: 976
Schwartz: 1254

Comments: Simple appendectomy and resection of the mesoappendix is considered adequate treatment for carcinoids of the appendix that do not have regional nodal metastases and that have been completely resected by appendectomy. If nodes are involved, then right hemicolectomy should be performed. Chemotherapy with a combination of 5-fluorouracil and streptozocin has provided some palliation from the carcinoid syndrome in patients with unresectable metastatic disease. Various antiserotonin agents have also been employed for controlling symptoms in patients with the carcinoid syndrome.

Answer: A, C

19. When a mucocele of the appendix is found at the time of surgery, appropriate therapy would be:

A. Incisional biopsy with subsequent appendectomy if diagnosis is confirmed by frozen section
B. Right hemicolectomy with lymph node dissection
C. Needle aspiration of cystic fluid
D. Appendectomy
E. None of the above

Schwartz: 1255

Comments: Appendectomy is adequate treatment for mucocele, but care should be taken to avoid rupture, as pseudomyxoma peritonei has been reported following rupture and peritoneal dissemination of the appendiceal contents.

Answer: D

CHAPTER 28

Colon and Rectum

1. Which of the following statements is/are true regarding anatomy of the colon?

A. The inner circular and outer longitudinal muscle layers are complete
B. The haustra are separated by plicae circulares
C. The ascending and descending colon are normally fixed to the retroperitoneum
D. The anatomic rectum is partially intraperitoneal and partially extraperitoneal

Sabiston: 983

Comments: A thorough understanding of anatomy is integral to the surgical management of problems of the colon. The colon has both an inner circular and an outer longitudinal muscle layer, but unlike in the small bowel, the longitudinal layer is incomplete and grossly is recognized as three strips of muscle known as the taeniae coli. The haustra, located between the taeniae coli, are separated by crescentic folds known as plicae semilunares. This produces a characteristic radiologic pattern that permits differentiation of the colon from the small intestine, which has circular mucosal folds known as plicae circulares or valvulae conniventes. Knowledge of embryology of the colon in terms of its subsequent peritoneal relationships is prerequisite to operative dissection. Normally, the ascending and descending portions of the colon become fused to the retroperitoneum, whereas the transverse and sigmoid colon remain free. Developmental anomalies of fixation, as seen with malrotation and in some cases of volvulus, are not uncommon, however. The rectum lies beneath the peritoneal reflection and is, therefore, entirely extraperitoneal without a serosal layer.

Answer: C

2. Which of the following statements is/are true regarding the arterial blood supply to the colon and rectum?

A. The ileocolic, right colic, and middle colic arteries originate from the superior mesenteric artery
B. The middle colic and left colic arteries originate from the inferior mesenteric artery

C. The superior and middle hemorrhoidal arteries originate from the inferior mesenteric artery
D. The middle and inferior hemorrhoidal arteries originate from the internal iliac artery or its branches

Sabiston: 983
Schwartz: 1216

Comments: The colon is derived from both the embryologic midgut and hindgut. The right and transverse colon is supplied via the superior mesenteric artery and its ileocolic, right colic, and middle colic branches. The left colon and sigmoid are supplied by the left colic and the sigmoid branches originating from the inferior mesenteric artery. Generally, there are well-developed collaterals between these two circulations through a marginal arcade adjacent to the colon. The rectum is supplied by the superior hemorrhoidal arteries originating from the inferior mesenteric artery and by the middle and inferior hemorrhoidal arteries originating from the internal iliac or the internal pudendal branch of that vessel. The venous and lymphatic drainage of the colon and rectum generally parallel the arterial supply. Understanding these patterns is important in determining the extent of resection required for neoplastic processes and in the preservation of adequate blood supply to the remaining segments of colon to maintain viability.

Answer: A, D

3. Which of the following is/are the most effective method(s) for reducing risk of infection in colorectal operations?

A. Systemic antibiotics alone
B. Mechanical bowel cleansing alone
C. Mechanical cleansing plus systemic antibiotics
D. Mechanical cleansing plus nonabsorbable oral antibiotics
E. Mechanical cleansing plus nonabsorbable oral antibiotics plus systemic antibiotics

Sabiston: 991
Schwartz: 1200

Comments: The colon contains a higher concentration of bacteria than any area of the body and infectious complications constitute the major morbidity of colorectal operations. The benefit of intestinal antisepsis in decreasing these complications has been well established in numerous experimental and clinical studies, although there remain conflicting data on the best method of providing antisepsis. Mechanical cleansing of the colon can be achieved by the administration of a cathartic in combination with enemas or by peroral lavage with a large volume of solution. Such mechanical preparation is clearly important, but does not alone significantly alter bacterial flora. A combination of mechanical preparation with the administration of nonabsorbable oral antibiotics active against both aerobic and anaerobic colonic flora provides the most effective protection against infectious complications. Systemic antibiotics are often combined with oral antibiotics, but the combination has not been conclusively demonstrated to confer an advantage over the use of oral antibiotics alone. The use of systemic antibiotics in place of oral antibiotics is a less effective method of prophylaxis.

Answer: D, E

4. The most common cause of colonic obstruction in the United States is:

A. Adhesions
B. Diverticulitis
C. Cancer
D. Volvulus
E. Hernia

Sabiston: 996
Schwartz: 1034

Comments: Whenever a patient presents with signs and symptoms of intestinal obstruction, one first attempts to define the level of obstruction, i.e., small bowel or large bowel. Colonic obstruction is often suggested by the gas pattern on plain abdominal x-rays and can be confirmed by a carefully performed barium enema. Cancer is by far the leading cause of large bowel obstruction in this country. In adults, diverticular disease or volvulus may also produce obstruction, and in some parts of the world volvulus is the leading cause. Intussusception is a common cause of colon obstruction in the pediatric population. In contradistinction to obstruction of the small intestine, adhesive obstruction of the large bowel is extremely unusual. Other causes of large bowel obstruction include fecal impaction, especially in the elderly and infirm, and functional obstruction or so-called pseudo-obstruction. These latter two entities are not uncommonly encountered in postoperative patients. The importance of recognizing the presence and etiology of colonic obstruction cannot be overemphasized, since obstruction from any mechanism can lead to necrosis and perforation.

Answer: C

5. The most common cause of massive colonic bleeding is:

A. Cancer
B. Ulcerative colitis
C. Diverticulosis

D. Diverticulitis
E. Angiodysplasia

Schwartz: 1051, 1186

Comments: Although cancer is a common cause of occult lower intestinal bleeding, most **massive** hemorrhage is attributed to diverticulosis. This is to be differentiated from diverticulitis, in which significant bleeding is unusual. Acquired vascular ectasias are also a cause of massive bleeding, particularly when bleeding originates from the right colon. Bloody diarrhea is a frequent manifestation of ulcerative colitis, but the hemorrhage is generally mild to moderate; massive bleeding can occasionally occur.

Answer: C

6. An increased risk of colon cancer is associated with which one or more of the following?

A. Diet high in fiber
B. Diet low in animal fat and protein
C. Ulcerative colitis
D. Familial polyposis
E. Previous cholecystectomy

Schwartz: 1197

Comments: Colorectal cancer in the United States is second only to lung cancer as the leading cause of cancer deaths. Environmental factors, particularly dietary habits, may explain the wide variance in the geographical distribution of colon cancer. Diets low in fiber and high in animal fats and protein are associated with an increased risk of colon cancer. Mechanisms may include alterations in intestinal transit time and an increase in the formation of carcinogenic compounds as a result of bacterial metabolism of dietary components. A small but increased risk has also been identified in patients with prior cholecystectomy; in this physiologic setting, there is increased exposure of bile salts to metabolism by intestinal bacteria, perhaps producing carcinogenic agents. The role of genetic factors in the development of colon cancer is uncertain. The risk associated with inflammatory bowel disease and polyposis syndromes is well recognized but accounts for a small number of the total cases of colorectal malignancy.

Answer: C, D, E

7. The most useful screening test for colon cancer is:

A. Rigid proctoscopy
B. Flexible sigmoidoscopy
C. Colonoscopy
D. Testing for occult blood in the stool
E. Level of carcinoembryonic antigen
F. Barium enema

Sabiston: 989
Schwartz: 1206

Comments: Early detection of colonic neoplasms is facilitated by regular examination of the stool for occult blood. Although the test is not specific for malignant disease and a variety of colonic pathologies may cause detectable blood in the stool, the test is quite sensitive for breakdown products of hemoglobin. A single positive test in a patient on a red meat–free and peroxidase-free diet is significant and demands further investigation. Endoscopic examinations of the colon and rectum are extremely important diagnostically. Proctosigmoidoscopy does not examine a sufficient length of colon to be sensitive enough for a general screening procedure, however, and the time and cost of total colonoscopy limits its usefulness as a screening tool. Determination of CEA levels is important when following patients with colorectal malignancy for evidence of recurrent or metastatic disease, but is neither sensitive nor specific enough to be employed for screening purposes.

Answer: D

8. Select the most common mode of spread of colon cancer:

A. Hematogenous
B. Lymphatic
C. Direct extension
D. Peritoneal

Sabiston: 1007
Schwartz: 1198

Comments: Of the various mechanisms by which colon cancer may spread, the lymphatic route to regional mesenteric lymph nodes is the most common. This has important surgical implications as to the extent of resection necessary when operating with curative intent. Hematogenous spread occurs primarily to the liver, although lung and bone may also be involved. Direct extension to adjacent structures such as the prostate, bladder, or small bowel may occur without distant metastases and may require en bloc resection of portions of these organs. When tumor has broken through the serosal surface with cancer of the colon, or with other visceral malignancies, peritoneal dissemination may result, accounting for metastatic deposits in the rectovesical pouch (Blumer's shelf), of the umbilicus (Sister Mary Joseph nodule), and on the ovary (Krukenberg tumor). Intramural extension of disease occurs and this mode of spread has given rise to the traditional surgical dictum that at least 5 cm of colon distal to the tumor must be resected.

Answer: B

9. The most important prognostic determinant for colorectal malignancy is:

A. Lymph node involvement
B. Transmural extension
C. Tumor size
D. Histologic differentiation
E. DNA content

Sabiston: 1008
Schwartz: 1198

Comments: Of the many variables that have an impact upon long-term survival for colon cancer, lymph node status remains the most important. Long-term survival for node-positive patients is approximately half that achieved by node-negative patients. The other factors listed above as well as tumor location, extent of opera-

tion, and presence or absence of obstruction also influence outcome, but do not correlate as well as lymph node involvement.

Answer: A

10. Regarding colon cancer, list all of the structures (indicated by lower case letters in the diagram) that should be involved for each of the stages of the modified Astler-Coller (1978) staging system enumerated below.

A
B_1
B_2
B_3
C_1
C_2
C_3
D

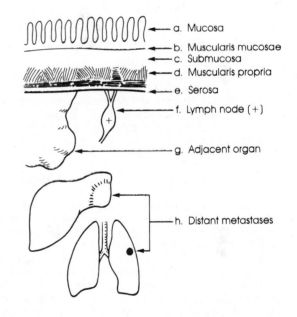

a. Mucosa
b. Muscularis mucosae
c. Submucosa
d. Muscularis propria
e. Serosa
f. Lymph node (+)
g. Adjacent organ
h. Distant metastases

Sabiston: 1009

Comments: Dukes' classification has long been the standard method of staging colon malignancy. Confusion arises, however, because of misunderstanding of Dukes' original classification and subsequent modifications. According to Cuthbert Dukes' original scheme proposed in 1932, an A lesion was confined to the bowel wall, a B lesion extended through the bowel wall but did not involve lymph nodes, and a C lesion implied regional node involvement. It is not uncommon to hear someone refer to a colon cancer with distant metastases as a Dukes' D lesion; this, however, was not part of the original classification. In 1949 Kirklin et al. modified Dukes' classification, describing an A lesion as one confined to mucosa, a B_1 lesion as one extending into the muscularis propria of the bowel wall, but not through it, and a B_2 lesion as one extending through the muscularis propria to the serosa. In 1954 Astler and Coller further modified the Kirklin classification by designating a C_1 lesion as one limited to the bowel wall, but with positive lymph nodes, and a C_2 lesion as one invading all layers of the bowel wall with positive lymph nodes. In 1978 it was modified even further: An A lesion is mucosal confinement. B_1 is involvement of muscularis, B_2 is involvement of serosa, and B_3 is involvement of an adjacent organ. The C lesions are the same with respect to local involvement but with positive lymph nodes. D is any of the above, to include distant metastases. So, as one can see, the number and extent of modifications have been such that it is something of a misnomer to refer to this as a modification of Dukes' classification. Rather, it is a classification that stands on its own and should be referred to as such. The American Joint Committee on Cancer has proposed a TNM classification which also stages tumor according to the extent of bowel wall involvement and the presence or absence of lymph node involvement.

Answer: A–a; B_1–a, b, c, d; B_2–a, b, c, d, e; B_3–a b, c, d, e, g; C_1–a, b, c, d, f; C_2–a, b, c, d, e, f; C_3–a, b, c, d, e, f, g; D–a, b, c, d, e, f, g, h

11. The minimum acceptable operation for a localized sigmoid cancer includes:

A. Segmental sigmoid resection
B. Resection of sigmoid and distal descending colon, sparing the main left colic artery
C. Resection of sigmoid and descending colon including the inferior mesenteric artery at its origin
D. Resection of the entire colon proximal to the lesion with ileorectostomy
E. Oophorectomy in women

Schwartz: 1202

Comments: The propensity of colon cancers to disseminate to the mesenteric lymphatics and the nature of the vascular supply to various areas of the colon determine the amount of resection necessary when one is operating for intended cure. At the minimum, resection for a localized sigmoid cancer should include the sigmoid and distal descending colon and accompanying mesentery including the sigmoidal and superior hemorrhoidal vessels. More extensive mesenteric dissection with ligation of the inferior mesenteric artery at its origin is advocated by some, although evidence that it improves survival is controversial. A more extensive resection of the entire intra-abdominal colon can be considered, particularly in younger patients who, for the remainder of their lives, will remain at risk of developing subsequent premalignant lesions or another colon cancer. Oophorectomy should be considered in postmenopausal women, as approximately 6% of patients will have drop metastases to the ovaries. Although it has not been established that routine oophorectomy improves survival (one third of these have microscopic involvement only), it may spare such patients the need for a later celiotomy to remove a symptomatic pelvic mass.

Answer: B

12. Which one or more of the following constitute(s) appropriate operative management of obstructing colon cancer?

A. Operation performed after adequate bowel preparation
B. Primary right colectomy and anastomosis for right-sided tumor
C. Initial decompressing colostomy only for left-sided tumor
D. Primary left colectomy and Hartmann's procedure for left-sided tumor
E. Primary subtotal colectomy and ileocolic anastomosis for left-sided tumor

Sabiston: 996
Schwartz: 1202

Comments: Cancer is the leading cause of colon obstruction, and left-sided tumors in particular are prone to obstruction. In the face of high-grade colonic obstruction, an adequate bowel prep cannot be performed and decompression is the treatment priority. The majority of right colon tumors presenting with obstruction can be safely treated by primary resection and anastomosis. For left-sided tumors producing obstruction, the traditional surgical approach has involved an initial decompressing transverse colostomy followed by a second-stage resection and possibly a third-stage operation for colostomy closure. Initial treatment by decompressing colostomy only is still appropriate, particularly for poor-risk patients, but primary resection of the obstructing pathology is more commonly performed today. A primary colocolostomy remains hazardous in the patient with an unprepared distended bowel. So for many patients with obstructing left-sided tumors, the preferred operation is **primary resection** accompanied by a Hartmann's procedure, or creation of a mucous fistula with reanastomosis at a second stage. A primary ileocolic anastomosis may be safer, and some advocate primary subtotal colectomy with an ileocolic anastomosis.

Answer: B, C, D, E

13. Indications for combined abdominoperineal resection in rectal cancer include:

A. Rectal cancer at any level
B. Rectal cancer in which a 5-cm distal margin cannot be obtained
C. Rectal cancer in which a safe low anterior resection cannot be performed
D. Anastomotic recurrence following low anterior resection
E. Palliation of obstructing rectal cancer with minimal liver metastases

Sabiston: 1008
Schwartz: 1202

Comments: The Miles abdominoperineal resection is the operation of choice for most distal rectal cancers. The price is a permanent colostomy and the potential surgical morbidity, including impotence and bladder dysfunction. Curative resection of lesions located 7 to 8 cm above the anal verge can be performed by low anterior resection without the need for permanent colostomy, depending upon the exact extent of the lesion, the size of the patient's pelvis, and the skill of the surgeon. The EEA stapling devices introduced through the rectum have greatly facilitated low resections. The traditional 5-cm distal margin may not be necessary; patients with margins of 2 cm have demonstrated equivalent survival. Several reports, however, have found higher rates of local recurrence following stapled low anterior anastomoses compared with hand-sewn anastomoses. This raises concern that the technical ability to perform low anastomoses may compromise the efficacy of operations for cure of cancer. Abdominoperineal resection is an operation that should be performed with curative intent. While it is not generally indicated as a palliative operation in patients with advanced disease, there are those with abundant local disease and minimal distant metastases in whom the operation can truly be palliative of local symptoms and thus justified.

Answer: C, D, E

14. Rectal cancer, as compared with cancer of the intraperitoneal colon, has a:

A. Lower overall survival rate
B. Higher overall survival rate
C. Lower local recurrence rate
D. Higher local recurrence rate

Schwartz: 1205

Comments: The rectum is an area with a rich vascular and lymphatic supply. Malignant disease can spread lymphatically to pararectal, pelvic, para-aortic, and even inguinal lymph nodes; it can spread hematogenously to the liver and other distant sites; and it can involve, by direct extension, adjacent pelvic organs. All in all, rectal cancers have a lower rate of resectability for cure than cancers of the intraperitoneal colon and thus a slightly lower overall survival. Local recurrence is also more common for rectal cancers. Both survival and local recurrence rates correlate with the site and stage of a rectal cancer. Lower lesions and those with lymph node involvement have a worse prognosis.

Answer: A, D

15. Adjuvant radiotherapy for locally advanced colorectal malignancy has most clearly been shown to:

A. Decrease local recurrence of rectal cancer
B. Increase survival of rectal cancer
C. Decrease local recurrence of intraperitoneal colon cancer
D. Increase survival of intraperitoneal colon cancer

Schwartz: 1203

Comments: There is a high rate of local recurrence following surgical treatment of rectal cancer. Radiotherapy is an established modality that decreases local recurrence rates by approximately 15 to 20%. The most effective method of utilizing radiotherapy, i.e., preoperatively, postoperatively, or in combination, is still being investigated. The evidence is conflicting as to whether radiotherapy improves survival in patients with rectal cancer.

Answer: A

16. Following resection for colon cancer, an asymptomatic patient is found to have a rise in his CEA from 3 ng/ml to 10 ng/ml. Which of the following statements is/are true?

A. This is a minor change and, in the absence of symptoms, not specific enough to warrant further investigation
B. If all diagnostic imaging modalities fail to demonstrate recurrence, laparotomy is indicated
C. Recurrent disease is more likely to be resectable than if detected owing to symptoms
D. The patient is more likely to have resectable disease if the interval between successive CEA determinations was 3 months rather than 12 months
E. The patient will likely be cured by operation and survive longer than if recurrent disease was detected owing to symptoms

Schwartz: 1206

Comments: Determination of carcinoembryonic antigen (CEA) has proved most useful as a marker for recurrent cancer in patients whose CEA was elevated prior to tumor resection, reverts to normal following resection, and subsequently rises. A rise above 5 ng/ml is highly significant and should prompt an evaluation for both recurrent intra-abdominal and extra-abdominal disease. If there is no evidence of extra-abdominal spread, a second-look laparatomy is warranted, even though contrast studies and CT scan may be negative. Studies of large groups of patients followed with routine CEA determinations suggest that recurrent disease is likely to be discovered on the average 2 to 3 months sooner by CEA determinations alone than if the patient develops symptoms. Patients are more likely to have resectable disease if the cancer is detected on the basis of a CEA rise alone and also are more likely to be resectable if CEA determinations are carried out at 3-month intervals. It is not clear, however, that overall patient survival is improved compared with that in patients who have recurrent disease detected on the basis of symptoms and are treated at that time.

Answer: B, C, D

17. Hamartomas are found in which of the following situations?

A. Juvenile polyps
B. Peutz-Jeghers syndrome
C. Familial polyposis
D. Gardner's syndrome
E. Chronic ulcerative colitis

Sabiston: 1024
Schwartz: 1190

Comments: Hamartomas are lesions in which normal tissue is found in an abnormal structural configuration. Since the cells themselves are not neoplastic, there is no malignant potential. Among the polypoid lesions of the gastrointestinal tract, those found with Peutz-Jeghers syndrome and in cases of juvenile polyps are hamartomas and therefore are not considered precancerous. Gastrointestinal cancers have been described in patients with Peutz-Jeghers syndrome, and occasionally these cancers have been related to the polypoid lesions; however, it is not clear that there is, in fact, a causal relationship, and the findings may be coincidental. The polypoid lesions observed in chronic ulcerative colitis are inflammatory "pseudopolyps"; the malignant potential of ulcerative colitis is not related to the presence of these lesions. The polyps found in cases of familial polyposis, Gardner's syndrome, and other polyposis syndromes are neoplastic adenomas with malignant potential.

Answer: A, B

18. Which of the following colorectal polyps is/are considered precancerous?

A. Hyperplastic polyps
B. Tubular adenoma
C. Tubulovillous adenoma
D. Villous adenoma

Sabiston: 1024
Schwartz: 1191, 1196

Comments: See Question 20.

19. For each statement in the left-hand column, select the appropriate response from the right-hand column.

Statement	Pathology
A. Most common type of intestinal polyp	a. Tubular adenoma
B. Children and adolescents	b. Hyperplastic polyp
C. Mitoses at depth of crypts	c. Both
D. Mitoses at surface of crypts	d. Neither
E. Differentiation into mature goblet cells	

Sabiston: 1024
Schwartz: 1191

Comments: See Question 20.

20. For each statement in the left-hand column, select the appropriate response in the right-hand column.

Statement	Pathology
A. Pedunculated	a. Tubular adenoma
B. Size usually less than 1 cm	b. Villous adenoma
C. Rectosigmoid most common location	c. Both
D. Malignant potential related to size	d. Neither
E. Malignant potential related to location	

Sabiston: 1026
Schwartz: 1191

Comments: Polypoid colorectal lesions can be considered as either neoplastic or non-neoplastic in origin. Hyperplastic polyps are by far the more common; they result from an imbalance between cell division and cell exfoliation. These lesions are small, multiple, and sessile and occur most frequently in the rectosigmoid; they are not neoplastic and have no malignant potential. Hyperplastic polyps are removed, however, in order to differentiate them from neoplastic adenomas, which have varying malignant potential depending upon their size, their histologic pattern, and the degree of cellular atypia. A histologic distinction between hyperplastic polyps and adenomatous polyps can readily be made on the basis of cellular differentiation and the location of cell division. In

normal colonic mucosa and in hyperplastic polyps, cell division is limited to the depths of the crypts of Lieberkühn, and differentiation into mature cells occurs as cells migrate up the crypt to the surface. In neoplastic polyps, on the other hand, cell division occurs at all levels of the crypt, including the surface, and the differentiation is incomplete. The most common type of neoplastic polyp is the tubular adenoma; these are generally asymptomatic, pedunculated lesions less than 1 cm in size and, like all colon polyps, are most commonly located in the rectosigmoid region. The likelihood of a neoplastic polyp containing cancer is directly related to polyp size. Only 1% of tubular adenomas less than 1 cm harbor malignancy; this figure increases to 10% for 1- to 2-cm tubular adenomas and exceeds 30% for larger lesions. Approximately 10% of neoplastic colon polyps are villous adenomas. As compared with tubular adenomas, these are larger sessile lesions that are more likely to present with symptoms such as rectal bleeding, mucous discharge, or diarrhea and that have a significantly higher risk of malignancy. Overall, approximately two thirds of villous adenomas contain cancer, and one half of these are invasive cancers. Approximately 15% of neoplastic colon adenomas contain a mixed histologic pattern with both tubular and villous elements and are referred to as tubulovillous adenomas. The risk of malignancy in tubulovillous adenomas is greater than that seen with tubular adenomas but less than that reported with villous adenomas.

Answer: Question 18: B, C, D
Question 19: A–b; B–d; C–c; D–a; E–b
Question 20: A–a; B–a; C–c; D–c; E–d

21. A pedunculated 1.5-cm tubular adenoma is removed endoscopically from the sigmoid colon and found to contain carcinoma extending to the muscularis mucosae. Select the best therapeutic option.

A. Observation and repeat endoscopic examination in 3 months
B. Endoscopic fulguration of polypectomy site
C. Operative colotomy and excision of polypectomy site
D. Sigmoid colectomy

Sabiston: 1027
Schwartz: 1191, 1196

Comments: By definition, carcinoma above the muscularis mucosae is carcinoma-in-situ. Benign colorectal polyps and polyps containing carcinoma-in-situ are adequately treated by total polypectomy. The polyp and the stalk must be inspected carefully for evidence of invasion, however. A lymphatic plexus exists just below the muscularis mucosae, so that lymphatic dissemination is possible when invasion has occurred beyond the muscularis mucosae. When a pedunculated polyp is found to have cancer in the lymphatics or invading the muscularis mucosae, a formal cancer resection is generally advocated, provided that the patient is an acceptable operative risk.

Answer: A

22. Biopsy of a 5-cm villous adenoma of the rectum reveals atypia. The most appropriate next step in management is:

A. Re-biopsy
B. Fulguration
C. Transanal excision
D. Abdominal perineal resection
E. Intracavitary radiotherapy

Sabiston: 1003, 1027
Schwartz: 1193

Comments: A villous adenoma of this size should be assumed to harbor malignancy until proved otherwise. The biopsy represents a very limited sample size and is not adequate proof of the lesion's benign nature. The finding of atypia, in fact, suggests a high probability of cancer elsewhere in the adenoma. For this reason, complete transanal excision should be performed. If there is no invasive cancer, then the patient is followed by interval endoscopic examination because of the risk of recurrence, even though the initial lesion was benign. If, on the other hand, invasive malignancy is found, then an appropriate cancer operation is performed. For a lesion in this location, abdominoperineal resection is the procedure of choice. Patients unfit to undergo such an extensive operation should be closely followed once the lesion has been completely excised, and consideration should be given to re-excision, fulguration, or radiotherapy for symptomatic local recurrence.

Answer: C

23. Concerning ulcerative colitis, correct statements include which one or more of the following?

A. In at least half of the cases, the entire colon is involved and the pattern of involvement is continuous, without skip areas
B. The characteristic histologic finding of crypt abscess is the sine qua non of ulcerative colitis, and is not seen in other inflammatory conditions of the bowel
C. The disease is most commonly a chronic relapsing illness; an acute and fulminant course is seen in only 10 to 15% of patients
D. Carcinomas arising in ulcerative colitis tend to be more evenly distributed throughout the involved colon, are more frequently multicentric, and usually are more aggressive than similar lesions arising from noncolitic colons

Sabiston: 1013
Schwartz: 1170

Comments: Ulcerative colitis is a disease usually limited to the mucosal and submucosal layers of the bowel. The rectum is almost always involved, with proximal continuous spread to varying lengths of colon. The entire colon is involved in at least half of the cases. The characteristic crypt abscesses consist of infiltration of neutrophils and eosinophils into the bases of the crypts of Lieberkühn. While crypt abscesses may be seen in other inflammatory conditions of the colon, they are always present in ulcerative colitis and usually in greater numbers. Ulcerative colitis is most commonly chronic and relapsing in character, but it runs an abrupt and fulminant course in 10 to 15% of the cases. Cancers arising from colons with past or present ulcerative colitis usually are diagnosed later because the signs and symptoms may initially be confused with a relapse of inflammation; for this reason,

these cancers are associated with a poor prognosis. Recent studies, however, have suggested that these cancers are not intrinsically more aggressive than those developing de novo in an otherwise normal colon.

Answer: A, C

24. A 25-year-old white woman presents with a history of repeated attacks of bloody diarrhea, cramping, lower abdominal pain, and weight loss. The presumed diagnosis is ulcerative colitis. Which of the following is/are true concerning the management of this patient?

A. A barium enema x-ray examination should be done early to assess the severity and extent of her disease
B. Hydrocortisone has been shown to induce remissions; however, such steroid-induced remissions are more likely to be followed by a relapse than are spontaneous remissions
C. Total parenteral nutrition, if administered early as part of the treatment, may delay or even prevent the need for colectomy
D. Maintenance, low-dose steroids are effective in preventing relapses
E. If medical therapy fails and a colectomy with ileorectal anastomosis is performed, there is a 15 to 20% chance that carcinoma will develop in the rectal remnant in the course of the next 20 years

Sabiston: 1017
Schwartz: 1173

Comments: Endoscopy with biopsy is perhaps the most reliable means of diagnosing ulcerative colitis. Barium enema examinations can be performed, but should be done with caution and should be avoided altogether during acute attacks because of the risk of precipitating toxic megacolon. Prednisone or hydrocortisone is very effective in treating acute phases of the illness; both drugs have sufficiently adverse side effects, however, that the dose should be tapered when this is possible. Administration of low-dose steroids is not very effective in preventing relapses. Recurrence following a steroid-induced remission is not any less likely than following a spontaneous remission. The optimal role of total parenteral nutrition in the treatment of these patients has not been well defined; it does not, however, appear to delay the need for surgical intervention. When an ileorectal anastomosis is performed, lifetime rectal surveillance is mandatory because of the subsequent risk of cancer, although the precise risk of cancer has varied among reports.

Answer: E

25. Match the clinical comment with the disease process.

Clinical Comment	Disease Process
A. Rectal involvement	a. Crohn's colitis
B. Small bowel involvement common	b. Ulcerative colitis
C. Chronic diarrhea, cramps, fever	c. Both
D. Curative surgery available	d. Neither

Schwartz: 1179

Comments: Rectal involvement is seen in both types of inflammatory bowel disease of the colon, although much more commonly in ulcerative colitis (95% vs. 50%). The small bowel is extensively involved in approximately 50% of patients with Crohn's colitis, whereas "backwash ileitis" occurs in perhaps only 10% of patients with ulcerative colitis. The clinical presentations are similar: chronic diarrhea, cramping, abdominal pain, and fever. Bloody stools, common with ulcerative colitis, are less commonly seen in patients with Crohn's disease. Total proctocolectomy eliminates the disease process in ulcerative colitis, but there is no curative operation for Crohn's disease. Indeed, even after total proctocolectomy for pancolonic involvement with Crohn's disease, recurrence rates may be as high as 50%; one third of patients will require additional surgery for such recurrence.

Answer: A–c; B–a; C–c; D–b

26. Match the clinical presentation with the clinical condition.

Clinical Presentation

A. The principal etiology is twisting of a short segment of bowel on its mesentery
B. Most common in elderly debilitated persons or in those with severe psychiatric or neurologic diseases
C. Nonoperative reduction is successful in 80 to 90% of patients
D. Abdominal distension, pain, and radiographic signs of a small bowel obstruction
E. Early recognition and prompt operation when strangulation is suspected has reduced operative mortality to 5%

Clinical Condition

a. Sigmoid volvulus
b. Cecal volvulus
c. Both
d. Neither

Sabiston: 994
Schwartz: 1211

Comments: The prerequisite for developing either a sigmoid or a cecal volvulus is the rotation of a mobile segment of bowel around a mesentery whose points of fixation are in close proximity. Otherwise, there are surprisingly few similarities between sigmoid and cecal volvulus. Volvulus of the cecum is most frequently seen in persons 25 to 35 years of age. Contrariwise, it is very unusual for sigmoid volvulus to occur in an active, otherwise healthy individual; usually it is seen in elderly debilitated persons or in those with psychiatric or neurologic disorders. Both varieties of volvulus of the colon typically cause abdominal distension and pain, but only in cecal volvulus may there be radiographic evidence of small bowel obstruction. Nonoperative reduction with endoscopy and insertion of a rectal tube is the preferred initial approach for sigmoid volvulus and should be done if the mucosa is not gangrenous. Similar nonoperative reduction of cecal volvulus is not very successful, and an operation is indicated as soon as the patient can be prepared for it. Even prompt operation for suspected stran-

gulation is associated with a mortality rate of about 50% for sigmoid volvulus and 10% for cecal volvulus.

Answer: A–c; B–a; C–a; D–b; E–d

27. With regard to diverticular fistulas, which of the following statements is/are true?

A. Colocutaneous fistulas frequently occur spontaneously
B. Colovesical fistulas normally present with urinary tract infections that may be accompanied by pneumaturia and fecaluria, and diagnosis is best confirmed by cystoscopy
C. Coloenteric fistulas may cause no symptoms whatsoever
D. Surgical correction must employ staged operations because of the hazards of primary anastomosis in the presence of extensive local inflammation.

Sabiston: 999
Schwartz: 1189

Comments: Fistula formation is a common complication of diverticulitis, second only to perforation in frequency. Fistulas usually form to adjacent viscera, i.e., bladder, uterus, vagina, or small bowel. Colocutaneous fistulas rarely form spontaneously; they are, however, a common postoperative complication, draining through operative wounds or drain tracts. Colovesical fistulas are most commonly the result of diverticular disease and first present with urinary tract symptoms such as fecaluria and pneumaturia. While a barium enema may give information regarding the extent and site of involvement of the colon with diverticulosis, actual demonstration of a fistula is better achieved with cystoscopy. Coloenteric fistulas may cause no symptoms or may present with diarrhea. Operative correction may be achieved safely in one stage in most patients; indeed this is the preferred choice. If bowel preparation is not adequate or if there is extensive local inflammation with abscess formation, then staged procedures are indicated.

Answer: B, C

28. Match the following features and locations of diverticula.

Characteristic Features

A. Are true diverticula and therefore are considered congenital in origin
B. May be clinically and radiographically indistinguishable from cancer
C. Resection and primary anastomosis may be hazardous in the presence of perforation with frank peritonitis
D. Incidental asymptomatic diverticula found on barium enema should be treated operatively because of the high incidence of complications

Location of Diverticula

a. Left-sided
b. Cecal
c. Both
d. Neither

Schwartz: 1190

Comments: Cecal diverticula contain all layers of the bowel wall and thus are true diverticula. Usually they are found in younger patients and are considered congenital in origin. The correct preoperative diagnosis rarely is made in cases of cecal diverticulitis; it is confused with acute appendicitis in 80%, and with cancer in approximately 5% of instances. If there have been repeated attacks of cecal inflammation with subsequent scarring and fibrosis, the radiographic and operative findings may be indistinguishable from carcinoma. Surgical options depend on the extent of inflammation; if it is limited to the diverticulum, then cecal diverticulectomy may be all that is necessary. If there has been perforation with frank peritonitis, then most surgeons would hesitate to perform a primary anastomosis, instead performing an ileostomy with transverse colon mucous fistula. For both types of diverticula, incidental asymptomatic diverticula are not treated.

Answer: A–b; B–c; C–c; D–d

29. With regard to radiation enterocolitis, which of the following statements is/are true?

A. The incidence of clinically significant radiation injury to the bowel is dose-dependent, usually occurring with administration of 3000 rads
B. The histologic changes include a progressive vasculitis of the submucosal arteries; subintimal foam cells are pathognomonic
C. The rectum is the most common site of injury
D. Barium enema and angiography show characteristic but nonspecific changes
E. Long segments of strictured bowel are best treated with resection

Schwartz: 1182

Comments: At tissue doses less than 4000 rads, significant bowel injury is uncommon. In addition to irradiation dosage, other factors that may predispose to injury include advanced age, hypertension, arteriosclerosis, diabetes, and adhesions that fix the bowel to one place. After cessation of therapy, denuded intestinal epithelium will regenerate; however, there is a progressive vasculitis that may lead to thickening of the vessel wall with luminal occlusion and/or thrombosis. The rectum is the most frequent site of involvement because of its proximity to target organs (e.g., cervix, uterus, prostate) and because of its fixed position. Rectal ulcers are seen on the anterior wall at about 4 to 6 cm from the dentate line, and rectal strictures usually occur at the 8 to 12 cm level. Barium enema and angiography show changes that are characteristic but not specific for radiation injury. In treating radiation enterocolitis, certain principles should be followed: avoid an operation unless no other option exists; resect short segments, bypass long segments of diseased bowel; avoid extensive adhesiolysis; protect anastomoses with a proximal colostomy.

Answer: B, C, D

30. Regarding pseudomembranous colitis, which of the following statements is/are true?

A. Diarrhea that begins after the antibiotics have been stopped cannot be pseudomembranous colitis

B. Administration of vancomycin or metronidazole is appropriate treatment
C. The relapse rate is 50% following a course of antibiotics
D. Diagnosis is made based on endoscopic appearance and cytotoxic assay for *Clostridium difficile*

Sabiston: 999
Schwartz: 1183

Comments: Enterocolitis, or pseudomembranous colitis, has been seen most frequently after the use of clindamycin and ampicillin. Almost all antibiotics, however, can cause the illness; diarrhea may begin as late as three weeks after discontinuance of the medication. Treatment with oral vancomycin or metronidazole is indicated in addition to cessation of other antibiotics.

Answer: B, D

31. Which of the following statements is/are true regarding carcinoid tumors of the colon and rectum?

A. They are rare and occur with equal frequency at these two sites
B. The incidence of invasive malignancy in carcinoids correlates poorly with size
C. They frequently cause the malignant carcinoid syndrome even in the absence of liver metastases
D. Rectal lesions may be excised transanally; if invasion is seen histologically, abdominal perineal resection is indicated

Sabiston: 1002
Schwartz: 1157, 1209

Comments: Carcinoid tumors of the colon and rectum are rare, but they do not occur with equal frequency; about 2% of gastrointestinal carcinoids occur in the colon, 17% in the rectum, and in these locations they rarely cause the carcinoid syndrome. The incidence of invasive malignancy correlates well with size. Rectal tumors less than 1 cm are rarely malignant; those larger than 2 cm are usually malignant and have nodal metastases. Rectal lesions may be excised transanally; abdominoperineal resection may be indicated if there is malignancy. Carcinoid tumors of the cecum and ascending colon are rare but highly malignant, two thirds having metastasized at the time of diagnosis.

Answer: D

32. Concerning amebiasis, which of the following statements is/are true?

A. In the United States, approximately 10% of the population are asymptomatic carriers
B. *Entamoeba histolytica* antibodies are detectable in the serum of over 90% of patients with active amebiasis
C. Acute amebic dysentery closely resembles fulminant ulcerative colitis; both should be treated aggressively with steroids
D. Amebic abscesses of the spleen are the most common complications of amebic colitis

Sabiston: 1000
Schwartz: 1184

Comments: Amebic dysentery is caused by the protozoan *E. histolytica*; it has been estimated that 10% of the American population are asymptomatic carriers. The disease can assume both an acute and a chronic form. Acute amebic dysentery has a presentation similar to that of acute ulcerative colitis, characterized by fever, cramps, and bloody diarrhea. Distinction between these two entities is important since steroids are contraindicated in amebic dysentery. Diagnosis is aided by serologic tests for *E. histolytica* antibodies, which are present in 90% of patients with active amebiasis. Perforation of the colon during the acute form of the disease is rare. Amebic abscesses of the liver are the most common complication of amebic colitis, and they may rupture into the pleura, pericardium, or peritoneum.

Answer: A, B

33. Match the following diseases with the appropriate drug(s) that may be used in their treatment.

Disease	Treatment
A. Pseudomembranous colitis	a. Hydrocortisone
B. Amebic colitis	b. Metronidazole
C. Actinomycosis	c. Penicillin
D. Lymphogranuloma venereum	d. Diloxanide furoate
E. Tuberculous enteritis	e. Vancomycin
F. *Yersinia* infection	f. Tetracycline
	g. Streptomycin

Sabiston: 999
Schwartz: 1152, 1183, 1250

Comments: Treatment of pseudomembranous colitis includes stopping the offending antibiotic and beginning vancomycin. Metronidazole may also be used and is much less expensive than vancomycin. Relapse rates of 20% have been reported. • Amebic colitis is an infection caused by *Entamoeba histolytica*. The acute dysentery is treated with metronidazole. Chronic mild amebic dysentery can be treated with diiodohydroxyquin or diloxanide furoate. Diiodohydroxyquin is effective in only 60 to 70% of patients and may cause optic neuritis. • Actinomycosis is a chronic fungal infection characterized by chronic inflammatory induration and sinus formation. Although the causative fungus is part of the normal oral flora, infections may occur in the cervicofacial area, thorax, or abdomen. The cecal region is the most frequent site of abdominal infection, producing a pericecal mass, abscesses, and sinus. Treatment consists of surgical drainage and penicillin or tetracycline. • Lymphogranuloma venereum is a transmissible disease affecting the colon, producing ulceration, sinus tracts, and fistulas. When the rectum is involved, strictures may occur. Diagnosis is made by the Frei intracutaneous test. This disease has been considered a premalignant condition because of the risk of adenocarcinoma developing in the rectosigmoid area and epidermoid cancer in the perianal region. Tetracycline is curative and steroids have been recommended. • The ileocecal region is the most frequent site of tuberculous enteritis, occasionally producing stenosis of the distal ileum, cecum, and ascending colon. Surgery is ill-advised unless there is obstruction. Triple drug therapy with isoniazid, para-aminosalicylic acid, and streptomycin usually heals intestinal lesions. • *Yersinia* infections are transmitted

through food contaminated by feces or urine, and they produce a clinical picture frequently indistinguishable from acute appendicitis. *Yersinia* is responsive to treatment with tetracycline, streptomycin, ampicillin, or kanamycin.

Answer: A–b, e; B–b, d; C–c, f; D–a, f; E–g; F–f, g

34. Which of the following statements is/are true concerning ischemic colitis?

A. The most frequent symptoms are lower abdominal pain and bright red rectal bleeding
B. Occlusion of the major mesenteric vessels is responsible for producing the ischemia
C. The splenic flexure and descending colon are the most vulnerable, although any segment of colon may be involved
D. Nonoperative management is not justified since, in a significant percentage of such cases, there will eventually develop perforation and peritonitis

Sabiston: 1000
Schwartz: 1181

Comments: Ischemic colitis may present as three distinct clinical syndromes depending on the extent and duration of vascular occlusion, the efficiency of collateral circulation, and the extent of septic complications. Mild or transient ischemia is compensated for by collateral blood flow; however, there may be partial reversible mucosal slough, which heals in 2 to 3 days. Healing occurs by mucosal regeneration, but if fibrosis of the bowel wall develops, stricture formation follows—the so-called stricturing ischemic colitis. If there is complete loss of blood flow with full-thickness infarction of the bowel wall perforation, peritonitis may follow. This entity has been called gangrenous ischemic colitis. Abdominal pain, either cramping or diffuse, and the passage of bloody stool are the most common signs. • Ischemic colitis appears to be a disease of the small arterioles and has been seen in patients with thromboangiitis obliterans, polyarteritis nodosa, and other collagen vascular diseases. Occlusion of the major mesenteric vessels does not adequately explain the etiology of this disease. For example, patients with frank ischemic colitis may have radiographic evidence of patent major arteries; moreover, ligation of these vessels (as in ligation of the inferior mesenteric artery during aortic aneurysmectomy) may not cause ischemic colitis. Although this disease can occur in any segment of the large bowel, it is most commonly seen in the splenic flexure or descending parts of the colon. • Diagnosis is made by endoscopy or by barium enema that may show the typical thumbprinting of the bowel wall. If gangrenous colitis is suspected, these studies are contraindicated. • Transient ischemic colitis responds to nonoperative management. Ischemic strictures may be electively resected with primary anastomosis after the initial ischemic episode has subsided.

Answer: A, C

35. Select the correct statement(s) regarding the operation of colectomy, mucosal proctectomy, and endorectal ileoanal anastomosis.

A. It is indicated for either ulcerative colitis or Crohn's disease, provided the rectum is minimally involved

B. Bladder and sexual function are preserved postoperatively
C. The need for an ileostomy is avoided
D. Construction of an ileal pouch proximal to the anastomosis increases intestinal storage capacity and decreases stool frequency

Sabiston: 1020
Schwartz: 1175

Comments: Patients who may require total proctocolectomy and permanent ileostomy frequently ask about sphincter-preserving alternative treatments. Colectomy, mucosal proctectomy, and endorectal ileoanal anastomosis offers advantages over more traditional surgical procedures in that not only is the diseased mucosa eliminated, but also the need for a permanent abdominal stoma is avoided. Initially described by Ravitch and Sabiston in 1947, the operative technique has undergone certain modifications, namely construction of an ileal pouch proximal to the ileoanal anastomosis. The pouch may be S-shaped or J-shaped, increasing intestinal storage capacity and decreasing stool frequency. A temporary diverting ileostomy is usually required for 2 to 3 months while the pouch heals. The procedure presently is recommended for selected patients with ulcerative colitis and polyposis syndromes, but is not indicated for Crohn's disease or indeterminate inflammatory bowel disease, or in patients with anal sphincter incompetence. Functional results are good, with preservation of the parasympathetic innervation to the bladder and genitalia. Rectal sensation and continence are retained in the majority of patients.

Answer: B, D

36. Regarding megacolon, which of the following statements is/are true?

A. The common denominator in congenital (Hirschsprung's disease) and acquired megacolon is chronic partial colon obstruction
B. Hirschsprung's disease is due to the congenital absence of ganglion cells in the myenteric plexus
C. There is a transition zone from dilated colon to normal-caliber aganglionic bowel
D. Acquired megacolon may be seen in patients whose colon is infested with *Trypanosoma cruzi* and in patients with neurologic disorders such as paraplegia and poliomyelitis
E. The surgical importance of megacolon is in its formation of chronic bowel dilatation, elongation, and a propensity to volvulus formation

Sabiston: 1273
Schwartz: 1213

Comments: **Megacolon,** or chronic dilatation of the colon, may be congenital or acquired. The common denominator is dilatation, elongation, and hypertrophy of the colon with resultant obstruction and increased risk of volvulus. **Hirschsprung's disease** is due to the congenital absence of ganglion cells in the myenteric plexus of the bowel. The rectosigmoid region is most frequently involved with variable extension of the disease proximally. There is a transition zone from normal, dilated bowel to

the aganglionic aperistaltic normal-caliber colon. Primarily a disease of infants and children, occasionally it may not become manifest until later in life. **Acquired megacolon** may result not only from protozoal infection with *Trypanosoma cruzi,* but also in patients with paraplegia, poliomyelitis, and psychotic disorders. In this latter group of patients, colonic dilatation is the result of constipation due to the loss of voluntary defecatory muscles, extreme inactivity, or voluntary inhibition of defecation. Colon resection may be justified in these patients; some surgeons advocate subtotal colectomy rather than "straightening out" the colon should operation be necessary for volvulus.

Answer: A, B, C, D, E

37. For each of the following characteristics, choose one or more syndromes in which it appears.

Characteristics	Syndrome
A. Malignant potential	a. Peutz-Jeghers syndrome
B. Extraintestinal manifestations	b. Familial polyposis
	c. Gardner's syndrome
C. Small bowel polyps	d. Turcot's syndrome
D. Mendelian dominant gene	e. Cronkhite-Canada syndrome

Sabiston: 1028
Schwartz: 1155, 1194

Comments: Of the conditions listed, the Peutz-Jeghers and Cronkhite-Canada syndromes do not have a significant malignant potential. In the former condition, the polyps are hamartomas and are found primarily in the jejunum and ileum, with involvement of the colon and rectum in one third and the stomach in one fourth of the cases. The polyps in the Cronkhite-Canada syndrome are dispersed throughout the gastrointestinal tract and do not undergo malignant transformation. This entity is also characterized by hyperpigmentation of the skin, alopecia, and atrophy of the fingernails and toes. Familial polyposis, Gardner's syndrome, and Turcot's syndrome may represent different expressions of the same disease. Familial polyposis lacks the extraintestinal manifestations of the other entities, namely the central nervous system tumors of Turcot's syndrome, and the osteomas, exostoses, and dermoid tumors of Gardner's syndrome. In addition to intestinal polyps, the Peutz-Jeghers syndrome is characterized by melanin spots of the oral mucosa, lips, palms of the hands, and soles of the feet. ● Small bowel polyposis is seen in all of the syndromes listed with the exception of familial polyposis and Turcot's syndrome. In the original report of the syndrome, Gardner described gastric polyps, and this finding has been reported in the Japanese literature as well. Periampullary carcinomas have also been described in patients with Gardner's syndrome. ● A familial pattern is frequently observed in these patients. An autosomal dominant gene has been proposed for Peutz-Jeghers syndrome, familial polyposis, and Gardner's syndrome, whereas it is believed that Turcot's syndrome is due to an autosomal recessive gene. No pattern of inheritance has been observed for the Cronkhite-Canada syndrome.

Answer: A–b, c, d; B–a, c, d, e; C–a, c, e; D–a, b, c

38. Which of the following statements is/are true regarding the polyposis coli syndromes?

A. These syndromes are unique to American and European Caucasians
B. Deaths from colon cancer occur at a significantly earlier age than in the general population
C. The risk of colon cancer developing approaches 100%
D. Abdominal colectomy and ileoproctostomy eliminates the risk of carcinoma

Sabiston: 1028
Schwartz: 1194

Comments: While it is true that most reports of polyposis syndromes reflect experience in American and European populations, these diseases have been identified in Africans and in Asians. There probably is no race or geographic location that is exempt. The polyposis syndromes occur in approximately one of every 12,000 births; thus, in the United States 300 new patients should have the disease each year. The polyps, which are not present at birth, first appear at about age 13 years, and gradually increase in number so that by age 21, the colon and rectum are carpeted by thousands of polyps. If the polyps are left untreated, the risk of developing cancer of the colon approaches 100% and the average age of death from colon cancer is 41.5 years. Subtotal colectomy with ileoproctostomy has been advocated as the procedure of choice, but close surveillance of the rectal remnant is mandatory. In the Mayo Clinic experience, the chance of rectal carcinoma developing after such a procedure is 5% by 5 years and increases to 59% at 23 years. Mucosal proctectomy with ileoanal anastomosis removes the neoplastic mucosa while avoiding the need for permanent ileostomy.

Answer: B, C

CHAPTER **29**

Anorectal Disease

1. Identify the anatomic structures indicated by capital letters in the following diagram by matching each with an item in the list below.

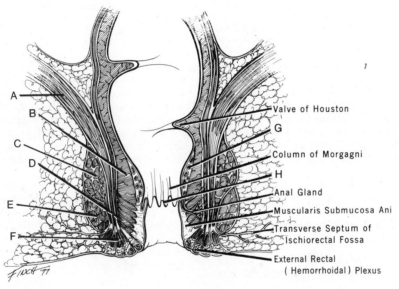

Modified from Storer EH, et al.: Chapter 28 in Schwartz SI, et al. (eds.): Principles of Surgery. 4th ed. Copyright © 1984 by McGraw-Hill, Inc. Used by permission of McGraw-Hill Book Company.

A. Internal sphincter
B. Conjoined longitudinal muscle
C. Levator ani
D. Subcutaneous external sphincter
E. Superficial external sphincter
F. Deep external sphincter and puborectalis
G. Internal hemorrhoidal plexus
H. Dentate line

Sabiston: 1035
Schwartz: 1214

Comments: See Questions 2 and 3.

Answer: A–c; B–a; C–f; D–b; E–e; F–d; G–g; H–h

2. Regarding the anal sphincteric mechanism, which of the following is/are true?

A. The teniae of the colon thicken to form the internal sphincter
B. The internal sphincter is made up of smooth muscle and surrounds the distal two thirds of the anal canal
C. The external sphincter is made up of striated muscle and is voluntary
D. The puborectalis is a part of the levator muscle
E. The anorectal ring is composed entirely of the palpable deep portion of external sphincter

Sabiston: 1035
Schwartz: 1214

Comments: The teniae of the colon form the conjoined longitudinal muscle. The circular muscle of the colon thickens to form the involuntary internal sphincter that surrounds the proximal two thirds of the anal canal. The external sphincter is formed of three parts—subcutaneous, superficial, and deep—which are striated muscles and voluntary. The puborectalis muscle is fused with the deep portion of the external sphincter and is not part of the levator muscle. The puborectalis muscle and the deep portion of the external sphincter along with the upper portion of the internal sphincter form the palpable anorectal ring.

Answer: C

3. Regarding the anatomy of the anal canal, which of the following is/are true?

A. The pectinate line lies above the column of Morgagni
B. Anal gland ducts open into the anal crypts
C. Anal glands extend into the ischiorectal space
D. The column of Morgagni overlies the internal hemorrhoidal plexus
E. The epithelium above the pectinate line is innervated by the autonomic nervous system

Sabiston: 1035
Schwartz: 1215

Comments: The pectinate line is at the level of the anal crypts; above it are the vertical mucosal folds that overlie the internal hemorrhoidal plexus. The anal mucosa proximal to the pectinate line is supplied by the autonomic nervous system and is physiologically painless; the anoderm distal to this is supplied by somatic nerves and is sensitive to painful stimuli. Anal glands, 6 to 10 in number, lie in the intersphincteric space and their ducts open into the anal crypts.

Answer: B, D, E

4. Of the following statements regarding perirectal spaces, which is/are true?

A. The pelvirectal space is situated above the levator muscle and is connected with the contralateral side anteriorly
B. The retrorectal space lies between the rectum and sacrum above the rectosacral fascia
C. The deep postanal space lies between the levator ani and superficial external sphincter posteriorly
D. The perianal space and the superficial postanal space lie deep to the superficial anal sphincter
E. The intersphincteric space lies within the conjoined longitudinal muscle

Schwartz: 1216

Comments: The pelvirectal space is located above the levator ani on both sides and communicates with the contralateral side posteriorly. The retrorectal space lies above the rectosacral fascia between the rectum and sacrum. The fascia runs downward and forward from the sacrum to the anorectal junction. The ischiorectal space lies distal to the levator muscle, proximal to the transverse septum of ischiorectal fossa, and between the external sphincter and lateral pelvic wall. The space communicates posteriorly through the deep postanal space that lies between the levator ani and the superficial sphincter. This communication allows a deep postanal space abscess to ex-

tend to both ischiorectal spaces (horseshoe abscess). The perianal space (the most common space involved in abscesses) lies superficial to the superficial anal spincter, and the intersphincteric space lies within the conjoined longitudinal muscle, where the anal glands also are located.

Answer: B, C, E

5. Regarding hemorrhoids, which of the following is/are true?

A. Internal hemorrhoids are vascular cushions above the dentate line and are covered by anoderm
B. Prolapsing hemorrhoids are external hemorrhoids covered by anoderm
C. Bleeding internal hemorrhoids are best managed by surgical excision
D. Thrombosed hemorrhoids are best treated by hemorrhoidectomy with the patient under general anesthesia
E. Recurrence is uncommon after surgical hemorrhoidectomy

Sabiston: 1042
Schwartz: 1222

Comments: **Internal** hemorrhoids are exaggerated vascular cushions normally located above the dentate line and therefore are covered by the mucous membrane of the anal canal and not by anoderm. **External** hemorrhoids are the dilated veins of the inferior hemorrhoidal plexus located below the dentate line and are covered by anoderm. **Prolapsing** hemorrhoids are internal hemorrhoids that prolapse beyond the dentate line. **Bleeding** is the main manifestation of internal hemorrhoids and is managed conservatively either by injection or by rubber banding and not by surgery. **Thrombosed** hemorrhoids are best treated by excision of the entire thrombosed hemorrhoid with use of local anesthesia. **Recurrence** should be rare after surgical hemorrhoidectomy and is related to inadequate removal of the rectal mucosa and hemorrhoidal tissue.

Answer: E

6. Which of the following is/are true regarding anal fissure?

A. It is located above the dentate line
B. It is located on the posterior midline in over 90% of patients
C. The operation of choice for a midline fissure is excision of the fissure and posterior sphincterotomy
D. Lateral partial subcutaneous sphincterotomy is the operation of choice for nonmidline fissures
E. Treatment should consist of fissurectomy and lateral partial subcutaneous external sphincterotomy

Sabiston: 1049
Schwartz: 1224

Comments: Anal fissure is a tear of the skin-lined part of the anal canal and is located at or below the dentate line; gentle spreading of the buttocks is frequently all that is necessary to reveal the fissure. About 90% of fissures (acute or chronic) are located at the posterior midline, an area of trauma during defecation. Fissures located laterally should arouse suspicion of Crohn's disease, ulcerative colitis, syphilis, tuberculosis, leukemia, or other causes. The initial treatment of fissure should be conservative, using lubricants and bulk laxatives. If conservative management fails, operative treatment should be a lateral subcutaneous partial internal sphincterotomy to relax the internal sphincter. A major reason of nonhealing is inadequate sphincterotomy. Posterior fissurectomy and sphincterotomy can lead to a keyhole deformity and constant soiling.

Answer: B

7. Regarding perirectal suppuration, which of the following is/are true?

A. The pathophysiology of perirectal abscess is related to infection of the perianal skin
B. A horseshoe abscess begins as a posterior midline infection
C. An intersphincteric abscess causes pain in the rectum but involves no external swelling
D. Most perianal abscesses can be drained using local anesthesia and without concern for subsequent formation of fistula in ano
E. Ischiorectal abscesses should be drained with the patient under general anesthesia and the fistula identified and treated

Sabiston: 1044
Schwartz: 1227

Comments: A **perirectal abscess** starts in the anal glands lying in the intersphincteric space. **Horseshoe abscesses** are bilateral ischiorectal abscesses communicating through the deep postanal space. These infections usually start from posterior midline anal glands. The patient should be treated in the operating room under regional or general anesthesia by draining the posterior midline through the rectum, and a counterdrain in each ischiorectal fossa but without a search for or treatment of a fistula. An **intersphincteric abscess** usually presents with pain and bulging inside the rectum but with no external swelling. Most **perianal abscesses** can be drained using local anesthesia without serious concern about subsequent fistula formation.

Answer: B, C, D

8. In the management of patients with fistula in ano, which of the following is/are true?

A. All internal openings of fistulas are located posteriorly according to Goodsall's rule
B. The most common type of fistula is intersphincteric
C. Excision of the entire fistulous tract is necessary for cure
D. High fistulas should be managed using the two-stage Seton procedure
E. A horseshoe fistula can be treated by posterior midline internal sphincterotomy combined with opening of the deep postanal space

Sabiston: 1047
Schwartz: 1228

Comments: Anal fistulas are classified as intersphincteric (the most common), transsphincteric, suprasphincteric, and extrasphincteric. Goodsall's rule states that if the external opening is anterior, the fistula usually runs directly into the anal canal, and if the external opening is posterior, the tract will curve to the posterior midline. Anal fistulotomy and establishment of adequate drainage is sufficient therapy; excision of the tract is unnecessary. High transsphincteric fistulas are best managed in two stages using a Seton procedure. A horseshoe fistula, starting with infection at the posterior midline anal glands, is best treated by opening the deep postanal space and an internal sphincterotomy in the posterior midline.

Answer: B, D, E

9. Anal incontinence associated with rectal prolapse is due primarily to which one of the following?

A. Anatomic defect associated with prolapse
B. Loss of rectal angle
C. Stretching of the anal sphincter
D. Stretching of pudendal nerve
E. Loose endopelvic fascia

Sabiston: 1040
Schwartz: 1232

Comments: Anal and urinary incontinence in advanced cases of prolapse is due to entrapment and stretching of the pudendal nerve resulting in neuromuscular dysfunction. It is very important, therefore, to repair rectal prolapse before incontinence develops. The other defects are associated with the prolapse but are not the cause of incontinence. Their correction, therefore, does not cure the problem of incontinence.

Answer: D

10. Regarding idiopathic ulcerative proctitis, which of the following is/are true?

A. It is a localized form of ulcerative colitis
B. Its course is characterized by remission and relapse
C. The disease usually progresses briskly to involve the entire colon within a period of 1 year
D. In almost half the patients, with time, the disease progresses to involve the entire colon
E. As with ulcerative colitis, it involves a negligible risk of developing a malignancy

Sabiston: 1040
Schwartz: 1235

Comments: Ulcerative proctitis is, by its designation, confined to the rectum and is a process that is inflammatory in nature. The feeling is that it is a localized variant of ulcerative colitis. As with ulcerative colitis, its cause is unknown. The fact that in about 1 in 10 patients the disease progresses to involvement of the entire colon may mean that the disease at original diagnosis was ulcerative colitis or that ulcerative proctitis has that potential. The risk of malignancy when the disease entity is confined to the rectum is very small. The symptoms and microscopic findings in this disease are those expected from an inflammation, namely rectal tenesmus from nonspecific rectal inflammation.

Answer: A, B

11. Select the most appropriate initial therapy for the following anal conditions.

Anal Condition	Most Appropriate Initial Therapy
A. Bowen's disease	a. Local excision
B. Paget's disease	b. Local excision and postoperative radiotherapy
C. Basal cell carcinoma	c. Abdominoperineal resection
	d. External beam radiotherapy
	e. Chemotherapy and radiation therapy

Sabiston: 1051
Schwartz: 1236

Comments: **Bowen's disease** is intraepidermal squamous cell carcinoma. It rarely metastasizes but can be locally recurrent. Local excision with adequate peripheral margins is quite adequate. **Paget's disease** of the perianal skin is a malignant neoplasm of the intraepidermal portion of the apocrine glands. It appears usually as an eczematoid perianal lesion in women and is intensely pruritic. Paget cells stain with periodic acid–Schiff stain, and this differentiates them from bowenoid cells. Invasion occurs late and metastasis is rare. Wide local excision with adequate margins is the procedure of choice. Both Bowen's and Paget's diseases are associated with other cutaneous or visceral malignancies. **Basal cell carcinoma** is usually noninvasive and nonmetastasizing. Local excision with adequate margins virtually assures a cure.

Answer: A–a; B–a; C–a

12. As compared with squamous cell cancers of the anal margin, squamous cell cancers of the anal canal generally are:

A. More common in women
B. More often associated with benign anal conditions
C. More advanced when diagnosed
D. More frequently associated with basaloid histology
E. Associated with a better prognosis

Sabiston: 1009
Schwartz: 1236

Comments: Squamous cell cancers of the anal canal are more common in women. Because they are often mistaken for benign anal disorders, they are usually advanced at the time of diagnosis and therefore have a worse prognosis. Basaloid carcinoma is a histologic variant seen with squamous cell cancer of the anal canal. Conversely, perianal squamous cell carcinoma is four times more common in men, and is usually slow-growing and late to metastasize. Basaloid features are uncommon. Wide local excision with a 2-cm margin may be adequate therapy for squamous cell cancers of the perianal skin, while squamous cell cancers of the anal canal require multimodality therapy including radiation and chemotherapy.

Answer: A, C, D

13. There is general agreement that survival after treatment for squamous cancer of the anus is related to which one or more of the following?

A. Tumor size
B. Depth of invasion
C. Basaloid versus squamous histology
D. Lymph node involvement

Sabiston: 1009

Comments: The poor prognosis of squamous cell carcinoma of the anal canal is related to delay in diagnosis. Therefore large (1.5 cm), deeply invading lesions that are associated with inguinal lymph node metastasis (in about 50% of cases) are generally associated with poor prognosis, irrespective of the histologic type. In basaloid cancers, there is good correlation between histologic differentiation and 5-year survival (90% for well differentiated, 50% for moderately differentiated, and 0 for anaplastic lesions). Basaloid histology vs. squamous histology alone, however, has not been conclusively shown to affect prognosis.

Answer: A, B, D

14. Select the true statement(s) regarding the management of inguinal lymph nodes in patients with squamous cell cancer of the anus:

A. Prophylactic groin dissection is indicated when abdominoperineal resection is performed
B. Groin dissection, whether for synchronous or for metachronously appearing nodes, yields equivalent survival rates
C. Metachronously appearing lymph nodes should be treated by radiation therapy, since surgical salvage is minimal
D. Combined radiation and chemotherapy may be curative without surgical lymph node dissection

Schwartz: 1236

Comments: The multimodality approach utilizing radiation and chemotherapy, but without inguinal node dissection, has been associated with a high cure rate. Even when treatment failures are subjected to abdominoperineal resection, there is no evidence that prophylactic groin node dissection increases the patient's survival sufficiently to justify the morbidity of the procedure. However, inguinal lymph node dissection for metachronous nodes prolongs the disease-free interval and in such instances, surgery is preferable to radiation therapy for curative purposes.

Answer: D

15. Which of the following may be appropriate initial therapy for a 3-cm cancer of the anal canal with invasion of the internal sphincter and no inguinal adenopathy:

A. Local excision
B. Abdominoperineal resection
C. Combined external beam and interstitial radiotherapy
D. Combined chemotherapy and radiotherapy

Sabiston: 1009
Schwartz: 1236

Comments: The optimal management of a small (<5 cm) squamous cell cancer of the anal canal without palpable groin lymph nodes is multimodal with radiation therapy and chemotherapy. As the effect of chemotherapy is believed to be radiopotentiating, recent protocols including external beam radiation and interstitial therapy have been tried with equal success. No randomized trial is available comparing these two protocols. The cure rate without AP resection approaches 80 to 85%.

Answer: C, D

16. Select the true statement(s) regarding the results of initial combined radiation therapy with 5-fluorouracil (5-FU) and mitomycin C for squamous cell cancer of the anus.

A. Complete regression of gross tumor has been observed in most patients
B. Patients may be followed without abdominoperineal resection if post-treatment biopsies reveal no tumor
C. Anal sphincter function may be preserved in at least one half of patients
D. Randomized prospective trials demonstrate improved survival compared to abdominoperineal resection alone.

Sabistion: 1009
Schwartz: 1236

Comments: Combination of radiation therapy and chemotherapy with 5-FU and mitomycin C results in regression of gross tumor in all cases and microscopic disappearance of tumor cells in over 80% of the patients. It is estimated that in 85% of the patients the anal sphincter can be saved. Therefore, abdominoperineal resection is reserved only for patients with gross or microscopic persistent tumors or for those with treatment failure and recurrent disease. Based on the excellent results of multimodal therapy, randomization with abdominoperineal resection alone is not justified.

Answer: A, B, C

CHAPTER 30

Morbid Obesity

1. True statements regarding intestinal bypass include:

A. End-to-side (Payne procedure) and end-to-end (Scott procedure) jejunoileal bypasses are the preferred operations for morbid obesity.
B. The operative mortality rate of intestinal bypass is 2 to 5%.
C. The late mortality rate of intestinal bypass is 10%.
D. Intestinal bypass for hypercholesterolemia successfully reduces serum cholesterol in 60% of patients
E. The appendix is not removed during these operations

Sabiston: 932
Schwartz: 1164

Comments: Jejunoileostomy has induced significant weight loss in the morbidly obese. However, it has been abandoned in favor of gastric partitioning for several reasons. More than 20%—in some series more than 80%—of patients having jejunoileal bypass require reversal of the operative procedure because of the development in these patients of hepatic failure, glomerulonephritis, cerebral failure, unmanageable electrolyte and metabolic imbalances, excessive weight loss, urinary calculi, polyarthritis, intractable diarrhea, and local anorectal problems. This list of complications is formidable, and the late mortality rate for this operation has been reported at 10%. For these reasons, jejunoileostomy has been abandoned in favor of gastrointestinal operations that can produce a similar weight loss with far fewer late complications and a much lower need for rehospitalization. Hypercholesterolemia is reduced by bypassing the ileum. The mortality rate of intestinal bypass is approximately 2%. The appendix should always be removed to simplify the diagnosis of any subsequent episodes of abdominal discomfort.

Answer: B, C, D

2. Which of the following conditions disqualify patients as candidates for morbid obesity surgery?

A. Presence of associated diseases such as diabetes, hypertension, myocardial infarction, and stasis ulcers

B. A weight of more than 100 pounds over the ideal body weight
C. Oxalate stones due to a jejunoileal bypass operation
D. Three failures of gastric restrictive surgery, at least one of them due to patient noncompliance
E. Patient had a C2 lesion of the left colon excised 6 months ago

Sabiston: 936

Comments: The permissive criteria for morbid obesity surgery include the following: a weight in excess of 100 pounds or twice the ideal body weight; this weight has existed for 3 to 5 years; the patient has made honest attempts to lose weight through dieting which resulted in loss of weight that has subsequently been regained; sufficient intelligence to follow postoperative orders; ability to understand the immediate and long-term complications of morbid obesity surgery; age between 12 and 65 years; and no associated conditions that would shorten or complicate the patient's life, such as ulcerative colitis or cancer. Associated conditions that can be improved by weight loss naturally make such an operation beneficial beyond that of the weight loss. Some such conditions are the pickwickian syndrome, congestive heart failure, diabetes, arthritis, panniculitis, hypertension, and infertility. Patients who have had repeated failures of surgery for morbid obesity are not good candidates for yet another operation because of the increased failure rate and the multiple associated complications. Thirty percent of patients with intestinal bypass develop oxalate stones. Such patients should have the bypass reversed at the same time that a gastric restrictive operation is performed. These stones form because the malabsorption of fat allows it to combine with calcium, therefore permitting the oxalate to remain in the colon as a soluble salt and be absorbed in increased amounts.

Answer: D, E

3. Which one or more of the following conditions must exist to allow a successful gastric restrictive operation?

A. A pouch size of less than 45 ml
B. Permanency of staple lines
C. A pouch outlet with a circumference of 1 cm
D. Absence of esophageal reflux
E. Absence of a fatty liver

Sabiston: 935

Comments: At the present time there are two gastric restrictive operations that are successful and still widely used: the **vertical band gastroplasty** and the **gastric bypass**. Experience has shown that for these operations to be successful, the pouch should be less than 45 ml in volume; the staple line must not disrupt; the gastric outlet must be approximately 1 cm in internal diameter. A gastric restrictive operation by its very design inhibits retrograde flow of acid formed in the distal stomach; for this reason they also are excellent antireflux operations. Approximately 80% of the patients with morbid obesity have a fatty liver, which regresses as the patient loses weight.

Answer: A, B, C

4. Complications of a loop-type gastric bypass include:

A. Bile reflux
B. Cirrhosis of the liver
C. Iron deficiency
D. Excluded, distal stomach
E. Vitamin B_{12} deficiency

Sabiston: 941

Comments: A loop-type gastric bypass results in a 20% incidence of bile reflux esophagitis in the course of a year. The reason probably is the distension of the gastric stump that occurs with time. Some surgeons view this as a favorable complication because it induces increased weight loss in patients. Many of the patients, however, are incapacitated and require a conversion of the loop-type gastric bypass to one utilizing a Roux-en-Y principle. Other surgeons prevent this complication by performing a Roux-en-Y type of operation initially. Vitamin B_{12} deficiency results in most of the patients with either type of gastric bypass and therefore, they require periodic B_{12} injections, or 100 mcg of B_{12} orally daily. About half of menstruating women will develop iron deficiency anemia; this can be corrected by administration of iron orally. Peptic ulceration in the distal stomach and proximal duodenum has been found in 1.8% of patients; this is the same incidence as in a normal population.

Answer: A, C, E

5. One of the most dreaded postoperative complications of gastric restrictive operation is perforation. It often presents as sudden cardiovascular collapse and may be misdiagnosed as pulmonary embolus. The presumptive diagnosis can be made from which one or more of the following?

A. An increased white blood count
B. A fever of 99.9° F
C. A pulse of 130
D. Coffee-ground emesis from the nasogastric tube on the second day
E. Left shoulder pain

Sabiston: 942

Comments: Patients who have a gastric bypass have approximately a 1 to 4% incidence of gastric leak or rupture; with vertical band gastroplasty it is less than 1%. Patients with an uncomplicated course following gastric restrictive operations recover quickly and have little discomfort. A presumptive diagnosis of a gastric leak may be made when, on the 4th to 6th day, the patient appears ill, anxious, and dyspneic and the pulse is over 120 per minute. Often the patient may have increased abdominal pain and referred pain to the shoulder. An elevated white blood count or an unexpectedly low white blood count with a left-shifted differential count, tachycardia, and fever should alert the surgeon to the presence of a leak and a subphrenic abscess despite initially minimal symptoms and physical findings. A diagnosis of leak is confirmed if swallowed Gastrografin is seen outside the stomach. Whether or not a leak can be proved, drainage by laparotomy or by a catheter inserted under the guidance of a CT scan is mandatory.

Answer: C, E

6. Which of the following is/are expected results of morbid obesity surgery?

A. Weight loss of 100% of the excess body weight
B. Reversal of hypertension and diabetes in over 90% of patients
C. Sustained weight loss in 100% of patients for at least 5 years
D. Serum cholesterol decreased by 40%
E. Reversal of any mental depression

Sabiston: 943

Comments: The expected weight loss after a gastric restrictive operation is approximately 60% of the excess body weight or approximately 30 to 40% of the patient's original body weight. Weight loss in terms of percentage of excess body weight is more meaningful because in heavier patients, a calculated weight loss based on the percentage of the entire body weight will still have patients excessively overweight. After weight loss, over 90% of patients who had hypertension become normotensive and those who were diabetic no longer require insulin. Also, cholesterol and triglyceride levels decrease by 40%. The failure rate of gastric bypass surgery is approximately 10 to 15% over a 5-year period, probably due to dilatation of the stomach, disruption of the staples, or conscious intake of easily swallowed high-calorie foods. In vertical band gastroplasty, the failure rate is approximately 1 to 2% per year. It has been shown repeatedly that when such patients lose weight they gain a great deal of self-respect, become outgoing and useful members of society, and overcome depression.

Answer: B, D, E

7. Which of the following morbid obesity operations has/have been shown to be safe and effective?

A. Payne intestinal bypass
B. Horizontal gastroplasty
C. Intragastric balloon
D. Vertical band gastroplasty
E. Scopinaro operation

Sabiston: 932

Comments: The **Payne and DeWind jejunoileal bypass** results in a 30% incidence of oxalate stone formation and a 3 to 5% death rate due to development of cirrhosis of the liver. Other complications include vitamin B_{12}, folate, vitamin K, potassium, magnesium, and calcium deficiencies; late bone resorption; arthritis; hemorrhoids; and a variety of gastrointestinal complaints. The **horizontal gastroplasty** was used extensively in 1979, but the frequent disruption of the horizontal staple line in more than 50% of the patients resulted in its abandonment. The **vertical band gastroplasty** has been employed since 1980 and is associated with little morbidity and mortality and a low failure rate. The **Scopinaro operation** is a biliary pancreatic bypass that currently is performed by Scopinaro and his associates in Italy and by Holian in the United States. This is a 75% gastric resection in combination with bypass of most of the intestine. Because the biliary and pancreatic fluids course through a greater length of intestine and are absorbed, diarrhea is not a great factor and the complications of development of cirrhosis and formation of oxalate stones are not prominent. This operation, however, has not as yet been evaluated completely.

Answer: D

8. Preoperative evaluation and preparation of a patient for morbid obesity surgery routinely includes which one or more of the following?

A. Antibiotics
B. Subcutaneous heparin
C. Treadmill test
D. Explanation of complications and expectations of the surgery
E. Dexamethasone suppression test

Sabiston: 936

Comments: Preoperative antibiotics do not reduce the incidence of leaks or intra-abdominal infection. Only subcutaneous infection is reduced in those cases that are clean-contaminated. Because of the risk of pulmonary emboli in obese patients (1 to 2% develop clinically apparent emboli), most surgeons use subcutaneous heparin and elastic stockings or intermittent pneumatic compres-

sion perioperatively. A treadmill test on these patients is performed only when indicated; it is not routine. Patients must be thoroughly informed of the indications, contraindications, complications, and expectations of surgery so that they are realistic about the results. Measurements of T3, T4, and plasma cortisol levels and a lateral skull x-ray (for sella turcica size) may be required by third party payers in order to screen out patients with hormonal obesity. However, patients who are truly hypothyroid or those who have actual Cushing's disease have a completely different appearance than those who have morbid obesity. Patients with Cushing's disease have small legs and arms and are extremely weak owing to lean tissue loss. A 400-pound patient presenting for this operation could not have Cushing's disease because they could not ambulate. Many obese patients have slightly increased cortisol levels, but if the stigmata of Cushing's disease are not evident, a dexamethasone suppression test is not indicated.

Answer: A, B, D

9. True or False: Intestinal bypass for hypercholesterolemia produces many of the complications associated with jejunoileal bypass for morbid obesity.

Schwartz: 1165

Comments: Intestinal bypass for hypercholesterolemia consists of bypassing the distal 200 cm or distal one third of the small intestine length (whichever is greater). Although some patients develop diarrhea, it does not cause significant weight loss and is not associated with the undesirable side effects of jejunoileal bypass. It lowers cholesterol by interfering with its absorption and by increasing bile acid excretion and causing micelle deficiency and decreased cholesterol absorption. It causes a 60% decrease in cholesterol absorption, a 40% reduction in the serum cholesterol levels, and a 50% reduction in plasma triglyceride levels. A significant number of patients with angina associated with hypercholesterolemia experience improvement or total remission of their symptoms following this operation.

Answer: False

CHAPTER 31

Liver

1. Which of the following statements about liver anatomy is/are true?

A. The left lobe extends to the right of the falciform ligament
B. The right lobe is divided into inferior and superior segments
C. The quadrate "lobe" is within the medial segment of the left lobe
D. The caudate "lobe" involves both the anatomic right and anatomic left lobes

Sabiston: 1054

Comments: Anatomically, the liver is divided into right and left lobes by a plane between the gallbladder fossa and the inferior vena cava. The left lobe is divided into medial and lateral segments by the falciform ligament. The right lobe is divided into anterior (ventral cephalad) and posterior (dorsal-caudal) segments, which do not have external landmarks. As defined by Couinaud, the liver is further divided into eight subsegments. The quadrate lobe, bounded by the ligamentum teres, gallbladder fossa, and portal triad, is contained within the anatomic medial segment of the left lobe. The caudate lobe is predominantly within the medial segment of the left lobe as well, but extends into the anatomic right lobe.

Answer: A, C, D

2. Which of the following statements is/are true about the hepatic arterial supply?

A. It provides 75% of blood flow to the liver
B. "Normal" arterial anatomy is present in only 50% of persons
C. It parallels the portal venous system intrahepatically
D. The most common variant is origin of the right hepatic artery from the gastroduodenal artery

Sabiston: 1056
Schwartz: 1257

Comments: The hepatic arterial supply normally is derived from the celiac axis by way of the proper hepatic artery, which becomes the common hepatic artery after giving off the gastroduodenal branch and subsequently bifurcates into right and left hepatic branches. There is, however, significant variability in hepatic arterial anatomy. In approximately 15 to 20% of persons, the right hepatic artery can arise from the superior mesenteric artery; in approximately 15%, the left hepatic artery may originate from the left gastric artery. These commonly encountered variants can have important surgical implications. The arterial blood supply accounts for only 25% of hepatic blood flow, with the remainder supplied by the portal vein.

Answer: B, C

3. Select the true statement(s) about hepatic veins from among the following:

A. They are valveless
B. The right, middle, and left veins drain the entire liver
C. The middle vein usually drains into the left vein
D. The hepatic veins parallel the hepatic arterial system intrahepatically

Sabiston: 1057
Schwartz: 1258

Comments: The hepatic veins begin in the liver lobules as the central veins and coalesce to form the right, left, and middle hepatic veins, which drain into the inferior vena cava and are of considerable surgical importance. The **right vein,** which is generally the largest, drains most of the right lobe. The **left vein** drains the lateral segment of the left lobe and a portion of the medial segment as well. The **middle vein,** which in 80% of individuals enters the left hepatic vein, drains the inferior anterior portion of the right lobe and the inferior medial segment of the left lobe. There are also **smaller veins,** particularly those draining the caudate lobe posteriorly, which enter directly into the vena cava.

Answer: A, C

4. Physiologic functions of the liver include which of the following?

217

A. Only site of albumin synthesis
B. During fasting, supplies glucose by glycogenolysis and gluconeogenesis
C. Active secretion of secondary bile acids
D. Primary site of cholesterol synthesis
E. Hydroxylation of vitamin D by cytochrome P-450

Sabiston: 1063

Comments: The liver performs a wide range of synthetic and metabolic functions and is an important component of the reticuloendothelial system. It is the principal site of synthesis of numerous plasma proteins, including albumin, urea, fibrinogen, and most coagulation factors. The liver also plays an integral role in glucose and lipid metabolism. During feeding it is a site of glycogen synthesis, and during fasting it provides energy substrates by glycogenolysis and gluconeogenesis as well as by formation of ketone bodies. The liver is the most active site of cholesterol synthesis; cholesterol is subsequently converted to bile salts or directly excreted into the bile. Primary bile acids are synthesized, conjugated, actively secreted, and effectively retrieved (enterohepatic circulation) by the liver. Bile is also the principal route of bilirubin excretion. The liver also plays a critical role in the metabolism of both fat- and water-soluble vitamins and is the site of initial 25-hydroxylation of vitamin D. The liver is responsible for the metabolism of many drugs and toxins by the oxidative reactions of the cytochrome P-450 system.

Answer: A, B, D

5. In typical obstructive jaundice, marked elevations might be expected in:

A. SGOT (AST)
B. SGPT (ALT)
C. Alkaline phosphatase
D. 5'-Nucleotidase
E. Leucine aminopeptidase

Sabiston: 1063
Schwartz: 1259

Comments: SGOT, SGPT, and LDH are markers of hepatocellular damage and usually are only mildly or moderately elevated in pure obstructive jaundice. On the other hand, enzymes including alkaline phosphatase, 5'-nucleotidase, leucine aminopeptidase, and gamma glutamyltranspeptidase are useful markers of cholestasis, and more pronounced elevations may be expected with biliary tract obstruction.

Answer: C, D, E

6. Which form(s) of viral hepatitis is/are usually transmitted parenterally?

A. Type A hepatitis
B. Type B hepatitis
C. Non-A, non-B hepatitis
D. Delta-associated hepatitis

Sabiston: 1123

Comments: Four types of viral hepatitis are recognized currently, each caused by a distinct etiologic agent. Hepatitis A virus is usually transmitted by a fecal-oral route and does not constitute a particular risk to the surgeon. Hepatitis B virus, non-A, non-B hepatitis, and delta-associated hepatitis (which requires the presence of hepatitis B virus) are usually transmitted by the parenteral route, although nonparenteral transmission may occur. The classic method of parenteral transmission has been by blood transfusion. Blood products do not all carry an equal risk of hepatitis. Most whole blood and its derivatives have a relatively small risk compared with products prepared from pooled plasma for the administration of clotting factors.

Answer: B, C, D

7. Select the true statement(s) regarding non-A, non-B hepatitis from among the following:

A. It is the most common cause of post-transfusion hepatitis
B. It results in chronic hepatitis more frequently than does type B hepatitis
C. It rarely leads to cirrhosis, even in chronic cases
D. Previous exposure to hepatitis B virus protects against non-A, non-B hepatitis infection
E. Active immunization is available

Sabiston: 1123

Comments: Non-A, non-B hepatitis is being recognized more frequently and accounts for approximately 20% of all cases. The specific virus or antigens responsible have not yet been identified. Consequently, there are no tests available to exclude non-A, non-B hepatitis from blood products, and it is the most common cause of post-transfusion hepatitis. Previous exposure to one type of hepatitis does not protect against subsequent infection with other types. It is thought that the non-A, non-B infection results in chronic hepatitis more frequently than does hepatitis B and that as many as 30% of patients with chronic active hepatitis may become cirrhotic. A vaccine is available for active immunization against hepatitis B, but not for non-A, non-B hepatitis.

Answer: A, B

8. Select the true statement(s) regarding an asymptomatic patient who is hepatitis B surface antigen–positive (HBsAg+).

A. The patient is a carrier and definitely infectious
B. If antibodies to HBsAg and hepatitis B$_e$ antigen (HB$_e$Ag) are present, the patient is in the incubating stage of acute illness and is more likely to be infectious
C. An accidental needle stick from this patient should be treated with immune serum globulin
D. An accidental needle stick from this patient should be treated with hyperimmune hepatitis B immune globulin
E. Elective surgery should be postponed if high titers of HB$_e$Ag are present

Sabiston: 1123

Comments: HBsAg can be detected both in patients with acute illness and in chronic carriers. The presence of this antigen does not indicate that the patient is necessarily infectious, but suggests that infectious virus may be present. This is more accurately detected by determination of core and core-related antigens. There is no test that conclusively determines whether or not a particular patient is infectious. *Guidelines:* Patients more likely to be infectious are those with a recent acute bacterial infection, those with higher titers of hepatitis B core antibody and HB$_e$Ag, and immunocompromised patients. Those less likely to be infectious are patients with antibodies to HBsAg or HB$_e$Ag. All patients who are surface antigen–positive should be considered potentially infectious, however, and appropriate precautions taken. Possible parenteral exposure to hepatitis B virus should be treated by administration of hepatitis B immune globulin within 7 days of exposure and repeated 1 month later. Exposure to hepatitis A virus or non-A, non-B virus and nonparenteral exposure to hepatitis B virus are treated by administration of immune serum globulin within 14 days of exposure.

Answer: D, E

9. Match the following disease states which produce jaundice with their appropriate pathophysiology.

Disease	Pathophysiology
A. Gilbert's disease	a. Bilirubin production exceeds excretory capacity
B. Hemolysis	b. Extrahepatic biliary obstruction
C. Physiologic neonatal jaundice	c. Deficient hepatocyte secretion
D. Crigler-Najjar syndrome	d. Deficient hepatocyte uptake
E. Dubin-Johnson syndrome	e. Deficient conjugation
F. Suppurative cholangitis	

Schwartz: 1052

Comments: It is useful to consider patients with jaundice in terms of the possible pathophysiologic mechanisms: excess bilirubin production, deficient hepatocyte uptake, deficient conjugation, deficient hepatocyte secretion, and deficient bilirubin excretion. These have been classically grouped as prehepatic, hepatic, and posthepatic causes. One of the first tests to be performed in the evaluation of the jaundiced patient is a fractionated bilirubin assessment to determine the relative proportion of conjugated and unconjugated bilirubin. **Hemolysis** is suggested by a predominance of unconjugated bilirubin, which indicates prehepatic causes, or hepatic deficiencies of uptake or conjugation of bilirubin. Predominance of conjugated bilirubin suggests defects in hepatocyte secretion into the bile ducts, or biliary excretion into the gastrointestinal tract. Combined conjugated and unconjugated hyperbilirubinemia usually suggests complex pathophysiology in which there has been acquired liver damage, or in which prehepatic or posthepatic causes have become associated with hepatocyte damage. **Gilbert's disease** is a relatively common abnormality of hepatic uptake of bilirubin and usually presents as a mild hyperbilirubinemia without other associated abnormalities. The **Crigler-Najjar syndrome** represents an inability to conjugate bilirubin within the hepatocyte due to a deficiency of glucuronal

transferase. **Physiologic neonatal jaundice** also represents a deficiency in conjugation; however, this is due to a self-correcting immaturity of bilirubin glucuronide synthesis. The **Dubin-Johnson syndrome** is caused by a deficiency in liver cell secretion and therefore presents as an intrahepatic form of obstructive jaundice. **Extrahepatic biliary obstruction** clearly is the most significant category of jaundice as relates to surgical practice. This is usually caused by gallstones, stricture, or neoplasm. Clinically, the patient may present with a spectrum of findings ranging from asymptomatic jaundice to the sepsis and moribund state of the patient with acute suppurative cholangitis. The latter is among the most urgent general surgical situations one may encounter.

Answer: A–d; B–a; C–e; D–e; E–c; F–b

10. Which of the following is/are appropriate in the management of hepatic trauma?

A. Hepatic arterial ligation if the patient is hypotensive and bleeding from a bilobar stellate laceration
B. Simple suture closure and drainage of nonbleeding lacerations
C. Right thoracotomy and placement of an atriocaval shunt for retrohepatic vena caval injury
D. Observation of a subcapsular hematoma
E. Routine T-tube drainage of the common bile duct

Sabiston: 314
Schwartz: 1261

Comments: The liver is the intra-abdominal organ most frequently injured by penetrating trauma and the second most frequently injured by blunt trauma. Many simple lacerations are not bleeding at the time of exploration and require drainage only; these lacerations should not be closed because of the risk of liver abscess. Simple bleeding lacerations can generally be controlled by direct suture ligation or the use of hemostatic collagen. The preferred method of controlling bleeding from deeper wounds is by direct ligation after adequate exposure is obtained. Compression of the portal vein and hepatic arterial inflow in the hepatoduodenal ligament (Pringle maneuver) may be useful in controlling bleeding from these deeper injuries. Extensive hemorrhage following inflow occlusion suggests hepatic venous or retrohepatic caval injury and requires control of the vena cava above and below the liver and possible placement of an atriocaval shunt; this is accomplished via sternotomy. Selective ligation of the right or left hepatic artery for control of hemorrhage is rarely necessary, but might be helpful in occasional deep wounds involving one lobe in which exposure of the wound would require extensive hepatotomy. Hepatic arterial ligation, particularly in the presence of hypotension, may produce hepatic necrosis. More extensive parenchymal injuries require resection or débridement to remove all necrotic or devitalized tissue. Resection rarely follows precise anatomic lines. Routine drainage is indicated following repair of hepatic injuries, but routine common duct drainage is not indicated, as it is associated with a higher rate of complications. Patients with documented subcapsular hematomas may be observed if they do not have signs of continuing hemorrhage or infection.

Answer: D

11. Select the type of hepatic abscess in the right-hand column that is best described by each statement on the left.

A. Usually single
B. Predominantly involves right lobe
C. Cultures usually sterile
D. Treatment primarily medical
E. Treatment primarily surgical

a. Amebic liver abscess
b. Pyogenic liver abscess
c. Both
d. Neither

Sabiston: 1068
Schwartz: 1264

Comments: Most hepatic abscesses are pyogenic or amebic. Although the clinical signs and symptoms may be similar, predominantly consisting of fever and pain, it is important to differentiate the two for therapeutic purposes. *Escherichia coli* or other gram-negative bacteria are the most commonly isolated organisms from pyogenic abscesses; *Staphylococcus* and *Streptococcus* species may also be involved, and anaerobes are becoming increasingly common. Today, the most common source of pyogenic abscess is contiguous infection in the biliary tract. Other sources include infectious foci within the portal venous drainage system, direct extension from perihepatic sites, and hematogenous spread. Approximately 20% of pyogenic abscesses are cryptogenic. The right lobe is most commonly involved with any hepatic abscesses; this has been attributed to a streaming effect in the portal vein. Diagnosis is based on clinical presentation and hepatic imaging and may be confirmed by fine needle aspiration. Treatment of pyogenic abscess generally requires surgical exploration and drainage, which allows assessment of associated intra-abdominal pathology. Abscesses may be successfully treated by percutaneous drainage alone, and in the occasional patient with multiple small abscesses, antibiotic therapy alone may suffice. Amebic abscesses are caused by the protozoan *Entamoeba histolytica*; diagnosis requires hepatic imaging and serologic tests. Hepatic amebiasis is treated primarily by the administration of amebicidal drugs, with metronidazole as the drug of choice. Percutaneous aspiration may be indicated if the patient does not respond to medical management; open surgical drainage is indicated only in the presence of secondary bacterial infection.

Answer: A–a; B–c; C–a; D–a; E–b

12. In a patient with a calcified cystic lesion of the liver and a positive Casoni test, appropriate treatment(s) may include:

A. Metronidazole
B. Percutaneous drainage
C. Transperitoneal surgical drainage
D. Cyst excision
E. Hepatic lobectomy

Sabiston: 1087

Comments: The helminth *Echinococcus granulosus* is responsible for most hydatid disease of the liver. This is usually a unilocular process involving the right lobe, although it may present as multiple cysts. Complications include intrabiliary, intraperitoneal, or intrapleural rupture, secondary infection, anaphylaxis, and mass replacement of the liver. These lesions often have a calcified wall and can be diagnosed serologically by indirect hemagglutination tests, complement fixation tests, and the Casoni skin test. Treatment is primarily surgical; percutaneous aspiration or drainage is contraindicated because of the risk of intraperitoneal dissemination. At the time of operation, the cyst is aspirated and scolicidal agents are injected. Alternatives for management of the cyst cavity include marsupialization and drainage, obliteration of the cyst cavity, and cyst excision in the form of pericystectomy or hepatectomy for larger lesions. Mebendazole may be useful in the treatment of some *Echinococcal* cysts.

Answer: C, D, E

13. Match the following characteristics with the appropriate hepatic pathologic finding(s).

Characteristics

A. Occurs predominantly in women
B. Associated with oral contraceptives
C. Involves risk of hemorrhage
D. Involves risk of malignancy
E. Forms a stellate scar

Hepatic Pathology

a. Focal nodular hyperplasia
b. Hepatic adenoma
c. Cavernous hemangioma
d. None of the above

Sabiston: 1085
Schwartz: 1271

Comments: Hemangioma, hepatic adenoma, and focal nodular hyperplasia are the most common benign hepatic neoplasms. Cavernous **hemangiomas** are usually small and asymptomatic and have a characteristic arteriographic appearance. These lesions may be very large, however, and occasionally may be complicated by rupture and hemorrhage, congestive heart failure, or consumptive coagulopathy. **Hepatic adenoma** is associated with the use of oral contraceptives and is composed of hepatocytes histologically. It may be quite large and may carry the risk of rupture and hemorrhage, particularly during pregnancy. **Focal nodular hyperplasia** has a characteristic histologic appearance, a central stellate scar, and lesions that are usually small and asymptomatic. These lesions are not associated with any particular risk of hemorrhage, although occasionally they may grow and produce symptoms. They too have an association with contraceptives and are composed of hepatocytes histologically. None of these common benign lesions is associated with an increased risk of malignancy.

Answer: A–a, b, c; B–a, b; C–b, c; D–d; E–a

14. A 25-year-old woman with right upper quadrant abdominal pain is found to have a 5-cm solid lesion in the right lobe of the liver. She takes oral contraceptives. She should be advised that:

A. The most likely diagnosis is focal nodular hyperplasia
B. Excision of the lesion is indicated

C. The symptoms will subside if oral contraceptives are discontinued
D. There is no future risk of hemorrhage if oral contraceptives are discontinued
E. Her symptoms are probably unrelated and no specific treatment of the lesion is necessary

Sabiston: 1086

Comments: Liver cell adenomas in women on oral contraceptives are often discovered because of pain or a palpable mass and are particularly prone to rupture and hemorrhage. Although hepatic adenomas have occasionally been reported to regress following cessation of oral contraceptives, this cannot be anticipated with any reliability. Even if oral contraceptives are discontinued, there is a considerable risk of rupture of a liver cell adenoma during subsequent pregnancy. For these reasons, resection is generally indicated.

Answer: B

15. Polycystic liver disease in adults:

A. Is associated with polycystic kidney disease
B. Is associated with hepatic fibrosis and portal hypertension
C. Does not usually require specific treatment
D. May be treated by percutaneous aspiration
E. Often requires hepatic resection

Sabiston: 1087
Schwartz: 1268

Comments: Adult polycystic disease of the liver is often associated with cystic involvement of the kidneys and other organs such as the pancreas or spleen. Complications of the liver disease per se are infrequent, so specific therapy is usually not necessary. If local pressure or pain develops, percutaneous aspiration, surgical unroofing, or excision of larger cysts may provide symptomatic relief. A childhood form of polycystic kidney disease may be associated with congenital hepatic fibrosis. Hepatic fibrosis also occurs in association with multiple dilatations of the intrahepatic biliary tree (Caroli's disease).

Answer: A, C, D

16. The most common primary tumor site associated with hepatic metastases is:

A. Lung
B. Colon
C. Pancreas
D. Breast
E. Stomach

Sabiston: 1083

Comments: Bronchogenic carcinoma is the primary malignancy most frequently associated with hepatic metastases. However, compared with patients with primary lung tumors, a greater percentage of patients with gastrointestinal primaries will develop hepatic metastases. The liver is the most common site of metastases for colorectal cancer. The presence of hepatic metastases is suggested by elevation of liver enzymes and specific tumor markers and is confirmed by hepatic imaging, radionuclide scans, ultrasonography, CT scan, or biopsy.

Answer: A

17. True or False: Survival of patients with solitary unresected hepatic metastases from colorectal cancer is the same as survival of patients with widespread hepatic metastases.

Sabiston: 1085

Comments: The effectiveness of treatment for hepatic metastases has often been judged by comparison with the natural survival history of patients with untreated hepatic metastases. The overall prognosis for untreated hepatic metastases from colorectal cancer has been poor, with most patients dying of cancer by 3 years after diagnosis. While it was formerly thought that patients with untreated solitary hepatic lesions did as poorly as the others, it has more recently been recognized that patients with solitary metastases have a 3-year survival of approximately 20%, which is better than survivals observed for patients with widespread metastases or multiple unilateral lesions.

Answer: False

18. Resection of hepatic metastases has most clearly benefited patients with which one or more of the following primary malignancies:

A. Colon
B. Breast
C. Stomach
D. Ovary
E. Wilms' tumor

Sabiston: 1085
Schwartz: 1275

Comments: Most of the experience with resection of hepatic metastases has involved those from colorectal cancer. Five-year survival following resection of solitary lesions is approximately 25–30%. Favorable results have also been reported among smaller groups of patients with Wilms' tumor. Results of resection of hepatic lesions metastasizing from stomach, pancreas, breast, gallbladder, ovary, melanoma, and head and neck tumors have not been as encouraging. Palliative resection of hepatic metastases has been useful in controlling symptoms due to metastatic carcinoid tumors, insulinomas, and gastrinomas.

Answer: A, E

19. Disease-free survival following resection of colorectal hepatic metastases is adversely influenced by which of the following?

A. Shorter time interval between resection of primary lesion and hepatic metastases
B. Hepatic metastases synchronous with primary tumors
C. Large hepatic metastases (greater than 5 cm)
D. Positive colonic lymph nodes in resected primary (Dukes' C classification)

E. Wedge resection of hepatic metastases rather than lobectomy

Sabiston: 1085

Comments: Among the more commonly employed treatment modalities for hepatic metastases are resection, systemic chemotherapy, and intra-arterial infusion of chemotherapeutic agents. Various criteria have been evaluated in order to identify the subset of patients who might best benefit from resection. Outcome has not been as favorable in patients with larger metastatic lesions. Moreover, no significant correlation has been identified between disease-free survival and synchronous vs. metachronous lesions, solitary vs. multiple lesions in the same lobe, shorter or longer time interval between primary resection and resection of metastases, wedge resection with adequate margin vs. lobar resection or presence or absence of involved mesenteric lymph nodes. More recently, it has been suggested that patients with fewer than four unilobar lesions do better than patients with four or more unilobar lesions or with bilobar disease.

Answer: C

20. Which of the following hepatic resection(s) involve(s) dissection in the plane of the umbilical fissure?

A. Right lobectomy
B. Right trisegmentectomy
C. Left lateral segmentectomy
D. Left lobectomy
E. None of the above

Sabiston: 1089
Schwartz: 1276

Comments: The umbilical fissure is the segmental plane between the medial and lateral segments of the left lobe of the liver. Within the fissure are vessels critical to both of these segments. Dissection is therefore never carried out directly in the segmental fissure. In the left lateral segmentectomy, the plane of parenchymal dissection is to the left of the fissure, while in the right trisegmentectomy, the parenchyma is divided to the right of the fissure. Both right and left lobectomies involve dissection well to the right of this plane.

Answer: E

21. Which of the following is/are true regarding the management of patients undergoing major hepatic resection?

A. Preoperative prothrombin time and serum albumin determinations accurately predict functional adequacy of the remaining liver
B. Postoperative hyperglycemia results from intraoperative release of glycogen stores and is best managed by continuous insulin infusion
C. Postoperative coagulopathy reflects vitamin K deficiency and is best treated by parenteral vitamin K
D. Transient postoperative elevations of serum ammonia levels are expected and are treated by lactulose and administration of branched-chain amino acids.
E. Postoperative hypoalbuminemia usually resolves within 7–10 days and is treated by daily administration of exogenous albumin

Sabiston: 1089
Schwartz: 1275

Comments: The operative mortality of major hepatic resection has been decreased to 5 to 10%, reflecting not only refinements in surgical technique but also advances in preoperative preparation and postoperative support. Preoperative preparation involves correction of reversible defects, such as anemia, malnutrition, and vitamin K deficiency. Unfortunately, there are no single tests of liver function that accurately predict the adequacy of the remaining liver. However, generalized abnormalities of hepatic function suggested by increased bilirubin and depressed synthetic parameters suggest that great care must be taken before performing major resections. Postoperative complications of major hepatic resection include hypoglycemia (which is treated by infusion of 10% dextrose), hypoalbuminemia (which is treated with exogenous albumin), and coagulopathy (which is treated by administration of fresh whole blood or platelets and fresh-frozen plasma). Transient elevations of alkaline phosphatase, bilirubin, or transaminases are not uncommon, but even with extensive hepatic resection, blood ammonia levels usually remain normal.

Answer: E

22. Which of the following is/are true regarding major hepatic resection?

A. 80% hepatectomy is incompatible with life
B. Hepatic regeneration is dependent on portal blood flow
C. Cirrhotic livers regenerate at the same rate as noncirrhotic livers
D. Uncontrolled regeneration in cirrhotic livers is associated with malignancy

Schwartz: 1275

Comments: An 80% hepatectomy is generally well tolerated if the liver is otherwise normal. Regeneration occurs rapidly and is dependent upon hepatotrophic factors such as insulin found in the portal venous blood. The presence of cirrhosis is a relative contraindication to major hepatic resection, since hepatic reserve is limited and hepatic failure may result. Little regeneration occurs after resection of cirrhotic liver.

Answer: B

23. Risk factor(s) for the development of hepatocellular carcinoma include(s):

A. Primary biliary cirrhosis
B. Alcoholic cirrhosis
C. Alpha-antitrypsin deficiency
D. Hepatitis B
E. Hemochromatosis

Sabiston: 1079

Comments: Primary hepatocellular carcinoma is one of the most common malignancies in the world. It has a particularly high prevalence in parts of Africa, Southeast Asia, and Japan. The incidence in the United States appears to be increasing. Although the etiology is uncertain, it appears to develop in association with underlying hepatic cirrhosis, particularly in low-incidence areas. Important risk factors include hepatitis B, alcoholic cirrhosis, hemochromatosis, alpha$_1$-antitrypsin deficiency, and blood group B. Aflatoxins, oral contraceptives, androgens, vinyl chloride, and Thorotrast have also been associated with hepatic malignancies. Although the malignancy is frequently found in patients with end-stage liver disease, it does not seem to occur in patients with primary biliary cirrhosis.

Answer: B, C, D, E

24. Elevations of alpha-fetoprotein (AFP) may be found with which one or more of the following?

A. A normal 6-week-old infant
B. Breast carcinoma
C. Hepatitis B
D. Teratocarcinoma
E. Gastric carcinoma

Sabiston: 1080
Schwartz: 1273

Comments: Determination of AFP levels is useful in the diagnosis and follow-up of patients with hepatocellular carcinoma. Approximately 75% of African or Asian patients with hepatocellular carcinoma have elevated AFP levels. In the United States, most patients with hepatocellular carcinoma and underlying cirrhosis also have elevated levels; approximately one third of patients with hepatocellular cancer in a noncirrhotic liver have elevated AFP. AFP is useful diagnostically in detecting malignant lesions of the liver and may be used to detect their recurrence following resection. AFP is normally present in the fetus, but it rapidly disappears several weeks after birth. Other conditions that may be associated with elevated AFP levels include testicular and ovarian embryonal malignancies, hepatitis B, and occasionally metastatic pancreatic or gastric carcinoma. Mild elevations may be found in patients with chronic liver disease.

Answer: C, D, E

25. Which of the following is/are true regarding the treatment of primary hepatocellular carcinoma?

A. Mean survival of untreated patients is 3–4 months from the time of onset of symptoms
B. Most lesions are amenable to resection by partial hepatectomy with a 5-year survival of approximately 30%
C. Most lesions are not amenable to partial hepatectomy and are best treated by irradiation
D. Both systemic chemotherapy and hepatic arterial chemotherapy produce a response rate of approximately 60%
E. Orthotopic liver transplantation has become the treatment of choice

Sabiston: 1081
Schwartz: 1273

Comments: Surgery remains the only definitive treatment for hepatocellular carcinoma. Overall, however, only 20 to 30% of patients can undergo resection because of the extent of tumor or the presence of cirrhosis. Five-year survival following resection approximates 30% and

may be somewhat better in the North American population. Orthotopic liver transplantation has been used in patients with hepatocellular carcinoma not resectable by conventional techniques. In general, recurrence following orthotopic transplantation has been the rule, although successful palliation has been achieved. Radiation therapy has not been of benefit. Most patients have not responded to chemotherapy, nor has chemotherapy, in general, been found to prolong survival.

Answer: A

26. Fibrolamellar hepatoma is a histologic variant of hepatocellular carcinoma associated with which of the following factor(s)?

A. Cirrhosis
B. Multicentricity
C. *Clonorchis sinensis*
D. Younger patients
E. Better prognosis

Sabiston: 1082

Comments: Fibrolamellar hepatocellular carcinoma is a histologic subtype that appears to have a better prognosis than other types of hepatic carcinoma. These tumors are usually solitary and occur in younger patients with otherwise normal livers. Long-term survival following resection has been reported, but it is not entirely clear whether the more favorable prognosis reflects the natural history of their disease or a higher resectability rate.

Answer: D, E

27. Which of the following study(ies) may be important in determining treatment in a patient with hepatic encephalopathy?

A. Serum ammonia level
B. Serum amino acid pattern
C. Electroencephalography (EEG)
D. Paracentesis
E. Angiography

Sabiston: 1112
Schwartz: 1286

Comments: Although the etiology of hepatic encephalopathy is not fully understood, current understanding focuses on toxic effects of ammonia, mercaptans, short-chain fatty acids, methane thiols, and false neurotransmitters. The mechanism involves hepatic dysfunction or portosystemic shunting or usually a combination of both. A number of situations can precipitate hepatic encephalopathy and should be sought in the initial evaluation of patients. These causes include gastrointestinal bleeding, infection, constipation, electrolyte or metabolic abnormalities, and diuretic and other drug therapy (particularly sedatives or hypnotic drugs). In evaluating patients for potential infection, it is important to recognize the possibility of spontaneous primary bacterial peritonitis in patients with ascites and to perform paracentesis to clarify this point. Some cases of hepatic encephalopathy have no identifiable precipitating cause other than the patient's inability to metabolize protein adequately or the presence of portosystemic shunting. In cases of refractory encephalopathy, angiographic assessment and therapeutic occlusion of a prior surgical shunt or of major collaterals may bring about improvement in the patient's condition. Although serum ammonia levels are usually elevated with encephalopathy and amino acid patterns are altered, these findings do not point toward a specific therapeutic approach. EEG may provide confirmatory diagnostic information.

Answer: D, E

28. Initial treatment of the patient in hepatic coma should include:

A. Lactulose
B. Nutritional supplementation with standard amino acid formulas
C. Nutritional supplementation with branched-chain amino acids
D. Systemic antibiotics
E. Ileostomy

Sabiston: 1113
Schwartz: 1286

Comments: The treatment of hepatic encephalopathy and coma is aimed at limiting the nitrogen that the liver must metabolize by eliminating nitrogen materials from the gastrointestinal tract and inhibiting their absorption. At the same time, precipitating causes are sought and treated. Lactulose acts as a cathartic and also inhibits absorption of ammonia by acidifying the colon. Intraluminal neomycin reduces the colonic flora and the production of ammonia. Although alterations in the balance of aromatic amino acids and branched-chain amino acids have been demonstrated in patients with hepatic disease and encephalopathy, there is no evidence that administration of branched-chain amino acids will significantly improve encephalopathy. Nutritional support is important and can be initiated with standard amino acids and restriction of dietary protein. Branched-chain amino acids can be reserved for patients with intractable encephalopathy despite these initial maneuvers. Systemic antibiotics may be useful in the treatment of specific infections precipitating encephalopathy, but are not indicated empirically. Since the colon is the major site of ammonia absorption, colonic resection or exclusion has been used to improve encephalopathy, but is not a widely employed therapeutic measure.

Answer: A, B

29. Which of the following is/are relative contraindication(s) to peritoneovenous shunting for intractable ascites?

A. History of variceal bleeding
B. Hepatorenal syndrome
C. Acute hepatitis
D. Uncorrectable coagulopathy
E. Malignant intra-abdominal disease

Sabiston: 1116

Comments: Patients with significant ascites due to cirrhosis or malignancy who do not respond to a medical regimen of sodium and fluid restriction and diuretics may be candidates for peritoneovenous shunting. These shunts decrease ascites and increase cardiac output and renal blood flow. Some degree of coagulopathy, usually transient, occurs in nearly all patients with cirrhotic ascites; uncorrectable coagulopathy is considered a contraindication to shunting. Patients with portal hypertension and previous variceal bleeding may rebleed following shunting because of the increase in circulating blood volumes; a side-to-side portacaval shunt is preferred for these patients. Other contraindications to shunting in patients with cirrhotic ascites include infection, acute hepatitis, and end-stage liver disease. Patients undergoing peritoneovenous shunts for malignancy have a higher incidence of shunt occlusion; relative contraindications include the presence of bloody ascitic fluid or fluid with high protein content.

Answer: A, C, D

CHAPTER 32

Biliary System

1. During cholecystectomy, a 3 mm bile duct in the triangle of Calot, which is not the cystic duct, is transected. This most likely represents:

A. The main right hepatic duct, which should be primarily reconstructed
B. The main right hepatic duct, which should be anastomosed to jejunum
C. A segmental right hepatic duct, which should be primarily reconstructed
D. A segmental right hepatic duct, which should be anastomosed to jejunum
E. A segmental right hepatic duct, which should be ligated

Sabiston: 1129
Schwartz: 1309

Comments: Variations in arterial and ductal anatomy of the biliary tract are common and are important to recognize because of the possibility of injury at operation and because they may have catastrophic long-term consequences. Usually, the anterior and posterior segmental ducts of the right lobe join intrahepatically to form the main right hepatic duct. However, either segmental duct may cross to join the left hepatic duct, and occasionally a segmental duct may join the cystic duct or common hepatic duct outside of the liver. It is in this location that the duct is subject to injury during cholecystectomy. If the segmental duct is 2 to 3 mm, anastomosis to the jejunum is recommended; smaller ducts can be ligated.

Answer: D

2. Intraoperatively, a replaced hepatic artery is most commonly found:

A. In the gastrohepatic ligament
B. Anterior to the common bile duct
C. Posterolateral to the common bile duct
D. Medial to the portal vein
E. Within the head of the pancreas

Schwartz: 1309

Comments: The most common variation in hepatic arterial anatomy is origin of the right hepatic artery from the superior mesenteric artery. This is a replaced hepatic artery and not simply an accessory vessel that can be sacrificed with impunity. Whenever an operation is being performed in the right upper abdomen, an assessment should be made of the size of the normal common hepatic artery in its expected location medial to the common duct. If the vessel is absent or small, one should be alerted to the possibility of a significant replaced hepatic vessel. When the right hepatic artery takes its origin from the superior mesenteric artery, it courses posterior to the head of the pancreas and portal vein and is usually identified posterolateral to the common bile duct. Only rarely does a replaced right hepatic artery actually course through the pancreas. A replaced left hepatic artery originating from the left gastric artery is identified in the gastrohepatic ligament. In addition to replaced vessels, it is important to recognize variations in the cystic artery and right hepatic artery, which could complicate cholecystectomy.

Answer: C

3. Which of the following inhibit(s) bile flow?

A. Secretin
B. Cholecystokinin
C. Bile salts
D. Vagal stimulation
E. Splanchnic stimulation

Schwartz: 1314

Comments: Up to 1,000 ml of bile is secreted daily in response to various neural, hormonal, and chemical stimuli. Bile flow is stimulated by vagal activity, by bile salts via the enterohepatic circulation, and by secretin, which is released predominantly from the duodenal mucosa in response to hydrochloric acid, protein, and fats. Gallbladder contraction is predominantly stimulated by cholecystokinin, which is released in response to duodenal fat. Sympathetic splanchnic nerve stimulation is inhibitory to both bile secretion and gallbladder motor function.

Answer: E

4. Which of the following is/are true regarding enterohepatic circulation of bile salts?

A. 95% of excreted bile salts are reabsorbed in the intestine
B. The secondary bile acids, cholic and chenodeoxycholic acid, are formed in the gallbladder
C. Primary bile acids are conjugated in the intestine to allow reabsorption
D. Interruption of enterohepatic circulation decreases bile salt secretion

Sabiston: 1147
Schwartz: 1321

Comments: Following their secretion in the liver, bile salts are concentrated in the gallbladder prior to excretion into the intestine. Most excreted bile salts are subsequently reabsorbed, predominantly in the ileum. Cholic and chenodeoxycholic acid are the primary bile acids. These are conjugated with taurine or glycine within the liver and subsequently deconjugated by the action of intestinal bacteria to form the secondary bile acids deoxycholic and lithocholic acid. Secondary bile acids are absorbed in the colon. Bile acids are potent choleretic agents, and interruption of enterohepatic circulation decreases the secretion of bile salts. This reduces cholesterol solubility and contributes to the formation of stones in patients with ileal disease or resection.

Answer: A, D

5. Cholecystectomy:

A. Decreases enterohepatic circulation of bile
B. Increases enterohepatic circulation of bile
C. Decreases bile salt secretion
D. Increases bile salt secretion

Sabiston: 1147
Schwartz: 1321

Comments: Cholecystectomy produces a more continuous flow of bile into the intestine. This increases the frequency of enterohepatic cycling and stimulates bile salt secretion. For these reasons, bile that is formed following cholecystectomy tends to be less lithogenic.

Answer: B, D

6. Most gallstones contain:

A. Cholesterol
B. Calcium
C. Bile pigment
D. Oxylates

Sabiston: 1147
Schwartz: 1320

Comments: Gallstones are usually composed of a combination of cholesterol, calcium, and bile pigments. In the United States, most gallstones are predominantly of cho-

lesterol, which form when the proportion of bile salts and lecithin in the bile are inadequate to form micelles to dissolve cholesterol. Pure cholesterol stones are rare, however, and most of these stones also contain calcium and pigment. Approximately 30% of patients in the United States have pigment stones, which are of two varieties: black pigment stones and brown pigment stones. Both contain calcium bilirubinate, although in somewhat different forms. Black pigment stones are associated with hemolysis, cirrhosis, and old age; brown pigment stones, the so-called earthy stones, are usually found in association with infection.

Answer: A, B, C

7. Pigment gallstones are associated with:

A. Obesity
B. Exogenous estrogens
C. Truncal vagotomy
D. Biliary tract infection
E. Total parenteral nutrition

Sabiston: 1148

Comments: Pigment stones all contain calcium bilirubinate. In pigment stones associated with infection, calcium bilirubinate is the main constituent, whereas black pigment stones, found in hemolysis and cirrhosis, are primarily composed of a polymer of bilirubinate (although calcium bilirubinate is present). The association of calcium bilirubinate stones with infection has been attributed to the activity of a bacterial enzyme, beta-glucuronidase, which deconjugates bilirubin, allowing it to form an insoluble complex with calcium. Sludge in the gallbladder is predominantly calcium bilirubinate, and an increased incidence of sludge and pigment gallstones has been found in patients on long-term parenteral hyperalimentation. There is an increased incidence of predominantly cholesterol gallstones associated with obesity, estrogens, pregnancy, and truncal vagotomy.

Answer: D, E

8. A healthy 30-year-old woman has asymptomatic gallstones. Recommended treatment is:

A. Observation
B. Cholecystectomy
C. Chenodeoxycholic acid
D. Ursodeoxycholic acid

Sabiston: 1151

Comments: The appropriate management of asymptomatic cholelithiasis has been controversial. First of all, one must determine whether the patient is in fact asymptomatic, since gastrointestinal complaints other than pain may be attributable to biliary tract disease. It was formerly thought that most patients with silent gallstones would eventually develop symptoms and that the risk of subsequent complications was high. More recent studies suggest that many patients will not develop symptoms and that serious complications are relatively infrequent. The morbidity, mortality, and cost of cholecystectomy in these patients may exceed that of expectant therapy. Currently, then, the incidental finding of asymptomatic gallstones does not mandate cholecystectomy. However, cholecystectomy should be considered even in the absence of symptoms in patients who are diabetic, immunosuppressed, or on long-term parenteral hyperalimentation. It has also been suggested that patients with nonvisualization of the gallbladder on oral cholecystography, those with stones larger than 2.5 cm, or with calcification of the gallbladder are at increased risk of complications and should also be considered for early cholecystectomy. Medical dissolution of gallstones is not appropriate for most patients.

Answer: A

9. Treatment of gallstones using chenodeoxycholic acid:

A. Produces complete dissolution of stones in one third of patients
B. Reduces symptoms of cholelithiasis even without complete dissolution
C. Works by inhibiting cholesterol synthesis
D. Reduces complications of cholelithiasis
E. Decreases recurrence of stones following cessation of therapy

Sabiston: 1151
Schwartz: 1321

Comments: Oral administration of the primary bile acid chenodeoxycholic acid expands the bile acid pool and inhibits cholesterol synthesis by reducing the activity of the enzyme HMG-CoA reductase. However, this therapy has not proved particularly effective in dissolving gallstones. The National Cooperative Gallstone Study (1981), which included over 900 patients, demonstrated that in only 14% were gallstones completely dissolved even when high doses of chenodeoxycholic acid were used; approximately 25% of patients had partial dissolution. Medical dissolution has not been shown to reduce symptoms or prevent complications of cholelithiasis, and even if dissolution is complete, recurrence occurs following cessation of therapy. The most common side effect is diarrhea; hepatotoxicity and elevation of serum cholesterol and low-density lipoproteins may also occur. Ursodeoxycholic acid is an epimer of chenodeoxycholic acid derived from the Japanese white-collared bear. It has fewer side effects, but has not been shown to be significantly more effective.

Answer: C

10. In which of the following situations would medical dissolution of gallstones most likely be successful?

A. Elderly, obese female
B. Young, thin female
C. Small, radio-opaque stones
D. Heriditary spherocytosis
E. Hepatic cirrhosis

Sabiston: 1151
Schwartz: 1321

Comments: The clinical application of chenodeoxycholic acid for treatment of gallstones would seem to be limited to patients with concomitant disease precluding operation. Results of dissolution therapy have been better in patients who were nonobese females and who had eleva-

tions of serum cholesterol. Bile acid therapy is not appropriate for treatment of radio-opaque stones or pigment stones.

Answer: B

11. A 40-year-old woman complains of recurrent postprandial attacks of colicky right upper quadrant pain. Ultrasonography does not demonstrate gallstones. She presently is pain-free. The next diagnostic test should be:

A. Oral cholecystography
B. Tc-99m iminodiacetic acid scan
C. CT scan of the gallbladder
D. Endoscopic retrograde cholangiopancreatography (ERCP)
E. Percutaneous transhepatic cholangiography (PTC)

Sabiston: 1150
Schwartz: 1316

Comments: In the patient with chronic cholecystitis, ultrasonography is approximately 95% accurate for the detection of gallstones and, for the most part, has replaced oral cholecystography as the initial method of diagnosis. Oral cholecystography is still useful, however, in the evaluation of patients with typical symptoms of chronic cholecystitis who have an equivocal or negative ultrasound. Radioisotope scanning with derivatives of technetium-99m iminodiacetic acid is most useful in the diagnosis of acute cholecystitis. CT scan can demonstrate gallstones, but is not appropriate for initial screening of patients with suspected calculous disease. Direct visualization of the bile ducts by PTC or ERCP is important in the evaluation of common duct obstruction; these tests have replaced intravenous cholangiography.

Answer: A

12. Which of the following is most accurate in the diagnosis of acute cholecystitis?

A. Plain abdominal x-ray
B. Ultrasonography
C. Oral cholecystography
D. Tc-99m iminodiacetic acid scan
E. Physical exam

Sabiston: 1139
Schwartz: 1326

Comments: Radionuclide scanning with technetium-99m iminodiacetic acid agents normally visualizes the liver, gallbladder, and extrahepatic biliary tree. In acute cholecystitis, the gallbladder fails to visualize because of cystic duct obstruction; this finding is approximately 98% reliable for the detection of acute cholecystitis. Ultrasonography may demonstrate gallstones, pericholecystic fluid, and thickening of the gallbladder, but is not as accurate in the diagnosis of acute cholecystitis as is isotope scanning. Oral cholecystography is not as accurate because of the frequency of false positive studies. Plain abdominal x-rays can reveal up to 15% of gallstones and demonstrate emphysematous cholecystitis but otherwise play no specific role in the diagnosis of acute cholecystitis. Physical examination may suggest the diagnosis, but again does not always discriminate other inflammatory upper abdominal conditions.

Answer: D

13. Which of the following may not differentiate acute cholecystitis from coronary artery disease?

A. Electrocardiography
B. Response to nitroglycerin
C. Coronary angiography
D. Tc-99m iminodiacetic acid scan

Sabiston: 1139
Schwartz: 1326

Comments: The differential diagnosis of acute cholecystitis includes other intra-abdominal conditions, such as perforated peptic ulcer, pancreatitis, appendicitis, and hepatitis, as well as extra-abdominal conditions such as myocardial ischemia and pleurisy. Oftentimes, these can be differentiated on the basis of a careful history and physical examination. Atypical or unclear cases, however, will require additional investigation. A chest x-ray and electrocardiogram are important for the evaluation of cardiopulmonary disease; however, electrocardiographic changes may be observed with acute cholecystitis, and nitroglycerin may ameliorate the pain of both biliary colic and myocardial ischemia.

Answer: A, B

14. Choose the most appropriate initial test for the evaluation of obstructive jaundice.

A. Tc-99m iminodiacetic acid scan
B. Ultrasonography
C. CT scan
D. Percutaneous transhepatic cholangiography (PTC)
E. Endoscopic retrograde cholangiopancreatography (ERCP)

Sabiston: 1132
Schwartz: 1058

Comments: All of the above imaging modalities may be useful in the evaluation of a patient with obstructive jaundice. Overall, ultrasonography is the most cost-effective initial examination; it permits confirmation of ductal dilatation and suggests the level of obstruction as well as providing information about the liver, pancreas, and presence or absence of calculous disease. PTC is the best method of visualizing the proximal extent of obstruction and of assessing the suitability of the proximal hepatic ducts for anastomosis. ERCP is particularly useful in cases of distal biliary tract obstruction and allows evaluation of the ampullary region. Both PTC and ERCP allow cytologic or histologic sampling, and both can be used for placement of catheters to decompress the obstructed biliary tract. Computerized tomography best delineates the anatomy of mass lesions in the hepatobiliary pancreatic region and assists in the preoperative assessment of resectability. Although technetium-99m iminodiacetic acid scan can demonstrate ductal obstruction, it does not provide sufficient anatomic definition to determine etiology or make therapeutic decisions.

Answer: B

15. Choose the most common cause of hydrops of the gallbladder:

A. Papillary mucinous adenocarcinoma
B. *Clonorchis sinensis*
C. Cholelithiasis
D. Choledocholithiasis
E. *Salmonella*

Sabiston: 1153
Schwartz: 1322

Comments: Hydrops of the gallbladder results when there is complete obstruction of the cystic duct, usually by a stone. The gallbladder remains distended with bile that gradually becomes clear and mucinous as the bile pigment is reabsorbed. At the time of cholecystectomy, preliminary decompression of the tense gallbladder facilitates a safe dissection.

Answer: C

16. In which situation will bile cultures least often yield bacteria?

A. Acute cholecystitis
B. Chronic cholecystitis
C. Choledocholithiasis
D. Bile duct stricture
E. Bile duct malignancy

Sabiston: 1151

Comments: The recognition of clinical situations in which bacteria are likely to be present in bile is important because the presence of bacteria in the bile correlates with the risk of postoperative infectious complications. Prophylactic antibiotics have decreased the infectious morbidity in patients over 50 years old and in those with jaundice, acute cholecystitis, or choledocholithiasis and cholangitis. Bile cultures are positive in approximately 5 to 40% of patients with chronic cholecystitis, 55% with acute cholecystitis, 60 to 80% with choledocholithiasis, and nearly all patients with bile duct stricture. Interestingly, bacteria are not usually cultured from the bile of patients with biliary tract malignancy if the bile ducts have not been manipulated. Nonetheless, prophylactic antibiotics are still usually given to these patients because of their age and the more complex nature of the biliary tract procedure being performed.

Answer: E

17. Choose the type of organism most commonly isolated from bile.

A. *Escherichia coli*
B. *Clostridium* species
C. *Bacteroides fragilis*
D. *Klebsiella* species
E. *Enterococcus* species

Sabiston: 1151
Schwartz: 1326

Comments: All of the above organisms are found in the biliary tract, but gram-negative enteric organisms with *E. coli* predominating are found most frequently. Other gram-negative bacteria that are commonly cultured include *Klebsiella*, *Proteus*, and *Enterobacter*. Gram-positive organisms, especially *Streptococcus faecalis*, are also frequently observed. Anaerobes are being recognized more frequently—most commonly *Bacteroides fragilis*, followed by *Clostridium* species. Polymicrobial infection is common. Effective prophylactic or therapeutic antibiotic therapy must be effective against the anticipated organisms. For prophylaxis, cephalosporins are usually favored. Serious biliary sepsis is usually treated with a combination of an aminoglycoside and antibiotics effective against anaerobes and enterococci.

Answer: A

18. Acute emphysematous cholecystitis is associated with:

A. Diabetes mellitus
B. Female patients
C. Acalculous gallbladder
D. Gangrene of the gallbladder

Sabiston: 1145
Schwartz: 1327

Comments: Acute emphysematous cholecystitis is a rare form of acute cholecystitis, manifested by air in the wall and lumen of the gallbladder and by a serious clinical course. It often is associated with diabetes and occurs most commonly in men, unlike nonemphysematous cholecystitis, which is more prevalent in women. Up to one half of cases are not associated with cholelithiasis. There is a high incidence of gangrene and prompt cholecystectomy is indicated. The usual offending gas-forming organisms are *E. coli*, *Klebsiella*, and *Clostridium perfringens*.

Answer: A, C, D

19. A young black woman is found at the time of cholecystectomy to have a firm, yellow nodule in the wall of the gallbladder. The likely diagnosis is:

A. Cholesterolosis
B. Carcinoid tumor
C. Adenocarcinoma
D. Granular cell myoblastoma

Sabiston: 1146

Comments: Granular cell myoblastomas are neuroectodermally derived benign tumors that tend to occur in the biliary tract of young black women. No treatment beyond excision is required. It is important always to examine the gallbladder carefully in the operating room at the time of cholecystectomy. Occasionally, an incidental malignancy may be detected and the patient may benefit from extension of the operative procedure.

Answer: D

20. Which of the following are absolute indications for common bile duct exploration without preliminary cholangiography?

A. Pancreatitis
B. Toxic cholangitis
C. Bilirubinate stones in the gallbladder

D. Multiple small stones in the gallbladder
E. Dilated common duct

Sabiston: 1133
Schwartz: 1322

Comments: Absolute indications for common bile duct exploration at the time of cholecystectomy include palpable or cholangiographic evidence of a stone in the duct and the presence of ascending cholangitis, classically manifested by jaundice, fever, and right upper abdominal pain. Even in this situation cholangiography may be useful in defining distal anatomy prior to exploration. Other findings that counsel the need for common duct exploration include a dilated common bile duct, elevated liver enzymes, pancreatitis, multiple small stones in the gallbladder, a single faceted stone in the gallbladder, an empty gallbladder with symptoms of biliary tract disease, and an enlarged cystic duct. In the presence of these relative indications, intraoperative cholangiography should be performed in order to determine whether common duct exploration is necessary. Cholangiomanometry and flow studies (debimetry) have also been useful in the detection of common duct pathology, but their use has not gained widespread acceptance.

Answer: B

21. Which of the following statements is/are true regarding choledocholithiasis?

A. Common duct stones are present in one third of patients undergoing cholecystectomy
B. The incidence of common duct stones is higher in older patients
C. Most common duct stones are composed of calcium bilirubinate
D. Common duct stones are more frequently found when cholecystectomy is performed for chronic cholecystitis than for acute cholecystitis

Sabiston: 1132, 1143
Schwartz: 1322

Comments: Common duct stones are present in 8 to 18% of patients with cholecystolithiasis, and their proper recognition is important because of the associated risk of biliary tract obstruction and cholangitis as well as the increased morbidity and mortality of common duct exploration. The incidence of choledocholithiasis increases with each decade over the age of 60. Most common duct calculi are thought to originate in the gallbladder and are, therefore, of the cholesterol variety. Friable "earthy" stones however, are composed of calcium bilirubinate thought to arise de novo in the common duct in association with biliary tract infection. Choledocholithiasis occurs as often in the setting of acute cholecystitis as it does with chronic cholecystitis, so thorough evaluation of the common duct is always mandatory.

Answer: B

22. Which of the following treatments is most appropriate for an elderly patient with multiple common duct stones and a dilated common duct 3 years following cholecystectomy?

A. Endoscopic sphincterotomy
B. Transhepatic infusion of mono-octanoin
C. Common duct exploration and placement of T-tube
D. Common duct exploration and sphincteroplasty
E. Common duct exploration and choledochoduodenostomy

Sabiston: 1133
Schwartz: 1323

Comments: By definition, common duct stones occurring more than 2 years after cholecystectomy are considered primary common duct stones. Usually these are associated with biliary tract infection and stasis. All of the listed choices of treatment may be appropriate for the treatment of common duct stones, depending upon the clinical setting. In order to achieve the most definitive treatment for the patient described, however, and to prevent recurrence, most surgeons would advocate operative duct exploration and choledochoduodenostomy. A Roux-en-Y choledochojejunostomy might also be successful, although the technical ease of performing choledochoduodenostomy makes it attractive. Sphincteroplasty is a more involved operation, but might be necessary if the patient has an impacted distal stone and a small nondilated duct. Endoscopic sphincterotomy and stone extraction can be successful if the patient is deemed unfit for operative intervention, but carries a mortality of approximately 1% and may not be as successful in the case of multiple stones. Mono-octanoin and other agents can dissolve cholesterol stones; primary common duct stones, however, are usually of the calcium bilirubinate variety.

Answer: E

23. Which of the following may contraindicate endoscopic treatment of retained common bile duct stones?

A. Multiple stones
B. Stones larger than 2 cm
C. Bile duct stricture
D. Duodenal diverticulum
E. Pancreatitis

Sabiston: 1134

Comments: Retained common bile duct stones are no longer as common or hazardous to manage as they once were. Intraoperative cholangiography and choledochoscopy have decreased the incidence of retained common duct stones. Small retained stones probably pass spontaneously in most instances and are of no clinical consequence. Persistent retained stones can be successfully removed in the radiology suite via a percutaneous T-tube tract or by endoscopic routes. Occasionally, dissolution of retained stones is possible. Although endoscopic approaches to biliary tract disease are becoming increasingly successful in a variety of circumstances, all of the above criteria have been considered relative contraindications to endoscopic sphincterotomy and removal of retained common duct stones.

Answer: A, B, C, D, E

24. The preferred management of the most common type of choledochal cyst is by:

A. Complete excision
B. Cyst duodenostomy
C. Cyst jejunostomy
D. External drainage
E. Endoscopic sphincterotomy

Sabiston: 1131
Schwartz: 1310

Comments: Cystic disease of the biliary tract may involve the intrahepatic or extrahepatic ducts, or both. The most common pattern of involvement is a dilatation of the extrahepatic bile duct with or without associated intrahepatic involvement. These lesions frequently produce jaundice or biliary obstruction. Furthermore, their association with biliary tract malignancy and with anomalous relationships between the pancreatic duct and bile duct are well recognized. For these reasons, complete cyst excision with Roux-en-Y hepaticojejunostomy is the preferred treatment. Internal drainage procedures are followed by a high rate of recurrent jaundice, cholangitis, and stricture. In some instances, because of the intrahepatic or retroduodenal extent of disease, or because of technical considerations, complete excision may not be feasible and the surgeon may have to settle for partial excision. Endoscopic sphincterotomy may occasionally be appropriate for the rare choledochocele if it is not associated with duodenal obstruction.

Answer: A

25. An elderly man who has previously undergone cholecystectomy presents to the emergency room with jaundice, fever, and right upper quadrant abdominal pain. Initial treatment should be:

A. Antibiotics
B. Percutaneous transhepatic drainage
C. Endoscopic sphincterotomy
D. T-tube decompression of the common bile duct
E. Choledochoduodenostomy

Sabiston: 1154
Schwartz: 1329

Comments: Charcot's triad, consisting of fever, jaundice, and upper abdominal pain, is the clinical hallmark of acute cholangitis. Cholangitis may be of varying severity. Initial treatment consists of fluid resuscitation and antibiotics to cover gram-negative organisms, anaerobes, and enterococci. In mild to moderate cases, a second- or third-generation cephalosporin may be adequate. In severe cholangitis, a combination of aminoglycoside with either clindamycin or metronidazole and high-dose ampicillin or penicillin is appropriate. If the patient improves with these measures, cholangiographic assessment of the biliary tract is carried out in order to plan definitive therapy. Most cases of acute cholangitis are caused by calculous disease, although benign strictures and malignancies must be excluded. If the patient does not respond to initial nonoperative therapy, prompt decompression of the biliary tract must be carried out. In most cases, this has consisted of common duct exploration and T-tube drainage, although both percutaneous transhepatic decompression and endoscopic decompression have been successful. Such therapy should be considered in situations in which it is preferable that an operation be avoided and the expertise and facilities for it are available. When the common bile duct is dilated (greater than 1.5 cm), choledochoduodenostomy at the time of bile duct exploration has been as successful as T-tube decompression alone.

Answer: A

26. A nondilated common bile duct is cleanly transected at the time of cholecystectomy. Preferred management at this time is:

A. Primary duct-to-duct anastomosis with a stent
B. Primary duct-to-duct anastomosis without a stent
C. Roux-en-Y choledochojejunostomy
D. Choledochoduodenostomy
E. Duct ligation, transhepatic drainage, and delayed repair

Schwartz: 1320, 1334

Comments: Benign bile duct strictures usually result from injury at the time of cholecystectomy. Most of these injuries are of the crushing type and are not recognized initially but discovered later when the patient develops a bile fistula, cholangitis, or jaundice. If the injury is recognized at the time of operation and consists of a clean transection (rather than a crushing injury of the duct or a segmental loss of duct), the preferred treatment is a primary duct-to-duct anastomosis over a T-tube stent. The principle of repair of bile duct injuries is to achieve mucosal approximation without tension. If the nature of the injury precludes this, anastomosis to a Roux limb of jejunum or to the duodenum may be appropriate.

Answer: A

27. In most cases delayed repair of bile duct stricture secondary to operative trauma involves:

A. Duct-to-duct anastomosis with a stent
B. Duodenal anastomosis without a stent
C. Duodenal anastomosis with stent
D. Roux-en-y jejunal anastomosis without stent
E. Roux-en-y jejunal anastomosis with stent

Sabiston: 1134
Schwartz: 1320

Comments: The best method of biliary reconstruction for a benign bile duct stricture depends upon the location of the stricture. Pancreatitis may produce distal strictures that can be adequately treated by choledochoduodenostomy. However, most strictures secondary to operative trauma are located in the proximal extrahepatic bile ducts. Principles of a tension-free, mucosa-to-mucosa anastomosis cannot be satisfied by direct ductal repair or by hepaticoduodenostomy. Most of these cases, therefore, will require a jejunal anastomosis, which is usually performed to a Roux limb and which has the additional theoretical advantage of minimizing the subsequent risk of enterobiliary reflux and cholangitis. In order to avoid devascularization, the proximal duct should not be dissected extensively. The anastomosis should be stented,

although there are no conclusive data as to how long the stent should be left in place; periods ranging from 3 to 12 months are often recommended. In experienced hands, successful outcome following repair of benign bile duct strictures can be expected in 85% of cases.

Answer: E

28. True statements regarding nonoperative injury of the gallbladder include:

A. The most common injury is avulsion from the liver bed secondary to blunt trauma
B. An isolated laceration of the gallbladder is best treated by suture and drainage
C. Intraperitoneal leak of sterile bile is usually well tolerated
D. The main prognostic consideration is the degree and duration of intraperitoneal bile leak

Schwartz: 1318

Comments: The gallbladder may be injured as a result of either blunt or penetrating trauma, but penetrating injury is by far the most common. Most injuries of the gallbladder and extrahepatic biliary tree are associated with involvement of other organs, such as the liver, small bowel, and colon. Penetrating injuries, however, may produce isolated injury of the gallbladder; the treatment in such instances usually is cholecystectomy. The consequences of intraoperative bile leak are largely dependent upon whether the bile is infected or not. Sterile bile may produce a chemical peritonitis that is relatively innocuous, but leakage of infected bile may be lethal. In general, the prognosis following nonoperative injury of the biliary tract is related to the significance of associated injuries.

Answer: C

29. The most common type of biliary enteric fistula is:

A. Cholecystocolic
B. Cholecystoduodenal
C. Choledochoduodenal
D. Choledochogastric

Sabiston: 1161
Schwartz: 1323

Comments: The most common cause of spontaneous biliary enteric fistula is calculous disease, although peptic ulcer disease and malignancy are sometimes responsible. Although fistulas can occur between various sites of the biliary tract and the alimentary tract, by far the most common is the cholecystoduodenal fistula.

Answer: B

30. Regarding the initial surgical management of gallstone ileus:

A. The stones should be removed by enterotomy at the site of impaction, if possible
B. Stone removal usually requires small bowel resection
C. Concomitant cholecystectomy and fistula repair are contraindicated

D. Cholecystostomy is the preferred initial treatment of the biliary tract
E. If cholecystectomy is not initially performed, interval removal is recommended, even in asymptomatic patients.

Sabiston: 1164
Schwartz: 1325

Comments: Gallstone ileus should be suspected in a patient with small bowel obstruction and a previous history suggestive of biliary tract disease, or the findings of air in the biliary tree, or an opaque stone on x-ray; most cases, however, are not diagnosed preoperatively. The most common site of obstruction is the terminal ileum. The stone should be removed by enterotomy proximal to the site of obstruction or milking of the stone retrogradely to the enterostomy. Concomitant cholecystectomy and fistula repair should be carried out if the patient is stable. These patients are usually elderly, however, and oftentimes have coexisting cardiac disease or diabetes. If the patient's condition is unstable, definitive biliary tract surgery should be delayed but interval operation is usually recommended, because of the risk of recurrent biliary tract infection or gallstones ileus.

Answer: E

31. Sclerosing cholangitis has been associated with:

A. Ulcerative colitis
B. Crohn's disease
C. Retroperitoneal fibrosis
D. Peyronie's disease

Sabiston: 1136
Schwartz: 1331

Comments: Sclerosing cholangitis is a disease of unknown etiology that produces progressive bile duct stenosis leading to biliary cirrhosis, portal hypertension, and hepatic failure. Immunologic, infectious, and toxic etiologies have been considered, and the disease has been associated with a number of conditions, particularly ulcerative colitis. Males are affected more commonly than females, and most patients present in their 30's or 40's with jaundice, pruritus, or cholangitis.

Answer: A, B, C, D

32. Which of the following is/are true regarding sclerosing cholangitis?

A. Definitive diagnosis depends upon demonstration of granulomatous lesions from bile duct biopsy
B. It characteristically involves only the extrahepatic bile ducts
C. Cholelithiasis usually is not associated
D. There is an increased incidence of biliary tract malignancy

Sabiston: 1136
Schwartz: 1331

Comments: The diagnosis of sclerosing cholangitis depends upon the clinical findings and typical cholangiographic appearance of narrow, beaded ducts. There are no specific histologic findings and, in fact, the differentiation from sclerosing carcinoma of the biliary tract can be difficult. Cholelithiasis and choledocholithiasis are not usually associated with sclerosing cholangitis, and it has been recommended that cholecystectomy not be performed in the absence of stones if operative intervention is required for sclerosing cholangitis.

Answer: C, D

33. Which of the following treatments have been shown to halt the progression of sclerosing cholangitis in patients with ulcerative colitis?

A. Corticosteroids
B. Antibiotics
C. Azothioprine
D. Colectomy
E. None of the above

Sabiston: 1136
Schwartz: 1331

Comments: All known treatments for sclerosing cholangitis, both medical and surgical, are palliative. The disease usually pursues a progressive course. The goal of treatment is to provide adequate biliary drainage and prevent cholangitis. Pharmacologic methods of inhibiting or reversing the sclerotic process or of improving bile flow have not altered the overall outcome. Surgical decompression in the form of biliary enteric anastomoses and transhepatic catheters may produce temporary improvement, but the inexorable course is one of recurrent cholangitis and obstruction.

Answer: E

34. An adenocarcinoma of the gallbladder invading the muscularis is discovered incidentally following cholecystectomy. Treatment should include:

A. Radiotherapy
B. Chemotherapy
C. Right hepatic lobectomy
D. Wedge resection of the liver
E. Regional lymphadenectomy

Sabiston: 1168
Schwartz: 1333

Comments: Although cancer of the gallbladder has a dismal prognosis, a small percentage of patients may be salvaged with appropriate initial surgical treatment. Based upon knowledge of the venous and lymphatic drainage of the gallbladder, this should include wedge resection of the gallbladder bed and removal of lymph nodes along the hepatoduodenal ligament. Gallbladder cancer confined to the mucosa is adequately treated by cholecystectomy alone. There is no conclusive evidence that either radiotherapy or chemotherapy is of benefit in cancer of the gallbladder or bile ducts, although effective palliation has been demonstrated with radiotherapy and adjuvant radiotherapy has been reported to improve survival. One should always be alert to the possible presence of cancer when operating for presumed calculus disease, and the gallbladder should always be examined after removal for the presence of coincidental neoplasm. Reports describe gallbladder cancer in 1 to 2% of biliary tract operations performed for calculous disease and in as many as 15% of those patients who are over the age of 70.

Answer: D, E

35. Which of the following is/are true regarding cancer of the extrahepatic bile ducts?

A. The natural history of rapid local growth and metastatic spread limits the benefit of palliative therapies
B. Proximal lesions, although less often resectable than distal lesions, have a more favorable prognosis
C. Survival following pancreatoduodenectomy for distal lesions exceeds that of pancreatic carcinoma
D. Effective decompression can be achieved by endoscopic or percutaneous catheters

Sabiston: 1135
Schwartz: 1333

Comments: The natural history of adenocarcinoma of the extrahepatic bile ducts is one of slow local growth; deaths generally occur as the result of hepatic failure and sepsis from biliary obstruction. These tumors are usually beyond the confines of surgical resection at the time of diagnosis and are, therefore, rarely curable. Significant palliation, however, can often be achieved by therapy directed at the relief of biliary obstruction. Prognosis is related to tumor location, resectability, and histologic pattern. Lesions occurring proximal to the cystic duct junction near the hepatic bifurcation are the most common but are also least often resectable and therefore have a less favorable prognosis. Distal lesions resectable by pancreatoduodenectomy have the best prognosis, with 5-year survival of approximately 30%. In some centers, aggressive resection of proximal lesions, usually including hepatic resection, has produced improved survival with morbidity not exceeding that of nonoperative treatment; there is, however, a distinct lack of data from any randomized prospective controlled clinical trials. Palliative decompression can be achieved by techniques of surgical anastomosis, surgical intubation, or endoscopic or percutaneous catheter placement. The most appropriate method of palliative decompression for a particular patient will depend upon tumor location and extent, the patient's underlying condition, the local expertise available, and the anticipated complications of each technique.

Answer: C, D

36. Which of the following are true regarding cholangiohepatitis?

A. Most commonly occurs in elderly Chinese
B. Usually presents with chronic weight loss and anemia
C. Etiologic factors include both pyogenic and parasitic infection and hemolysis
D. Surgical drainage effectively prevents recurrence

Schwartz: 1329

Comments: Cholangiohepatitis is a serious infectious process of the bile ducts, which is difficult to eradicate and frequently culminates in death from sepsis or end-stage hepatic failure. The disease is endemic in China, where it most frequently affects patients in their 30's and 40's. A number of etiologic factors have been implicated in initiating the inflammatory changes. Therapy includes antibiotics and biliary decompression, predominantly by means of intestinal anastomosis. In patients in whom the infection is localized to one side of the liver, partial hepatectomy may be successful.

Answer: C

37. Postcholecystectomy syndrome:

A. Refers specifically to symptoms caused by a long cystic duct remnant
B. Is a synonym for biliary dyskinesia
C. Is a nonspecific term incorporating both biliary and extrabiliary pathology
D. Usually is caused by retained or recurrent common duct stones
E. Can be successfully treated by sphincteroplasty in most cases

Schwartz: 1328

Comments: Postcholecystectomy syndrome is a nonspecific term for persistent or recurrent symptoms that might be attributable to biliary tract disease in a patient who has previously undergone cholecystectomy. Obviously, this includes a wide range of pathologic states, both biliary and nonbiliary in origin. With current diagnostic techniques, most organic causes of the so-called postcholecystectomy syndrome can be diagnosed. Diagnosis of functional biliary tract disorders, known as biliary dyskinesia, remains difficult, however. Various tests have been used in an attempt to define these conditions and to select patients for operative therapy. In general, the results of provocative pharmacologic testing, with or without dynamic imaging studies, have not been consistent. Increasing experience with endoscopic manometric evaluation of the biliary tract may make some of these functional disorders more accessible.

Answer: C

38. Advantages of cholecystostomy in acute biliary tract disease include:

A. It can be performed using local anesthesia
B. It allows stabilization of critically ill patients
C. It does not require removal of impacted gallbladder stones
D. It usually constitutes adequate definitive treatment

Sabiston: 1143
Schwartz: 1335

Comments: In patients with biliary tract sepsis who are judged to be too ill to withstand a definite operation, or in whom the severity of the inflammatory process precludes safe cholecystectomy, cholecystostomy may be used as a temporizing procedure. It also can be performed as a planned procedure with the patient under local anesthesia. When cholecystotomy is performed, attempts should be made to remove stones from the gallbladder, since they might prevent effective drainage.

Cholecystostomy is not a definitive method of correcting biliary tract disease, and definitive operation should be carried out when patients are stable.

Answer: A, B

39. Match the following:

A. Cystic duct obstruction
B. Empyema
C. Requires immediate operation
D. Rokitansky-Aschoff sinuses
E. Tc-99m iminodiacetic acid scan specific diagnostic test

a. Acute cholecystitis
b. Chronic cholecystitis
c. Both
d. Neither

Sabiston: 1137, 1149
Schwartz: 1326

Comments: Cholecystitis is considered as acute or chronic, depending upon the clinical presentation. The pathophysiology of both implies cystic duct obstruction usually caused by gallstones. In acute cholecystitis, persistent obstruction of the cystic duct leads to a chemical and bacterial inflammation of the gallbladder wall itself and potential complications of empyema, gangrene, perforation, and fistula formation. Tc-99m iminodiacetic acid scan is considered a specific test for acute cholecystitis because of the low rate of false positive studies. Acute cholecystitis requires cholecystectomy but the timing of operation has been more controversial. Early cholecystectomy prevents complications and recurrent symptoms, and has been shown to be as safe in terms of morbidity and mortality as delayed operation when symptoms resolve. Proponents of delayed cholecystectomy have suggested that since most bouts of acute cholecystitis resolve and since operation may typically be more difficult in the face of an acute inflammatory process, that operation is more appropriately carried out later. Most surgeons favor early operation. In chronic cholecystitis, intermittent cystic duct obstruction produces biliary colic; the diagnosis is usually made on the basis of symptoms and an ultrasound demonstrating cholelithiasis. Chronic cholecystitis is treated by elective cholecystectomy. The histologic findings of mucosal crypts (Rokitansky-Aschoff sinuses) is a typical feature of chronic cholecystitis but is often found in association with acute cholecystitis as well, since many patients with acute cholecystitis have had prior symptoms.

Answer: A–c; B–a; C–d; D–c; E–a

CHAPTER **33**

Pancreas

1. Concerning the surgical anatomy of the pancreas, which of the following statements is/are true?

A. The uncinate process lies just ventral to the junction of the splenic and superior mesenteric veins
B. The duct of Santorini is ventral to the duct of Wirsung
C. The main pancreatic and common ducts rarely unite to form a common channel
D. The body and tail cross the aorta, left adrenal gland, and upper pole of the left kidney
E. The arterial supply is derived primarily from the splenic artery

Sabiston: 1170
Schwartz: 1345

Comments: The pancreas has relationships to the common bile duct, stomach, duodenum, spleen, left adrenal, and left kidney as well as to vascular structures. The arterial supply arises from a pancreaticoduodenal arcade (from the gastroduodenal artery and superior mesenteric artery), a dorsal pancreatic artery (variable origin), and the pancreatica magna artery (from the splenic artery). The main pancreatic duct (Wirsung) occupies a more central position in the parenchyma as the distance from the head of the gland increases; this is an important consideration during pancreaticojejunostomy. The minor pancreatic duct (Santorini) is more ventral and subject to injury on this surface of the gland. There are numerous variations in the anatomic relationship between the common bile duct and pancreatic duct. In 85% of cadavers examined by endoscopic retrograde cholangiopancreatography (ERCP), there was a common channel uniting the ducts. The uncinate process is dorsal to the superior mesenteric artery and vein.

Answer: B, D

2. Concerning *pancreas divisum*, which of the following is/are true?

A. It is an embryologic failure of rotation of the ventral pancreas
B. It may be associated with pancreatitis

C. It is a frequent cause of pancreatitis
D. The main ductal drainage is via the duct of Wirsung
E. It is best diagnosed by CT scan

Sabiston: 1172
Schwartz: 1345

Comments: In *pancreas divisum*, the major and minor ductal systems fail to fuse, so that the duct of Santorini drains the main portion of the pancreas into the minor papillae, whereas the duct of Wirsung drains only a portion of the caudal head and uncinate process. Approximately 10% of the population has *pancreas divisum*, and although pancreatitis may be associated with this, a causal relationship is not clear. *Pancreas divisum* itself produces no CT abnormalities; the diagnosis depends upon pancreatography. Injection of the ampulla fills a short duct of Wirsung, whereas injection of the minor papilla fills the long duct of Santorini.

Answer: B

3. Concerning annular pancreas, which of the following statements is/are true?

A. Invariably it presents in newborn infants
B. The anomalous ductal drainage frequently produces pancreatitis
C. Usually it presents with duodenal obstruction
D. It is best treated by resection of the annular portion
E. It is associated with an increased risk of adenocarcinoma

Sabiston: 1175
Schwartz: 1347

Comments: Incomplete migration of the ventral pancreatic anlagen produces the annular pancreas, which may present with duodenal obstruction or jaundice at any age. Often, the finding is incidental; pancreatitis is unusual. The recommended treatment is bypass, in the form of duodenojejunostomy. Resection of the annular tissue is contraindicated and carries a high morbidity.

Answer: C

4. Concerning heterotopic pancreas, which of the following statements is/are true?

A. It may be a submucosal lesion of stomach
B. Often it is associated with pancreatitis
C. It is associated with an increased risk of adenocarcinoma
D. It requires resection because of the risk of hemorrhage

Sabiston: 1175
Schwartz: 1347

Comments: Heterotopic pancreas is a submucosal nodule of normal pancreatic tissue usually found in the stomach or duodenum or in a Meckel's diverticulum. The lesions usually are not clinically significant, although bleeding may occur from mucosal erosion.

Answer: A

5. Which of the following is/are true regarding exocrine pancreatic physiology?

A. An increase in the rate of secretion of pancreatic juice results in a higher concentration of bicarbonate
B. Vagal stimulation results in water and bicarbonate secretion
C. Secretin is a strong stimulant of pancreatic enzyme secretion
D. Pancreatic digestive enzymes are all secreted as inactive precursors
E. Pancreatic polypetide and glucagon inhibit exocrine secretion

Sabiston: 1175
Schwartz: 1348

Comments: The exocrine pancreas secretes bicarbonate, water, and digestive enzymes. Ductal and centroacinar cells secrete a bicarbonate-rich juice by an active transport mechanism in response to secretin and vasoactive intestinal peptide. As secretory rates increase, bicarbonate concentration increases and chloride concentration decreases. Digestive enzymes are secreted from acinar cells in response to cholecystokinin-pancreozymin, gastrin, and vagal stimulation. Amylase and lipases are secreted in their active forms, whereas the proteolytic enzymes are activated in the duodenum. Pancreatic polypeptide, glucagon, and somatostatin inhibit exocrine secretion.

Answer: A, E

6. Pancreatic exocrine insufficiency may be associated with:

A. Fat malabsorption
B. Gastric hyposecretion
C. Impaired absorption of vitamin B_{12}
D. Peptic ulcer disease
E. Protein-losing enteropathy

Schwartz: 1349

Comments: The nutritional consequences of pancreatic exocrine insufficiency may be ameliorated by the oral ad-

ministration of exogenous pancreatic enzymes. Efficacy of exogenous supplements may be improved by concomitant use of H2 receptor antagonists or antacids by minimizing their acid degradation. Experimental pancreatic diversion causes gastric hypersecretion, which, with pancreatic buffer deficiency, may result in peptic ulceration.

Answer: A, C, D

7. Regarding endocrine function of the pancreas:

A. Alpha cells, the most common islet cell type, produce glucagon
B. The blood glucose level is the primary stimulant to insulin release from beta cells
C. Pancreatic endocrine function is completely independent of its exocrine function
D. Somatostatin released from delta cells stimulates the release of various intestinal hormones

Sabiston: 1177
Schwartz: 1349

Comments: The islets of Langerhans contain various cell types. Beta cells, which compose 75% of the islets, release insulin primarily in response to blood glucose levels. Glucagon, which is released from alpha cells, has a primary catabolic action opposing insulin. Delta cells are the source of gastrin, pancreatic polypeptide, and somatostatin; the latter inhibits hormone secretion and various biologic activities. Pancreatic endocrine hormones play a role in regulating exocrine function.

Answer: B

8. Regarding the etiology of acute pancreatitis:

A. Gallstone pancreatitis is caused by reflux of sterile bile into the pancreatic duct
B. Alcohol and hyperparathyroidism are the most common causes in the United States
C. Simple pancreatic ductal obstruction by various mechanisms is the basic cause
D. A vascular etiology has been suspected in pancreatitis following cardiopulmonary bypass
E. Hyperlipemia may be seen as both a cause and an effect of pancreatitis

Sabiston: 1178
Schwartz: 1350

Comments: Alcohol ingestion and biliary tract disease account for 80 to 90% of acute pancreatitis, although the mechanisms of each have not been fully elucidated. Neither the common channel theory proposed by Opie nor simple bile reflux adequately explains most cases associated with biliary disease. Alcohol stimulates pancreatic secretion, produces ductal obstruction by protein precipitation, and increases ampullary resistance; a direct toxic effect has also been postulated. Numerous other causes of acute pancreatitis include hypercalcemia, hyperlipidemia, drugs, toxins, infection, autoimmune disorders, and an idiopathic familial form. Hyperlipidemias may produce pancreatitis by conversion of triglycerides to toxic free fatty acids; patients with alcoholic pancreatitis may have secondary hyperlipemia due to inhibition of li-poprotein lipase.

Answer: D, E

9. Which of the following is/are pathognomonic of acute pancreatitis?

A. An alcoholic patient with fever, tachycardia, leukocytosis, and abdominal pain
B. Serum amylase level over 1,000 Somogyi units
C. Elevated serum lipase
D. Amylase creatinine clearance ratio greater than 5
E. An ultrasound or CT demonstrating fluid in the lesser sac
F. None of the above

Sabiston: 1180
Schwartz: 1351

Comments: Although serum amylase levels may be markedly elevated in acute pancreatitis, variable elevations are observed and elevations may result from pathologic processes other than pancreatitis. The amylase/creatinine clearance ratio has been considered to be of greater diagnostic accuracy but is certainly not pathognomonic. Hyperlipasemia has been recorded in patients without pancreatic disease. The overlap of clinical, biochemical, and radiologic findings may preclude differentiation from another intra-abdominal catastrophe by any means short of laparotomy.

Answer: F

10. In the management of acute gallstone pancreatitis:

A. Immediate cholecystostomy is indicated at the time of diagnosis
B. The mortality of biliary surgery correlates with the severity of the pancreatitis
C. The risk of recurrent pancreatitis is minimal following nonoperative treatment
D. Supportive initial management is indicated unless the patient's condition deteriorates
E. Endoscopic papillotomy is contraindicated

Sabiston: 1182
Schwartz: 1352

Comments: The timing of operation for acute gallstone pancreatitis is controversial. In general, supportive care is instituted and definitive biliary tract operation undertaken when the acute pancreatitis has subsided. Some have advised urgent cholecystectomy and common duct exploration in all patients with pancreatitis and known biliary tract disease, but this is not universally accepted. In critically ill patients with cholangitis, prompt surgical or endoscopic decompression of the biliary tract is mandatory. The mortality from biliary surgery correlates with the severity of the pancreatitis rather than with the timing of operation. Delayed definitive operation following resolution of acute biliary pancreatitis is associated with a significant risk of recurrence.

Answer: B, D

11. Unfavorable prognostic criteria in acute pancreatitis include:

A. A WBC greater than 16,000/μl
B. A serum calcium level of less than 8 mg/100 ml during the initial 48 hours
C. A serum amylase on admission of over 1,000 Somogyi units
D. A serum lipase level greater than twice normal
E. A familial etiology of the pancreatitis

Sabiston 1185
Schwartz: 1353

Comments: A retrospective review of a large number of cases of acute pancreatitis by Ranson delineated 11 parameters present at the time of admission or developing during the initial 48 hours of hospitalization that were of prognostic value. These criteria reflect the patient's underlying status, the severity of the intra-abdominal inflammatory process, and effects on distant organs such as the kidneys and lungs.

Answer: A, B

12. A 45-year-old alcoholic presents with abdominal pain, vomiting, and tachycardia. The serum amylase is 1,000. He is not jaundiced. The initial evaluation and treatment should include:

A. Nasogastric decompression
B. Abdominal films
C. Immediate laparotomy and peritoneal drainage
D. Ultrasonography
E. Closed peritoneal lavage

Sabiston: 1182

Comments: Initial evaluation requires abdominal films to rule out bowel obstruction. Volvulus of the small bowel presents in this manner, and a clue may be gleaned by the films. Ultrasound will include the biliary system and pancreas. The initial treatment of acute pancreatitis focuses on supportive measures such as fluid and electrolyte resuscitation and respiratory support as well as evaluation of potential etiology. Immediate laparotomy may be indicated diagnostically in order to exclude gangrenous cholecystitis, intestinal infarction, perforated ulcer, or some other intra-abdominal catastrophe. Early therapeutic laparotomy in severe pancreatitis has a higher morbidity and mortality than does medical management. Nasogastric decompression usually is instituted to relieve vomiting due to gastric dilatation and perhaps to decrease pancreatic stimulation, although randominized trials have not proved that it affects the course of alcoholic pancreatitis. Routine antibiotic administration is sometimes advocated but has not been demonstrated to decrease the incidence of subsequent septic complications.

Answer: A, B, D

13. The patient described in Question 12 experiences progressive clinical deterioration with renal and respiratory insufficiency and requires intubation. Appropriate management at this point might include:

A. Administration of pancreatic enzyme inhibitors

B. Pancreatic débridement and drainage
C. Percutaneous placement of catheters for peritoneal lavage
D. Total pancreatectomy
E. Antibiotics and continued respiratory support to forestall acute respiratory distress syndrome

Sabiston: 1182
Schwartz: 1352

Comments: Progressive deterioration despite optimum medical management is an indication for operation. Peritoneal lavage decreases the early mortality related to cardiovascular and respiratory complications, but it does not prevent late peripancreatic sepsis or improve overall survival. Débridement of necrotic tissue and wide drainage of the retroperitoneum is indicated for patients whose clinical condition is deteriorating or who do not respond promptly to peritoneal lavage. Inhibitors of pancreatic enzymes such as the trypsin inhibitor or aprotinin (Trasylol) or the administration of glucagon and atropine have not been effective.

Answer: B, C

14. Concerning intra-abdominal complications of acute pancreatitis:

A. Pancreatic abscess, the most common complication, usually manifests itself within the first week
B. Pseudocyst formation is more common with alcoholic pancreatitis than with biliary pancreatitis
C. Hemorrhage may occur from associated pseudoaneurysms
D. Splenic vein thrombosis may require splenectomy
E. Paracentesis of pancreatic ascites yields fluid with a high amylase and low albumin content

Schwartz: 1353

Comments: Intra-abdominal complications of acute pancreatitis include pseudocyst (most common), pancreatic abscess, hemorrhage, splenic or portal vein thrombosis, pancreatic fistula with ascites, and, less commonly, common duct or duodenal obstruction or perforation of adjacent viscera such as the colon or stomach. Pancreatic abscess, frequently a lethal complication, occurs in up to 9% of patients with acute pancreatitis, depending on the severity and etiology of the pancreatitis and the effectiveness of early treatment. The diagnosis is based primarily on the clinical course of a patient who fails to improve or whose condition improves and subsequently deteriorates; pancreatic abscess is usually manifested 2 to 3 weeks following an episode of acute pancreatitis. Splenic vein thrombosis may require splenectomy in patients who develop left-sided portal hypertension with bleeding esophageal varices or hypersplenism. Pancreatic ascitic fluid has a high amylase and albumin content.

Answer: B, C, D

15. The Marseilles classification of pancreatitis includes which of the following categories?

A. Acute
B. Recurrent acute
C. Subacute
D. Chronic relapsing
E. Chronic

Sabiston: 1177

Comments: The currently accepted but ineffective clinical classification of pancreatitis was established at the Marseilles symposium in 1963. Acute pancreatitis indicates a single episode in a previously normal gland. In acute relapsing pancreatitis, the gland is normal between attacks. Chronic relapsing pancreatitis has pain-free intervals but persistent damage. In chronic pancreatitis, there is constant pain and irreversible glandular injury. Other classifications have been suggested to replace the Marseilles classification.

Answer: A, B, D, E

16. Clinical manifestations of chronic alcoholic pancreatitis include:

A. Diabetes mellitus in the majority of patients
B. Steatorrhea and malabsorption
C. Hypoglycemic episodes due to alterations in the glucagon/insulin ratio
D. Hepatic cirrhosis and portal hypertension
E. Pain and weight loss

Sabiston: 1185
Schwartz: 1354

Comments: Abdominal pain, nausea, anorexia, and weight loss are hallmarks of chronic pancreatitis. Exocrine insufficiency is said to occur when pancreatic function has been reduced to 10% or less. Fifteen to 40% of patients will have an abnormal glucose tolerance test. Interestingly, hepatic cirrhosis and portal hypertension are unusual despite the alcoholic etiology.

Answer: B, E

17. Prior to operation for chronic alcoholic pancreatitis, the most helpful imaging modality is:

A. Plain abdominal roentgenogram
B. Ultrasonography
C. Arteriography
D. ERCP
E. CT scan

Sabiston: 1186
Schwartz: 1354

Comments: The presence or absence of pancreatic ductal dilatation and the site of obstruction are the major determinants for selecting appropriate surgical therapy. Plain abdominal x-rays may demonstrate pancreatic calcification. Ultrasonography should be used to exclude biliary tract disease and for the evaluation of a possible pseudocyst. A CT scan may demonstrate glandular enlargement or adenopathy suggestive of malignancy. Arteriography may demonstrate pseudoaneurysms and arteriographic findings may correlate with resectability in pancreatic malignancy.

Answer: D

18. Surgical treatment of chronic pancreatitis:

A. Is justified only after failure of an adequate trial of aprotinin
B. Is indicated primarily for pain relief
C. Is indicated only for patients with pancreatic ductal dilatation or pseudocyst
D. Effectively prevents progression of endocrine insufficiency
E. Reverses exocrine insufficiency

Sabiston: 1186

Comments: Persistent disabling pain is the main indication for operation in chronic pancreatitis; the mechanism of pain may include ductal obstruction, chronic inflammation, or perineural fibrosis. Operation involves correction of primary biliary disease when present, pancreatic ductal drainage if obstruction and dilatation are present, or resective procedures in the absence of ductal dilatation. Operation itself does not alter the natural history of the disease, and success in terms of pain relief tends to decline with longer follow-up. Prior to operation for chronic pancreatitis, the surgeon must consider ductal anatomy and current pancreatic function, the role of continued alcohol or drug use, the anticipated endocrine and exocrine consequences of surgical therapy, the patient's ability to manage endocrine insufficiency, and the chance of achieving adequate pain relief. Occasionally, operation is indicated because of a question of adenocarcinoma, which may occur in 10% of patients with chronic pancreatitis. There is no role in these patients for pancreatic enzyme inhibitors.

Answer: B

19. Regarding the results of surgical treatment of chronic pancreatitis, which of the following is/are true?

A. Splanchnicectomy is as effective for pain relief as are resective procedures
B. Long-term pain relief can be anticipated in most patients following sphincteroplasty
C. Pancreaticojejunostomy itself accelerates the development of endocrine insufficiency
D. Total pancreatectomy produces good long-term beneficial results but has a high immediate operative mortality
E. Diabetes is a major source of morbidity after resective procedures

Sabiston: 1187
Schwartz: 1355

Comments: Although results are variable, reflecting patient selection, pain relief at 5-year follow-up occurs in approximately 50% of patients treated by sphincteroplasty or distal pancreatic resection, with somewhat better results in patients treated by pancreaticoduodenectomy or pancreaticojejunostomy. Splanchnicectomy has a lower long-term success rate. Patients having 95% or total pancreatectomy have better pain relief but a high incidence of endocrine insufficiency, which directly contributes to a high late death rate.

Answer: E

20. Which of the following statements is/are true about pancreatic trauma?

A. It most often occurs with blunt abdominal injury
B. It is the most common cause of pancreatic pseudocyst
C. Hyperamylasemia is pathognomonic
D. Negative peritoneal tap effectively excludes significant pancreatic injury
E. Exclusion requires exploration of all central retroperitoneal hematomas

Sabiston: 1192
Schwartz: 1355

Comments: Most pancreatic injuries are the result of penetrating trauma, although the gland is vulnerable to blunt trauma because of its fixed position over the vertebral column. The presence of significant pancreatic injury following blunt trauma is not always immediately apparent. Hyperamylasemia in the serum or peritoneal fluid suggests the diagnosis, but a negative peritoneal tap does not exclude significant retroperitoneal injury. Retroperitoneal hematomas in the upper abdomen should be explored to exclude pancreatic ductal injury. Pancreatitis is the most common cause of pseudocyst, although about 25% occur as a result of trauma.

Answer: E

21. During surgical exploration for blunt abdominal injury, a patient is found to have a complete transection of the pancreas in the neck region overlying the mesenteric vessels. There are no associated injuries. Appropriate treatment might include:

A. Drainage alone
B. Distal pancreatectomy, oversewing of proximal duct
C. Roux-en-Y pancreaticojejunostomy to distal pancreas, oversewing of proximal duct
D. Roux-en-Y pancreaticojejunostomy to both proximal and distal segments
E. Pancreaticoduodenectomy with Roux-en-Y pancreaticojejunostomy to distal duct

Sabiston: 1193
Schwartz: 1356

Comments: Pancreatic contusions or lacerations without ductal disruption are managed by drainage alone. The pancreatic neck is a frequent site of pancreatic injury when it occurs with blunt trauma. Distal pancreatectomy with identification and closure of the proximal duct and drainage is safe, and resections involving up to 80% of an otherwise normal gland can be accomplished without subsequent endocrine insufficiency. Roux-en-Y pancreaticojejunostomy to the distal pancreas may be considered when the distal segment itself is not severely damaged, resection would likely produce diabetes, and there are no significant associated injuries. Anastomoses to both proximal and distal segments have no particular advantage if the proximal duct is intact and add the morbidity of an additional pancreaticojejunostomy. Pancreaticoduodenectomy may occasionally be indicated in patients with combined duodenal, pancreatic, and bile duct injuries.

Answer: B, C

22. True cysts of the pancreas:

A. Are epithelial-lined structures
B. May be congenital or acquired
C. Usually grow rapidly
D. Are more common than pseudocysts
E. Require excision

Sabiston: 1188
Schwartz: 1358

Comments: True pancreatic cysts are rare, usually incidental lesions that require no specific therapy as long as their appearance does not suggest cystadenoma or cystadenocarcinoma. So-called retention cysts are pancreatic ductal dilations resulting from pancreatitis.

Answer: A, B

23. Most pancreatic pseudocysts are:

A. Epithelial-lined
B. Single and unilocular
C. Located in the head of the gland
D. Subject to a high rate of complications, usually within the first 3 weeks of acute pancreatitis
E. Best treated by resection

Sabiston: 1189

Comments: Pancreatic pseudocysts are most often unilocular and located in the lesser sac in the region of the body or tail. These are not true cysts, but are collections of pancreatic juice and necrotic tissue with a fibrous wall, usually resulting from pancreatitis or trauma; they are associated with ductal disruption. Serial evaluation with ultrasonography reveals that many fluid collections disappear with time. When a pseudocyst occurs in conjunction with acute pancreatitis, surgical treatment, which generally involves internal drainage, is delayed for about 6 weeks to allow formation of an adequate capsule essential for an anastomosis and to assure that the fluid collection will not resolve. Beyond 6 weeks, there is an increased incidence of infection, hemorrhage, and rupture. Occasionally, pseudocysts may cause duodenal or biliary tract obstruction.

Answer: B

24. Pancreatic cancer:

A. Usually arises from acinar cells
B. Occurs more frequently in diabetic patients
C. Is usually associated with lymph nodal metastases
D. Is usually associatedwith perineural invasion
E. Is often multicentric

Sabiston: 1194
Schwartz: 1360

Comments: Ninety percent of pancreatic malignancies are adenocarcinomas arising from the ductal cells. Lymph nodal metastases and perineural invasion are frequently present and hepatic metastases less so. About 30% of pancreatic adenocarcinomas may be multicentric. Cancer occurs twice as frequently in diabetic patients. Increased incidence with alcohol, coffee, or smoking has not been confirmed.

Answer: B, C, D, E

25. Regarding the clinical manifestations of pancreatic adenocarcinoma:

A. Lesions in the body of the pancreas usually first present with painless jaundice
B. Pain and weight loss are present in most patients
C. Malignancy often is heralded by the new onset of diabetes
D. Steatorrhea may be the first symptom of lesions involving the uncinate process
E. Migratory thrombophlebitis is a common finding

Sabiston: 1195
Schwartz: 1361

Comments: Dull, vague pain and weight loss are the most common presenting symptoms of pancreatic cancer, regardless of its location. Lesions of the pancreatic head may present earlier because of the development of painless jaundice and must be differentiated from lesions of the distal common bile duct, ampulla, or duodenum. Jaundice is a late finding in body or tail lesions, which often present with advanced local disease and back pain or with metastatic disease. Tumors of the uncinate process may obstruct the pancreatic duct prior to producing biliary obstruction and thus manifest themselves with steatorrhea. Migratory thrombophlebitis can occur, but is uncommon. Pruritus from subclinical jaundice can be another complaint of patients with pancreatic cancer. Cholangitis is rare.

Answer: B, D

26. Regarding the surgical treatment of pancreatic adenocarcinoma:

A. Only 10% of lesions are potentially resectable for cure
B. Resection of lesions of the body or tail yields a better cure rate than resection of lesions of the head
C. Total pancreatectomy has a better 5-year survival rate than does partial resection because of the multicentric nature of the disease
D. Portal vein or superior mesenteric vascular involvement generally indicates nonresectability

Sabiston: 1195
Schwartz: 1362

Comments: Survival in pancreatic adenocarcinoma is related to the site, size, and stage of the tumor. Metastatic cancer to the regional nodes or to the liver, or invasion of the portal vein, superior mesenteric vessels, or hepatic artery are frequent causes of nonresectability. Extensive resections involving critical vascular structures have been performed, but are not of proven benefit in the treatment of pancreatic adenocarcinoma. Total pancreatectomy has the advantage of one less anastomosis but has not produced greater survival than pancreaticoduodenectomy. In turn, it has a greater incidence of late complications related to endocrine insufficiency and bleeding postoperatively.

Answer: A, D

27. Regarding pancreaticoduodenectomy for pancreatic adenocarcinoma:

A. It is contraindicated without a histologic or cytologic diagnosis of malignancy
B. It is rarely associated with significant nutritional consequences
C. The pancreatic and biliary anastomoses should be proximal to the gastroenterostomy
D. It is associated with an operative mortality of 20%
E. Pancreatic fistula postoperatively is the most common fatal complication

Schwartz: 1362

Comments: It may be extremely difficult to differentiate between chronic pancreatitis and adenocarcinoma when dealing with a mass in the head of the gland. Cytologic diagnosis, based on intraoperative aspiration, has been useful in centers where this is available. However reluctantly, the surgeon must be prepared to carry out resection even in the absence of a confirmed diagnosis of malignancy, when the clinical setting is appropriate and the lesion is otherwise resectable. Pancreaticoduodenectomy today in major centers should have a mortality of 5% or less. Pancreatic and biliary anastomoses are performed proximal to the gastrojejunostomy to minimize the chance of marginal ulceration. Some advocate a vagotomy as well. Preservation of the stomach and pylorus may have nutritional benefit without compromising survival. Postoperative pancreatic fistulas usually close spontaneously.

Answer: C

28. A nonalcoholic 45-year-old woman presents with an asymptomatic, septated 10-cm cystic mass in the body of the pancreas. She should be advised that:

A. The lesion probably is benign and requires observation only
B. Drainage by Roux-en-Y jejunostomy is indicated
C. It is cancerous and she will likely die from it in 12 months
D. Complete excision of the lesion is indicated
E. Total pancreatectomy is the preferred surgical management

Sabiston: 1188

Comments: Cystadenoma and cystadenocarcinoma are cystic neoplasms of the pancreas that most commonly present as a mass lesion in middle-aged women. Cystadenoma is more common than the malignant variant, but malignant transformation may occur; short of operation, differentiating it from malignancy is difficult. Drainage or partial excision is inadequate. Complete excision should be carried out whenever possible; 5-year survival after resection of cystadenocarcinoma is approximately 50%.

Answer: D

29. Whipple's triad includes:

A. Fasting hypoglycemia (less than 50 mg/100 ml)
B. Symptoms of hypoglycemia
C. Jaundice
D. Hyperamylasemia
E. Symptoms of hypoglycemia relieved by glucose administration

Sabiston: 1197
Schwartz: 1366

Comments: Such a clinical setting establishes hypoglycemia. The differential diagnosis of the many causes of hypoglycemia will depend on complete history and laboratory evaluation.

Answer: A, B, E

30. In establishing a diagnosis of insulinoma:

A. Whipple's triad is pathognomonic
B. Blood sugar and serum insulin levels should be determined during a prolonged fasting test
C. An oral glucose tolerance test permits differentiation from reactive hypoglycemia
D. The tolbutamide test is useful in excluding factitious hyperinsulinemia
E. A CT scan is the most accurate preoperative method of tumor localization

Sabiston: 1198
Schwartz: 1366

Comments: The biochemical diagnosis of insulinoma is based on the findings of fasting hypoglycemia (less than 50 mg/dl) and hyperinsulinemia (greater than 20μU/ml), yielding an insulin/glucose ratio greater than 0.3. The use of tolbutamide or leucine as a provocative test to release insulin may be dangerous and is not required. C-peptide is cleaved from insulin prior to its release, and determination of C-peptide levels may be useful in excluding factitious hyperinsulinemia. Most insulinomas are small; arteriography or selective venous sampling may be useful in their preoperative location.

Answer: B, C

31. Regarding the treatment of insulinoma:

A. Diazoxide, which inhibits insulin release, is the preferred initial method of treatment
B. Simple enucleation is acceptable for localized pancreatic lesions
C. Since most lesions are multiple or diffuse, near total pancreatectomy is routinely indicated
D. Since most lesions are malignant, adjuvant streptozotocin is usually indicated
E. Parathyroid adenoma should be excluded or treated prior to pancreatic resection

Sabiston: 1198
Schwartz: 1367

Comments: Insulinomas are usually single and benign and are rarely ectopic. While localization of an insulinoma can be difficult, in addition to preoperative imaging, thorough mobilization and exploration of the pancreas is mandatory; intraoperative ultrasonagraphy has been reported as useful. For localized lesions, simple enucleation is the preferred method of treatment, but the pancreatic duct integrity must be ascertained. If the lesion cannot be identified and the biochemical basis of the diagnosis is firm, blind distal pancreatic resection with careful histologic examination of the specimen is generally advised. Diazoxide inhibits insulin release from beta cells and is occasionally used for preoperative control or

242 of 450 / Chapter 33

in patients with recurrent postoperative hypoglycemia. For patients with metastatic malignant insulinoma, tumor debulking may be beneficial as is the use of streptozotocin and 5-fluorouracil. Gastrinoma, not insulinoma, is the most common pancreatic adenoma associated with multiple endocrine adenomatosis, type I (MEA-1) syndrome. Parathyroid disease should be treated prior to surgical intervention for gastrinoma.

Answer: B

32. Appropriately match the items in the two columns.

A. Diarrhea	a. Zollinger-Ellison syndrome
B. Decreased gastric acid secretion	b. Verner-Morrison syndrome
C. Increased gastric acid secretion	c. Both
D. Hypercalcemia	d. Neither
E. Malignancy	

Sabiston: 1199
Schwartz: 1368

Comments: Both of these syndromes are produced by islet cell tumors, which, in the case of Zollinger-Ellison syndrome, secretes gastrin and, in the case of Verner-Morrison syndrome, vasoactive intestinal peptide. Zollinger-Ellison syndrome is associated with a marked increase in gastric acid secretion as well as with diarrhea; hypercalcemia may occur owing to associated parathyroid abnormalities. The Verner-Morrison syndrome is characterized by watery diarrhea, hypokalemia, and achlorhydria. Hypercalcemia may occur, but the parathyroids are usually normal. Both syndromes are frequently associated with malignant adenomas.

Answer: A–c; B–b; C–a; D–c; E–c

33. The clinical syndrome associated with glucagonomas includes:

A. A characteristic skin rash
B. Diabetes
C. Seizures
D. Hypoglycemia
E. Anemia

Sabiston: 1197
Schwartz: 1369

Comments: Glucagon-secreting tumors present with diabetes, anemia, weight loss, venous thrombosis, glossitis, and a characteristic cutaneous lesion known as necrolytic migratory erythema. The lesion is rare and often metastatic at the time of diagnosis.

Answer: A, B, E

CHAPTER 34

Spleen

1. Regarding the spleen, which of the following statements is/are true?

A. Accessory spleen(s) is/are present in 15 to 30% of people and may have a significant role in patients with hematologic disorders
B. Splenic pulp pressure reflects the pressure throughout the portal venous systems
C. In normal circumstances, the spleen has an important immunologic as well as a reticuloendothelial function
D. The spleen removes aged red and white blood cells and platelets from the blood of normal individuals

Sabiston: 1203
Schwartz: 1373

Comments: Although accessory spleens are present in up to 30% of individuals, they may be important only in patients with hematologic disorders. In decreasing order of frequency, their locations are the hilus of the spleen, the gastrosplenic, splenocolic, gastrocolic, and splenorenal ligaments, and the greater omentum. They may also occur in the pelvis of the female and the left peritesticular region in the male. • While a precise description of splenic circulation has yet to be developed, it is felt that splenic pulp pressure reflects the pressure throughout the portal venous system. • The spleen has an important function in immunologic function; its most important one from a surgical standpoint is the activity of the splenic reticuloendothelial system. • The spleen is the most important site of selective erythrocyte sequestration; alterations in the red blood cells make them sensitive to splenic destruction after 100 to 120 days in circulation. The spleen is also capable of removing nuclear remnants from circulating erythrocytes. It is not clear what role the spleen has in the destruction of neutrophils under normal conditions. Augmented destruction can occur secondary to splenic enlargement or in immune neutropenias. Normally one third of the total platelet pool is sequestered in the spleen; with splenomegaly, this may increase to as high as 80%. The role of the spleen in the

final removal of platelets is not defined. Following splenectomy, however, thrombocytosis frequently occurs.

Answer: A, B, C

2. Concerning the ruptured spleen, which of the following statements is/are true?

A. It is the organ most frequently injured as a result of blunt trauma to the abdomen or lower thorax
B. Spontaneous rupture is almost always associated with hematologic as opposed to infectious disease
C. Injury most commonly involves transverse tears through the parenchyma
D. Delayed rupture of the spleen following blunt trauma occurs within 2 weeks of injury in the majority of patients

Sabiston: 1208
Schwartz: 1376

Comments: The spleen is the most frequently injured organ with blunt trauma to the abdomen or lower thorax. In 70% of cases, there is associated injury to other organ systems, including, in decreasing order of frequency, the ribs, kidney, spinal cord, and liver. Malaria and infectious mononucleosis are the most common causes of spontaneous rupture, but it also can occur with sarcoidosis, leukemia, hemolytic anemia, and polycythemia vera. Most lacerations of the spleen are transverse because the internal architecture of the organ is arranged in a transverse plane; in some instances this is relevant to the ability to salvage or repair the spleen. Delayed rupture of the spleen occurs in 10 to 15% of cases of blunt splenic trauma. The length of delay, known as the "latent period of Baudet," is less than 2 weeks in 75% of these cases.

Answer: A, C, D

3. Which of the following statements is/are true regarding splenectomy for hemolytic anemias?

243

A. Splenectomy is the sole therapy for hereditary spherocytosis
B. Hereditary elliptocytosis becomes symptomatic and is treated by splenectomy when ovalocytes constitute 50 to 90% of the red cell population
C. Splenectomy may be worthwhile in severe cases of pyruvate kinase deficiency but is not indicated for patients with glucose-6-phosphate dehydrogenase (G6PD) deficiency
D. Splenectomy is the primary treatment for patients with idiopathic autoimmune hemolytic anemia

Sabiston: 1219
Schwartz: 1379

Comments: **Hereditary spherocytosis** is transmitted as an autosomal dominant trait and is characterized by anemia, reticulocytosis, jaundice, and splenomegaly; cholelithiasis is seen in up to 60% of patients. An erythrocyte membrane defect causes increased osmotic fragility and susceptibility to splenic destruction. Splenectomy is the sole therapy but generally can be delayed until the fourth year of life. Preoperative cholecystography should be performed because of the high incidence of bilirubin stones in the gallbladder and bile ducts. **Hereditary elliptocytosis** usually is harmless, but can become symptomatic when ovalocytes constitute 50 to 90% of the red cell population; in such cases splenectomy is indicated. **Pyruvate kinase (PK) deficiency** and **G6PD deficiency** render red blood cells susceptible to increased hemolysis; in severe cases of PK deficiency, splenectomy is sometimes worthwhile. **Idiopathic autoimmune hemolytic anemia** is produced when there are antibodies against normal red blood cells and occurs most frequently in women over 50 years of age. Splenectomy is considered under the following conditions: when therapy with steroids is ineffective; when steroids are required in excessive doses; and when splenic sequestrations can be demonstrated by injecting chromium-tagged red blood cells. In approximately 80% of such cases, patients achieve a good response to splenectomy.

Answer: A, B, C

4. Regarding thalassemia and sickle cell disease, which of the following statements is/are true?

A. Thalassemia is transmitted as an autosomal trait and occurs in a major (homozygous) and a minor (heterozygous) form
B. A characteristic feature of thalassemia major is replacement of normal hemoglobin A with abnormal hemoglobins, leading to increased splenic sequestration of red blood cells and necessitating splenectomy
C. Except for rare cases in which excessive splenic sequestration of red blood cells can be demonstrated, splenectomy is not indicated for sickle cell disease
D. When splenic abscess occurs in patients with sickle cell disease, drainage of the abscess cavity within the parenchyma of the spleen may be necessary

Sabiston: 1220
Schwartz: 1380

Comments: **Thalassemia major** (homozygous thalassemia), transmitted as an autosomal trait, becomes apparent in the first year of life and is characterized by pallor, retarded body growth, and enlargement of the head. The characteristic feature of this disease is persistence of hemoglobin-F and reduction in hemoglobin A. In thalassemia major, occasionally splenectomy may reduce the hemolytic process. In a few patients, splenomegaly or symptomatic repeated splenic infarction constitutes an indication for splenectomy. **Thalassemia minor** permits most affected patients to lead normal lives and to accommodate to a slightly reduced level of hemoglobin. In **sickle cell disease,** normal hemoglobin A is replaced by abnormal sickle hemoglobin (hemoglobin S). Under conditions of reduced oxygen tension, hemoglobin S undergoes crystallization producing sickling of red cells; this leads to increased blood viscosity and circulatory stasis. Repeated episodes of stasis produce splenic infarction leading eventually to autosplenectomy. Rarely, in patients with sickle cell anemia (homozygous state for hemoglobin S) excessive splenic sequestrations of red cells can be prevented by splenectomy. ● Whenever possible, splenectomy should be avoided in patients younger than 5 years of age because of the increased short- and long-term risk of severe infectious complications.

Answer: A, C, D

5. Concerning idiopathic (immune) thrombocytopenic purpura (ITP), which of the following statements is/are true?

A. The male/female ratio is 3:1
B. The diagnosis is suggested when there is a thrombocytopenia with adequate, normal-appearing megakaryocytes and no history of ingestion of drugs capable of producing thrombocytopenia
C. One of the most common symptoms is bleeding gums; the bleeding time is prolonged but the clotting time is normal
D. Splenectomy is reserved for those patients who fail initial therapy with steroids

Sabiston: 1210
Schwartz: 1381

Comments: Although there is no established etiology, it is believed that idiopathic (immune) thrombocytopenic purpura (ITP) is an autoimmune disease. The ratio of women to men affected is 3:1. ITP is characterized by thrombocytopenia in the presence of marrow containing normal or increased megakaryocytes. The bleeding disorder is manifested most commonly by petechia and/or ecchymosis; bleeding gums, hematuria, or vaginal or gastrointestinal tract bleeding may also occur. Splenomegaly to a degree that it can be palpated is unusual. The platelet count is usually less than $50,000/\mu l$ and the bleeding time may be prolonged. About 80% of patients under 16 years of age have a spontaneous complete recovery without specific therapy. In adults, the initial treatment is with steroids for a 6- to 8-week period. If such patients fail to respond, or if the disorder recurs after discontinuation of steroids, splenectomy is indicated. Platelet transfusions are indicated in patients who continue to bleed after splenectomy. The results of splenectomy are excellent in 80% of patients. Usually a good initial response to steroid therapy foretells a good response to splenectomy. Up to 10% of patients will relapse after benefitting from a splenectomy.

Answer: B, C, D

6. Concerning thrombotic thrombocytopenic purpura (TTP), which of the following statements is/are true?

A. Clinical presentation includes the classic pentad of fever, purpura, hemolytic anemia, neurologic manifestations, and signs of renal disease
B. Fragmented red blood cells are often seen on peripheral smear
C. Mortality from the disease is approximately 25%
D. Splenectomy together with steroid therapy has been reported to be successful in some cases

Sabiston: 1213
Schwartz: 1382

Comments: Thrombotic thrombocytopenic purpura is a disease of arterioles or capillaries resulting in their widespread occlusion by a hyaline membrane. The classic presentation is a pentad of fever, purpura, hemolytic anemia, neurologic manifestations, and signs of renal disease. The peripheral blood smear shows fragmented, distorted red blood cells. Unchecked, the disease runs a fulminating course, resulting in death, most commonly secondary to intracerebral hemorrhage or to renal failure. Some patients have been cured by steroid therapy and splenectomy. Approximately 5% of cases of thrombocytopenia occur during pregnancy and must be distinguished from idiopathic thrombocytopenia that can be corrected by termination of the pregnancy.

Answer: A, B, D

7. As regards primary and secondary hypersplenism, which of the following statements is/are true?

A. Both are best treated by splenectomy alone
B. Both are usually caused by hepatic disease or by extrahepatic portal vein obstruction
C. They are dissimilar in that primary hypersplenism is a diagnosis of exclusion and splenectomy is curative
D. Both are best treated by corticosteroids and splenectomy

Sabiston: 1213
Schwartz: 1383

Comments: **Primary hypersplenism** can produce any combination of neutropenia, anemia, or thrombocytopenia, with the spleen being the primary site of cellular sequestration. Most patients are women, and symptoms depend on the cell type that is sequestered. The diagnosis is one of exclusion and is confirmed by clinical response to splenectomy; corticosteroids rarely affect the course of the disease process. **Secondary hypersplenism** is due either to hepatic disease or to extrahepatic portal vein obstruction leading to anemia, leukopenia, or thrombocytopenia, singly or in any combination. In this clinical setting, no correlation exists between the degree of cellular depression and symptoms; splenectomy therefore usually is not necessary, although occasionally it is indicated in patients with portal hypertension. Thrombocytopenia is often improved following a portacaval shunt.

Answer: C

8. Match the anatomic involvement with Hodgkin's disease and the clinical stage of the disease.

Anatomic Involvement	Stage
A. Right axillary lymph nodes	a. Stage I
B. Epigastric lymph nodes; liver	b. Stage II
C. Left cervical lymph nodes; right mediastinal lymph nodes	c. Stage III
D. Left cervical lymph nodes; epigastric lymph nodes; spleen	d. Stage IV

Sabiston: 1215
Schwartz: 1384

Comments: The prognosis and treatment of Hodgkin's disease is related to the histologic type and clinical stage at the time of presentation. Hodgkin's disease is commonly staged as follows: Stage I—One area or two contiguous areas of lymp node involvement on the same side of the diaphragm; Stage II—Two noncontiguous areas on the same side of the diaphragm; Stage III—Involvement on each side of the diaphragm (for purposes of this classification, the spleen is considered a lymph node); Stage IV—Involvement of liver, bone marrow, bone, lung, or any other non–lymph nodal tissue, besides the spleen. In addition to staging the disease anatomically, the system is modified to allow the distinction between patients who are asymptomatic ("A" patients) and those who have constitutional symptoms such as night sweats, fever, or weight loss ("B" patients). Since treatment involves radiation therapy or chemotherapy, given alone or in combination, accurate staging is necessary if one is to avoid the complications of over- or undertreatment.

Answer: A–a; B–d; C–b; D–c

9. Of the following statements regarding staging laparotomy in patients with Hodgkin's disease, which is/are true?

A. Lymphangiography and computed tomographic scanning used together have eliminated the need for staging laparotomy
B. Staging laparotomy consists of wedge biopsy of the liver; splenectomy; careful sampling of lymph nodes from multiple, specific intra-abdominal sites; and oophoropexy in premenopausal women
C. Staging laparotomy is more likely to be positive in patients with involvement of the right cervical lymph nodes than in those with involvement of the left cervical lymph nodes
D. Splenectomy enhances the quality and duration of response to chemotherapy

Sabiston: 1215
Schwartz: 1384

Comments: Accurate staging is critical if one is to avoid the complications of over- or undertreatment. Unfortunately, noninvasive means of clinical staging frequently are inaccurate. This is particularly true in assessment of the upper abdominal lymph nodes, the spleen, and the liver. In most reported clinical series, there is a 30 to 40% change in stage of the disease following laparotomy; slightly more patients are up-staged (and need more aggressive therapy) than down-staged. Several groups of patients do not require a staging laparotomy, an example being Stage I patients whose involvement is isolated lymph nodes high in the right neck. Left neck disease, however, is associated with a high enough incidence of occult splenic and/or upper abdominal lymph node disease to warrant staging laparotomy. Patients with clearly advanced disease (Stage III or IV) as determined by lymphangiography and CT scan likewise do not require a staging laparotomy, since their treatment includes systemic chemotherapy. Patients with Stage I or II disease and who are symptomatic ("B" patients) require staging laparotomy to search for occult visceral or intra-abdominal involvement, if they are to avoid systemic therapy (chemotherapy). Similarly, patients with an equivocal lymphangiogram or CT scan probably should be staged by laparotomy. The controversy centers on patients with Stage 1A or 2A disease (other than those with isolated high right neck involvement). In this group, laparotomy provides the most accurate staging but, unless there is symptomatic splenomegaly, carries with it the risk of an unnecessary operation. The need for splenectomy is not an indication for a staging laparotomy since, in most series, the morbidity of radiation therapy and chemotherapy in nonsplenectomized patients is not significantly increased.

Answer: B

10. Hypersplenism requiring splenectomy may occur in:

A. Felty's syndrome
B. Sarcoidosis
C. Gaucher's disease
D. Porphyria erythropoietica

Sabiston: 1214
Schwartz: 1385

Comments: **Felty's syndrome** is a triad of rheumatoid arthritis, splenomegaly, and neutropenia. Response of the neutropenia to steroids is not long-lasting and the salutary effects of splenectomy generally are excellent. **Sarcoidosis** leads to hepatosplenomegaly in approximately 25% of the cases; 20% of patients so affected develop signs and symptoms of hypersplenism, particularly thrombocytopenic purpura. Splenectomy is indicated for patients experiencing the complications of hypersplenism. **Gaucher's disease** is characterized by abnormal retention of glycolipid cerebrosides in reticuloendothelial cells, often leading to splenomegaly. When this results in hypersplenism, splenectomy is almost uniformly beneficial. **Porphyria erythropoietica** is a congenital disorder of erythrocyte pyrrole metabolism; it leads to premature destruction of red cells in the spleen. When this disorder is complicated by hemolysis or splenomegaly, splenectomy is followed by marked improvement.

Answer: A, B, C, D

11. Regarding myeloid metaplasia, which of the following statements is/are true?

A. It is rarely accompanied by splenomegaly
B. It generally affects young females
C. Symptoms usually are related to anemia and progressive splenomegaly
D. The peripheral blood smear has a characteristic appearance
E. Splenectomy alters the course in about half the patients

Sabiston: 1223
Schwartz: 1383

Comments: Myelofibrosis with myeloid metaplasia is an unusual illness with no known cause, affecting middle-aged or older persons. It is characterized by progressive impairment of hematopoiesis as a result of fibrosis and sclerosis of the bone marrow. The peripheral smear characteristically shows immature red cells, anisocytosis, poikilocytosis, and numerous teardrops and elongated shapes. Immature granulocyte forms are present as well. The panproliferative process also involves the liver, spleen, and long bones. The consequent extramedullary hematopoiesis commonly results in moderate to marked splenomegaly; therapy is directed mainly toward stemming the anemia and the accompanying splenomegaly. This may include the giving of transfusions, corticosteroids, androgens, chemotherapy, and splenic irradiation. Splenectomy normally is performed for thrombocytopenia, the continuing need for a large number of transfusions, high-output cardiac failures, and symptoms from the enlarged spleen; it does not, however, alter the course of the disease.

Answer: C, D

CHAPTER 35

Hernias—Abdominal

1. Match the items in the two columns.

Abdominal Wall Layers	Corresponding Spermatic Cord Layers
A. Subcutaneous tissue	a. Cremasteric muscle
B. Transversalis fascia	b. Internal spermatic fascia
C. External oblique	c. Obliterated processus vaginalis
D. Internal oblique	d. Dartos muscle (in the scrotum)
E. Parietal peritoneum	e. External spermatic fascia

Sabiston: 1232
Schwartz: 1458

Comments: During descent of the testicle from its original retroperitoneal position to the scrotum, it passes through the abdominal wall. Understanding of the anatomic continuations of the abdominal wall layers onto the spermatic cord is essential for the proper performance of herniorrhaphy.

Answer: A–d; B–b; C–e; D–a; E–c

2. The iliopubic tract:

A. Extends from the anterior superior iliac spine to the pubis
B. Is a condensation of the transversalis fascia
C. Is of anatomic interest but has little clinical significance
D. Is synonymous with the shelving portion of Poupart's ligament
E. None of the above

Sabiston: 1237

Comments: The transversalis fascia is the portion of the endoabdominal fascia that underlies the transversus abdominis muscle. It has several thickenings, the most important of which is the iliopubic tract arising from the iliopectineal arch, inserting on the anterior superior iliac spine, and extending over the femoral vessels to the pubis. Proper utilization of the transversalis fascia in the re-

pair of inguinal hernia is important to the success of the operation.

Answer: A, B

3. The anatomic boundaries of the orifice of the femoral canal include:

A. Cooper's ligament
B. Inguinal ligament
C. Iliopubic tract
D. Femoral vein
E. Lacunar ligament

Sabiston: 1238
Schwartz: 1470

Comments: Femoral hernias are situated in the femoral canal, the entrance to which is bounded superiorly and medially by the iliopubic tract, inferiorly by Cooper's ligament, and laterally by the femoral vein. The inguinal ligament is more superficial; it is a common misconception that the medial boundary of the femoral canal is formed by the recurved fibers of the inguinal ligament known as the lacunar ligament.

Answer: A, C, D

4. Hesselbach's triangle:

A. Defines the boundaries of a low lumbar hernia
B. Defines the inguinal floor in the region of a direct inguinal hernia
C. Is found in a single plane of the inguinal floor and is bound by the inferior epigastric artery, inguinal ligament, and rectus sheath
D. Is bounded medially by the inferior epigastric vessels
E. None of the above

Sabiston: 1235
Schwartz: 1459

Comments: A direct inguinal hernia projects through the inguinal floor in the region of Hesselbach's triangle. The boundaries of this anatomic triangle are generally consid-

247

ered to be the inguinal ligament inferiorly, the inferior epigastric artery laterally, and the lateral border of the rectus sheath medially; this definition is not anatomically precise, however, since none of the borders are in the same abdominal wall layer and all are superficial to the floor of the inguinal canal. The inferior epigastric vessels may be a useful landmark for differentiating groin hernias, since indirect hernias originate lateral to these vessels and direct hernias originate medial to them. Very large indirect hernias disrupt the posterior inguinal wall medial to the epigastric vessels, thus extending to the region of Hesselbach's triangle. Large indirect hernias require repair of the posterior floor, as in direct hernia repair.

Answer: B

5. Which of the following statements is/are true regarding the incidence of abdominal wall hernias?

A. The indirect inguinal hernia is the most common hernia in either sex
B. Femoral hernias are more common in females than in males
C. Direct hernias are unusual in females
D. Hernias in general occur with approximate equal frequency in males and females
E. None of the above

Sabiston: 1239
Schwartz: 1458

Comments: Approximately three quarters of all abdominal wall hernias occur in the groin region, and roughly two thirds of these are indirect inguinal hernias. In general, hernias are considered to be at least five times more common in males than in females, and it has been estimated that approximately 5% of the total adult male population is affected. Hernias, therefore, constitute a significant economic problem in terms of loss of time from work.

Answer: A, B, C

6. Concerning recurrence after repair of groin hernias:

A. Most indirect recurrences are attributed to an inadequate repair of the inguinal floor
B. Indirect hernias at any age have a lower recurrence rate than either direct or femoral hernias
C. Most recurrent hernias are direct, occurring after the repair of an indirect inguinal hernia
D. Recurrence rates are higher following bilateral simultaneous herniorrhaphy
E. None of the above

Sabiston: 1241
Schwartz: 1473

Comments: Recurrence rates for groin hernias vary between 2% and approximately 30%; 3 to 10% is a reasonable estimate. True recurrence rates are difficult to establish because of inadequate patient follow-up. Recurrence is more common with direct or femoral hernias than with indirect hernias. Repair of recurrent hernias is associated with even higher rates of recurrence. Higher recurrence rates have been associated with failure to recognize and treat chronic respiratory problems, urinary tract obstruc-

tion, chronic constipation, anorectal disease, and ascites. Since most recurrences occur after 1 year, the etiology is probably tissue dysfunction related to excessive tension. Relaxing incisions may be very helpful in reducing tension on repairs involving fascial tissue. With attenuated tissue and very large defects, the selective use of prosthetic materials has been demonstrated to result in low recurrence rates. The most popular prosthetic material is Marlex (polypropylene) with promising early results from Gore-Tex (polytetrafluorethylene). Recurrence of an indirect inguinal hernia is due to failure to remove the hernia sac or failure in repairing the dilated internal ring.

Answer: B, C, D

7. Which of the following statements is/are true concerning direct inguinal hernias?

A. The etiologic mechanism may involve a congenital defect
B. Direct hernias should be repaired promptly because of the risk of incarceration
C. A direct hernia may be a sliding hernia involving a portion of the bladder wall
D. A direct hernia may pass through the external inguinal ring
E. None of the above

Sabiston: 1241
Schwartz: 1459, 1461, 1468

Comments: Although direct inguinal hernias are generally acquired, they may result from a congenital anatomic defect in the support of the lower inguinal canal or abnormalities in collagen. Since generally there is a diffuse weakness in the area of Hesselbach's triangle without a narrow-necked sac, the risk of incarceration is low. Rarely incarceration may result when the direct hernia passes through the external ring posterior to the cord structures. The involvement of the urinary bladder as a sliding component on the medial wall of a direct hernia sac usually does not cause a problem because the sac can simply be reduced unopened.

Answer: A, C, D

8. A sliding inguinal hernia on the right side is likely to involve:

A. Ileum composing the posterior wall of the sac
B. Ovary and fallopian tube in a female infant
C. A loop of small bowel fixed by adhesions
D. Cecum composing the posterior wall of the sac
E. Cecum composing the anteromedial wall of the sac

Sabiston: 1248
Schwartz: 1468

Comments: A sliding hernia is one in which the visceral peritoneum of an organ makes up a part of the wall of the hernia sac. If the hernia is indirect, this most commonly involves the cecum on the right or the sigmoid colon on the left. In females, especially infants and children, portions of the female genital tract are often involved. Recognition of the presence of a sliding hernia and the position of the visceral component is important in order to avoid injury of the involved organs during repair.

Answer: B, D

9. Which of the following statements is/are true regarding groin hernias in females?

A. Femoral hernias are more common than inguinal hernias
B. A mass within a hernia in a female infant is usually a nonfunctioning ovary
C. An ovary present within a hernia should be returned to the abdominal cavity before repair is completed
D. In repair of an indirect inguinal hernia, the round ligament should be preserved
E. Biopsy should be performed on any abnormal-appearing gonad found in a hernia sac

Sabiston: 1248
Schwartz: 1462

Comments: Although femoral hernias are found more often in females than in males, inguinal hernias are still more common than femoral hernias. The round ligament is usually adherent to the hernial sac when an indirect hernia is present; the round ligament can simply be divided, and recurrence of an indirect hernia in females is extremely unusual. A solid mass palpable within the hernia of a female infant is usually a normal ovary that simply is returned to the abdominal cavity. The internal ring can be closed completely after returning the ovary and fallopian tube to the abdominal cavity. If the gonad appears abnormal or resembles a testicle, however, biopsy must be performed in order to rule out testicular feminization. Most patients with this syndrome have inguinal hernias.

Answer: C, E

10. Appropriate management of an incarcerated groin hernia might include:

A. Intravenous sedation and attempted reduction of an inguinal hernia
B. Intravenous sedation and attempted reduction of a femoral hernia
C. Operation only after repeated attempts at reduction have failed
D. If reduction is successful, delayed repair in 2 to 3 days
E. Opening of the hernial sac prior to reduction at the time of operation

Sabiston: 1247
Schwartz: 1463

Comments: Incarceration and subsequent strangulation of small bowel is a serious complication of groin hernias, particularly of femoral hernias. If the patient has an incarcerated inguinal hernia and strangulation is not suspected, an attempt at reduction using sedation, Trendelenburg positioning, and gentle sustained pressure over the groin mass is appropriate. Because of the narrow neck and greater risk of strangulation with a femoral hernia, attempted reduction of an incarcerated femoral hernia is not indicated. Vigorous attempts at reduction of an incarcerated hernia may produce "reduction en masse" wherein the entire hernial sac and its contents are reduced so that even though the external bulge is gone, the incarceration within the sac remains. If there is any indication of strangulation, reduction should not be attempted preoperatively. Rather, the sac should first be opened prior to reduction to inspect the viability of the contents. Delayed repair following successful reduction may permit resolution of edema.

Answer: A, D, E

11. Which of the following statements about the management of inguinal hernias in infants and children is/are true?

A. Repair should be delayed until the child is 2 years of age
B. Repair requires only high ligation of the hernial sac
C. The distal sac should be removed to prevent formation of a secondary hydrocele
D Contralateral inguinal exploration is routinely indicated because of the high risk of bilaterality
E. None of the above

Sabiston: 1293
Schwartz: 1471

Comments: Inguinal hernias in infants and children are nearly always indirect, resulting from failure of obliteration of the processes vaginalis. Effective treatment requires only high ligation and transection of the sac with or without excision of the distal component. Repair need not be delayed unless the infant has associated medical problems. The role of exploration of the opposite side in children who present with a unilateral inguinal hernia is controversial. The incidence of a contralateral hernia appearing following unilateral inguinal herniorrhaphy in children has been reported to be as high as 30%. However, there is a poor correlation between the number of children found to have a patent processus vaginalis at the time of routine contralateral exploration and the number who subsequently develop clinically significant inguinal hernias.

Answer: B

12. True statements concerning umbilical hernias include:

A. They are the embryologic equivalent of a small omphalocele
B. Prompt repair of even small defects in infants is indicated because of the risk of incarceration
C. Repair in asymptomatic adults is not indicated
D. The "vest-over-pants" type of repair is stronger than simple approximation of fascial margins
E. They are most common in black infants

Sabiston: 1249
Schwartz: 1472

Comments: Umbilical hernias are the result of a patent umbilical ring, whereas an omphalocele is due to failure of abdominal wall closure in the midline in early intrauterine life. Umbilical hernias are said to be present in 40 to 90% of black infants. Incarceration is rare in infants; unless the defect is very large, most surgeons would defer repair until approximately 4 years of age, since spontaneous closure does occur. In adults, however, repair should be carried out promptly because of the risk of incarceration. There is no convincing evidence that a "vest-over-pants" type of repair is structurally superior to simple approximation of fascial margins. Repair in adults may require use of a prosthetic material such as Marlex or Gore-Tex if the fascial defect is large.

Answer: E

13. Match the items in the two columns:

Repair	Characteristic Features
A. Cooper's ligament repair	a. Restoration of transversalis fascia around spermatic cord
B. Bassini's repair	b. Transversus abdominis approximated to Cooper's ligament to include sutures into femoral sheath
C. Shouldice repair	c. Imbrication of multiple layers of inguinal wall with continuous suture
D. Plastic repair of internal ring	d. Transversus abdominis aponeurosis approximated to Poupart's ligament
	e. None of the above

Sabiston: 1241
Schwartz: 1469

Comments: The classic Bassini type repair is the most widely utilized operation for reconstituting the floor of the inguinal canal. Various modifications have been introduced over the years and are well known. Excellent results have been reported using the Shouldice technique, although use of this method has not become widespread. A relaxing incision should always be used in the Cooper repair. Risk of femoral vein injury has dissuaded many surgeons from using this repair routinely. Femoral hernias may be repaired through the groin by Cooper's ligament repair, by preperitoneal repair, or by "repair from below." The Shouldice Clinic has reported excellent results with the latter. This repair may be especially useful in incarcerated femoral hernias in the elderly, utilizing local anesthesia only. The expert hernia surgeon utilizes various techniques, selecting the repair most appropriate for the individual hernia. The repair may include the use of a prosthetic material. The choice is based on a sound knowledge of anatomy and the principles of hernia surgery.

Answer: A–b; B–d; C–c; D–a

14. Which of the following statements is/are true regarding the preperitoneal or posterior approach for the repair of groin hernias?

A. It may be appropriate for repair of both direct and indirect inguinal hernias
B. It may be appropriate for repair of femoral hernias

C. It is performed through the same skin incision as the anterior approach
D. In performing a Cooper's ligament repair via a preperitoneal approach, a transition suture is not required
E. None of the above

Sabiston: 1244

Comment: The preperitoneal approach, utilizing a horizontal skin incision three fingerbreadths above the pubic tubercle, has been especially successful in the repair of femoral hernias. Both direct and indirect inguinal hernias can also be approached in this manner, although many have reported higher recurrence rates for direct hernias when using this approach. A Cooper's ligament repair is carried out in the same way as it is with an anterior approach: Cooper's ligament is approximated to the transversus abdominis aponeurosis medially with a transition suture between the transversus aponeurosis, the iliopubic tract, and Cooper's ligament, and completion laterally by approximation of the iliopubic tract and transversus aponeurosis. This repair has not achieved widespread use. General or spinal anesthesia is necessary. Postoperative ileus is not infrequent.

Answer: A, B

15. Match the following hernias with the most appropriate response:

A. Spigelian hernia	a. Noncircumferential incarceration of bowel wall
B. Richter's hernia	b. Latissimus dorsi, external oblique, iliac crest
C. Littre's hernia	c. Incarcerated Meckel's diverticulum
D. Petit's hernia	d. Howship-Romberg sign
E. Grynfeltt's hernia	e. Twelfth rib, internal oblique
F. Obturator hernia	f. Lateral border of rectus at linea semicircularis

Sabiston: 1248

Comments: All of the above refer to more unusual anatomic locations of abdominal or lumbar hernias except for Richter's and Littre's, which represent incarceration of a limited portion of the small bowel. It is important to recognize these two types of hernias because vascular compromise may occur without evidence of intestinal obstruction.

Answer: A–f; B–a; C–c; D–b; E–e; F–d

16. Most umbilical hernias are associated with a:

A. Patent urachus
B. Patent omphalomesenteric duct
C. Patent vitelline duct
D. Patent ligamentum venosum
E. None of the above

Sabiston: 1249
Schwartz: 1460

Comments: Umbilical hernias result when the umbilical ring remains patent after birth. Other abnormalities may be present at the umbilicus in the form of draining si- nuses, fistulas, or cysts due to the persistence of embryo- logic structures such as the urachus or the omphalomes- enteric (vitelline) duct. This association with umbilical hernia, however, is coincidental rather than causal.

Answer: E

CHAPTER 36

Abdominal Wall, Omentum, Mesentery, and Retroperitoneum

1. Which of the following is/are true regarding hematomas of the rectus sheath?

A. They usually result from rupture of the epigastric vessels
B. The only recognized etiologic factor is trauma
C. They are characterized by a palpable mass that is not influenced by tensing of the rectus abdominis muscle
D. Their treatment is usually nonoperative

Sabiston: 781
Schwartz: 1421

Comments: While hematomas most commonly follow trauma, they can also occur as a result of certain infectious diseases (e.g., typhoid fever), collagen vascular diseases, blood dyscrasias, coagulopathies, and anticoagulation therapy. In addition to Fothergill's sign (answer C), a bluish discoloration to the skin is also diagnostic; however, this may take a few days to develop. Sonography can be helpful in establishing the diagnosis. Although treatment is usually nonoperative, operation may be indicated in cases of an expanding hematoma or significant local symptoms, or if the diagnosis is in doubt.

Answer: A, C, D

2. Which of the following statements is/are true regarding desmoid tumors?

A. They occur more commonly in women
B. These are benign fibrous growths often found within or deep to the lower anterior abdominal musculature
C. Because of their benign nature, they are unlikely to recur
D. The treatment of choice is wide resection

Sabiston: 781
Schwartz: 1423

Comments: Desmoid tumors fall in the middle of a spectrum of fibromatoses ranging from benign fibroma to aggressive fibrosarcoma. Although considered "benign,"
252

when excised incompletely they have a propensity to recur and invade local structures. Although local radiation may have a role in the therapy of some desmoid tumors, wide resection (including the contiguously invaded structures) is the treatment of choice.

Answer: A, B, D

3. Which of the following is/are true regarding omental torsion?

A. Secondary torsion is more common than primary
B. The diagnosis should be considered in any patient with serosanguinous peritoneal fluid in the presence of a normal gallbladder, appendix, and pelvic organs
C. The associated pain is most often on the left side
D. Proper treatment involves detorsion of the involved omentum with resection only if it is not viable

Sabiston: 786
Schwartz: 1424

Comments: Primary or idiopathic torsion of the omentum is rare as compared with secondary torsion, which involves two points of omental fixation (frequently related to abdominal adhesions). Patients present clinically with epigastric pain which later radiates to the right lower quadrant, causing this entity to be confused with appendicitis. The correct treatment is resection of the involved omentum as well as correction of any predisposing conditions.

Answer: A, B

4. Which of the following statements characterize retroperitoneal fibrosis?

A. A hypersensitivity reaction to the antiserotonin drug methysergide has been implicated
B. It is two to three times more common in women
C. Symptoms are generally related to partial inferior vena caval obstruction

D. The most definitive noninvasive diagnostic test is an intravenous pyelogram (IVP)

Sabiston: 787
Schwartz: 1447

Comments: Retroperitoneal fibrosis is one of a constellation of processes of "systemic idiopathic fibrosis." A hypersensitivity to methysergide is one of the few identified etiologic factors. Its incidence in men is two to three times that in women. Although the inferior vena cava may be compressed by the fibrotic stage of the process, symptoms usually relate to genitourinary tract involvement and lymphatic obstruction. The characteristic finding of medial deviation of both ureters on IVP is highly diagnostic of this entity.

Answer: A, D

5. Which of the following statements is/are true regarding mesenteric lymphadenitis?

A. It occurs more commonly in children than in adults
B. It is easily distinguished from appendicitis clinically
C. Cultures taken at the time of operation usually show the presence of coliform bacteria
D. The disease process tends to be self-limiting and it rarely recurs

Sabiston: 974
Schwartz: 1443

Comments: A disease primarily of children and adolescents, mesenteric lymphadenitis is characterized by vague and at times migratory abdominal pain. It is frequently difficult to distinguish from appendicitis; however, the inability to exactly localize the site of maximum tenderness and the change in site of maximum tenderness is frequently a helpful sign. The small amount of free peritoneal fluid found in these patients is usually sterile. The disease process is self-limiting, but approximately one fourth of patients will have additional episodes during their childhood years.

Answer: A

6. Tumors of the mesentery are characterized by which of the following statements?

A. Primary and metastatic tumors of the mesentery occur with approximately equal frequency
B. Of the primary mesenteric tumors, the majority are cystic
C. Of the solid primary tumors of the mesentery, the majority are malignant
D. Malignant mesenteric tumors tend to occur near the root of the mesentery, while benign tumors are more likely peripheral in location.

Schwartz: 1444

Comments: Most of tumors within the mesentery represent metastases to the mesenteric lymph nodes. Primary mesenteric tumors are rare and are more often cystic rather than solid, frequently representing developmental defects of embryonic rests. Among the solid primary tumors, the majority are benign; these frequently are found

in the periphery of the mesentery, closer to the intestine. Malignant mesenteric tumors (most often liposarcoma and leiomyosarcoma) are usually found near the root of the mesentery, which significantly increases both the hazards of resection and the consequent likelihood of recurrence.

Answer: B, D

7. Regarding retroperitoneal tumors in general, which of the following statements is/are correct?

A. These are tumors of young adulthood
B. Malignant tumors predominate, the most common of which is rhabdomyosarcoma
C. Complaints are usually vague, but on clinical examination, a palpable mass is almost always present
D. Ultrasonography and/or CT scanning gives valuable information

Sabiston: 788
Schwartz: 1449

Comments: Considering all histologic types of retroperitoneal tumors, this tends to be a disease of the fifth and sixth decades, although 15% are found in children. Malignancies predominate over benign conditions, the most common being lymphoma, followed by liposarcoma and fibrosarcoma and then the other sarcomas. The clinical history usually is one of vague back or abdominal pain. Since the tumor itself is palpable only when it reaches significant size, one relies heavily on radiographic assessment. CT scanning and ultrasonography have been valuable in delineating the extent of the tumor and its relationship to contiguous structures.

Answer: D

8. Which of the following statements accurately characterize retroperitoneal sarcomas?

A. The operative approach is best achieved through a flank incision
B. These tumors have a well-defined capsule; they can be easily shelled out of the tumor bed with excellent results
C. Fewer than 25% can be resected totally
D. Local recurrence rates range from 30 to 50%
E. Five-year disease-free survival is in the range of 10%

Schwartz: 1449

Comments: Retroperitoneal sarcomas can grow to a very large size and typically invade contiguous structures. They are surrounded by a pseudocapsule; although the tumors can be shelled out along this capsular plane, in such instances there is virtually always residual tumor. Avoiding this necessitates wide excision, frequently en bloc with the attached organs (e.g., kidney, bowel, abdominal wall). Because of the frequent proximity of these tumors to nonresectable structures, complete excision is possible in only about 25% of patients. For these same reasons, local recurrence rates may be as high as 50%; this, and their potential for distant metastasis, results in 5-year disease-free survival rates that can be as low as 10%. Current investigations of adjuvant external beam and intraoperative radiation therapy to reduce the recurrence rate are in progress.

Answer: C, D, E

9. An idiopathic disease process characterized by inflammatory and fibrotic thickening of the root of the small bowel mesentery associated with abdominal pain, nausea, vomiting, and malaise and occasionally benefiting from use of steroids or irradiation is known as:

A. Mesenteric panniculitis
B. Retractile mesenteritis
C. A variant of retroperitoneal fibrosis
D. No such disease entity exists in this isolated form

Schwartz: 1444

Comments: The disease entity described above can occur in an isolated manner or in conjunction with other fibrotic reactions including retroperitoneal fibrosis. It is of uncertain etiology and tends to be a self-limiting process. At operation, multiple biopsies should be taken to exclude the diagnosis of malignancy; rarely, colostomy or intestinal bypass is needed to relieve symptoms of obstruction.

Answer: A, B, C

10. Tumors of the omentum are characterized by which of the following statements?

A. All omental cysts are postinflammatory in nature
B. Omental cysts usually are asymptomatic
C. The most common solid omental tumor is metastatic carcinoma
D. Primary solid tumors of the omentum are fairly common and most often malignant
E. Omentectomy for metastatic carcinoma has a role in the management of certain tumors

Sabiston: 786
Schwartz: 1426

Comments: Omental cysts may be "true cysts," presumably caused by congenital lymphatic obstruction or neoplastic dermoid cysts, or they may be pseudocysts resulting usually from fat necrosis, trauma, or a foreign body reaction. Unless they undergo torsion, the majority are asymptomatic and the rest produce vague nondescript symptoms. The preponderant majority of solid omental tumors represent metastatic carcinoma, and in the case of ovarian carcinoma omentectomy can contribute to improved disease control despite the presence of metastases elsewhere. Primary solid omental tumors are exceedingly rare, and only one third are malignant. Ultrasound can be valuable in bolstering a clinical diagnosis and in determining their cystic or solid status. At present, percutaneous needle/catheter drainage of presumed omental cysts is too hazardous.

Answer: B, C, E

CHAPTER 37

Vascular—Brachiocephalic

1. The most common cause of cerebral ischemia involves which one of the following?

A. Extracranial arterial stenosis
B. Intracranial arterial thrombosis
C. Arterioarterial embolization
D. Cardioarterial embolization

Sabiston: 1847
Schwartz: 942

Comments: Atherosclerosis is the most common cause of ischemic stroke. Neurologic injury may result from progressive stenosis of the internal carotid artery near the carotid bifurcation, but it is felt that the most common mechanism of neurologic injury in atherosclerosis is embolization from atherosclerotic plaques at the carotid bifurcation. The embolizing particles may consist of plaque fragments or platelet fibrin aggregates. This mechanism accounts for cerebral ischemic events in patients with nonstenotic ulcerated lesions. A small proportion of ischemic strokes may be caused by processes other than atherosclerosis, such as emboli from cardiac sources, fibromuscular hyperplasia, occlusive arteritis of the aortic arch vessels, dissecting thoracic aortic aneurysms, and trauma.

Answer: C

2. What percentage of patients with cerebral ischemia have a surgically accessible lesion?

A. 95%
B. 75%
C. 50%
D. 25%
E. 5%

Schwartz: 942

Comments: If patients with cerebrovascular ischemia are studied by four-vessel angiography, 75% of the group will be found to have significant extracranial disease that is surgically accessible. In the carotid vessels, lesions characteristically involve the carotid bifurcation and the

proximal 1 to 2 cm of the internal carotid artery. In patients with vertebral basilar insufficiency, plaques or stenotic lesions characteristically occur near the origin of the vertebral arteries from the subclavian vessels. Since stroke is the third leading cause of death in the United States and since the responsible lesions are often surgically accessible, endarterectomy benefits a significant proportion of patients with symptoms of cerebral ischemia.

Answer: B

3. In which one or more of the following situations is carotid endarterectomy a generally accepted form of treatment?

A. Acute stroke, ulcerated carotid plaque
B. Acute stroke, totally occluded internal carotid artery
C. Transient neurologic deficit (less than 24 hours)
D. Completed stroke, mild deficit, ulcerated carotid plaque
E. Completed stroke, totally occluded internal carotid artery

Sabiston: 1850
Schwartz: 946

Comments: Among patients with symptoms of cerebrovascular ischemia, those with transient ischemic attacks are optimal candidates for carotid endarterectomy, since their risk of subsequent stroke is significantly decreased by operative intervention. Endarterectomy may also benefit patients with a completed stroke, if their neurologic deficit is not severe and they have an ulcerated plaque that could serve as the source of continued emboli. There is no benefit to performing endarterectomy for a completed stroke with total occlusion of the internal carotid artery, since restoration of flow will not restore neurologic function. The role of carotid endarterectomy in an acute or evolving stroke is controversial. Restoration of flow is usually not indicated in patients with fixed deficits and may in fact worsen symptoms and produce death by causing hemorrhage in the area of infarction. In

255

patients with an evolving stroke and fluctuating neurologic deficit, emergent endarterectomy may be of benefit.

Answer: C, D

4. Presence of a cervical bruit correlates with which one or more of the following?

A. Risk of unilateral stroke
B. Presence of carotid stenosis
C. Degree of carotid stenosis
D. Presence of ulcerated carotid plaque
E. Risk of death from coronary artery disease

Schwartz: 944

Comments: Cervical bruits reflect disturbances of flow and may result from carotid or noncarotid sources such as cardiac valvular disease. The presence of a bruit is not a reliable indicator of hemodynamically significant stenosis or the risk of cerebral ischemia. Only one half of patients with hemodynamically significant lesions have a cervical bruit, and only approximately one third of patients with bruits have hemodynamically significant lesions. In some studies, the stroke rate has been higher than expected when bruits were detected, but strokes have often involved the contralateral side. Studies have demonstrated, however, a correlation between cervical bruits and subsequent risk of coronary artery disease. Despite the poor correlation between the mere presence of a cervical bruit and ipsilateral cerebral ischemia, bruits should not be ignored and should prompt a noninvasive evaluation to exclude significant carotid lesions.

Answer: E

5. Which of the following is the best screening test for significant carotid stenosis in the patient with an asymptomatic bruit?

A. Oculoplethysmography and supraorbital Doppler monitoring
B. Four-vessel cerebral angiography
C. Digital subtraction angiography
D. CT brain scan with infusion
E. Electroencephalography

Sabiston: 1849
Schwartz: 945

Comments: Because of their sensitivity, safety, and repeatability, noninvasive cerebrovascular studies provide the best means of screening patients with asymptomatic bruits for the detection of significant stenotic lesions. Oculoplethysmography and supraorbital Doppler monitoring are about 90% accurate in the detection of significant stenotic lesions, although they cannot quantify the degree of stenosis. Real time "B" mode ultrasonography or duplex scanning (combines ultrasonography and frequency spectrum analysis) provide noninvasive methods of quantifying the degree of stenosis and of assessing morphologic characteristics. The definitive method of evaluating carotid anatomy in most centers remains angiography. The study is not without risk, however, and so is not advocated as a screening procedure. Digital subtraction angiography has been evaluated as a screening

tool in asymptomatic patients, but has been found to have limited usefulness.

Answer: A

6. Which of the following statements is/are true regarding asymptomatic carotid stenosis?

A. If symptoms eventually develop, they invariably will involve transient ischemic attacks (TIA's), not stroke
B. Incidence of subsequent TIA's is increased compared with that in patients without stenosis
C. Incidence of subsequent stroke is increased compared with that in patients without stenosis
D. Cerebral ischemic events can be decreased by prophylactic carotid endarterectomy

Sabiston: 1852
Schwartz: 945, 947

Comments: The value of prophylactic carotid endarterectomy in asymptomatic stenosis is predicated upon a progressive natural history of the disease process and the ability to perform endarterectomy with low morbidity and mortality. Several studies indicate that asymptomatic patients with hemodynamically significant carotid stenosis (reduction of at least 50% of the arterial diameter) have a higher percentage of cerebral ischemic events than patients without stenosis, and that carotid endarterectomy in a prophylactic setting decreases the expected risk of cerebral ischemic events. There is controversy, however, about the precise relationship of carotid stenosis to subsequent cerebral ischemic events, the initial manifestation of those events, and the efficacy of prophylactic endarterectomy in reducing the risk of stroke.

Answer: B, C, D

7. A patient with symptomatic carotid stenosis is found to have a 50% stenosis of the contralateral carotid artery. Appropriate initial treatment includes which of the following?

A. Simultaneous bilateral carotid endarterectomy
B. Staged bilateral carotid endarterectomy with a 1-week interval
C. Carotid endarterectomy on the symptomatic side only
D. Carotid endarterectomy on the side with the greatest stenosis regardless of symptoms

Sabiston: 1852
Schwartz: 945, 947

Comments: The long-term risk of asymptomatic carotid stenosis, whether associated with contralateral symptomatic disease or not, is not fully defined. Evaluation of patients with symptomatic disease who are found to have asymptomatic stenosis on the contralateral side suggests that 10 to 15% of patients may develop TIA's related to the asymptomatic lesion and approximately 1% will suffer stroke. This is for lesions with 50 to 75% stenosis. The risk for patients with more significant narrowing is not known and may be higher. It would appear, therefore, that patients with asymptomatic contralateral disease can be managed expectantly and that cerebral ischemic symptoms, when they do develop, will predominantly be in the form of TIA's, which can be treated when they become manifest.

Answer: C

8. Which of the following statements is/are true regarding the asymptomatic patient with an ulcerated carotid plaque?

A. Cerebral ischemia may occur even in the absence of significant associated stenosis
B. TIA's are more likely to develop than in patients with asymptomatic stenosis
C. Stroke is more likely to develop as the first manifestation of cerebral ischemia than in patients with asymptomatic stenosis
D. Treatment with aspirin or antiplatelet drugs decreases the risk of stroke

Schwartz: 945

Comments: The increasing recognition of arterioarterial emboli from ulcerated atherosclerotic plaques as the cause of cerebral ischemic events has generated interest in pharmacologic alteration of blood coagulability as a means of preventive treatment. Studies have suggested that aspirin and antiplatelet drugs may be of benefit in certain patients with TIA's, but there are no data demonstrating the benefit of these medicines in patients with asymptomatic carotid disease. Treatment of asymptomatic patients by these measures is therefore entirely empiric. Likewise, the natural history of asymptomatic ulcerated carotid plaques is not defined, and there are no prospective trials from which absolute treatment guidelines can be formulated. Risk of subsequent stroke does seem to correlate with size and multiplicity of ulcerated lesions, so prophylactic operative treatment of patients with large or multiple lesions has been advocated.

Answer: A

9. True statements about the technique of carotid endarterectomy include which one or more of the following?

A. The hypoglossal and superior laryngeal nerves are preserved
B. An intra-arterial shunt is routinely required to prevent ischemic injury
C. Arterial patch grafts are strictly avoided owing to the increased risk of thrombosis
D. The procedure may be performed using a local anesthetic

Sabiston: 1849
Schwartz: 947

Comments: Carotid endarterectomy is generally performed via an incision at the anterior border of the sternocleidomastoid muscle. The hypoglossal, vagus, and superior laryngeal nerves are immediately adjacent to the surgical field and must be preserved. Cerebral flow may be maintained during the procedure by the use of an intra-arterial shunt; some surgeons employ this routinely, others selectively based upon assessment of adequacy of collateral cerebral flow according to measurement of stump pressure in the occluded internal carotid artery

and monitoring of electroencephalographic changes or neurologic changes experienced by the patient when the procedure is carried out with use of a local anesthetic. Following endarterectomy, a patch graft of saphenous vein or prosthetic material should be used if the vessel is narrowed.

Answer: A, D

10. True statements regarding long-term results of carotid endarterectomy include which of the following?

A. Rate of restenosis is 10 to 15%
B. Restenosis most commonly presents as stroke
C. Ischemic cerebral events are the main cause of late death
D. Restenosis rates are higher when endarterectomy is performed for symptomatic disease than when it is performed for asymptomatic disease

Schwartz: 947

Comments: The operative morbidity and mortality rates for carotid endarterectomy approximate 5% and 1%, respectively. Coronary artery disease is the main cause of both immediate and late postoperative deaths. A significant rate of restenosis is recognized following carotid endarterectomy, although many of these lesions are asymptomatic and not hemodynamically significant. Nevertheless, the risk of restenosis must be considered when recommending prophylactic endarterectomy for asymptomatic patients.

Answer: A

11. Choose the correct statement(s). Symptoms of vertebral basilar ischemia:

A. Include diplopia, dysarthria, vertigo, and tinnitus
B. Are usually indistinguishable from those of carotid insufficiency
C. Usually reflect unilateral vertebral disease
D. Most commonly are caused by emboli

Schwartz: 944, 948

Comments: Stenosis of the vertebral artery usually involves a localized segment near the origin from the subclavian. Unlike carotid plaques, the stenotic lesions are usually smooth and nonulcerated, and ischemia is generally attributed to decreased flow rather than an embolic phenomenon. Unilateral vertebral stenosis is unusual. Symptoms generally reflect bilateral disease; associated atherosclerotic involvement of the basilar artery is also common. Symptoms of vertebral basilar insufficiency are those of brain stem ischemia and produce a characteristic clinical syndrome quite distinct from the cerebral hemispheric ischemia produced by carotid disease.

Answer: A

12. The majority of patients with "subclavian steal" syndrome have:

A. Reversal of flow in the involved vertebral artery
B. Disabling neurologic symptoms
C. Upper extremity claudication

D. Decreased systolic blood pressure in the ipsilateral arm

Sabiston: 1854
Schwartz: 944, 948

Comments: "Subclavian steal" syndrome refers to reversal of flow in the ipsilateral vertebral artery distal to occlusion of the left subclavian artery or, less commonly, the innominate artery. Most patients with this phenomenon are asymptomatic, although limb weakness and paresthesias or symptoms of vertebral basilar insufficiency may occur. Patients with subclavian disease alone do not develop strokes. However, most affected patients have associated atherosclerotic disease of other extracranial arteries, particularly the carotid vessels, which may contribute to symptoms of cerebral ischemia.

Answer: A, D

13. Which of the following is/are appropriate treatment(s) for symptomatic "subclavian steal" syndrome?

A. Subclavian endarterectomy
B. Carotid-subclavian bypass
C. Axilloaxillary bypass
D. Intra-arterial streptokinase

Sabiston: 1856
Schwartz: 948

Comments: Since most patients with the abnormal flow phenomena demonstrated in "subclavian steal" are asymptomatic, surgical treatment is not required. Furthermore, some patients with subclavian steal have symptoms on the basis of other extracranial arterial disease and benefit from therapy directed at carotid disease. For patients whose symptoms are attributed to the subclavian steal phenomenon, a variety of surgical procedures have been proposed. Currently, carotid-subclavian and axilloaxillary bypass are both considered acceptable.

Answer: B, C

14. A patient with a carotid bruit is about to undergo abdominal surgery. In which of the following situations is the risk of perioperative stroke clearly increased?

A. Any patient with a carotid bruit
B. Symptomatic bruits only
C. Asymptomatic bruits without significant stenosis revealed by noninvasive studies
D. Asymptomatic bruits with significant stenosis revealed by noninvasive studies
E. None of the above

Sabiston: 1849
Schwartz: 945

Comments: The risk of perioperative stroke in patients undergoing general surgical procedures is not related to the mere presence of a carotid bruit. Furthermore, although the data are conflicting, it appears that there is no increase in the perioperative stroke rate among patients with significant carotid stenosis demonstrated by noninvasive studies. Although it has long been speculated that the mechanism of perioperative stroke is related to hypotension in the presence of carotid occlusive disease, this mechanism has not been substantiated and, in fact, many perioperative strokes may result from embolic phenomena. There are insufficient data to draw firm conclusions about the perioperative risk of stroke in patients who are symptomatic or who have severe carotid stenosis. These patients are often selected for prophylactic endarterectomy prior to other surgical procedures. There is an increased incidence of late TIA's among patients with asymptomatic carotid lesions discovered preoperatively. For these reasons, preoperative patients with incidental carotid bruits should be evaluated for the presence of significant lesions and considered for carotid endarterectomy prior to elective abdominal surgery according to the same criteria used to select patients with asymptomatic bruits discovered under other circumstances. In addition, it is important to note that patients with carotid stenoses discovered preoperatively have a higher incidence of postoperative myocardial infarction, and the possibility of coexistent coronary artery disease should be assessed.

Answer: E

15. Select the true statement(s) regarding carotid artery aneurysms.

A. Most are false aneurysms resulting from carotid endarterectomy
B. The main risk is cerebral embolism
C. They are usually bilateral
D. Resection and ligation are equally acceptable treatments

Sabiston: 1821
Schwartz: 956

Comments: Carotid artery aneurysms are rare; atherosclerosis is the primary cause of them. Less frequently they result from cystic medial necrosis, trauma, or infection. Most commonly, the lesions involve the common carotid bifurcation and are unilateral. The primary risk and indication for operation is the threat of cerebral ischemia due to embolism of thrombotic material from the aneurysm. Occasionally, rupture or symptoms due to compression of adjacent neural structures (hoarseness, dysphagia, tongue weakness, Horner's syndrome) may occur. The treatment of choice is resection with reconstruction, either by direct anastomosis or by graft interposition. An important consideration during resection is the maintenance of cerebral flow to prevent ischemic injury. In patients who require ligation, an extracranial-intracranial bypass may be necessary.

Answer: B

16. Carotid body tumors most commonly present with:

A. Hypertension
B. Painless neck mass
C. Cranial nerve deficit
D. Horner's syndrome
E. Cerebral ischemia

Sabiston: 1824
Schwartz: 588

Comments: Carotid body tumors are the most common form of chemodectoma, which is a paraganglionoma arising from neural crest tissue. The lesions are located at the carotid bifurcation, where these cells normally function as chemoreceptors. Often these are slow-growing tumors, but they may display malignant behavior because of histology, local growth or recurrence, or lymphatic and hematogenous metastases. Most commonly, they present as a painless neck mass, although symptoms may result from compression of the vagus, hypoglossal, glossopharyngeal, or sympathetic nerves. Arteriography is the definitive method of diagnosis. Excision is the recommended treatment and is indicated for symptomatic lesions, enlarging lesions, and suspected malignancy and in young patients. Observation may be appropriate for elderly patients with asymptomatic, stable lesions.

Answer: B

17. A patient with a carotid bruit is about to undergo elective abdominal surgery. In which of the following situations is the risk of perioperative stroke clearly increased?

A. Any patient with a carotid bruit
B. Symptomatic bruits only
C. Asymptomatic bruits without significant stenosis on noninvasive studies
D. Asymptomatic bruits with significant stenosis on noninvasive studies
E. None of the above

Sabiston: 1849
Schwartz: 945

Comments: The risk of perioperative stroke in patients undergoing general surgical procedures is not related to the mere presence of a carotid bruit. Furthermore, although the data are conflicting, it appears that there is no increase in the perioperative stroke rate among patients with significant carotid stenosis demonstrated by noninvasive studies. Although it has long been speculated that the mechanism of perioperative stroke is related to hypotension in the presence of carotid occlusive disease, this mechanism has not been substantiated and, in fact, many perioperative strokes may result from embolic phenomenon. There are insufficient data to draw firm conclusions about the perioperative risk of stroke in patients who are symptomatic or who have severe carotid stenosis. These patients are often selected for prophylactic endarterectomy prior to other surgical procedures. There is an increased incidence of late TIA's among patients with asymptomatic carotid lesions discovered preoperatively. For these reasons, preoperative patients with incidental carotid bruits should be evaluated for the presence of significant lesions and considered for carotid endarterectomy prior to elective abdominal surgery according to the same criteria used to select patients with asymptomatic bruits discovered under other circumstances. In addition, it is important to note that patients with carotid stenoses discovered preoperatively have a higher incidence of postoperative myocardial infarction, and the possibility of coexistent coronary artery disease should be assessed.

Answer: E

CHAPTER 38

Vascular—Thoracic

1. True statements regarding ascending aortic aneurysms include:

A. They are most often caused by atherosclerosis
B. They may be related to earlier venereal disease
C. Most dissecting aneurysms begin in the ascending aorta
D. The connective tissue of the aortic wall is normal in the majority of cases

Sabiston: 1795, 1797
Schwartz: 873

Comments: Etiologic factors involved in aortic aneurysms vary in their frequency according to the location of the aneurysm. In the ascending aorta, a connective tissue abnormality recognized histologically as cystic medial necrosis is the most common underlying abnormality and is the defect seen in aneurysms associated with Marfan's syndrome. Syphilitic aneurysms are steadily decreasing in frequency, and atherosclerotic aneurysms of the ascending aorta are relatively uncommon. Most dissecting aneurysms do originate in the ascending aorta.

Answer: B, C

2. Which of the following statements is/are true regarding the clinical characteristics and management of ascending aortic aneurysms:

A. The most common clinical presentation is that of a pulsatile substernal mass
B. Bruits heard over the aneurysm are quite common; valvular murmurs, however, are rare
C. Aortography is contraindicated because of the risk of causing dissection of the aneurysm with the catheter
D. Operative management with placement of a composite graft of aortic conduit and aortic valve is the treatment of choice for all ascending aortic aneurysms
E. None of the above

Sabiston: 1795
Schwartz: 873

Comments: Although the relatively uncommon saccular ascending aortic aneurysm may present as a mass in the anterior chest wall, patients are often asymptomatic and their aneurysms frequently are detected on routine chest x-ray. When symptoms are present, frequently they relate to congestive heart failure that is caused by dilatation of the aortic annulus, resulting in aortic insufficiency and its characteristic murmur. Aortography confirms the diagnosis and is important in defining the extent of the aneurysm as well as its relationship to the rest of the aorta, its major branches, and the coronary ostia. Although surgical correction is clearly the treatment of choice, debate persists over the routine use of a composite valve/conduit graft. It is widely used, however, when the aneurysm is associated with massive dilatation of the aortic annulus or is of the Marfan variety.

Answer: E

3. The superior vena cava syndrome is characterized by which of the following:

A. The majority of cases are due to obstruction from malignant tumors
B. Venous pressures rarely exceed 15 mmHg
C. Acute obstruction is rarely clinically significant because of the large number of collateral vessels available
D. The fully developed syndrome is difficult to differentiate clinically from congestive heart failure or from constrictive pericarditis
E. Surgical correction is rarely indicated

Sabiston: 1728
Schwartz: 892

Comments: Greater than 90% of cases of superior vena caval obstruction are due to malignant tumors, most often mediastinal invasion by bronchogenic carcinoma. When obstruction occurs, venous pressures rise to levels of between 20 and 50 mmHg. Acute complete obstruction can produce fatal cerebral edema as well as significant edematous laryngeal obstruction. A more gradual onset of obstruction results in the characteristic clinical picture of facial swelling and dilatation of the collateral veins of the head and neck, arm, and upper thoracic areas. In such circumstances, the clinical differentiation from congestive heart failure or constrictive pericarditis is usually obvious. The treatment of choice for obstruction due to associated malignancy is prompt radiation therapy. Surgery is rarely indicated in the management because of the technical difficulties associated with vena caval grafts, the underlying poor prognosis in malignant conditions, and the usual adequacy of collateral venous circulation in the rare instances of slowly developing obstruction from benign conditions.

Answer: A, E

4. Match the aneurysms with their most common associated etiology:

Aneurysm	Etiology
A. Ascending aorta	a. Atherosclerosis
B. Transverse aortic arch	b. Connective tissue disorder
C. Descending thoracic aorta	c. Syphilis
D. Thoracoabdominal	d. Trauma

Sabiston: 1793
Schwartz: 873

Comments: Atherosclerosis is the most common etiologic factor associated with transverse, descending, and thoracoabdominal aortic aneurysms. It is relatively uncommon as a cause of ascending aortic aneurysms, which are most often due to cystic medial necrosis. Transverse thoracic and thoracoabdominal aortic aneurysms are rarely due to causes other than atherosclerosis; however, descending thoracic aortic aneurysms may be seen as a result of trauma or of syphilitic degeneration.

Answer: A–b; B–a; C–a; D–a

5. Match the items in the two columns:

A. Aortogram should be performed in most cases	a. Penetrating chest injury
B. Tamponade poses a life-threatening problem	b. Deceleration chest injury
C. Fatal hemorrhage is sometimes prevented by the aortic adventitia	c. Both
D. Thoracotomy may be indicated	d. Neither

Sabiston: 300
Schwartz: 888

Comments: Both penetrating and deceleration injuries of the thoracic aorta frequently are fatal. When the patient is in extremis from exsanguination, thoracotomy in the emergency room to control hemorrhage may be indicated even though frequently it is unsuccessful. In the clinically stable patient, aortography is indicated in both types of injury to define the anatomy of the injury as it may influence the surgical approach. In penetrating injuries, pericardial tamponade, in addition to exsanguination, is a major cause of death. In deceleration injuries, complete disruption of the aorta is nearly always fatal. In some instances, however, the adventitia remains intact, confining the hemorrhage and allowing time for surgical correction.

Answer: A–c; B–a; C–b; D–c

6. Traumatic thoracic aortic aneurysms are characterized by which of the following:

A. They almost invariably arise from partial aortic transection due to closed chest trauma
B. Survival without repair beyond 2 months from the injury is extremely rare
C. Most arise just distal to the origin of the left subclavian artery
D. Hoarseness may be a presenting complaint

Sabiston: 305
Schwartz: 876

Comment: Traumatic thoracic aortic aneurysms are false aneurysms, most commonly resulting from horizontal deceleration injury. Fixation of the aorta within the chest cavity at the ligamentum arteriosum is thought to explain the common location of aneurysms at this site, which corresponds to the origin of the left subclavian artery. Unlike aneurysms from other causes, traumatic thoracic aneurysms may enlarge slowly and present 10 to 20 years after the traumatic event. Enlargement of the aneurysm may result in compression of the left recurrent laryngeal nerve, the left main stem bronchus, or the esophagus, producing hoarseness, dyspnea, or dysphagia. Although elective excision is recommended in the majority of patients, an asymptomatic small aneurysm discovered later than 10 years after the injury may, in select circumstances, be observed.

Answer: A, C, D

7. Match the items in the two columns:

Clinical Feature	Type of Aortic Dissection
A. Related to Marfan's syndrome	a. Type A
B. Readily accessible to surgical excision	b. Type B
C. Arises distal to the left subclavian artery and extends into the abdomen	c. Type C1
D. Involves entire thoracic and abdominal aorta	d. Type C2

Sabiston: 1797
Schwartz: 886

Comments: Aortic dissections have been classified according to their site of origin and degree of aortic involvement. **Type A** originates in the ascending aorta and dissects throughout the entire thoracic and abdominal aorta. **Type B** originates in the ascending aorta but is confined to that segment of the aorta and is the type commonly seen in Marfan's syndrome. **Type C1** originates distal to the left subclavian artery but remains confined to the descending thoracic aorta, making it accessible for total excision via left thoracotomy. **Type C2** originates distal to the left subclavian artery but dissects down into the abdominal aorta, which complicates its surgical repair. There are other very similar classifications whose focus is to help the surgeon with clinical judgment or choice of operative technique.

Answer: A–b; B–c; C–d; D–a

8. Which of the following statements regarding thoracoabdominal aneurysms is/are correct:

A. They are considerably less common than aortic aneurysms occurring below the renal arteries
B. They are usually palpable owing to large size
C. They usually expand at a rapid rate with frequent spontaneous rupture
D. A stable aneurysm in an asymptomatic patient does not require repair
E. Paraplegia is a recognized complication of repair

Sabiston: 1816, 1834
Schwartz: 881

Comments: Thoracoabdominal aneurysms occur primarily in older patients with extensive atherosclerosis and are rare compared with infrarenal aortic aneurysms. The cephalad location of the abdominal component frequently precludes palpation. These aneurysms usually enlarge at a very slow rate, with symptoms being caused by the gradual compression and displacement of adjacent structures. Technical difficulties in surgical repair, including the need to reimplant the celiac, superior mesenteric, and renal arteries, increase the risk of this operation sufficiently that repair is usually warranted only for symptomatic or significantly enlarging aneurysms. Paraplegia due to temporary or permanent loss of spinal cord blood flow can occur.

Answer: A, D, E

9. Correct statements regarding transverse aortic arch aneurysms include:

A. Syphilitic medial necrosis was formerly a major cause
B. Repair of these aneurysms is associated with the highest operative mortality of any of the aortic aneurysms
C. Differentiation from mediastinal tumors is easily done on standard chest x-ray

D. Hypothermia/low-flow techniques and cardiopulmonary bypass have significantly reduced the mortality of repairing these aneurysms

Sabiston: 1818
Schwartz: 875

Comments: Transverse aortic arch aneurysms are almost always the result of atherosclerosis. In the asymptomatic individual, frequently they are detected on routine chest x-ray. Aortography or computed tomography is required, however, to differentiate them from mediastinal tumors and to define the vascular anatomy prior to repair. Concomitant association with coronary and cerebrovascular disease together with the need to temporarily disrupt flow to the brain during repair have resulted in an operative mortality exceeding that of other aortic aneurysms. The introduction of cardiopulmonary bypass and low-flow hypothermia technique has significantly reduced this operative mortality.

Answer: B, D

10. The most common site of rupture of the aorta in patients who sustain blunt trauma to the chest is:

A. Ascending aorta at cardiac junction
B. Below the left subclavian artery at the point of insertion of the ligamentum arteriosus
C. At the level of the diaphragm
D. At or immediately before the takeoff of the innominate artery

Sabiston: 305
Schwartz: 890

Comments: Eighty-five to 90% of patients who sustain an aortic rupture die at the scene. In the vast majority of the patients who survive, the rupture is located at the aortic isthmus (immediately distal to the origin of the left subclavian). Of these survivors, 20% will die within 6 hours and 72% will die within 1 week. Patients who sustain rupture of the ascending aorta rarely survive to reach the hospital.

Answer: B

CHAPTER 39

Vascular—Abdominal Aorta

1. Which one or more of the following may be acceptable treatment(s) for occlusive aortoiliac disease?

A. Thromboendarterectomy
B. Aortofemoral bypass
C. Axillofemoral bypass
D. Percutaneous balloon angioplasty

Sabiston: 1860, 1874
Schwartz: 904

Comments: The basic principle of arterial revascularization is to provide adequate inflow and outflow. In patients with occlusive aortoiliac disease requiring surgery, a variety of techniques are applicable depending upon the site and extent of obstruction, the presence or absence of aneurysmal disease, and the patient's underlying medical condition. The majority of patients are managed by aortofemoral bypass grafting with excellent results in terms of immediate and long-term patency and relief of claudication. Thromboendarterectomy, although contraindicated by concomitant aneurysmal disease, is appropriate for some patients and has produced comparable results to bypass grafting. In some instances, aortofemoral bypass and localized endarterectomy are combined. For patients in whom an abdominal operation may pose excessive risk, extra-anatomical bypass grafts (axillofemoral, femorofemoral) have been successful. Percutaneous balloon angioplasty has been used to reconstitute blood flow at numerous sites in the arterial tree and has been particularly successful for isolated segmental lesions of the iliac artery with 3-year patency rates of 80 to 90%. Angioplasty has also been used as an adjunct to surgical revascularization where dilatation of an iliac stenosis can provide inflow for a more distal femoral popliteal bypass. Disadvantages of percutaneous angioplasty include a lower rate of initial success (compared with conventional bypass techniques) and a higher rate of embolic complications.

Answer: A, B, C, D

2. Which of the following statements is/are true regarding the late complications of aortic bypass grafts?

A. Most late deaths are due to complications of progressive peripheral vascular disease
B. Most late deaths are due to coronary artery disease
C. The most frequent late complication is graft occlusion due to anastomotic thrombosis
D. The most frequent late complication is graft occlusion due to progressive atherosclerosis of the graft

Schwartz: 904, 910

Comments: The long-term patency rates of aortofemoral bypass grafts are reported to range from approximately 65 to 90%. The most frequent late complications are graft infection and false aneurysms, which occur at the suture line. Associated coronary artery disease is the leading cause of late death following aortic reconstruction. Since atherosclerosis is a diffuse process, patients presenting with signs or symptoms of occlusive peripheral vascular disease require thorough evaluation for associated coronary or cerebrovascular atherosclerosis.

Answer: B

3. Which of the following is the most common clinical manifestation of an abdominal aortic aneurysm?

A. Chronic peripheral ischemia
B. Peripheral embolization
C. Acute rupture
D. Back pain
E. Most are asymptomatic

Sabiston: 1830
Schwartz: 949

Comments: Most abdominal aortic aneurysms are discovered incidentally and, therefore, are asymptomatic. Occasionally, patients may note low back pain or epigastric pain. When complications related to an abdominal aortic aneurysm ensue, a variety of manifestations are possible. Rupture may mimic other acute intra-abdominal conditions and present with vascular collapse. Signs and symptoms of acute ischemia to the lower extremities may follow thrombosis or embolization from an abdominal aneurysm.

Answer: E

4. Which of the following is the most common associated manifestation of atherosclerotic disease seen in patients with abdominal aortic aneurysms?

A. Thoracic aortic aneurysm
B. Occlusive peripheral vascular disease
C. Coronary artery disease
D. Carotid stenosis
E. Renovascular hypertension

Sabiston: 1830
Schwartz: 949

Comments: Atherosclerosis is the etiology of most abdominal aortic aneurysms; rare causes include syphilis, trauma, and Marfan's syndrome. Since atherosclerosis is a generalized process, patients with abdominal aortic aneurysm frequently have vascular pathology in other areas as well, particularly involving the coronary arteries. Nearly one half of patients with untreated abdominal aortic aneurysms die from related atherosclerotic problems such as cardiac, cerebral, or renal disease. For these reasons, it is important to carefully evaluate patients with abdominal aortic aneurysms for evidence of associated atherosclerotic problems.

Answer: C

5. Which of the following best summarizes indications for operation on an abdominal aortic aneurysm?

A. Any abdominal aortic aneurysm
B. Only symptomatic aneurysms
C. Only symptomatic aneurysms greater than 5 cm in diameter
D. Any aneurysm greater than 5 cm in diameter

Schwartz: 950

Comments: The natural history of an abdominal aortic aneurysm is progressive enlargement, and the risk of rupture is directly related to the size of the aneurysm. One half to two thirds of deaths in patients with untreated abdominal aortic aneurysms are due to rupture. The risk of rupture in patients with 5- to 6-cm aortic aneurysms is approximately 20% per year. Rupture commonly occurs in asymptomatic aneurysms, although the presence of acute back, flank, or abdominal pain suggests impending rupture and is an indication for operation on an emergency basis. Ultrasonography provides a reliable and noninvasive method of following patients with small asymptomatic aneurysms. In otherwise healthy patients with enlarging aneurysms, even if they are smaller than 5 cm, surgical intervention should be considered.

Answer: D

6. Arteriography is the best method for defining which one or more of the following in regard to abdominal aortic aneurysms?

A. Presence of an aneurysm when suspected clinically
B. Aneurysm size
C. Patency of tributary vessels
D. Distal occlusive disease

Sabiston: 1832
Schwartz: 950

Comments: An abdominal aortic aneurysm should be suspected in a patient in whom the abdominal aortic pulsation is palpated to be larger than 1 inch in diameter. Radiologic confirmation and delineation of anatomic characteristics can be accomplished with ultrasonography, CT scan, or arteriography. Since it is reliable, noninvasive, and relatively inexpensive, ultrasonography is the preferred method for initial radiologic diagnosis and for following patients with small aneurysms. Arteriography is most useful in evaluation of associated distal occlusive disease, suprarenal extent of the aneurysm, and the patency of renal, celiac, and mesenteric vessels. All of these are important considerations at the time of operation. Since a thrombus may be present within the aneurysm, contrast visualization of the lumen alone may not give an accurate assessment of the true size of the aneurysm.

Answer: C, D

7. Select the true statement(s) regarding operative technique in repair of abdominal aortic aneurysms.

A. Bifurcation grafts are preferred to straight grafts even if the iliac vessels are uninvolved
B. The aneurysm should be excised as completely as possible
C. Bleeding lumbar vessels are routinely ligated
D. The inferior mesenteric artery is routinely reimplanted in elderly patients

Sabiston: 1834
Schwartz: 953

Comments: Although details of operative technique will vary somewhat depending upon individual circumstances, several general principles are followed to minimize complications. Proximal and distal control are established, with care taken to identify the left renal vein and to clamp the proximal aorta distal to the renal vessels. The aneurysm is opened and the thrombus evacuated. The lumbar vessels are ligated. The inferior mesenteric artery can usually be safely ligated at its origin; however, flow to at least one hypogastric artery should be preserved in order to maintain the collateral flow to the colon via the middle hemorrhoidal arteries. In some instances in which the aneurysm is extensive, the celiac, superior mesenteric, and renal arteries may be involved and require more complex revascularization procedures. Following graft placement, proper techniques of aortic flushing and sequential unclamping are important so as to minimize the risk of hypotension and of distal embolization. The aneurysm sac is not extensively resected and is closed over the prosthetic graft in order to isolate the graft from the duodenum and minimize the risk of late aortoduodenal fistula.

Answer: C

8. Two days following repair of an abdominal aortic aneurysm, a patient who is still on antibiotics develops bloody diarrhea. The differential diagnosis includes:

A. Inadequate heparin reversal
B. Pseudomembranous colitis
C. Ischemic colitis
D. Aortoenteric fistula
E. Acute hepatic failure

Sabiston: 1836
Schwartz: 954

Comments: The main concern in this situation is that the patient has developed ischemic colitis as a result of interruption of flow to the inferior mesenteric artery and inadequate collateral supply to the sigmoid colon. Pseudomembranous enterocolitis associated with antibiotic use is also a consideration. Aortoenteric fistula is a late complication of aortic aneurysm repair, resulting from erosion of a false aneurysm at the suture line into the duodenum or sigmoid colon. Proctosigmoidoscopy is important in the initial evaluation of such a patient in order to assess mucosal viability. If the mucosa is nonviable or if the patient has signs and symptoms of abdominal sepsis, immediate laparotomy is warranted with resection of compromised bowel and colostomy. Evaluation for the possibility of pseudomembranous colitis includes proctosigmoidoscopy and examination of stool for *Clostridium difficile* titers and enteric pathogens. Treatment in the latter case involves supportive measures and the administration of vancomycin or metronidazole.

Answer: B, C

9. Which of the following complications occurs most commonly following repair of an abdominal aortic aneurysm?

A. Impotence
B. Ischemic colitis
C. Renal failure
D. Peripheral embolization
E. Paralysis

Sabiston: 1836
Schwartz: 954

Comments: All of these complications may occur following repair of an abdominal aortic aneurysm. With appropriate operative technique, most of these are uncommon except for disturbance in sexual function manifested as impotence, which has been reported to occur in 25 to 65% of male patients. Disturbance in sexual function results from injury to the autonomic nerve fibers overlying the anterior aorta near the origin of the inferior mesenteric artery and aortic bifurcation. Avoiding excessive aortic dissection in this region should minimize this complication.

Answer: A

10. Rupture is the most common complication of aneurysms involving which of the following vessels?

A. Carotid
B. Subclavian
C. Abdominal aorta
D. Femoral
E. Popliteal

Sabiston: 1832, 1839
Schwartz: 956

Comments: Whereas rupture is the most common complication of an abdominal aortic aneurysm, it is an unusual event when aneurysms involve these other sites. The main hazard of aneurysms of peripheral vessels is distal ischemia as a result of embolism or thrombosis. This risk constitutes an indication for operation when aneurysmal involvement of peripheral arterial sites is discovered.

Answer: C

11. Which of the following statements is/are true regarding rupture of an abdominal aortic aneurysm?

A. It is the most common cause of late death in patients with untreated abdominal aortic aneurysms
B. Associated mortality is 30 to 50%
C. The highest salvage rate is obtained by prompt left thoracotomy for proximal control
D. Renal failure is the leading cause of late postoperative death

Sabiston: 1830, 1836
Schwartz: 954

Comments: Rupture is a catastrophic complication of abdominal aortic aneurysms which may be heralded by abdominal, back, or flank pain and vascular collapse. It is the most common single cause of death among patients with untreated abdominal aneurysms, although patients also frequently die of associated atherosclerotic conditions. The mortality of a ruptured abdominal aneurysm is high compared with the mortality of 5% or less when elective operations are performed. Renal failure is a leading cause of death; mortality also correlates with hypotension, transfusion requirements, operative time, and the time interval prior to operative intervention. Immediate operation is mandatory to save these patients; proximal control generally is obtained in the abdomen just below the diaphragm and above the stomach. Since left thoracotomy is occasionally required for control, access to the chest as well as the abdomen should be provided for when preparing the patient in the operating room.

Answer: A, B, D

CHAPTER 40

Vascular—Peripheral

1. Which of the following statements is/are true about the manifestations of occlusive arterial disease of the lower extremities?

A. Claudication is virtually diagnostic of chronic arterial occlusion
B. Rest pain usually occurs in the same muscle groups affected by claudication
C. Nutritional changes such as hair loss and brittle nails generally precede symptoms of claudication
D. Tissue necrosis is more likely in the presence of distal arterial disease
E. Arterial ulcerations, like those of venous insufficiency, characteristically begin near the malleoli

Sabiston: 1863
Schwartz: 898, 901

Comments: Chronic arterial occlusion of the lower extremities is the result of atherosclerotic disease of the aorta and its branches and can be diagnosed by characteristic signs and symptoms. The classic symptom of intermittent claudication refers to cramping pain in specific muscle groups that occurs when blood flow is inadequate to meet the demands of exercise. The pain usually occurs below the level of occlusion, so that claudication of the buttock and thigh muscles suggests aortoiliac obstruction and calf claudication suggests femoral artery obstruction. As chronic ischemia progresses, trophic changes such as hair loss, brittle nails, and muscular atrophy occur. Ischemic rest pain is a manifestation of end-stage disease and characteristically involves the more distal aspects of the arterial circulation such as the toes and feet. Associated physical findings include exacerbation of pain with extremity elevation and dependent rubor due to reactive hyperemia. Tissue necrosis usually signifies disease of the distal arterial tree, since chronic proximal occlusion alone is associated with the development of collaterals often adequate to prevent necrosis and gangrene. Most ulcers from arterial insufficiency involve the toes or plantar surface of the foot and are painful, whereas venous ulcers are less painful and typically occur near the malleoli.

Answer: A, D

2. The most common site for atherosclerotic occlusion in the lower extremities is the:

A. Aortic bifurcation
B. Common femoral artery
C. Profunda femoris artery
D. Proximal superficial femoral artery
E. Distal superficial femoral artery

Schwartz: 910

Comments: Although atherosclerotic disease frequently involves the area of arterial bifurcations such as the aortic, iliac, and common femoral, the most common site of occlusion in the lower extremities is the distal superficial femoral artery. This occurs in the adductor canal proximal to the popliteal fossa and may be related to the anatomic relationship of the artery to the adductor magnus tendon at this site. Patients frequently have disease at multiple levels, however, emphasizing the need for accurate angiographic assessment prior to revascularization procedures. Involvement of the superficial femoral artery alone is associated with intermittent claudication but not generally with more serious signs of ischemia. This is because the profunda femoris artery is not usually occluded and serves as an important source of collateral blood flow. Distal tibioperoneal disease is characteristically found in diabetics.

Answer: E

3. A 55-year-old male complains of inability to maintain an erection and of thigh claudication after walking 3 blocks. Examination is likely to reveal which one or more of the following?

A. Absent femoral pulses
B. Pulsating abdominal mass
C. Toe ulceration or gangrene
D. Lower extremity hair loss and brittle nails

Sabiston: 1859
Schwartz: 902

Comments: Leriche is credited with describing chronic aortoiliac occlusive disease and its characteristic manifestations. Often, there is a significant thrombotic component associated with the atherosclerotic process, particularly in younger patients. The common clinical manifestations are intermittent claudication of the thigh or buttock and impotence due to decreased hypogastric blood flow. Femoral, popliteal, and pedal pulses are diminished or absent and there may be lower limb atrophy. With aortoiliac involvement alone, however, trophic changes are not present because collateral flow originating from the lumbar arteries is preserved. Nutritional changes, when present, signify additional distal disease. Although necrotic lesions also suggest additional distal occlusion, the possibility of emboli from atherosclerotic plaques in the aortoiliac vessels must always be considered. This has been referred to as the blue toe syndrome and can occur even in the absence of occluding lesions. Approximately 10% of patients with occlusive aortoiliac disease may have an associated aortic aneurysm.

Answer: A

4. Any patient who presents with intermittent calf claudication should be advised that:

A. Angiography is indicated to determine extent of arterial disease
B. Surgical reconstruction should be performed to prevent progression of disease
C. Surgical reconstruction is not indicated at present but will likely be required in the future owing to progression of disease
D. Nonoperative treatment will be sufficient for 75% of patients

Sabiston: 1864
Schwartz: 903

Comments: The goals of therapy for occlusive arterial disease of the lower extremities are to relieve pain, prevent limb loss, and maintain bipedal gait. Most patients who present with intermittent claudication alone will remain stable or even improve with appropriate conservative management. Prophylactic surgical intervention is therefore not indicated. The risk of developing gangrene in a limb where intermittent claudication is the only symptom is approximately 5% at 5 years. In contradistinction, patients with rest pain, ulceration, or gangrene have threatened limb loss and should be evaluated for revascularization procedures. Surgical intervention may be indicated in the presence of claudication alone for patients whose life style or livelihood is impaired by their symptoms and who do not otherwise have limiting cardiac disease. Arteriography is indicated only for patients who are considered candidates for operation.

Answer: D

5. Which of the following statements is/are true regarding nonoperative treatment of occlusive atherosclerotic disease of the lower extremities?

A. Exercise to claudication will promote development of collaterals
B. Cessation of cigarette smoking will reduce claudication

C. Foot protection is important since trivial trauma may lead to gangrene
D. Anticoagulant therapy with Coumadin or heparin promotes healing of arterial ulcers

Sabiston: 1865
Schwartz: 903

Comments: The majority of patients with intermittent claudication as their only manifestation of peripheral vascular disease will respond to conservative measures consisting of abstinence from tobacco and a graduated exercise program. Continued tobacco use has been associated with an increased risk of gangrene as well as a higher rate of premature graft failure following reconstructive procedures. For patients with more advanced ischemia, protection of the lower extremity is critical. The patient should avoid temperature extremes, improper foot wear, or overly aggressive trimming of nails and callouses. It is not uncommon for relatively minor trauma to result in gangrene and eventual amputation of an ischemically compromised foot. There is evidence that regular low-dose therapy with acetylsalicylic acid may be of benefit in preventing thrombosis in patients with atherosclerotic disease, but therapy with heparin or warfarin sodium has not proved beneficial.

Answer: A, B, C

6. Which of the following statements is/are true regarding axillofemoral bypass grafts?

A. The left subclavian artery is more often involved with atherosclerosis than the right
B. When the aortic bifurcation is occluded, bilateral axillofemoral grafts rather than unilateral grafts are required to reconstitute flow adequately
C. Operative mortality is lower than that of aortofemoral grafts
D. Unilateral axillofemoral grafts combined with a femoral-femoral graft have a higher patency rate than unilateral axillofemoral grafts alone
E. Unilateral axillofemoral grafts combined with femoral-femoral grafts have a higher patency rate than bilateral axillofemoral grafts

Schwartz: 908, 910

Comments: Extra-anatomic, axillofemoral bypass grafts have been useful in patients with aortoiliac occlusion who are unable to undergo an abdominal procedure and in patients with infection of a previously placed intra-abdominal graft. Although experience with axillofemoral grafts has not been reported as widely as that with aortofemoral bypass, data suggest equivalent short- and long-term patency rates and lower operative mortality in comparable patients. It has also been suggested that the addition of a femoral-femoral graft to a unilateral axillofemoral graft produces better patency rates by providing more adequate arterial outflow. Prior to an axillofemoral graft procedure, the axillary vessels must be evaluated for patency by comparison of upper extremity blood pressure and possibly angiography. Atherosclerotic involvement of the axillary arteries is observed more commonly on the left, and for this reason some prefer to use the right axillary artery.

Answer: A, C, D, E

7. Occlusive tibioperoneal disease occurs most commonly in patients with:

A. Buerger's disease
B. Raynaud's phenomenon
C. Diabetes mellitus
D. Arterial emboli
E. Hyperlipidemia

Schwartz: 912

Comments: Whereas the common pattern of atherosclerotic occlusive disease involves the femoral artery or the more proximal aortoiliac system, diabetic patients characteristically develop a pattern of distal occlusive disease involving the popliteal artery and its branches. This type of distal involvement may also be seen in patients with Buerger's disease or arterioarterial embolism. The reason for this particular distribution of arterial occlusion is unknown. Patients with tibioperoneal involvement often present with more advanced ischemia rather than simple claudication, and arterial reconstruction may require grafts extended to the ankle, which are not as successful as more proximal reconstructions.

Answer: C

8. Which of the following statements is/are true about the diabetic foot?

A. Foot pain due to diabetic neuropathy usually is relieved by dependent positioning
B. Trophic ulcers rarely occur if pedal pulses are palpable
C. Extensive débridement of infected tissue should be avoided because of the risk of nonhealing
D. Surgical revascularization may be required to control infection if there is arterial occlusion

Sabiston: 154
Schwartz: 900, 913, 917

Comments: The diabetic foot is at risk owing to diabetic neuropathy, occlusive arterial disease, and infection. Diabetic neuropathy commonly produces analgesia, rendering the foot susceptible to complications of trivial trauma and trophic ulceration. Trophic ulcers often occur on the plantar surface over the metatarsal heads as the result of pressure necrosis. Such lesions provide entry sites for infection, to which the diabetic foot is markedly susceptible. Control of infection requires aggressive treatment by débridement of all necrotic tissue, systemic antibiotics, and arterial revascularization if there is significant large vessel occlusion. Trophic ulceration and infection can occur in the presence of patent vessels. Arterial reconstruction in diabetic patients with occlusive arterial disease plays an important role in limb salvage. Diabetic neuropathy may also cause pain that is difficult to distinguish from ischemic rest pain. Ischemic pain, however, may be relieved by dependent positioning of the foot, whereas the pain of neuropathy is not.

Answer: D

9. Which of the following statements is/are true regarding femoropopliteal bypass?

A. Reversed saphenous vein autografts have higher long-term patency rates than prosthetic grafts both above and below the knee
B. Patency rates are higher when bypass is performed for claudication rather than for limb salvage
C. Continued cigarette smoking adversely affects graft patency
D. Diabetes adversely affects graft patency
E. Patency rates are unaffected by vein size

Sabiston: 1782, 1868

Comments: The reversed saphenous vein autograft has been the most successful arterial bypass graft below the inguinal ligament and is the standard against which the success of prosthetic grafts is measured. Patency rates for saphenous vein grafts are approximately 80 to 90% at 1 year and approximately 75% at 5 years. Limb salvage rates generally exceed graft patency rates. Patency is adversely affected by grafts performed below the knee, by continued tobacco use, by poor distal runoff, and by small vein size (less than 4 mm). Associated risk factors, such as diabetes, hypertension, and coronary artery disease, have not been shown to exert a detrimental effect on long-term graft patency.

Answer: A, B, C

10. Which one or more of the following may be used for femoropopliteal bypass as an alternative to reversed saphenous vein graft?

A. Polytetrafluoroethylene (PTFE) graft
B. Cephalic vein autograft
C. In-situ saphenous vein graft
D. Umbilical vein allograft
E. Endarterectomy and multiple vein roof patches

Sabiston: 1781, 1866
Schwartz: 911

Comments: In approximately 25% of people, the saphenous vein is inadequate for use as an arterial bypass graft owing to small size, previous disease, or removal. In this setting, a number of different techniques have been used, although none have proved superior to saphenous vein grafting. PTFE grafts have patency rates at 36 months equivalent to those obtained with saphenous vein for above-knee femoropopliteal bypass but are less successful distal to the popliteal artery. In-situ saphenous vein grafting allows a smaller vein to be used as a bypass conduit, and encouraging results have been reported. Uncontrolled reports indicate that in-situ saphenous vein grafts performed distal to the popliteal artery may have higher patency rates than conventional reversed saphenous vein grafts. The best results reported with umbilical vein allografts (modified by glutaraldehyde tanning and covered with a polyester mesh) indicate that they are comparable to the saphenous vein for above-knee sites, but inferior to saphenous vein for more distal grafting. Uniform success has not been reported with umbilical vein grafts, however, and their role is not yet clear. Revascularization by endarterectomy and vein roof patching has been reported to produce results comparable to those of venous bypass. Cephalic vein autografts have generally produced inferior results compared with saphenous vein.

Answer: A, B, C, D, E

11. Indications for tibioperoneal bypass grafting include which one or more of the following?

A. Necrotizing infection
B. Foot claudication
C. Rest pain
D. Ischemic ulceration
E. Gangrene extending proximal to the mid-tarsal level

Schwartz: 913

Comment: Revascularization procedures performed below the knee to the level of the proximal calf or to the ankle are not as successful as more proximal reconstructions and are indicated only for limb salvage. Intermittent foot claudication alone is not an acceptable indication. Revascularization should be considered, however, when there is ischemic rest pain, progressive ischemic gangrene of the forefoot, necrotizing infection (in combination with débridement) or a nonhealing wound. A foot in which gangrene of the sole extends proximal to the mid-tarsal level is not generally considered suitable for weight bearing, and amputation is therefore favored over distal arterial reconstruction. Stable dry gangrene involving single toes also is not alone a sufficient indication for distal arterial reconstruction.

Answer: A, C, D

12. Long-term patency of bypass grafts to the tibioperoneal vessels is influenced by which one or more of the following?

A. Diabetes
B. Level of distal anastomosis
C. Concomitant endarterectomy
D. Previous attempts at revascularization
E. Presence of a patent pedal arch

Sabiston: 1869
Schwartz: 913

Comment: Bypass graft procedures distal to the knee are less successful than proximal procedures, with 5-year patency rates below 50%. Patency is better when the pedal arch is intact angiographically. Grafts to the anterior or posterior tibial arteries are therefore preferred rather than grafts to the peroneal artery because of the usual continuity between these former vessels and the pedal arch. Anastomoses in the proximal calf have better long-term patency rates than those performed at the malleolar level. Concomitant endarterectomy of vessels in the upper calf has produced results similar to those of venous bypass alone. Diabetes has been associated with inferior long-term patency rates, but limb salvage following tibioperoneal bypass is the same as in nondiabetics. Previously performed operative procedures have not adversely affected early or long-term patency rates or limb salvage. The role of sequential grafts, the addition of an arteriovenous fistula to a bypass graft, and the use of postoperative antiplatelet drugs or anticoagulants in improving graft patency rates are difficult to assess. The role of in-situ saphenous vein grafts and PTFE prostheses for distal arterial reconstruction remains under evaluation.

Answer: A, B, E

13. A patient with a history of coronary artery disease and atrial fibrillation develops sudden pain and weakness of the left leg. Examination reveals a cool, pale extremity with absent pulses below the groin and a normal contralateral leg. The most likely diagnosis is:

A. Cerebrovascular accident
B. Arterial thrombosis
C. Arterial embolism
D. Acute thrombophlebitis
E. Dissecting aortic aneurysm

Sabiston: 1907
Schwartz: 919

Comments: See Question 15.

14. Which of the following tests is/are a mandatory part of the initial evaluation?

A. Electrocardiogram
B. Venography
C. Arteriography
D. Abdominal ultrasonography
E. CT head scan

Sabiston: 1908
Schwartz: 919

Comments: See Question 15.

15. If this patient had a history of intermittent left calf claudication and examination showed, in addition, trophic skin changes, then which of the following would be true?

A. Arteriography mandatory to differentiate thrombosis from embolism
B. Venography mandatory to exclude phlegmasia alba dolens
C. Prompt surgical intervention not likely to be required
D. Indications for surgical intervention unchanged
E. Extent of surgical procedure unchanged

Sabiston: 1908
Schwartz: 920, 923

Comments: The classic signs of acute arterial occlusion are pain, pallor, pulselessness, paralysis, and paresthesia (the 5 P's). The common causes of acute arterial occlusion are embolism, thrombosis, and trauma. In the patient presented in Question 13, the history of atrial fibrillation coupled with the classic findings of acute arterial occlusion make embolism the most likely diagnosis. Clinical findings that suggest arterial thrombosis rather than embolism as the cause include an absence of cardiac disease, symptoms of underlying occlusive atherosclerotic disease, and physical findings suggestive of chronic ischemia. It can be difficult, however, to differentiate embolism from thrombosis purely on clinical grounds; certainly, embolism can occur in patients with underlying peripheral vascular disease. Prompt operative intervention is indicated regardless of etiology where there is acute limb-threatening ischemia. It is important, however, to differentiate embolism from primary thrombosis because the extent of operation may vary considerably. Whereas embolism may be successfully treated by simple embolectomy and extraction of the thrombus that forms distal to the embolism, effective treatment of arterial thrombosis can be much more difficult, sometimes requiring arterial reconstruction. Arteriography is helpful in differentiating between embolic and thrombotic occlusions. A careful history and physical examination permit a diagnosis of embolic occlusions in most cases; arteriography is not always necessary and should not be performed if it will delay operative re-establishment of blood flow. Patients with arterial embolism should have electrocardiography and x-ray of the chest because of the high association with intrinsic cardiac disease and its potential for myocardial infarction. Acute arterial occlusion can be differentiated from acute thrombophlebitis, since thrombophlebitis is usually associated with edema, preservation of peripheral pulses, and superficial venous distension. Severe venous obstruction produces phlegmasia cerulea dolens; when this is associated with arterial thrombosis and spasm, phlegmasia alba dolens ensues. Rarely a dissecting aortic aneurysm may mimic acute embolism by producing loss of peripheral pulses, but the diagnosis may be suspected because of the presence of back or chest pain and hypertension. Acute arterial occlusion that rapidly produces paralysis and paresthesia may be mistaken for a stroke; the physical examination will direct attention toward the compromised extremity and eliminate stroke from the differential diagnosis. Prompt diagnosis of arterial occlusion is critical, since irreversible muscular necrosis necessitating amputation may occur within 4 to 6 hours.

Answer: Question 13: C
Question 14: A
Question 15: A, D

16. Appropriate initial treatment of an acute arterial embolus to the lower extremity may include:

A. 10,000-unit IV heparin bolus
B. 30,000-unit IV heparin bolus followed by continuous infusion of 2,000 to 3,000 units per hour
C. Delay heparinization until operative embolectomy is completed
D. Routine preoperative trial of intravenous nitroglycerin
E. Intravenous streptokinase

Sabiston: 1909, 1914
Schwartz: 921

Comments: Successful treatment of arterial embolism must be initiated promptly in order to prevent irreversible ischemic damage. Intravenous heparin should be administered to prevent formation and propagation of thrombus distal to the embolus; prompt embolectomy is necessary. In some patients who are extremely debilitated, or who present in delayed fashion and are tolerating their ischemia, high-dose heparinization alone has been advocated. Heparinization should not be delayed, because the degree of distal thrombus is an important determinant of surgical success and limb salvage. Although arterial spasm accompanies acute arterial occlusion, the value of routine use of vasodilators is not established. These agents carry a potential risk of dilating

constricted distal arterial beds, allowing extension of thrombus into smaller vessels that would not otherwise be involved. Fibrinolytic agents have been used in primary arterial thrombosis, but are not the recommended treatment of arterial embolism. Since patients with arterial embolism often have associated cardiac disease and may be compromised further by the metabolic effects of ischemic tissue, preoperative attention must be given to fluid and electrolyte status, arterial blood gases, and central venous or Swan-Ganz monitoring.

Answer: A, B

17. Which of the following statements is/are true regarding operative management of lower extremity arterial embolism?

A. Most emboli can be removed under local anesthesia
B. Aortoiliac emboli can be removed through bilateral groin arteriotomies
C. Removal of aortoiliac emboli generally requires laparotomy
D. Brisk back-bleeding is a reliable indicator of successful distal embolectomy
E. Wide fasciotomy should be avoided in heparinized patients because of the risk of hemorrhage

Sabiston: 1906, 1910
Schwartz: 921

Comments: In most cases, thromboembolectomy can be performed using balloon catheters introduced through arteriotomies proximal to the embolic site. Aortoiliac emboli can be removed successfully in retrograde fashion through the femoral vessels. Back-bleeding does not necessarily indicate adequate removal of the embolus distally since it may originate from an arterial branch proximal to the thrombus that still remains; distally, discontinuous thrombus is present in approximately one third of cases. For this reason, restoration of distal pulses and intraoperative arteriography are used to assess completeness of thromboembolectomy. Fasciotomy is an important concomitant procedure if the limb has been subjected to ischemia for 4 to 6 hours or longer or if increased muscle turgor is present preoperatively.

Answer: A, B

18. In the recovery room following femoral embolectomy, a palpable pedal pulse disappears. The patient's leg is pale and swollen. Appropriate treatment may include:

A. Venography
B. Intra-arterial streptokinase
C. Arteriography
D. Repeat thromboembolectomy
E. Fasciotomy

Sabiston: 1913
Schwartz: 922

Comments: In the immediate postoperative period, therapy focuses on maintenance of peripheral perfusion, treatment of the patient's underlying cardiac disease, and treatment of the potential metabolic complications following resumption of perfusion of an ischemic limb.

Frequent evaluation of peripheral pulses by palpation and by Doppler ultrasound and of limb temperature and color is mandatory. Any change that indicates ischemia warrants arteriography to assess the need for re-exploration. If swelling threatens the viability of peripheral musculature, fasciotomy is indicated. Intra-arterial streptokinase has been used for arterial thrombosis, but is contraindicated in patients who have had a recent operation because of the risk of hemorrhage at the operative site.

Answer: C, D, E

19. Following femoral embolectomy and fasciotomy, a patient with mitral stenosis and atrial fibrillation becomes oliguric and the urine is red. Immediate treatment includes:

A. Cessation of intravenous heparin
B. Determination of serum potassium
C. Intravenous sodium bicarbonate and mannitol
D. Renal arteriography
E. Emergency mitral valve replacement

Sabiston: 1907, 1913

Comments: When an extremity has been subjected to ischemia and muscular necrosis occurs, reperfusion can result in metabolic acidosis and profound hyperkalemia. Rhabdomyolysis releases myoglobin, which precipitates in acid urine, producing renal tubular obstruction and renal failure. Myoglobinuria produces a red urine that is free of red blood cells. Treatment of the patient in this situation requires at least the following: prompt reversal of hyperkalemia to prevent cardiac arrest (intravenous insulin and glucose); administration of sodium bicarbonate to alkalinize the urine and to treat the systemic metabolic acidosis; osmotic diuresis with mannitol to prevent renal tubular obstruction. Fasciotomy is indicated if it has not already been performed. Continuation of anticoagulation therapy is critical because the patient remains at significant risk of recurrent embolism from the underlying cardiac disease. Definitive cardiac surgery may be required, but it is not the initial focus of treatment in the described situation. Only 25% of arterial emboli involve the renal vessels.

Answer: B, C

20. The majority of arterial emboli originate from which one of the following sites?

A. Cardiac valves
B. Left atrium
C. Left ventricle
D. Thoracic aorta
E. Abdominal aorta

Sabiston: 1904
Schwartz: 918

Comments: By far the majority of arterial emboli originate in the heart, the most frequent intracardiac site being the left atrium. Left atrial thrombi form as the result of stasis in patients with atrial fibrillation and/or mitral valvular disease. A rare source of left atrial emboli is a left atrial myxoma. Left ventricular thrombi are a poten-

tial source of embolism in patients with myocardial infarction, left ventricular aneurysm, congestive heart failure, or cardiomyopathy. Valvular sources of emboli include vegetative endocarditis and thrombi formed on mechanical prosthetic heart valves. Noncardiac sources of arterial emboli include ulcerated atherosclerotic plaques in the aorta, or the carotid or subclavian arteries.

Answer: B

21. Cardioarterial emboli most frequently produce occlusion of which one of the following?

A. Cerebral vessels
B. Distal aorta
C. Common femoral artery
D. Superficial femoral artery
E. Popliteal artery

Sabiston: 1904
Schwartz: 918

Comments: Arterial emboli usually lodge proximal to arterial bifurcations and most commonly involve the lower extremities. One third to one half of arterial emboli obstruct the common femoral artery. This tendency for obstruction to occur proximal rather than distal to major bifurcations results in significant interruption of potential collateral flow and dangerous ischemic consequences.

Answer: C

22. Following brachial artery catheterization for coronary angiography, a patient complains of hand numbness and his radial pulse is noted to be absent. Appropriate treatment is:

A. Administration of systemic vasodilators
B. Surgical exploration and topical application of papaverine
C. Percutaneous balloon dilatation of brachial artery
D. Brachial artery excision and direct anastomosis
E. Venous bypass of brachial artery

Sabiston: 1897

Comments: Iatrogenic arterial injuries result from needles and catheters placed for radiographic studies or monitoring purposes. Arterial occlusion usually occurs as the result of thrombus in association with intimal injury. Treatment consists of prompt exploration with arteriotomy and thrombectomy. Intimal damage is usually treated by segmental excision with direct anastomosis. Surgery should not be delayed by attributing ischemia associated with arterial injury to arterial "spasm."

Answer: D

23. Which one or more of the following causes of arterial occlusion occur more commonly in the upper extremities than in the lower extremities?

A. Atherosclerosis
B. Embolism
C. Aneurysm
D. Vasospastic disorders
E. Arteritis

Sabiston: 1933

Comments: Only about 1% of patients with peripheral vascular disease have symptomatic involvement of the upper extremities. The adequacy of collateral circulation and the more limited oxygen demand of smaller muscle mass engaged in intermittent work make frank ischemic manifestations less common. Nevertheless, claudication and gangrene can occur related to a variety of etiologies. Inflammatory vascular disease, vasospastic disorders, and trauma occur more commonly in the upper extremities than in the lower extremities. Atherosclerotic occlusions, when they do occur in the upper extremity, most commonly involve the subclavian or innominate vessels. Emboli usually arise from the heart and may occlude the axillary or brachial arteries, although only a small percentage of cardioarterial emboli lodge in the upper extremities.

Answer: D, E

24. The most common symptom of thoracic outlet syndrome is:

A. Raynaud's phenomenon
B. Pain/paresthesia in ulnar nerve distribution
C. Pain/paresthesia in radial nerve distribution
D. Ischemic pain due to arterial compression
E. Arm edema due to venous obstruction

Sabiston: 2076
Schwartz: 937

Comments: Anatomic compression of the brachial plexus and/or subclavian-axillary vessels may occur at the thoracic outlet by a variety of mechanisms at several specific sites. The primary symptoms will depend upon which anatomic structures are compressed. The majority of patients present with pain or paresthesias as a result of brachial plexus compression. Pain and paresthesias may affect any part of the shoulder or upper extremity but most commonly are noted in the distribution of the ulnar nerve. Symptoms of arterial compression, such as ischemic pain, fatigue, and decreased temperature are less common. Embolic events may produce digital gangrene or Raynaud's phenomenon. Symptoms of venous compression occur even less frequently than those of arterial compromise and may include edema, venous distension, and discoloration. Rarely, so-called effort thrombosis of the subclavian vein (Paget-Schroetter syndrome) may occur. Nerve conduction studies and arteriography may aid in diagnosis of thoracic outlet syndrome; physical maneuvers aimed at detecting a pulse deficit have a low specificity. Both first rib resection and scalenectomy have provided successful decompressive treatment.

Answer: B

25. Which one of the following has proved to be the most effective component in the treatment of Buerger's disease?

A. Cessation of tobacco use
B. Anticoagulant treatment
C. Sympathectomy
D. Vasodilating drugs
E. Steroids

Sabiston: 1924
Schwartz: 926

Comments: Buerger's disease (thromboangiitis obliterans) is an inflammatory process of uncertain etiology that produces thrombosis of medium-sized to small arteries and veins. The disease typically affects young adult males who are heavy smokers. Both upper and lower extremities are affected and ischemic gangrene frequently results. Complete cessation of tobacco use is the most important aspect of treatment and may produce remission. Arterial reconstruction usually is not possible. Cervical or lumbar sympathectomy may be useful in management of pain in patients with associated vasospasm. No pharmacologic treatment has proved widely successful.

Answer: A

26. A 20-year-old football player presents with intermittent claudication and diminished foot pulses on the left side. The most likely diagnosis is:

A. Atherosclerotic occlusion
B. Popliteal aneurysm
C. Popliteal entrapment syndrome
D. Spontaneous knee subluxation

Schwartz: 930

Comments: An abnormal anatomic relationship between the popliteal artery and the leg muscles may predispose to arterial compression by the medial head of the gastrocnemius muscle. This should be suspected in any young patient with typical symptoms or signs of distal ischemia. Sometimes the findings are elicited only with dorsiflexion of the foot. Atherosclerotic aneurysms or occlusions occur in a much older age group. Popliteal arterial injury may occur with traumatic dislocation of the knee, and these injuries require arteriographic assessment.

Answer: C

27. Appropriate management of a popliteal aneurysm includes which one or more of the following?

A. Arteriography to search for associated aneurysms
B. Observation if the aneurysm is small, asymptomatic, and stable
C. Prophylactic anticoagulation with Coumadin
D. Excision and arterial reconstruction
E. Proximal and distal ligation with bypass graft

Sabiston: 1841
Schwartz: 956

Comments: Popliteal aneurysms present a high risk of acute limb ischemia and potential limb loss as a result of thrombosis or embolism. Operation is therefore recommended for all popliteal aneurysms regardless of size and symptoms. Isolation of the aneurysm by proximal and distal ligation and bypass grafting using autologous saphenous vein when possible is the procedure of choice. Aneurysm excision is not generally recommended because of risk of injury to the popliteal vein. Popliteal aneurysms are often bilateral and associated with proximal aortoiliac aneurysms. Patients, therefore, require thorough arteriographic assessment in a search for other correctable lesions.

Answer: A, E

28. Match the vascular disorder in the left-hand column with the typical clinical manifestations in the right-hand column.

Vascular Disorder	Clinical Manifestations
A. Raynaud's syndrome	a. Painful, cold, cyanotic hands and feet
B. Acrocyanosis	b. Painless, cold, cyanotic hands and feet
C. Livedo reticularis	c. Sequential pallor, cyanosis, rubor of fingers and hands
D. Erythromelalgia	d. Red, warm, painful extremities
	e. Reddish-blue, mottled legs and feet

Sabiston: 1925, 1936
Schwartz: 961, 963

Comments: Raynaud's syndrome is the most common vasospastic disorder and the most important in terms of the potential for digital gangrene. The condition is caused by intermittent spasm of arteries and arterioles in response to cold or emotional stimuli. It may exist as a primary disorder (Raynaud's disease) or it may occur secondarily in association with a variety of disorders including immunologic and connective tissue diseases and obstructive arterial diseases such as arteriosclerosis, thromboangiitis obliterans, and thoracic outlet syndrome. Avoidance of cold and tobacco is adequate treatment for most patients; treatment with vasodilating drugs or sympathectomy may benefit some of those more severely affected. Other vasospastic disorders include acrocyanosis and livedo reticularis; erythromelalgia appears to be a manifestation of vasodilatation rather than vasospasm. These latter conditions are rare, and conservative treatment usually suffices.

Answer: A–c; B–b; C–e; D–d

29. Appropriate initial treatment of frostbite includes:

A. Rapid rewarming in warm water
B. Rapid rewarming with dry heat
C. Slow rewarming at room temperature
D. Thorough débridement of blisters and devitalized tissue
E. Sympathectomy

Sabiston: 238
Schwartz: 965

Comments: The cold-injured extremity is best treated by rapid rewarming in warm water (40 to 42° centigrade). This results in less tissue damage than treatment by slow rewarming. Dry heat or water at warmer temperature risks additional thermal injury owing to decreased sensation of the injured part. The extremity should be elevated and exposed. Antibiotics are given if there is an open wound and tetanus prophylaxis is administered as indicated. Opening of blisters and débridement of apparently devitalized tissue are contraindicated. True demarcation of nonviable tissue requires many weeks and should be allowed to develop spontaneously. The initial use of vasodilating drugs or antithrombotic agents such as heparin and low molecular weight dextran have not conclusively been shown to be effective. Intra-arterial reserpine and sympathectomy may be useful in the treatment of the chronic sequelae of frostbite.

Answer: A

Vascular—Renal

1. True statements regarding the pathophysiology of renovascular hypertension include:

A. The relationship between unilateral renal artery stenosis and hypertension was established by Goldblatt
B. Activation of the renin-angiotensin system depends on intact aortic and carotid arch baroreceptors
C. In response to reduced renal blood flow and pressure, the juxtaglomerular apparatus produces angiotensin I
D. Angiotensin II elevates blood pressure by increasing peripheral vascular resistance and aldosterone production
E. Saralasin competitively inhibits angiotensin II and is routinely used to screen for patients with hypertension due to renin excess

Sabiston: 1943, 1946
Schwartz: 1010

Comments: Renovascular hypertension is the elevation of diastolic and systolic pressures associated with renal artery occlusive disease. This relationship was first defined by Goldblatt and today is explained in terms of the renin-angiotensinogen system. In renovascular hypertension due to renal artery stenosis, decreased renal artery pressure or flow stimulates the release of renin from the juxtaglomerular apparatus. Renin reacts with renin substrate (synthesized in the liver) to produce angiotensin I. Converting enzymes (located primarily in the lung) convert angiotensin I to angiotensin II. Angiotensin II increases blood pressure by its direct vasoconstrictor effect and by stimulating the release of aldosterone. Establishment of normal renal artery blood flow can restore normal levels of renin production. Parenchymal lesions due to infarction (secondary to emboli, thrombus, or trauma), disease of the distal renal artery branches, arteriolar nephrosclerosis, intrarenal aneurysms, and renal artery occlusion with insufficient collateralization can also produce hypertension via renin-angiotensin stimulation. Saralasin is a specific inhibitor of angiotensin II at the level of the arteriolar receptor site, but has not proved reliable for screening patients with presumed renovascular hypertension.

Answer: A, D

2. True statements regarding surgically correctable hypertension include:

A. Surgically correctable hypertension, by definition, represents disease of the renal blood vessels and parenchyma
B. It should be suspected when there is the sudden onset of severe hypertension before the age of 35 or when it develops after age 55 in the absence of a family history of hypertension
C. It should be suspected when easily controllable hypertension becomes labile
D. It should be suspected in children, adolescents, and premenopausal women with hypertension

Sabiston: 1944
Schwartz: 1004

Comments: Approximately 5 to 15% of cases of hypertension are surgically correctable. While lesions of the renal artery are the most common cause of surgically correctable hypertension, a number of other causes amenable to surgical correction exist. These include pheochromocytoma, various causes of Cushing's syndrome (adrenal hyperplasia, cortical adenoma, adrenal carcinoma), primary hyperaldosteronism, coarctation of the aorta, and unilateral renal parenchymal disease such as renal cell carcinoma associated with renin production. The nonrenovascular causes may be diagnosed by appropriate hormone assays and radiographs.

Answer: B, C, D

3. True statements regarding atherosclerosis and renovascular hypertension include:

A. It accounts for up to 80% of renal artery occlusions producing hypertension
B. It occurs equally in men and women between the ages of 55 and 75
C. The lesions are most commonly located near the origin of the renal artery, are segmental, and often are shorter than 1 cm in length

D. These lesions are the most common source of emboli to the kidney
E. Up to one third of these patients will have bilateral disease

Sabiston: 1943
Schwartz: 1008

Comments: Atherosclerosis is the most common cause of renovascular hypertension. It primarily affects males between the ages of 55 and 75 and is often a segmental defect of the proximal renal artery. Up to one third of these patients will have bilateral disease. Renal artery atherosclerosis may be associated with renal artery aneurysms and renal emboli. Most renal emboli, however, originate from the heart. Hypertension that appears suddenly or hypertension that is difficult to control in patients with other stigmata of atherosclerosis is highly suggestive of the diagnosis. Bruits over the kidneys are common but may represent transmission of sounds from nonrenal arterial stenosis. Renal bruits in essential hypertension are unusual.

Answer: A, C, E

4. A 14-year-old child who complains of headaches presents with marked diastolic hypertension and a soft to-and-fro bruit heard at the right costovertebral angle. The most likely diagnosis (diagnoses) is/are:

A. Coarctation of the aorta
B. Spontaneous segmental renal infarction
C. Intimal fibromuscular dysplasia
D. Medial fibromuscular dysplasia

Sabiston: 1944
Schwartz: 1008, 1010

Comments: Most asymptomatic children with mildly elevated blood pressure have essential hypertension. However, children with symptoms and a diastolic blood pressure above 100 to 110 mm Hg usually have secondary hypertension due to either a renal parenchymal disorder (such as glomerulonephritis) or a neurovascular lesion. One of the common causes of renovascular hypertension in children is fibromuscular dysplasia. Fibrodysplasia causes approximately 20% of all cases of renovascular hypertension. It is primarily a disease of children and premenopausal women. The lesions are classified according to the site (intimal, medial, adventitial) and type of involvement. The most common lesions in children are intimal and medial dysplasias of unclear etiology. In females, medial fibrodysplasia is most common and may be due to repeated renal artery stretching during pregnancy, causing damage to the vasa vasorum, or to the effect of estrogens, which are known to cause medial degeneration. The right renal artery is affected 85% of the time. The lesions frequently are multiple, creating the "string of beads" phenomenon often seen on arteriogram. Medial fibrodysplastic lesions may lend themselves to dilatation, while intimal and adventitial lesions do not. In 15% of patients the lesions progress or new lesions are formed after treatment. Coarctation is usually associated with brachial femoral pulse discrepancies and a chest x-ray showing rib notching.

Answer: C, D

5. True or False: Renal artery aneurysms produce renovascular hypertension through the mechanisms of blood turbulence within the aneurysmal sac.

Sabiston: 1828
Schwartz: 1009

Comments: Renal artery aneurysms themselves do not cause renovascular hypertension. However, they are often associated with fibromuscular dysplasia or atherosclerosis, which cause secondary narrowing of the renal artery. Aneurysms may occasionally be the source of emboli or thrombi that lead to parenchymal ischemia and secondary hypertension.

Answer: False

6. Which of the following statements is/are true regarding the work-up of patients suspected of having renovascular hypertension?

A. Split-renal function studies provide the most accurate assessment for the presence of renovascular hypertension
B. Renal artery stenosis demonstrated on arteriogram is sufficient indication for surgical correction in the hypertensive patient
C. IVP is considered the diagnostic procedure of choice in the evaluation of patients suspected of having renovascular hypertension
D. Systemic renin assays are the screening procedure of choice in patients suspected of having renovascular hypertension
E. Renal vein renin ratios are presently the best means of localizing the site of physiologically significant renal artery stenosis

Sabiston: 1944
Schwartz: 1011

Comments: The goal of the work-up for renovascular hypertension is to establish a relationship between an identifiable renal abnormality and altered renin-angiotensin function. The use of IVP to screen these patients has some drawbacks. There is a 75% false negative rate in children and a 20% false negative rate in adults with atherosclerosis. Delayed opacification, reduction of kidney size, and ureteral notching are considered positive findings. IVP is limited in identifying segmental or arterial branch lesions, bilateral parenchymal disease of unequal severity, or bilateral arterial disease. Intravenous digital subtraction angiography may become the preferred screening procedure. Arteriography remains the definitive procedure for localization of the renal artery lesions in patients suitable for operation. Because peripheral venous renin activity is quite variable, it is not considered a reliable screening test. Bilateral renal vein renin activity used alone or in combination with peripheral vein renin activity (the renal systemic renin index) is of central importance in the preoperative evaluation. A renal vein renin ratio greater than 1.5 is considered positive. The patient must be on a normal sodium diet and off diuretics before renin levels are determined. Captopril may be used to amplify the difference in renin activity between the normal and abnormal kidney. Before renin assays were available, split-renal function studies were used to assess the physiologic significance of renal lesions; they are no longer in wide use because of the high incidence of technical failure, complications, and unreliability.

Answer: E

7. True statements regarding the selection and preparation of patients for surgery to correct renovascular hypertension include:

A. Most patients with renovascular hypertension are hypovolemic and require careful preoperative hydration
B. Surgery clearly is superior to medical management of hypertension due to renal artery occlusive disease
C. Patients with renin levels that are nonlateralizing should not be operated upon
D. Patients with generalized atherosclerosis and renovascular hypertension do best with surgery, since hypertension is least well tolerated in this group

Sabiston: 1946
Schwartz: 1012

Comments: Many patients with renovascular hypertension are hypovolemic and hypokalemic, usually owing to diuretic therapy. These deficits must be carefully corrected before surgery. The importance of discontinuing antihypertensive therapy before operation is debatable. A diagnosis of renovascular hypertension can truly be made only in retrospect when correction of a renal artery stenosis leads to correction of the hypertension. Most patients with unilateral stenosis and lateralizing renin values are helped by surgery. (False negative results may be due to problems with the screening technique or the presence of unsuspected bilateral disease.) Medical therapy may control renovascular hypertension, but patients managed medically require close supervision and compliance since they seem to have a more aggressive course of any underlying atherosclerosis. It is clearly established that renal artery reconstruction provides long-term correction of hypertension. The same is true in women with fibrodysplastic disease. It is the patients with atherosclerosis whose disease is confined to the renal artery who do best with reconstruction. In patients with generalized atherosclerosis and involvement of other organs, surgery may be best reserved for those who fail medical manage-

ment or develop renal failure due to progressive renal artery occlusion.

Answer: A

8. True statements regarding the choice of procedure for correction of renovascular hypertension include:

A. Endarterectomy is rarely indicated because of the risk of emboli causing parenchymal ischemia and further renin activation
B. The internal iliac artery is the most common graft used for aortorenal bypass
C. Partial nephrectomy rather than revascularization may be curative for hypertension caused by segmental infarction, renal artery branch lesions, intrarenal aneurysms, or isolated arteriovenous malformations
D. Medial fibrodysplasia and renal artery occlusion by plaques originating in the aortic wall next to the renal artery are lesions most amenable to transluminal angioplasty

Sabiston: 1947
Schwartz: 1013

Comments: There are many surgical options available for the treatment of renovascular hypertension. The most frequent is aortorenal bypass using the saphenous vein. There is a tendency for the vein graft to dilate in children, so internal iliac artery grafts are often used in this setting. Selected atherosclerotic lesions are amenable to transaortic endarterectomy with good results. A growing experience with the technique of transluminal renal angioplasty suggests a technical success rate of up to 90%. Fibrodysplasia responds best to dilatation, while occlusion by atheromas originating in the aorta is least amenable. Restenosis after dilatation occurs more frequently in the atherosclerotic group. Small branch disease may be treated by bench-work surgery using cold perfusion and ex vivo surgical repair followed by reimplantation. In general, surgical treatment of carefully selected patients with renovascular hypertension is 80 to 90% successful.

Answer: C

CHAPTER 42

Vascular —Visceral

1. Which of the following features is/are true of the mesenteric circulation?

A. Splanchnic vascular blood flow receives 25 to 30% of cardiac output
B. Normal portal venous pressure is greater than 50 cm of water due to valves in the portal system
C. The ileum has more numerous vascular arcades than the jejunum
D. The abundance of collateral sources of blood supply to the superior mesenteric system minimizes the risk of bowel infarction with acute occlusion of the superior mesenteric artery

Schwartz: 1428

Comments: Under resting conditions, the splanchnic vascular bed receives up to 30% of the cardiac output and represents a large potential reservoir of blood from which the patient is "auto-transfused" in situations of severe hypovolemia. Normal portal venous pressure is between 12 and 15 cm of water. The portal vein contains no valves, and therefore blood flows within the portal vein according to the pressure gradient between the portal and systemic venous systems. Blood from the superior mesenteric artery reaches the small bowel via numerous arterial arcades, which become progressively greater in number and complexity in the more distal portion of the bowel. Although collateral flow does exist between the superior mesenteric system and the celiac and inferior mesenteric systems, these sources of collateral flow would only rarely be sufficient to maintain bowel viability in the event of acute occlusion of the superior mesenteric artery.

Answer: A, C

2. Which of the following statements is/are true regarding mesenteric vascular occlusion?

A. Inferior mesenteric artery occlusion usually causes severe colonic ischemia
B. Occlusion of the superior mesenteric artery occurs most often at its origin or at the origin of the middle colic artery

C. Clinically significant intestinal infarctions more often are due to arterial rather than to venous occlusion
D. Venous occlusions most often are embolic rather than thrombotic

Sabiston: 1937
Schwartz: 1431

Comments: Although acute occlusion of the inferior mesenteric artery can produce symptoms of colonic ischemia, collateral supply from the superior mesenteric system via the marginal artery of Drummond is usually sufficient to preserve viability of the left colon. Both acute and chronic occlusion of the superior mesenteric artery occur most often at its origin or near its first major branch, the middle colic. Approximately 20% of clinically significant mesenteric vascular accidents are due to primary venous thrombosis and 50% to primary arterial occlusion. The remaining cases occur in the absence of major vascular occlusion and may be related to spasm.

Answer: B, C

3. Which of the following statements accurately characterize(s) acute occlusion of the superior mesenteric artery?

A. Sudden complete occlusion more often is due to embolism than to thrombosis
B. Emboli most commonly arise from atheromatous plaques within the aorta
C. One third of affected patients have a history of intestinal angina
D. Pain classically is out of proportion to physical findings

Sabiston: 1939
Schwartz: 1433

Comments: Arterial emboli are the most common cause of sudden complete occlusion of the superior mesenteric artery. These emboli most often arise from the heart, either as mural thrombi from recent myocardial infarction or as auricular thrombi in patients with atrial fibrillation. The initial pain is extremely severe, often refractory to narcotics, and often out of proportion to physical findings. The physical signs of peritonitis, when present, represent a very late stage in the evolution of this process.

Answer: A, C, D

4. Which of the following statements is/are true regarding the diagnosis and management of acute occlusion of the superior mesenteric artery?

A. Early arteriography can both be diagnostic and offer therapeutic access
B. The majority of patients can avoid operation if arterial infusion of papaverine is begun early in the clinical course
C. Papaverine is extremely effective because it both lyses thrombus and dilates the smaller mesenteric vessels
D. As much as 70% of the small intestine can be resected without creating incapacitating digestive problems

Sabiston: 1940
Schwartz: 1433

Comments: Early arteriography not only confirms the diagnosis and assists in determining the etiology, it also provides a route by which intra-arterial papaverine can be administered. Papaverine, a potent vasodilator, may assist in dilating the more peripheral mesenteric bed, which frequently is severely constricted as a reflex response to the more proximal mechanical occlusion. Despite its use, the majority of patients will require laparotomy. Serious gastrointestinal disturbances are uncommon if more than 30% of the small bowel can be preserved; the likelihood of a good result is enhanced if the terminal ileum and ileocecal valve are preserved as well.

Answer: A, D

5. Which of the following statements correctly characterize(s) a nonocclusive mesenteric infarction?

A. It occurs more frequently than occlusive mesenteric infarction
B. It is usually related to a low cardiac output state
C. It is exacerbated by isoproterenol, which induces vasoconstriction
D. It is often accompanied by a markedly elevated hematocrit due to polycythemia
E. Treatment includes correcting the low-flow state as well as administering vasodilators

Schwartz: 1436

Comments: Small bowel infarction is due to nonocclusive phenomena in only 20 to 30% of cases. The "final common pathway" of nonocclusive infarction appears to be a low cardiac output state, which may accompany numerous processes including primary cardiac disease, as well as septicemia and hypovolemia. Isoproterenol is a vasodilating agent and may be therapeutically beneficial when accompanied by efforts to correct the low-flow state. Often, however, laparotomy is mandatory because of refractory hypotension or signs of peritonitis. The elevated hematocrit frequently seen in this disease process

is due to third-space loss of serum rather than to polycythemia.

Answer: B, E

6. Which of the following statements is/are true regarding mesenteric venous occlusion?

A. Inflammatory conditions such as appendicitis or diverticulitis can be predisposing factors
B. Patients with polycythemia vera, patients who have had a splenectomy, and patients on oral contraceptives may be at increased risk
C. Bloody diarrhea is less frequently seen with venous occlusion than with arterial occlusion
D. Shorter segments of intestine are usually involved in venous occlusion as compared with arterial occlusion

Schwartz: 1439

Comments: Mesenteric venous occlusion may be idiopathic or secondary to a number of conditions including appendicitis, diverticulitis, pelvic abscess, hematologic conditions, the postsplenectomy state, use of oral contraceptives, extrinsic compression by tumor, venous trauma, acute portal vein thrombosis, and many others. Bloody diarrhea tends to be a later finding and is seen more frequently with venous occlusion. The site of venous occlusion tends to be more peripheral within the mesentery than is arterial occlusion, and therefore shorter segments of bowel are involved.

Answer: A, B, D

7. Which of the following statements is/are true regarding splanchnic artery aneurysms?

A. Medial degeneration or disorders of connective tissue are the usual etiologic factors in adults
B. Most patients with these aneurysms are hypertensive
C. The splenic artery is the most common site of involvement, with the majority occurring in men
D. About 40% of splenic artery aneurysms are multiple

Sabiston: 1228
Schwartz: 1441

Comments: In adults, atherosclerosis, most often associated with hypertension, appears to be the commonest etiologic factor. Medial degeneration, connective tissue disorders, and mycotic embolization are less frequent causes. The splenic artery is the most common site for splanchnic artery aneurysms, and multiple splenic artery aneurysms are seen in as many as 40% of patients. These aneurysms usually are asymptomatic and occur much more commonly in women than in men. Pregnancy appears to be a significant risk factor for their rupture.

Answer: B, D

8. In which of the following clinical situations would surgical correction of the splanchnic artery aneurysm be indicated?

A. A 25-year-old man with an asymptomatic 3-cm splenic artery aneurysm
B. A 20-year-old pregnant woman with a splenic artery aneurysm

C. A 30-year-old ballet dancer with an asymptomatic hepatic artery aneurysm

D. A 50-year-old woman about to have a hysterectomy who has an asymptomatic calcified splenic artery aneurysm

Sabiston: 1228, 1827
Schwartz: 1441

Comments: Since rupture occurs in fewer than 10% of splenic artery aneurysms, the majority of such patients can be managed conservatively. Patients who are symptomatic, however, should have aneurysmectomy, as should women who are likely to become pregnant because of the increased hazard of rupture during pregnancy. Aneurysms of the other splanchnic arteries should be repaired when they are diagnosed, regardless of the absence of symptoms.

Answer: B, C

9. Which of the following statements is/are true regarding intestinal angina?

A. This term is a misnomer since it bears no pathophysiologic similarity to cardiac angina

B. It is characterized by cramping abdominal pain following meals

C. The diagnosis is primarily a clinical one, and arteriography has a minimal role in the evaluation of this problem

D. Operative correction, which is almost always indicated, is most easily achieved by excision of the stenotic segment of vessel

Sabiston: 1936
Schwartz: 1436

Comments: As with angina pectoris and claudication, intestinal angina represents an imbalance between the metabolic needs of an organ (the intestines) and the blood supply available to meet these needs. Postprandial abdominal cramping is characteristic and is often accompanied by a malabsorption syndrome. Although the diagnosis is suggested clinically, arteriography (particularly lateral views) is essential, delineating the arterial anatomy prior to operation. Because of the difficulty in exposing the origins of the superior mesenteric and celiac arteries, most surgeons prefer to use bypass grafting in operative correction of these vascular abnormalities.

Answer: B

10. The median arcuate ligament syndrome is characterized by which of the following statements?

A. It is always caused by an embryologic anomaly of the diaphragmatic fibers of the median arcuate ligament

B. A bruit is frequently heard over the upper abdomen

C. Vague abdominal pain, diarrhea, weight loss, and occasional nausea are the usual presenting symptoms

D. Initial treatment consists of transection of the median arcuate ligament

Sabiston: 1938
Schwartz: 1440

Comments: Compression of the celiac artery by the median arcuate ligament may be due to an abnormal proximal origin of the celiac artery or an abnormally low positioning of the median arcuate ligament. The symptoms described above are characteristic, and the weight loss may be severe as patients stop eating to avoid the fairly predictable postprandial pain. If initial transection of the median arcuate ligament does not result in restoration of proper blood flow, direct arterial reconstruction may be necessary.

Answer: B, C, D

11. Accepted principles of management of traumatic injury to the visceral blood vessels include:

A. Isolated mesenteric vascular injuries are common findings in stab wounds of the abdomen

B. Clinical evidence of ongoing hemorrhage is the principal indication for operating on patients with penetrating abdominal trauma

C. When indicated, ligation of the inferior mesenteric artery and smaller branches of the superior mesenteric artery and veins can be carried out, usually with impunity

D. If at all possible, the hepatic artery and portal vein should be repaired rather than ligated

Schwartz: 1442

Comments: It is generally accepted that all gunshot wounds of the abdominal cavity should be explored. Almost all stab wounds reaching the abdominal cavity should be explored. In such wounds, injuries to the bowel or solid viscera are often associated with the vascular injury. While smaller branches of the superior mesenteric artery can be ligated, the trunk of the superior mesenteric artery must be repaired. Collateral flow through the marginal artery is usually sufficient to permit ligation of the inferior mesenteric artery. Arterial and portal venous blood flow to the liver should be preserved if at all possible.

Answer: C, D

CHAPTER 43

Vascular—General

1. Blood pressure is under the influence of many factors. True statements regarding blood pressure include:

A. Blood pressure is primarily a function of cardiac output and peripheral vascular resistance
B. Normally, precapillary sphincter baroreceptors mediate blood pressure through sympathetic neural signals
C. Catecholamines influence blood pressure at the level of the renal medulla
D. Angiotensin II affects blood pressure primarily through its stimulation of adrenal medullary catecholamine excretion

Sabiston: 1943
Schwartz: 1003

Comments: The major determinants of blood pressure are cardiac output (heart rate × stroke volume) and peripheral vascular resistance; blood viscosity and vessel compliance play lesser roles. Right atrial stretch receptors and carotid and arotic arch baroreceptors affect blood pressure via sympathetic and parasympathetic stimulation. Many humoral mechanisms influence blood pressure; catecholamines increase small vessel tone; steroids lead to salt and water retention and potentiate the effects of epinephrine and norepinephrine; angiotensin II elevates blood pressure by its powerful vasoactive effect as well as by stimulating aldosterone secretion with resultant expansion of the intravascular volume.

Answer: A

2. Which one of the following is the most common cause of late failure of saphenous vein grafts?

A. Technical error
B. Arterial atherosclerosis
C. Vein graft atherosclerosis
D. Vein graft fibrous hyperplasia
E. Vein graft valve stenosis

Sabiston: 1782

Comments: Whereas early failure of saphenous vein grafts is attributed to technical error, late failure is usually related to progressive atherosclerotic disease of the native arterial vessels proximal or distal to the graft. The vein graft itself, however, can be the cause of late failure due to various mechanisms. All venous autografts develop some degree of fibrointimal and medial hyperplasia, which may progress to luminal occlusion. This has been related to vein trauma and in particular endothelial injury. Other pathologic changes that may occur in vein grafts and cause late failure include atherosclerosis, transmural fibrosis, valve stenosis, and the formation of venous aneurysms.

Answer: B

3. Which of the following is/are characteristic of prosthetic arterial graft healing in man?

A. Viable neo-intima forms
B. Lumen lined by fibrin
C. Platelet survival shortened
D. Eventual dynamic compliance equivalent to that of normal arteries

Sabiston: 1787

Comment: Whereas studies of prosthetic graft healing in experimental animals have demonstrated an organized process of luminal healing culminating in a living neo-intimal layer, a similar process does not occur in man. In humans, the luminal lining of prosthetic grafts is primarily composed of compacted fibrin. This limited luminal organization is associated with platelet deposition on prosthetic grafts and decreased platelet survival. Compliance of synthetic grafts is less than that of the normal arterial system. This results in localized turbulence, which may contribute to intimal damage and thrombosis.

Answer: B, C

4. Which of the following statements is/are true regarding complications of prosthetic arterial grafts?

A. Neo-intimal fibrous hyperplasia may be decreased by the use of antiplatelet drugs
B. Graft infection has an overall mortality of approximately 30%
C. False aneurysms are usually caused by graft fiber disruption
D. Anastomotic false aneurysms do not usually require operative repair

Sabiston: 1789

Comments: The more frequent complications of prosthetic arterial grafts include fibrous hyperplasia, infection, graft failure, and anastomotic false aneurysm formation. Fibrous hyperplasia is similar to that seen in venous autografts and tends to occur near the anastomotic sites. Local trauma and platelet deposition have been implicated in the etiology of this phenomenon; studies have suggested that the use of antiplatelet drugs may inhibit fibrous hyperplasia and improve graft patency. Graft infection is a serious complication best prevented by use of antibiotics, meticulous technique, and avoidance of prosthetic material in contaminated fields. Anastomotic false aneurysms result from anastomotic disruption or commonly from a tear in the native artery adjacent to a suture line. Repair is usually indicated when a false aneurysm is discovered. Graft failure due to fiber degeneration or diffuse dilatation is not a common problem.

Answer: A, B

5. Match the situation in the left-hand column with the most appropriate type of graft in the right-hand column.

A. Elective repair of abdominal aneurysm
B. Ruptured abdominal aortic aneurysm with transfusion coagulopathy
C. Pediatric renal artery reconstruction
D. Femoropopliteal bypass

a. Venous autograft
b. Woven Dacron graft
c. Knitted Dacron graft
d. Arterial autograft
e. Arterial allograft

Sabiston: 1778

Comments: A variety of natural tissues and prosthetic materials have been used for arterial bypass grafting. Saphenous vein autografts are preferred for replacement of small and medium-sized arteries. Clinical uses include lower extremity revascularization, coronary artery bypass, and less frequently, upper extremity bypass and visceral or renal artery bypass. Replacement of larger arteries such as the aorta usually is done with prosthetic textile grafts of Dacron or Teflon. Because of their handling characteristics, knitted grafts are widely used. Knitted textile grafts are more porous than their woven counterparts, however, and must be pre-clotted prior to insertion. In the presence of a coagulopathy, effective pre-clotting of knitted grafts may not be possible, so that a woven prosthesis is preferred in order to avoid excessive bleeding from the graft interstices. Clinical applications of arterial autografts include the use of the internal mammary artery for coronary artery bypass and the internal iliac artery for renal artery bypass. The use of the internal mammary artery for coronary artery revascularization has been quite successful, and it has been sug-

gested that this may be preferable to the use of the saphenous vein as a bypass graft. Because of the high incidence of venous aneurysm formation when the saphenous vein is used for renal revascularization in children, arterial autografts may be preferred. Arterial allografts are not used clinically because of the high incidence of complications and the availability of more satisfactory arterial substitutes.

Answer: A–c; B–b; C–d; D–a

6. A patient underwent bilateral aortofemoral bypass grafting 1 month ago and now presents with purulent drainage from the left groin. Along with the administration of intravenous antibiotics, appropriate treatment may include which of the following?

A. Drainage of the left groin
B. High ligation and excision of the left limb of the graft and, if necessary, extra-anatomic bypass
C. Removal of the entire prosthesis and bilateral axillofemoral bypass
D. Ligation of the left femoral artery and, if necessary, amputation

Sabiston: 1789
Schwartz: 909

Comments: The general approach to the treatment of infected prosthetic grafts involves antibiotics, removal of the entire prosthesis, and re-establishment of vascular continuity through noncontaminated fields. In select circumstances, local drainage and intravenous antibiotics alone may be adequate to control infection, particularly if the anastomotic suture line is not involved and viable tissue can be rotated to cover the exposed prosthetic material. The options available depend critically on the extent of infection along the prosthesis and the previous operative sites. Extra-anatomic routes of axillofemoral or femoral-femoral grafts permit revascularization through a clean field distal to the original operative site, but often are not applicable when the femoral artery anastomosis is infected. In the case at hand, infection at the femoral anastomosis precludes repeat common femoral artery grafting. If the graft above the inguinal ligament is noninvolved, the aortic and right limb portions of it could be left in place. Reconstruction to avoid limb loss could be accomplished by either obturator bypass from the right graft limb to the left superficial femoral artery or an axillo–superficial femoral artery bypass brought laterally to avoid the contaminated groin. Occasionally, in situations requiring revascularizing vessels to traverse through a contaminated area, autologous tissue can be used. Autologous tissue, however, can also become infected, and for that reason a route for revascularization that avoids the area of contamination is always preferable.

Answer: A, B, C

7. Which of the following statements is/are true regarding noninvasive vascular testing?

A. Patients without arterial disease generally have ankle-brachial indices greater than 1
B. Patients with advanced ischemia generally have ankle-brachial indices less than 0.5

C. Doppler ultrasound measures blood velocity and flow volume
D. Proximal obstruction produces a biphasic or uniphasic Doppler wave form
E. Plethysmography can determine changes in arterial or venous blood flow

Sabiston: 1864
Schwartz: 909

Comments: Information obtained by Doppler ultrasonography and plethysmography can provide information that is an important complement to the vascular physical examination. Also, these tests provide an objective method of assessing therapeutic results. Doppler ultrasound measures blood velocity, not flow. The Doppler instrument allows determination of segmental pressures and wave forms at different levels of the lower extremity and thus yields information about the location of arterial occlusion. Under normal conditions, the arterial wave form is triphasic, but the signal distal to an obstruction becomes biphasic and uniphasic according to the degree of obstruction. Plethysmography measures volume changes during the cardiac cycle and is useful in the evaluation of peripheral arterial, cerebrovascular, and venous disease. Pressure values measured by noninvasive techniques are standardized by comparison with the brachial arterial pressure (the ankle-brachial index), which is normally greater than 1 and declines with advanced degrees of ischemia. The sensitivity of noninvasive vascular testing can be increased by measuring changes in response to exercise that produces vasodilatation distal to a site of arterial obstruction and, therefore, a fall in the distal segmental pressure.

Answer: A, B, D, E

8. Which of the following is the most important factor in preventing infection in a patient with a contaminated arterial injury?

A. Adequate débridement and secondary wound closure
B. Avoidance of synthetic materials for arterial repair
C. Nature of wound contaminant
D. Prompt institution of systemic antibiotics
E. Antibiotic wound irrigation

Schwartz: 929

Comments: Infection is best prevented by adequate débridement of devitalized tissue at the time of initial repair. Every attempt should be made to cover the arterial anastomosis with viable muscle, and in some situations this may require use of a musculocutaneous flap. Skin closure is dictated by the nature of the wound; in severely contaminated cases, secondary closure is appropriate. If a graft is required, autologous vein is preferred in order to minimize the risk of infection. Antibiotic and tetanus prophylaxis are important, but do not supersede adequate local wound treatment.

Answer: A

9. Expected results of lumbar sympathectomy performed for peripheral vascular disease include improvements in:

A. Cutaneous circulation
B. Muscle circulation
C. Claudication
D. Skin ulceration
E. Patency rates of arterial reconstructions

Schwartz: 904, 907, 911, 914

Comments: Lumbar sympathectomy may benefit certain patients with peripheral vascular disease not amenable to arterial reconstruction. The primary effect of sympathectomy is to increase skin circulation. This may provide some protection against skin ulceration in patients with trophic changes; however, objective responses are not demonstrated in the majority of patients. Sympathectomy does not increase muscular blood flow and has not proved beneficial in patients with intermittent claudication as their only symptom. Bilateral lumbar sympathectomy has been performed in conjunction with arterial reconstruction, but has not clearly been demonstrated to improve graft patency.

Answer: A, D

10. Which of the following statements is/are true regarding the effects of aspirin in the treatment of atherosclerotic disease?

A. Antithrombotic effect is mediated by inhibition of thromboxane and prostacyclin production
B. High blood levels are required to inhibit platelet aggregation
C. High blood levels may promote thrombosis
D. Aspirin may cause detrimental intraplaque hemorrhage

Schwartz: 945

Comments: The benefit of aspirin in atherosclerotic disease is based upon its inhibition of platelet aggregation. This aggregation is controlled by a balance between thromboxane and prostacyclin. Very low levels of aspirin inhibit the conversion of arachidonic acid to thromboxane A-2 and, therefore, have an antithrombotic effect. Higher levels, however, also interfere with prostacyclin production in the vascular endothelium, and therefore may paradoxically predispose to thrombosis. An additional concern has been the role of aspirin in promoting hemorrhage into atherosclerotic plaques, which might contribute to subsequent ulceration and stenosis.

Answer: C, D

11. Which of the following statements is/are true regarding dissecting aneurysms?

A. They are three to four times more common in males
B. They occur predominantly in patients over age 50
C. A history of hypertension is present in the majority of cases
D. Mortality may reach 30% within 24 hours of diagnosis
E. Mortality is higher if the dissection begins in the ascending aorta

Sabiston: 1796
Schwartz: 883

Comments: The term "dissecting aneurysm" is misleading in that the actual process is an "aortic dissection" with the development of an aneurysm being a late sequela of the process. The majority are in males beyond the fifth decade of life. The underlying pathology relates to disease of the aortic wall in combination with hypertension, which may be present in as many as 75% of cases. Atherosclerosis, which is a disease of the intima, is not etiologically related. Once the presence of aortic dissection is confirmed, the mortality in untreated cases is high (30% within 24 hours; 75% within 2 weeks). This mortality increases when the ascending aorta is the site of original dissection. The characteristic clinical presentation is that of sudden excruciating pain in the chest and back, which may migrate caudally as the dissection continues. Emergency aortography followed by appropriate surgical repair is the appropriate management.

Answer: A, B, C, D, E

CHAPTER 44

Vascular—Portal Venous System

1. The portal vein:

A. Is valveless
B. Is formed by the junction of the inferior mesenteric vein and splenic vein
C. Commonly has variations of branching pattern
D. Has multiple portal-systemic collaterals

Sabiston: 1055
Schwartz: 1257

Comments: The portal vein is formed by the junction of the superior mesenteric vein and splenic vein, provides 75% of hepatic blood flow, and has a relatively constant pattern of branching within the liver. Portal hypertension is a common sequela of hepatic diseases that produce portal venous obstruction; prominent clinical manifestations are often due to increased blood flow through the many portal-systemic collateral pathways that are available. The portal venous system has no valves, and this permits measurement of portal venous pressure from any point in the system.

Answer: A, D

2. Which of the following is/are appropriate for the management of portal vein injury?

A. Direct venorrhaphy
B. Portal vein ligation
C. End-to-end anastomosis
D. Graft interposition
E. Portal vein ligation with portosystemic shunt

Sabiston: 315
Schwartz: 1264

Comments: Portal vein injuries generally result from penetrating trauma and have a high fatality rate. The preferred method of management is some form of repair, either by lateral venorrhaphy when possible or by reanastomosis or graft interposition. If repair is not possible, the portal vein may be ligated. Portosystemic shunt-

284

ing is not advocated; it is more dangerous than ligation alone and poses a risk of hepatic encephalopathy.

Answer: A, B, C, D

Sabiston: 1082

3. In which of the following disorders does the pathophysiology of portal hypertension involve presinusoidal intrahepatic obstruction?

A. Budd-Chiari syndrome
B. Cavernomatous transformation of the portal vein
C. Hemochromatosis
D. Alcoholic cirrhosis
E. Congenital hepatic fibrosis

Sabiston: 1100
Schwartz: 1279

Comments: Portal hypertension may result either from increased portal blood flow or increased resistance to flow. By far the most common cause is increased resistance due to some form of obstruction. The site of obstruction is most frequently intrahepatic but may be extrahepatic, as seen in the Budd-Chiari syndrome or portal vein thrombosis. It is useful to consider the site of obstruction as either presinusoidal or postsinusoidal, since patients with presinusoidal obstruction may have normal hepatocyte function, whereas patients with postsinusoidal obstruction usually have hepatocellular damage. By far the most common intrahepatic cause of obstruction is cirrhosis, which produces postsinusoidal obstruction. Presinusoidal obstruction involving fibrosis of the terminal radicles of the portal vein is produced by schistosomiasis and congenital hepatic fibrosis.

Answer: E

4. Which of the following is/are true regarding the angiographic evaluation of patients with portal hypertension?

A. Both venous anatomy and portal pressure can be determined by transhepatic portography, umbilical vein catheterization, or splenoportography

B. Indirect portography is inadequate for assessment of the portal vein
C. Wedged hepatic vein pressure is elevated with presinusoidal obstruction
D. The degree of portal hypertension measured during angiography correlates with the risk of variceal bleeding

Sabiston: 1097

Comments: Angiographic evaluation of patients with portal hypertension permits both visualization of the venous anatomy and measurement of portal pressures. The first approach to visualization of the portal venous anatomy is usually indirect portography performed by percutaneous injection into the splenic and superior mesenteric arteries. Direct portography via transhepatic or transsplenic routes is usually reserved for cases that cannot be visualized by indirect methods. A number of approaches allow direct measurement of portal venous pressures. Wedged hepatic vein pressure reflects sinusoidal pressure and is usually normal with presinusoidal obstruction. Although manometric studies are of interest in patients with portal hypertension, the degree of pressure elevation has not been found to correlate with the subsequent risk of variceal hemorrhage or ascites.

Answer: A

5. Following resuscitation of a patient with acute hemorrhage from esophageal varices, the next therapeutic measure(s) should be:

A. Intra-arterial vasopressin
B. Intravenous vasopressin
C. Endoscopic sclerotherapy
D. Portacaval shunt
E. Gastroesophageal devascularization

Sabiston: 1101
Schwartz: 1283

Comments: The approach to acute upper gastrointestinal hemorrhage in a patient with portal hypertension must focus on resuscitation followed by confirmation of the bleeding site and therapeutic measures directed at hemostasis. In general, the least invasive therapies are initiated first. Vasopressin can be administered via a peripheral vein as a bolus of 20 units/20 minutes followed by continuous infusion of up to 0.4 unit/minute. This controls hemorrhage in 50–70% of patients. There is no particular advantage to intra-arterial administration of vasopressin. If vasopressin does not control bleeding, endoscopic sclerosis of acute variceal hemorrhage is effective in achieving initial control in 80–90% of cases and results in a lower mortality than that achieved in patients managed medically without sclerosis. Balloon tamponade is no longer the preferred initial treatment for acute variceal hemorrhage, but it may be useful as a temporizing measure in patients who continue to bleed. Transhepatic variceal embolization may be useful in controlling hemorrhage, but rebleeding is not uncommon, and complications are significant. Emergency surgery in the form of either a shunting procedure or gastroesophageal devascularization is required in patients who continue to bleed.

Answer: B

6. The effect(s) of vasopressin include(s):

A. Esophageal variceal vasoconstriction
B. Splanchnic arteriolar vasoconstriction
C. Coronary arterial vasoconstriction
D. Cramping abdominal pain
E. Dilutional hyponatremia

Sabiston: 1101
Schwartz: 1283

Comments: Vasopressin produces generalized vasoconstriction. It is effective in reducing variceal hemorrhage because of constriction of splanchnic arteriolar beds and a secondary fall in portal pressure. It does not directly affect the bleeding varices which do not have smooth muscle. Vasopressin also may cause coronary vasoconstriction, contraindicating its use in patients with ischemic heart disease. Raynaud's phenomenon is also sometimes observed. Contraction of intestinal smooth muscle may produce cramping pain and diarrhea. Dilutional hyponatremia may occur as a result of the antidiuretic effect of vasopressin.

Answer: B, C, D, E

7. Which of the following treatment(s) may decrease recurrence of variceal bleeding?

A. Total portosystemic shunt
B. Selective variceal shunt
C. Gastric devascularization and portal-azygous disconnection
D. Endoscopic variceal sclerosis
E. Propranolol

Sabiston: 1103

Comments: The natural history of variceal hemorrhage in cirrhotic patients indicates that 60% will rebleed within 1 year of their initial hemorrhage, which is associated with significant mortality. Several therapeutic options are available and have been shown to decrease the incidence of recurrent variceal hemorrhage, although the criteria by which patients are selected for one treatment or another are not unequivocally defined. Both total and selective portosystemic shunts effectively prevent recurrent hemorrhage. Some favor selective shunts on the basis that they preserve hepatic blood flow and prevent hepatic failure and encephalopathy. Portal-azygous disconnection usually involves esophageal transection, splenectomy, and gastric devascularization; this approach may be useful in patients with compromised hepatic function or in those in whom shunting procedures cannot be performed for technical reasons. Repeated endoscopic sclerotherapy has been shown to decrease re-bleeding and improve survival of patients compared with those treated only medically. Long-term survival following sclerotherapy has not yet been demonstrated to be superior to that from shunting procedures. Pharmacologic measures to decrease portal pressure, such as treatment with the beta-adrenergic blocker propranolol, have been shown to decrease rebleeding in one randomized controlled trial.

Answer: A, B, C, D, E

8. Which of the following is/are true concerning prophylactic shunts in patients with cirrhosis and varices?

A. They decrease risk of hemorrhage compared with medical therapy
B. They improve survival compared with medical therapy
C. They increase risk of encephalopathy compared with therapeutic shunts
D. They increase risk of hepatic failure compared with therapeutic shunts

Sabiston: 1104

Comments: Clinical trials of portosystemic shunts performed prophylactically in patients with cirrhosis and documented varices (and who have not yet bled) have not demonstrated any advantage compared with standard medical therapy. Although the risk of bleeding is decreased, these patients are at risk both for encephalopathy and for hepatic failure and survival has not been improved. As a consequence, prophylaxis is not currently considered an indication for portosystemic shunting. In this regard, it should be noted that Sugiura's experience with portal-azygous disconnection and Inokuchi's experience with coronary-caval shunts, both of which report superior results, have included a significant proportion of patients for whom the procedures were performed prophylactically.

Answer: A

9. Which of the following is/are considered to be a total portosystemic shunt?

A. End-to-side portacaval
B. Side-to-side portacaval
C. Central splenorenal
D. Distal splenorenal
E. Coronary-caval

Sabiston: 1104
Schwartz: 1288

Comments: Physiologically, portosystemic shunts eventually function either as total shunts, which deprive the liver of blood flow, or selective shunts, which are performed with the goal of maintaining portal perfusion of the liver. End-to-side portacaval shunts function as Eck's fistulas with complete diversion of portal hepatic blood flow. However, even shunts that maintain portal-hepatic continuity, such as the side-to-side, mesorenal, central splenorenal, and mesocaval shunts, effectively produce a total physiologic shunt, since the portal vein acts as an outflow tract from the high-pressure system. The distal splenorenal shunt and coronary-caval shunt, however, are examples of selective shunts, which decompress the gastroesophageal region while maintaining portal hepatic flow. Adequate division of collateral pathways during creation of a selective shunt may be important to prevent its eventual function as a total shunt.

Answer: A, B, C

10. Total portosystemic shunts effectively:

A. Control acute variceal bleeding
B. Prevent recurrent variceal bleeding
C. Improve patient survival compared with medical management
D. Prevent hepatic encephalopathy

Sabiston: 1104

Comments: There is no question that total portosystemic shunts are effective in controlling acute variceal hemorrhage and in preventing recurrence of bleeding. The price, however, is the risk of encephalopathy and hepatic failure due to diversion of hepatic blood flow. Neither prophylactic nor therapeutic total shunts have been shown to improve overall survival significantly compared with nonshunting therapy.

Answer: A, B

11. In patients with alcoholic cirrhosis, distal splenorenal shunts, as compared with portacaval shunts, have been shown to:

A. Improve survival
B. Prevent hemorrhage more effectively
C. Reduce the risk of encephalopathy
D. Be technically easier

Sabiston: 1110
Schwartz: 1290

Comments: Randomized prospective trials comparing the selective splenorenal shunt with total portosystemic shunts in the treatment of portal hypertension due to alcoholic cirrhosis have demonstrated equivalent effectiveness for both types in controlling hemorrhage and in allowing long-term survival. In most studies, encephalopathy has been less common following selective shunts. Technically, an end-to-side portalcaval shunt is easier to perform.

Answer: C

12. Which of the following is/are incorporated in Child's classification of hepatic dysfunction?

A. Bilirubin determination
B. SGOT (AST) determination
C. Prothrombin time
D. Serum albumin determination
E. Assessment of ascites

Sabiston: 1097
Schwartz: 1291

Comments: Child's classification incorporates a combination of clinical and laboratory parameters that correlate with the early mortality of shunting operations. These prognostic factors include clinical assessment of ascites, encephalopathy, and nutritional status and laboratory determinations of serum bilirubin and albumin. Patients are designated as Class A, B, or C; respective operative mortality rates for shunting procedures are approximately <2%, 10%, and 50%. Prolongation of prothrombin time to more than 4 seconds above control (after vitamin K has been replaced) also suggests significant hepatic dysfunction. Elevations of SGOT may suggest hepatitis and warrant delay of operation until this diagnosis can be excluded.

Answer: A, D, E

13. Which of the following vein(s) is/are ligated during distal splenorenal shunt?

A. Left adrenal vein
B. Inferior mesenteric vein
C. Superior mesenteric vein
D. Coronary vein
E. Pancreatic branches of splenic vein

Sabiston: 1106

Comments: The selective distal splenorenal shunt is performed by end-to-side anastomosis of the distal end of the divided splenic vein to the left renal vein, thus decompressing gastroesophageal collaterals through the short gastric vessels. The left adrenal vein and inferior mesenteric vein are ligated during dissection of the splenic vein. It has additionally been recognized that pancreatic branches of the splenic vein should be divided in order to prevent the late development of peripancreatic collaterals, which would divert hepatic portal blood flow and negate the selectivity of the shunt. For this same reason, the left gastric vein (coronary vein) and right gastroepiploic vein are disconnected from the portal system.

Answer: A, B, D, E

14. Which of the following technical consideration(s) might preclude construction of a portacaval shunt?

A. Portal vein thrombosis
B. Large caudate lobe of liver
C. Previous splenectomy
D. Previous operations for biliary stricture

Schwartz: 1290

Comments: Selection of the appropriate type of shunting operation for a particular patient must consider etiology of the portal hypertension, clinical manifestations, status of the liver, and the technical demands of each operation. Portacaval shunts cannot be performed when there is portal vein thrombosis and may be difficult when there are extensive adhesions from previous right upper quadrant operations. The presence of a large caudate lobe may prevent direct approximation of the portal vein and inferior vena cava; this can sometimes be circumvented by placement of an interposition graft or by resection of the caudate lobe. Previous splenectomy has no bearing on technical construction of a portacaval shunt but would preclude the performance of a selective distal splenorenal shunt.

Answer: A, B, D

15. Which of the following is/are true regarding portal hypertension in children?

A. Congenital hepatic fibrosis is the most common cause

B. Variceal bleeding is the most common cause of massive hematemesis in children
C. Acute variceal hemorrhage usually requires operation
D. Portosystemic shunts are contraindicated because of the long-term risk of encephalopathy

Sabiston: 1290
Schwartz: 1282, 1284, 1293

Comments: Unlike portal hypertension in adults, most portal hypertension in children is caused by extrahepatic obstruction of the portal vein, usually as the result of portal vein thrombosis. Variceal hemorrhage constitutes the most common cause of massive upper gastrointestinal bleeding in the pediatric age group and is often the first manifestation of portal hypertension. Most episodes of acute variceal hemorrhage in children will stop without invasive therapeutic measures. Survival following shunting procedures in children with extrahepatic portal vein obstruction is better than that in adults with hepatic compromise. This has influenced some to suggest an aggressive approach to shunting procedures in children with recurrent hemorrhage. Since bleeding episodes are generally well tolerated, however, others advocate a conservative attitude and note that shunting procedures in children carry the risk of thrombosis and encephalopathy or of hepatic dysfunction. Total shunts, such as the mesocaval or central splenorenal type, have been performed in children with portal vein thrombosis; if the splenic vein is of sufficient size to avoid thrombosis, a selective distal splenorenal shunt may be preferable. Endoscopic sclerotherapy for variceal hemorrhage may be successful; patients may eventually demonstrate spontaneous regression of varices as they grow and collaterals develop.

Answer: B

16. Which of the following shunt(s) may be appropriate for the treatment of Budd-Chiari syndrome?

A. End-to-side portacaval
B. Side-to-side portacaval
C. Mesocaval
D. Mesoatrial
E. Distal splenorenal

Comments: Budd-Chiari syndrome is characterized by obstruction of the hepatic veins, which produces heptomegaly, ascites, and pain and progresses to hepatocyte necrosis with liver failure. Since the hepatic outflow tract is occluded, surgical decompression can be achieved only by some form of side-to-side shunt. The evaluation of patients with Budd-Chiari syndrome should include radiographic and manometric assessment of the inferior vena cava, since obstruction or thrombosis of the inferior vena cava may also be present. This situation would preclude a simple portacaval shunt and necessitate some form of portal-atrial or caval-portal-atrial shunt. A number of shunts have been proposed for this particular situation; mesoatrial interposition grafts have been successful, but have a significant incidence of thrombosis. These cases are unusual and experience in treating them has been limited.

Answer: B, C, D

CHAPTER 45

Vascular—Peripheral Venous and Lymphatic Disease

1. A 28-year-old overweight woman comes to the Emergency Room with a slightly reddened, painful "knot," 8 cm above the medial malleolus. Examination in the standing position demonstrates a distended vein above and below the mass. There are no other abnormalities on physical examination. The most likely diagnosis is:

A. Early deep vein thrombosis
B. Superficial venous thrombosis
C. Insect bite
D. Cellulitis
E. Subcutaneous hematoma

Sabiston: 1718
Schwartz: 975

Comments: Venous thrombi may be associated with an acute, nonbacterial inflammation producing pain, redness, and swelling, a condition known as thrombophlebitis. Thrombi, however, may form without producing any signs or symptoms. Superficial thrombophlebitis usually occurs as a localized process over the known course of a superficial vein. Distended varicosities above and below the lesion aid in the diagnosis. The diagnosis of cellulitis, insect bite, subcutaneous hematoma, and traumatic ecchymosis must be considered when evaluating these lesions. Some aids to the differential diagnosis are the location of the lesion, itching, and a history of trauma. The presence of increased redness, pain, fluctuance, fever, and leukocytosis is more typical of a bacterial infection and not superficial thrombophlebitis.

Answer: B

2. The treatment plan for the patient in Question 1 should include:

A. Hospitalization, venogram, heparinization
B. I-125–labeled fibrinogen scan, hospitalization, heparinization
C. Ligation of the vein proximal and distal to mass, bed rest, intravenous antibiotics
D. Bed rest, elastic support hose, leg elevation, antibiotics
E. Warm, moist packs, elastic support hose, ambulation but no sitting or standing, re-examination in 48 hours

Sabiston: 1719
Schwartz: 975

Comments: The usual aim of treatment of superficial thrombophlebitis is the relief of symptoms. The inflammation is nonbacterial and antibiotics are not necessary unless there is evidence of secondary infection. These thrombi rarely embolize to the lungs unless they have propagated to the deep venous system. Anticoagulation, therefore, need not be used. Ligation is reserved for superficial lesions in the greater saphenous system above the knee near its junction with the femoral vein and for lesions of the lesser saphenous system near the popliteal fossa. The risk of propagation of the thrombus is lessened by preventing venous stasis. This is accomplished by walking, using elastic stocking support, and by keeping the leg elevated above the level of the heart when in the supine position; sitting and standing still should be avoided whenever possible. Superficial thrombophlebitis is an acute problem and symptoms from it usually resolve in several days. Anti-inflammatory drugs are of variable effectiveness; aspirin usually suffices. Recurrent superficial thrombophlebitis may respond to proximal ligation followed at a later time by vein stripping.

Answer: E

3. The patient in Question 1 returns for examination after spending 2 days in bed with her leg elevated. She had felt better with partial resolution of her symptoms, but now notices a crampy pain in her calf when walking and a feeling of heaviness in the calf. Which of the following should the physician do?

A. Reassure her because the absence of pain while resting in bed precludes the diagnosis of deep venous thrombosis (DVT)

B. Begin antibiotics, since the most likely cause of her pain is secondary bacterial infection
C. Instruct her to begin ambulation and to avoid prolonged bed rest so that her muscle cramping can resolve
D. Become concerned about the presence of DVT, check for swelling, tenderness, and Homan's sign and obtain an impedance plethysmogram (IPG)
E. Obtain an emergency venogram and begin heparin if it is abnormal

Sabiston: 1719
Schwartz: 976

Comments: When treating superficial venous thrombosis, one must always examine for deep venous thrombosis, especially if the process is near the groin or popliteal fossa. Swelling remote from the site of the superficial thrombus, a positive Homan's sign, or calf, popliteal, or groin pain all are suggestive of concomitant DVT. However, in many large series, clinical examination alone has been shown to be incorrect in greater than 50% of cases. Noninvasive tests, including Doppler ultrasound, impedance plethysmography (IPG), and phleborheography (PRG), are accurate techniques for diagnosing DVT in the thigh but less dependable in the calf. Emergency venography performed on an outpatient basis remains the most accurate and cost-effective technique for diagnosing DVT in calf veins. DVT can occur anytime, and patients confined to bed often experience few, if any, symptoms. Because 85% of pulmonary emboli arise from the lower extremity, early diagnosis and aggressive treatment are important. An aching type of pain in the calf or thigh aggravated by muscular activity, cramps, or a feeling of heaviness accentuated by standing, all suggest the diagnosis. Swelling is variable and depends on the site and size of the thrombus. The swelling is often minimal and may be demonstrable only by actually measuring the diameter of the limb. The degree of swelling can be a very reliable sign of the course of DVT. Tenderness often is present and is elicited by palpation of the calf, popliteal space, adductor canal, and groin. Homan's sign is useful if positive, but may be less reliable than the presence of swelling and tenderness.

Answer: E

4. Match the items in the two columns.

Site of Thrombosis	Signs and Symptoms
A. Calf vein	a. Left side more frequently involved; swelling associated with cyanosis
B. Femoral vein	
C. Ileofemoral vein	b. No swelling
D. Pelvic vein	c. Ankle and calf swelling; venous pressure two to five times normal
	d. Minimal swelling; venous pressure normal

Sabiston: 1719
Schwartz: 977

Comments: The signs and symptoms of DVT vary according to the vein involved. The most frequent site of thrombus is the calf, usually arising in the sinuses of the soleus muscle. **Calf** vein thrombi usually produce pain and tenderness, but swelling is absent in 30% of patients. When there is swelling it usually is minimal (generally less than 1.5 cm diameter difference between the calves), and venous pressure is normal. **Femoral** vein thrombi produce pain in the calf, popliteal region, or adductor canal. Swelling is usually present up to the midcalf, and venous pressure is elevated. **Ileofemoral** thrombi are often localized but may extend to the calf. The left leg is involved three to four times more often than the right, probably because of the longer course of the left iliac vein and its compression by the right iliac artery. Swelling of the entire leg is often present and the venous pressure is elevated, producing bluish discoloration of the leg early in the course of the disease. Pain and cyanosis are often present. Extensive ileofemoral venous thrombosis can obstruct all venous drainage and impair arterial inflow, producing ischemia and eventually venous gangrene. This condition, phlegmasia cerulea dolens, is a surgical emergency. **Pelvic** vein thrombus can occur in women with pelvic inflammatory disease or in men with prostatic infections. The condition is detected by pelvic examination; there are few leg signs. **Upper extremity** DVT usually occurs in patients with heart failure or cancer. In normal patients, it has been termed the "Paget-Schroetter syndrome" or "effort thrombosis." It is due to subclavian vein thrombosis and presents as arm swelling and tenderness over the axillary vein.

Answer: A–d; B–c; C–a; D–b

5. True statements regarding the work-up of deep venous thrombosis include which of the following?

A. Venography has been replaced by the combined use of isotope scans and impedance tests
B. Isotope scans are associated with a risk of hepatitis
C. Doppler ultrasound and impedance plethysmography are equally useful in diagnosing femoral, popliteal, and major calf-vein thrombosis
D. Doppler ultrasound and impedance plethysmography are equally useful in diagnosing ileofemoral venous occlusion
E. Isotope scans cannot differentiate between active thrombosis and inflammatory fibrous exudate

Sabiston: 1726
Schwartz: 977

Comments: **Isotope scans** with I-125–labeled human fibrinogen are used to detect clot formation or thrombus propagation. Studies of even the sickest patient are possible by using portable instrumentation. It is not useful in patients with superficial thrombophlebitis, recent incisions, traumatic injuries, hematomas, cellulitis, active arthritis, or primary lymphedema, because it cannot differentiate between active inflammatory fibrous exudate and thrombus formation. Upper thigh and pelvic lesions can often be confused by the high background counts from the pelvic organs. An isotope scan can be 90% accurate in detecting the onset of thrombus when performed serially (daily) in high-risk patients. It is 80% accurate in testing for suspected established venous thrombosis. **Doppler ultrasound** is useful in detecting occlusions of major venous channels. It can also detect incompetence of the deep and perforator veins, but it cannot differentiate between old and new thrombi, nor diagnose small, nonobstructing thrombi. **Impedance plethysmography** is more accurate than Doppler ultrasound in the diagnosis of femoral popliteal and major calf vein thromboses. Venography is still considered the definitive test for the diagnosis of deep venous thrombosis and is used to resolve equivocal results obtained by the noninvasive techniques.

Answer: B, D, E

6. True statements regarding the prevention of venous thrombosis include:

A. There is no direct evidence that elastic stockings influence the incidence of thrombus formation
B. To be effective, pneumatic calf compression must be used for at least 3 days after an operation
C. Mini-heparinization remains the most effective means to prevent DVT in the surgical patient
D. Injury to the intima of veins is an important cause of venous thrombosis
E. Sequential pneumatic calf compression devices are as effective as mini-heparinization in preventing venous thrombosis

Sabiston: 1741
Schwartz: 980

Comments: Prophylaxis is critical in avoiding venous thrombosis. Attention to technical detail when handling veins so as not to injure their intima and avoidance of leg veins when infusing hypertonic or irritating solutions are but several examples of ways to help minimize the risk of thrombosis. Leg elevation and leg exercises in the postoperative period decrease venous stasis and its predisposition to thrombus formation. I-125–labeled fibrinogen scans have demonstrated the usefulness of pneumatic compression stockings in decreasing the incidence of thrombus formation. Extending their use into the postoperative period has no advantage over their use during operation and in the recovery room only. Sequential pneumatic devices are more effective than nonsequential devices and in at least one study have been shown to be as effective as mini-heparinization. Mini-heparinization given 2 hours preoperatively and continued until the seventh postoperative day has been shown to decrease the incidence of deep venous thrombosis. There is evidence, however, that it may increase the rate of bleeding and wound complication postoperatively; its impact on the incidence of postoperative pulmonary emboli has not been clearly defined. While no one method of prophylaxis has been shown to be clearly superior, some form of prophylaxis is important, whether it be aimed at preventing venous stasis physically or by the use of anticoagulants.

Answer: D, E

7. True statements regarding the medical treatment of deep venous thrombosis include:

A. Bed rest is recommended in order to allow the thrombi to become securely attached to the venous wall
B. Heparin is given to prevent thrombus attachment to the venous wall

C. Platelet counts lower than 75,000/µl imply active clot formation and inadequate levels of heparin
D. Anticoagulation should be continued for 1 to 6 months after the acute event, depending on the site of involvement
E. Streptokinase and urokinase are contraindicated within 10 days of major operations or trauma

Sabiston: 1740
Schwartz: 982

Comments: The prevention of embolization from existing thrombi and the inhibition of new thrombus formation are the goals of medical therapy. Bed rest with leg elevation for approximately 7 days decreases venous pressure and prevents fluctuations of pressure in the deep venous system. This allows the thrombus already present to become firmly attached to the vessel wall, minimizes venous distension, and reduces edema and pain. Elastic support is not needed with adequate elevation, but should be used when ambulation is started. Heparin prevents propagation of the thrombus by inhibiting thromboplastin formation and by inactivating thrombin in the presence of heparin cofactor. A partial thromboplastin time that is two times normal indicates adequate heparinization. Giving heparin by continuous intravenous infusion is the preferred method, but intravenous or subcutaneous bolus administration can be used. Heparinization is continued for at least 7 days. Some patients on heparin develop platelet clots in the arterial system, which can be a catastrophic complication. Therefore, a platelet count that falls to less than 75,000/µl is considered a reason to discontinue heparin. Coumadin derivatives are begun prior to stopping the heparin, to allow anticoagulant therapy to be continued on an outpatient basis. Treatment is usually continued for 4 weeks until the risk of recurrence diminishes. In cases of ileofemoral thrombosis, anticoagulation is continued for 6 months to allow time for the development of adequate collateral circulation, which decreases the risk of recurrence. **Streptokinase** and **urokinase** are both capable of lysing thrombi by the activation of plasminogen to plasmin. Their use in combination with heparin significantly reduces the incidence of late postphlebitic complications as compared with heparin alone. Pyrogenic, allergic, and bleeding complications occur with both agents, and their use is contraindicated within 10 days of major operations or injury. The value of antiplatelet drugs like aspirin is still undefined.

Answer: A, D, E

8. True or False: The major indication for deep venous thrombectomy is recurrent pulmonary emboli.

Sabiston: 1721
Schwartz: 982

Comments: The role of surgery in the treatment of acute venous thrombosis is limited for several reasons: the effectiveness of medical management, and the high incidence of residual or recurrent venous obstruction and valvular incompetency after surgery. Operation usually is reserved for major obstruction of the subclavian, iliac, or femoral vein and when the immediate or long-term function of the limb is in jeopardy. There are some who believe thrombectomy should be considered with any ileofemoral thrombosis, since there is considerable late morbidity in those patients treated with heparin alone. Progression of ileofemoral thrombosis to the stage of near-total occlusion with tenderness, massive edema, and cyanosis (phlegmasia cerulea dolens) may lead to venous gangrene. In this setting, failure to respond immediately to leg elevation and heparinization is an indication for thrombectomy. Operations for subclavian vein thrombosis should include resection of the first rib or clavicle, since most thrombi originate at the point where the clavicle crosses the first rib; failure to resect is associated with a high incidence of postoperative recurrence.

Answer: False

9. True statements regarding the evaluation of patients with suspected pulmonary emboli include:

A. The triad of dyspnea, pain, and hemoptysis is present in 60% of patients
B. The findings of a normal SGOT in the presence of an elevated serum bilirubin and LDH is present in over 50% of patients
C. Pulmonary arteriography requires cardiac catheterization
D. The arterial alveolar CO_2 gradient is increased in pulmonary embolism
E. Ventilation-perfusion scans must be compared with a recent chest x-ray to be of value

Sabiston: 1738
Schwartz: 983

Comments: One must have a very low threshold for suspecting pulmonary emboli in postoperative patients. Eighty-five per cent of pulmonary emboli arise from the lower extremity, 10% from the right atrium, and 5% from the pelvic veins, vena cava, or arms. Up to 30% of patients with pulmonary embolism are without symptoms, and only one third of patients with pulmonary emboli have physical evidence of deep vein thrombosis at the time of diagnosis. Emboli produce symptoms either by the direct effects of arterial obstruction or by secondary bronchospasm and vasoconstriction. The most common symptoms are dyspnea and chest pain and the most common signs are tachycardia, tachypnea, and rales. The classic triad of dyspnea, pain, and hemoptysis is present in less than 25% of patients. The classic biochemical triad of a normal SGOT with elevated LDH and bilirubin is now considered unreliable. Few patients will show diagnostic EKG changes other than tachycardia. Wedge-shaped defects on chest x-ray are seen only if infarction occurs. Decreased vascularity, pulmonary artery distension, and pleural fluid may be detected. Pulmonary arteriograms are the most specific way to make a diagnosis and may be performed either by contrast infusion via a right atrial or main pulmonary artery catheter or by simultaneous right and left arm superficial vein injection. On ventilation-perfusion scans, areas of the lungs that are normally ventilated but not perfused and that appear normal on chest x-ray should be considered to have pulmonary emboli. These scans are safe, convenient, and reliable and in most patients are generally preferred over arteriograms.

Answer: D, E

10. True statements regarding the treatment of pulmonary embolism include:

A. The primary treatment for confirmed pulmonary embolism is systemic anticoagulation
B. The primary treatment for confirmed pulmonary embolism is systemic anticoagulation and thrombolytic therapy
C. Caval interruption eliminates recurrent pulmonary embolus but is associated with a high incidence of continued thrombophlebitic symptoms
D. Partial caval interruption is performed in patients with pulmonary embolism and confirmed deep venous thrombosis
E. The use of thrombolytic agents has eliminated the need for pulmonary embolectomy

Sabiston: 1742
Schwartz: 984

Comments: The primary therapy for pulmonary emboli in most patients is anticoagulation. The precise role of thrombolytic agents is still in evolution. For certain patients, caval interruption may be indicated. These include patients in whom heparin therapy is contraindicated, those with recurrent emboli while on anticoagulation therapy, and those with free-floating ileofemoral thrombi; it may be used prophylactically in high-risk patients (e.g., prior to major pelvic surgery in those with a history of previous deep vein thrombosis or pulmonary emboli). Additionally, it includes some patients with septic pulmonary emboli who are refractory to heparin and to antibiotics. Caval interruption may be complete or partial; recurrence of pulmonary emboli after complete interruption is possible, though rare, and results from thrombi arising from the ovarian veins, the cava between the ligature and the renal veins, the right atrium, the right ventricle, and veins of the head and neck. Chronic leg swelling, recurring phlebitis, and the sequelae of deep venous obstruction (edema, discoloration, and ulceration) are more common after complete caval interruption and have been reported to occur with a frequency as high as 35%. However, experience with the Hunter balloon, a transvenous method for total occlusion, has shown the incidence of these complications to be low (5%) in patients who can be maintained on anticoagulants after caval interruption. Also, the presence of pre-existing deep venous obstruction and chronic venous insufficiency strongly influences late results after caval interruption. Partial interruption with such devices as the Greenfield filter or Miles clip result in a lower incidence of postphlebitic sequelae, a higher incidence of nonfatal emboli (7 vs. 4%), and a similar incidence of fatal emboli (about 1%). Caval filters can migrate and have also been associated with injury to adjacent retroperitoneal structures. Patients with massive pulmonary emboli producing hypotension who survive the acute event are candidates for pulmonary embolectomy. This is performed using a median sternotomy, cardiopulmonary bypass, and open clot extraction. An alternative to median sternotomy may be percutaneous catheter embolectomy.

Answer: A

11. Match the location and blood flow patterns with the appropriate superficial venous system.

Location and Flow Pattern

A. Ultimately joins the femoral vein in the thigh
B. Ultimately joins the popliteal vein behind the knee
C. Anterior and posterior branch in the calf, lateral and medial branch in the thigh
D. Receives blood from the deep system via perforators
E. Blood flows into the deep system via the perforators
F. Perforators are located posterior and superior to the malleoli

Venous System

a. Greater saphenous system
b. Lesser saphenous system
c. Both
d. Neither

Sabiston: 1710, 1724
Schwartz: 988

Comments: An understanding of normal venous anatomy and blood flow is essential when considering chronic venous insufficiency and its sequelae. Normal veins of the lower extremity contain valves that direct the flow of blood centrally toward the heart and from the superficial into the deep venous system. Competent valves resist the force of gravity that, in the erect position, tends to pool blood at the ankle. Forward flow is provided by the action of the left ventricle and compression of the veins as a result of muscular contraction. During muscular relaxation, deep venous pressure falls, leading to increasing emptying of the superficial veins into the deep veins with a resultant fall in superficial venous pressures to below-resting levels. Incompetence of the valves of the deep veins (usually the result of previous venous thrombosis) allows blood pooling and ineffective muscular pumping. Incompetence of the perforator valves (as a direct result of venous thrombosis or due to dilatation by back pressure from a valveless deep system) allows transmission of this increased deep venous pressure to the superficial system. When this occurs, the sequelae of venous stasis (brawny, nonpitting edema, brown pigmentation, dermatitis, and finally venous ulceration) develop. Venous ulcers usually occur over the perforators, which are located dorsal and cephalad to the medial and lateral malleoli. Superficial venous incompetency, perforator incompetency, and deep vein abnormalities all have the potential of causing these changes, and each may occur alone or in combination with the others.

Answer: A–a; B–b; C–a; D–d; E–c; F–c

12. A 56-year-old man presents with a history of heaviness, tiredness, and aching of the left lower leg for the past several months. The symptoms are relieved by leg elevation. He also mentions that he is awakened from sleep because of calf and foot cramping, but it is relieved by walking or massage. On physical examination, he has obvious varicosities, nonpitting edema bilaterally and a superficial ulcer 2 cm in diameter, 5 cm above and behind the medial malleolus, that is slightly painful. The differential diagnosis should include:

A. Arterial insufficiency with ulceration

B. Isolated symptomatic varicose veins
C. Varicose veins associated with incompetent perforator veins
D. Deep venous insufficiency with incompetent perforator veins

Sabiston: 1724
Schwartz: 989, 991

Comments: The most common symptoms associated with venous insufficiency are aching, swelling, and night cramps of the involved leg; the symptoms often occur after periods of sitting or inactive standing. Leg elevation frequently provides relief. While the **edema** of venous insufficiency can occur with varicose veins alone, usually it is associated with deep venous abnormalities and incompetent perforating veins. **Night cramps** are due to sustained contractions of the calf and foot muscles and are relieved by massage, ambulation, and proper management of the underlying venous insufficiency. The **brawny, nonpitting edema** is due to increased connective tissue in the subcutaneous tissue. **Brown discoloration** is due to hemosiderin deposition. **Ulceration** is most common in patients with deep venous abnormalities and incompetent perforators. In such cases ulcers usually are located above and posterior to the malleoli, reinforcing their relationship with perforator abnormalities. When patients with a history of DVT are followed beyond 10 years, up to 80% ultimately develop ulcers. The pain of arterial insufficiency often is increased with leg elevation. Ulcers associated with arterial insufficiency occur anywhere on the lower leg and eventually penetrate the fascia. Arterial ulcers have an associated blue erythematous border and are more painful than venous ulcers.

Answer: B, C, D

13. You have performed a Trendelenburg test on the patient described in Question 12 and determine he has incompetent varicose veins associated with incompetent perforating veins. You interpret this as a:

A. Negative/negative Trendelenburg test
B. Negative/positive Trendelenburg test
C. Positive/negative Trendelenburg test
D. Positive/positive Trendelenburg test

Sabiston: 1712
Schwartz: 990

Comments: There are several tests for diagnosing venous insufficiency. The **Trendelenburg test** is a two-part test used to delineate the competency of the superficial and perforating veins. While in the supine position, the patient elevates the legs until the superficial veins empty. The saphenofemoral junction is then occluded digitally and the patient is asked to stand. The superficial veins are observed for 30 seconds (part I) and then the saphenofemoral occlusion is released while the veins are kept under observation (part II). Part I assesses the competency of the perforator veins: slow, ascending, incomplete filling of the superficial veins during compression is a negative (normal) result, while rapid filling is a positive result, indicating incompetency. Part II assesses the competency of the superficial veins. Continued slow ascending filling after saphenofemoral release is a negative (normal) result. Rapid retrograde filling is a positive result indicating incompetency of the valves of the superficial system. The **percussion test** is performed by tapping the superficial veins near the saphenofemoral junction while palpating over the knee for transmitted pulses. It can also be used to examine the lesser saphenous system. Transmission of a pulse suggests incompetent valves. **Venous pressure** studies help delineate abnormalities in the normal venous pressure relationships during exercise. **Functional phlebography** is performed in patients before and after a standard active exercise and can demonstrate important pathologic and physiologic abnormalities. The **Perthes test** involves the application of elastic wraps to a leg with varicosities (so as to occlude the superficial venous system) before the patient is asked to exercise; pain during exercise suggests obstruction of the deep venous system.

Answer: D

14. Your therapeutic plan for the patient in Question 12 should include:

A. Varicose vein ligation and stripping as soon as possible
B. Ligation of his medial perforating veins as soon as possible
C. Initial treatment with appropriate leg wraps, leg elevation, and ambulation without sitting or standing still
D. Ulcer débridement, vein stripping, and skin graft

Sabiston: 1712, 1724
Schwartz: 991

Comments: Operative treatment of venous insufficiency in most instances is an adjunct to aggressive conservative management. Leg elevation, active exercise, and elastic compression form the cornerstones of nonoperative management. The goals of compression are to relieve symptoms and to reduce swelling. When ulcers are present, local medications should be avoided unless evidence of infection exists. Ulcers less than 3 cm in diameter will often heal with the above treatment. The indications for superficial vein ligation and stripping are moderate to severe symptoms without other signs of venous insufficiency, venous insufficiency with recurrent ulceration in spite of aggressive medical management, and, occasionally, severe varicosities without symptoms. Ligation of incompetent perforators can be an important addition to the treatment of venous insufficiency, particularly if done before ulceration develops. Ligation is most often performed through a longitudinal incision placed posterior and superior to the malleoli as first described by Linton. When present, incompetent superficial veins should be stripped as part of the procedure. Postoperatively, conservative measures must be continued aggressively. Obstructions of the ileofemoral or femoropopliteal veins have been bypassed using the ipsilateral (femoropopliteal occlusions) or contralateral (ileofemoral occlusions) saphenous veins. The saphenous vein has also been used to replace segments of valveless postphlebitic femoral veins in an attempt to restore competency.

Answer: C

15. Which of the following statements is/are true regarding lymphatic anatomy?

A. The limb vessels are valveless
B. The lymphatic system begins just below the dermis as a network of fine capillaries
C. Red blood cells, bacteria, and proteins readily enter lymphatic capillaries
D. Extrinsic factors (muscle contraction, arterial pulsations, respiratory movement, and massage) aid in the movement of lymph flow

Sabiston: 1697
Schwartz: 995

Comments: The lymphatic system begins as a network of capillaries in the superficial dermis. There is a second plexus in the deep or subdermal layer that joins with the first to form the lymphatic vessels, whose course parallels the major blood vessels. The vessels are valved, and lymph flow to the heart is aided by massage, arterial pulsations, respiratory movement, and muscle contraction. Intradermal lymphatics can be evaluated by the intradermal injection of patent blue dye. The capillaries normally become visible as a fine network 30 to 60 seconds after injection. Lymphangiography is used to visualize the lymphatic vessels. Unlike veins, these vessels appear of uniform caliber throughout their course. Lymphatic vessels are readily entered by proteins present in the extracellular fluid. Measurement of the protein content of edema fluid (normally less than 1.5 mg/dl) can be used to assess the status of lymphatic function in the edematous extremity.

Answer: C, D

16. True statements regarding the etiology and complications of lymphedema include:

A. Lymphedema praecox appears at birth and is more common in females
B. Primary lymphedema may be due to aplasia, hypoplasia, or varicosities of the lymphatic vessels
C. A lymphangiogram usually will demonstrate a point of obstruction of the lymphatics in primary lymphedema
D. Lymphedema usually is nonpitting and at times becomes woody secondary to the increase in fibrous tissue in the subcutaneous tissue
E. The major complication of lymphedema is the later development of lymphangiosarcoma

Sabiston: 1701
Schwartz: 996

Comments: Primary lymphedema is caused by abnormal development resulting in either aplasia, hypoplasia, or varicosities of the lymphatic vessels. Congenital lymphedema is present at birth. Lymphedema praecox usually appears during the teens, more commonly in females, and often develops insidiously. It is bilateral in 50% of cases and often follows minor trauma or infection. Secondary lymphedema is due to obstruction or destruction of normal lymphatic channels and can be caused by tumor, repeated infection, or parasitic infection, particularly filiriasis, or can occur following lymph node dissection. Lymphangiography will often demonstrate a discrete obstruction. Recurrent infections of venous stasis ulcers can destroy lymphatic vessels and lead to lymphedema. The inability to clear proteins leads to edema formation that gradually increases over time and becomes woody owing to fibrous tissue in the subcutaneous tissue. Repeated infection hastens the formation of this fibrous tissue accumulation. Some patients develop blisters containing edema fluid or chyle. The major complication of lymphedema is recurrent attacks of cellulitis or lymphangitis, often following minor injury. Beta-hemolytic streptococci are the responsible organisms, and the infection spreads rapidly because the protein-containing edema fluid is an excellent culture medium. Lymphangiosarcoma is a rare complication of long-standing lymphedema, most frequently described in patients following radical mastectomy (Stewart-Treves syndrome). It presents as a blue or purple nodule with satellite lesions. Metastases develop early, primarily to the lung. Rarely patients with lymphedema develop a protein-losing enteropathy that has been attributed to lymphatic obstruction of the small bowel.

Answer: B, D

17. True statements regarding the treatment of lymphedema include:

A. Greater than 50% of patients will ultimately require an operation
B. Diuretics have a crucial role in the conservative management of early lymphedema
C. Pneumatic compression devices can damage remaining lymphatics and should not be used
D. The two general categories of surgical treatment are excisional and physiologic

Sabiston: 1702
Schwartz: 998

Comments: The mainstay of management of lymphedema is conservative and nonoperative; only 15% of patients require an operation. The goals of therapy are the prevention of infection and the reduction of subcutaneous fluid volume. Fluid volume is reduced by elevation of the extremity during sleep, the use of pneumatic compression devices, and carefully fitted elastic support stockings. Diuretics are not used routinely but may be useful in women who retain fluid during the premenstrual period. Patients prone to recurrent lymphangitis require intermittent long-term antibiotic therapy at the first sign of infection. The drug of choice is penicillin, since streptococci are the usual infesting organisms. Secondary lymphedema requires treatment of the underlying cause, such as giving diethylcarbamazine for filariasis and appropriate antibiotics for tuberculosis or lymphogranuloma venereum. Edema that is excessive and interferes with normal activity and severe recurrent cellulitis are indications for operation. Excisional procedures include removal of the skin, subcutaneous tissue, and fascia followed by split thickness skin graft reconstruction (the Charles operation); excision of strips of skin and subcutaneous tissue followed by primary closure; and the creation of buried dermal flaps. Physiologic procedures to restore or enhance lymphatic drainage include insertion of silk, Teflon, or polystyrene threads into the subcutaneous tissue; construction of pedicle grafts from the involved limb to the trunk; and microsurgical lymphovenous shunts using dilated lymphatics or the capsule and efferent channels of isolated lymph nodes anastomosed to neighboring veins.

Answer: D

CHAPTER 46

Pediatric Surgery

1. Which fluid regimen provides the most appropriate fluid and electrolyte maintenance for a 6-kg infant?

A. Lactated Ringer's at 15 ml per hour
B. D5 0.5 normal saline + 30 mEq/l KCl at 15 ml per hour
C. D5 0.25 normal saline + 30 mEq/l KCl at 25 ml per hour
D. D5 0.5 normal saline + 15 mEq/l KCl at 25 ml per hour
E. D5 0.25 normal saline + 15 mEq/l KCl at 50 ml per hour

Sabiston: 1255
Schwartz: 1638

Comments: Understanding of maintenance fluid and electrolyte requirements is critical in the management of infant surgical patients. Maintenance free water requirements include replacement of insensible losses from the skin and lungs and the free water of solution necessary to clear metabolic solutes in the urine. Note that this does not include pre-existing deficits or ongoing fluid losses. There are numerous formulas applicable to the calculation of maintenance requirements. Based upon body weight, 24-hour requirements are approximately 100 ml/kg up to 10 kg, plus an additional 50 ml/kg from 10 to 20 kg, plus an additional 20 ml/kg over 20 kg. Estimations based on body surface area give equivalent results. Daily electrolyte requirements include 3 to 5 mEq/kg of sodium and 2 to 3 mEq/kg of potassium. Dextrose is administered to provide a glucose substrate; complete caloric support requires parenteral nutrition solutions.

Answer: C

2. A 28-day-old male presents with nonbilious vomiting. One week ago, he weighed 4 kg; his current weight is 3.6 kg. On examination his anterior fontanelle is flattened and his mucous membranes are dry. Between episodes of crying an olive-sized epigastric mass is palpable. Laboratory data include Na 133, K 3.6, Cl 93, CO_2 28, and capillary pH 7.51. The most likely diagnosis is:

A. Meningitis
B. Hypertrophic pyloric stenosis
C. Antral web
D. Intestinal atresia
E. Hiatal hernia

Sabiston: 1269
Schwartz: 1648

Comments: The age, sex, and clinical presentation of this infant are classic for hypertrophic pyloric stenosis. The olive-sized epigastric mass is virtually pathognomonic and is not seen with medical causes of vomiting or other causes of mechanical gastrointestinal obstruction in infancy. The child is too old for the first presentation of intestinal atresia, in which case bilious vomiting would also be expected. It is important to recognize gastroesophageal reflux as the cause of recurrent spitting up or vomiting in infants, since it usually responds to appropriate conservative measures.

Answer: B

3. The infant's laboratory data described in Question 2 reflect:

A. Normal acid-base balance
B. Metabolic alkalosis
C. Respiratory alkalosis
D. Combined metabolic and respiratory alkalosis
E. Compensated metabolic alkalosis

Sabiston: 68

Comments: Gastric outlet obstruction with sufficient loss of gastric contents produces a hypochloremic, hypokalemic metabolic alkalosis. The ability to compensate by hypoventilation is limited; in fact, infants and children who are crying are hyperventilating and have an additional respiratory alkalosis. A capillary pH of 7.51 indicates significant alkalosis; under normal acid-base balance, determination of capillary or venous pH would be expected to yield a more acidotic result than arterial pH.

Answer: D

4. Which of the following is/are appropriate for initial intravenous therapy?

A. Lactated Ringer's at 25 ml/hr
B. D5 0.5 normal saline + 20 mEq/l KCl at 15 ml/hr
C. D5 0.25 normal saline + 30 mEq/l KCl at 30 ml/hr
D. D5 0.5 normal saline + 30 mEq/l KCl at 25 ml/hr
E. D5W + 0.1 normal HCl at 30 ml/hr

Sabiston: 1256, 1269
Schwartz: 1648

Comments: Appropriate fluid therapy in this situation requires maintenance plus replacement of estimated deficit plus ongoing losses. Estimated initial volume replacement for the first 24 hours includes maintenance of 100 ml/kg plus replacement of approximately half of the estimated deficit. Based on actual weight loss or on estimation of 10% dehydration, the infant's total deficit is approximately 400 ml. The initial rate of fluid replacement is only an estimate, however, and should be adjusted to maintain urine output of 1 to 2 ml/kg/hr. An initial bolus of 20 ml/kg of normal saline may be appropriate for severely dehydrated patients. In terms of electrolytes, sodium, potassium, and chloride must be supplied both for maintenance and for replacement of gastric losses. These can be supplied by a solution of 5% dextrose with 0.5 normal saline and approximately 30 mEq/l of potassium chloride. Ongoing assessment of serum electrolytes should be performed and electrolyte replacement adjusted as necessary. After appropriate fluid and electrolyte correction, the infant requires myotomy for treatment of his pyloric stenosis.

Answer: D

5. The most common complication of a cystic hygroma is:

A. Infection
B. Hemorrhage
C. Respiratory distress
D. Malignancy

Sabiston: 1291
Schwartz: 1639

Comments: Cystic hygroma is a lymphangioma commonly occurring in the posterior neck region or the axilla, groin, or mediastinum. These lesions can reach large size, and all of the complications listed above have been described except malignant degeneration. Infection, however, is the most common complication.

Answer: A

6. Treatment of cystic hygromas should be:

A. Percutaneous aspiration
B. Excision
C. Radical neck dissection
D. Irradiation
E. Thoracic duct drainage

Sabiston: 1291
Schwartz: 1639

Comments: Excision is the preferred treatment of cystic hygroma. Because of their multiloculated and sometimes extensive nature, complete excision of cystic hygromas can be difficult and recurrence is not unusual. Repeat excision, even if partial, is the recommended treatment. Extensive neck dissection with sacrifice of vascular and neurologic structures is not advocated, as these are benign lesions.

Answer: B

7. The internal opening of the most common branchial cleft anomaly is located at the:

A. External auditory canal
B. Nasopharynx
C. Tonsillar fossa
D. Piriform sinus

Sabiston: 1291
Schwartz: 1640

Comments: The most commonly encountered branchial cleft anomaly is a persistent cyst or sinus tract involving the second pharyngeal pouch. The cyst or sinus tract is noted externally along the anterior border of the sternocleidomastoid muscle. When there is a complete fistula, the tract extends through the carotid bifurcation to the area of the tonsillar fossa. Cure is effected by complete excision. First branchial cleft anomalies extend to the external auditory canal with an external opening in the pretragal area. Third branchial cleft fistulas open internally at the piriform sinus, although the external opening may be similar to that of a second branchial fistula.

Answer: C

8. Thyroglossal duct cysts:

A. Are usually noted at birth
B. (Like branchial cleft cysts) occur along the anterior border of the sternomastoid muscle
C. Are usually asymptomatic
D. Should be excised because of the risk of malignancy
E. Require hyoid resection for complete removal

Sabiston: 1291
Schwartz: 1640

Comments: The differential diagnosis of midline neck masses includes thyroglossal duct cysts, dermoid cysts, and enlarged lymph nodes. Thyroglossal duct cysts are embryologic remnants of the thyroid, deposited during its descent from the foramen cecum through the hyoid to its position in the lower anterior neck. Most are discovered as asymptomatic masses in young children following disappearance of infantile subcutaneous fat. Occasionally, they may become infected. Successful excision requires removal of the central portion of the hyoid bone (Sistrunk procedure) if the tract extends proximally.

Answer: C, E

9. Which of the following characteristically present(s) with respiratory distress at birth?

A. Diaphragmatic hernia
B. Pulmonary sequestration

C. Tracheoesophageal fistula
D. Congenital lobar emphysema

Sabiston: 1259, 1262
Schwartz: 1641

Comments: Persistence of the pleuroperitoneal canal of Bochdalek produces the most common congenital diaphragmatic hernia. Displacement of the abdominal contents into the chest results in pulmonary hypoplasia and high-resistance pulmonary arterioles. Infants often present with poor Apgar scores and respiratory distress at birth. Some of these infants may remain stable initially, and then deteriorate. Other causes of immediate respiratory distress following delivery include pneumothorax, airway obstruction, and aspiration. In congenital lobar emphysema, progressive respiratory distress may develop owing to overexpansion of the affected lobe. Patients with tracheoesophageal fistula may have difficulty handling salivary secretions because of esophageal atresia and frequently develop respiratory symptoms with attempted feeding. The usual complication of pulmonary sequestration is infection.

Answer: A

10. Which of the following may be required in the treatment of an infant with congenital diaphragmatic hernia?

A. Tube thoracostomy
B. Extracorporeal membrane oxygenation (ECMO)
C. Priscoline
D. Repair via thoracic approach
E. Repair via abdominal approach

Sabiston: 1261
Schwartz: 1641

Comments: The primary physiologic disturbance in infants with respiratory distress due to congenital diaphragmatic hernia is related to pulmonary hypoplasia and the high resistance that develops in the pulmonary vasculature because of constriction of pulmonary arterioles. Initial resuscitation must be rapid to avoid stresses such as hypoxia, hypercarbia, acidosis, and hypothermia, which increase pulmonary vasoconstriction. High resistance in the pulmonary circulation produces right-to-left shunting via the patent ductus arteriosus, further compromising the infant's cardiopulmonary status. Initial treatment involves endotracheal intubation, placement of an orogastric tube, and maintenance of adequate vascular volume. These infants are prone to develop pneumothorax, and tube thoracostomy may be required; some advocate bilateral prophylactic chest tubes. Vasodilators that affect the pulmonary vascular bed, such as tolazoline (Priscoline), may be useful. The use of ECMO has salvaged infants who have remained critically ill despite conventional ventilator support. Definitive surgical repair is usually carried out via an abdominal approach, but a thoracic approach can also be used.

Answer: A, B, C, D, E

11. Which of the following fetal anomalies is/are associated with maternal polyhydramnios?

A. Esophageal atresia
B. Duodenal atresia
C. Jejunal atresia
D. Pyloric stenosis
E. Renal agenesis

Sabiston: 1263

Comments: The normal fetus swallows amniotic fluid, which is resorbed in the gastrointestinal tract and is excreted by the kidneys. In the presence of gastrointestinal obstruction, this circuit is interrupted and hydramnios results. Approximately 20% of mothers with hydramnios will have infants with gastrointestinal obstruction. Infants born to mothers with hydramnios should therefore have an orogastric tube passed and an evaluation for possible gastrointestinal atresias. Pyloric stenosis usually presents with evidence of gastric outlet obstruction in older infants and is not associated with polyhydramnios. Renal dysfunction produces oligohydramnios because of the inability to secrete the absorbed amniotic fluid.

Answer: A, B, C

12. Identify the most common type of esophageal atresia and tracheoesophageal fistula.

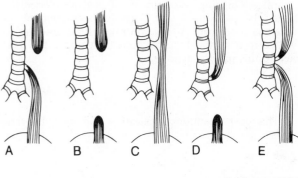

A   B   C   D   E

Sabiston: 1264
Schwartz: 1644

Comments: Eighty-five to 90% of patients with esophageal atresia and tracheoesophageal fistula have a blind proximal pouch with a distal tracheoesophageal fistula. Esophageal atresia without an associated fistula is the second most common form. Esophageal atresia is suggested when the infant has excess saliva or spitting up with attempted feedings. In the presence of esophageal atresia, a fistula is manifested by the findings of air in the gastrointestinal tract and/or respiratory symptoms with feedings. When an orogastric tube is passed in an infant with esophageal atresia, a chest x-ray will show it coiled in the blind pouch. Contrast studies and bronchoscopy may be useful in confirming the diagnosis and demonstrating the location of a tracheoesophageal fistula. Recognition of the anatomy of the anomaly is important for the establishment of appropriate initial treatment and definitive repair.

Answer: A

13. Which of the following is the preferred treatment for a 3,000-gm infant with esophageal atresia and distal

tracheoesophageal fistula, if there is no respiratory distress or associated anomaly?

A. Gastrostomy, cervical esophagostomy, delayed repair
B. Gastrostomy, sump tube drainage of proximal pouch, delayed repair
C. Fistula ligation, delayed esophageal repair
D. Take-down of fistula with primary esophageal anastomosis
E. Primary repair with colon interposition

Sabiston: 1264
Schwartz: 1644

Comments: The timing of surgical intervention for esophageal atresia and tracheoesophageal fistula is influenced by the maturity of the infant and the presence or absence of associated cardiorespiratory problems or other congenital anomalies. Mortality of primary repair is directly related to the risk group into which the infant falls. Otherwise healthy infants, weighing over 2,500 gm, are treated by primary repair with fistula division and closure of its tracheal end and end-to-end anastomosis of the esophageal segments. Infants who are not well enough for primary repair are treated by gastrostomy and drainage of the blind proximal pouch. Repair is carried out after complicating cardiorespiratory problems have been corrected. The presence of the tracheoesophageal fistula can cause problems with dissipation of ventilatory pressure into the stomach or allow aspiration of gastric contents into the lung. In some situations, occlusion of the fistula with a Fogarty balloon is helpful. Formerly, infants undergoing staged repairs were initially subjected to thoracotomy with fistula ligation to prevent these problems.

Answer: D

14. Which of the following is/are the complications of tracheoesophageal fistula repair?

A. Esophageal stricture
B. Anastomotic leak
C. Gastroesophageal reflux
D. Recurrent fistula
E. Empyema

Sabiston: 1265
Schwartz: 1647

Comments: Gastroesophageal reflux is a very frequent complication following operation in these infants that may ultimately and frequently require later fundoplication. The etiology of reflux may relate to underlying esophageal dysmotility and to dysfunction of the lower esophageal sphincter, which is often displaced proximally following repair. Stricture or anastomotic leak and subsequent fistula recurrence can also occur, but are less common. The morbidity of a potential anastomotic leak can be minimized by use of an extrapleural approach; if a leak does occur, it remains extrapleural.

Answer: A, B, C, D, E

15. In repair of an H-type tracheoesophageal fistula, which approach should be used?

A. Cervical
B. Thoracic
C. Abdominal
D. Endoscopic

Sabiston: 1267
Schwartz: 1646

Comments: This type of fistula is uncommon, composing only 1 to 2% of all tracheoesophageal fistulas. Symptoms include respiratory problems due to aspiration and abdominal distension. Since most of these lesions are located in the subglottic area, they are amenable to division and closure via a transcervical approach and do not require thoracotomy. Endoscopy is important in the diagnosis and localization of the fistula, but is not a method of definitive therapy.

Answer: A

16. The most common cause of duodenal obstruction in the neonate is:

A. Duodenal atresia
B. Duodenal web
C. Malrotation
D. Annular pancreas

Sabiston: 1270
Schwartz: 1649

Comments: Bilious vomiting in the newborn is the hallmark of intestinal obstruction. Vomiting within the first 24 hours of life and the absence of abdominal distension suggest high obstruction. The commonest cause of duodenal obstruction in the neonate is duodenal atresia. Among the various causes of duodenal obstruction beyond neonatal age, malrotation is the most common and potentially the most serious. The duodenal obstruction generally is from the extrinsic compression by the peritoneal bands that extend from the abdominal wall to the anomalously located cecum in the right upper quadrant. The catastrophic complication of malrotation is midgut volvulus and intestinal infarction, which may occur because of the narrow mesenteric pedicle by which the midgut is suspended. For this reason, any duodenal obstruction in the newborn should be considered malrotation until proven otherwise and requires prompt surgical attention.

Answer: A

17. Radiographs of a newborn infant demonstrate a "double-bubble" sign and a small amount of scattered gas in the midabdomen. Which of the following should be performed next?

A. Barium upper GI x-ray
B. Gastrografin upper GI x-ray
C. Barium lower GI x-ray
D. Gastrografin lower GI x-ray
E. Laparotomy

Sabiston: 1270
Schwartz: 1651

Comments: With duodenal obstruction, the dilated proximal duodenum and stomach produce the classic double-bubble sign. The presence of generalized abdominal distension and air in the distal gut, however, excludes duodenal atresia and should alert the physician to the possibility of malrotation with duodenal obstruction and midgut volvulus. The possibility of intestinal infarction in such a situation makes prompt laparotomy mandatory. Infants with duodenal obstruction not due to malrotation should be operated upon after decompression and appropriate resuscitation. If operation is best delayed because of compelling associated problems and if malrotation is not probable, a barium enema may be useful in excluding the diagnosis of malrotation and permitting delay of surgery. Radiographic assessment of high obstruction in neonates can be performed with simple injection of air into the stomach; contrast dyes are usually not necessary.

Answer: E

18. Operation for midgut volvulus with viable bowel should include detorsion and:

A. Cecopexy in the right lower quadrant
B. Appendectomy
C. Repositioning the small bowel in the right abdomen
D. Repositioning the colon in the left abdomen

Sabiston: 1270
Schwartz: 1652

Comments: The operative management of malrotation involves counterclockwise reduction of midgut volvulus when present; nonviable bowel is resected. If the viability is in question, or necrosis not certain, the bowel may be returned to the abdomen in the hope that some or all of it will survive and thus preserve bowel length. Even if the patient looks well, a "second-look" laparotomy should be performed 24 hours later, with the intestine reassessed and treated as necessary. Peritoneal bands (Ladd bands) between the cecum and the abdominal wall are divided and the duodenum is mobilized so that the small bowel can be positioned in the right abdomen and the colon in the left abdomen. Appendectomy is routinely performed. Intraluminal duodenal obstruction can occur with malrotation as a result of an associated web or stenosis. This is excluded by gastrotomy and passage of a balloon catheter through the proximal bowel.

Answer: B, C, D

19. True statements regarding jejunoileal atresia include:

A. Etiology is failure of embryologic recanalization of the gut, and therefore the atresias usually are multiple
B. Diagnosis is excluded by passage of transitional stool
C. Associated anomalies are more frequent than with duodenal atresia
D. Disparity in lumen size is common, but rarely presents a technical problem

Sabiston: 1272
Schwartz: 1650

Comments: Intestinal atresia is felt to result from an in-utero vascular accident; approximately 10% of cases have multiple atresias. A variety of forms may be seen, ranging from a simple web to stenosis, to complete separation of bowel ends with varying degrees of mesenteric

defect. In the most severe type (Christmas tree deformity) most of the small bowel mesentery is absent and the remaining distal small bowel is supplied by the ileocolic artery. Intestinal atresia usually presents with bilious vomiting and abdominal distension. The passage of transitional stool containing food establishes gastrointestinal patency. There may be a considerable disparity in size between the proximal and distal bowel. This has led to the development of a number of operative techniques for achieving a functional anastomosis. Associated anomalies are not seen as commonly as they are with duodenal atresia, which in as many as one third of cases is associated with trisomy 21 (Down's syndrome).

Answer: B

20. A newborn infant develops progressive abdominal distension and bilious vomiting. X-ray reveals distended bowel loops of varying size with a mottled appearance and with only a few air-fluid levels. What should be performed next?

A. Laparotomy
B. Sweat chloride test
C. Gastrografin lower GI x-ray
D. Gastrografin upper GI x-ray
E. Paracentesis

Sabiston: 1272
Schwartz: 1652

Comments: The postnatal development of signs of intestinal obstruction with the classic x-ray findings described above suggests a diagnosis of meconium ileus. Nearly all affected infants have cystic fibrosis with a deficiency of pancreatic enzymes, producing a thick, tenacious meconium that causes obstruction in the distal ileum. In-utero perforation may produce meconium peritonitis and is one of the few situations in which abdominal distension may be present at birth. In uncomplicated meconium ileus, as described in this clinical presentation, administration of a Gastrografin enema may be both diagnostic and therapeutic. The detergent and hyperosmolar effects of the contrast material may relieve the obstruction. Operation is indicated if the obstruction does not respond to Gastrografin enema or if complications such as peritonitis or perforation are present. In such instances, the usual operative treatment entails resection of impaired bowel and the creation of an external vent to allow postoperative irrigations with acetylcysteine (Mucomyst); later gastrointestinal continuity is re-established. A sweat chloride test should be performed on all of these infants. Paracentesis or lavage may be helpful in making the diagnosis of necrotizing enterocolitis, a condition mandating prompt operation.

Answer: C

21. The most common cause of colon obstruction in infants is:

A. Imperforate anus
B. Hypoplastic left colon
C. Meconium plug syndrome
D. Hirschsprung's disease

Sabiston: 1273
Schwartz: 1656

Comments: The differentiation of large bowel from small bowel obstruction in infants based on plain radiographs can be difficult because of the lack of haustral markings. Hirschsprung's disease is caused by congenital absence of colonic ganglion cells and should be suspected whenever an infant fails to pass meconium within the first 24 hours of life. The rectum and rectosigmoid areas are the regions most commonly affected, although longer segments may be involved; rarely, total colonic aganglionosis may be present. Both hypoplastic left colon syndrome and meconium plug syndrome may have clinical and radiographic characteristics similar to those of Hirschsprung's disease but usually can be treated with Gastrografin enemas. The diagnoses of Hirschsprung's disease and cystic fibrosis need to be considered in patients with hypoplastic left colon or meconium plug syndrome. Anorectal anomalies are rare causes of neonatal intestinal obstruction.

Answer: D

22. Which of the following is/are true regarding Hirschsprung's disease?

A. It is more common in males
B. It may be complicated by pseudomembranous enterocolitis
C. Barium enema studies may be normal
D. It may be diagnosed by rectal biopsy or anal manometry
E. The initial treatment usually involves colostomy

Sabiston: 1274
Schwartz: 1656

Comments: The primary clinical manifestation of Hirschsprung's disease is that of intestinal obstruction with failure to pass meconium in the newborn male infant or chronic constipation in older infants and children. Infants with Hirschsprung's disease are prone to develop pseudomembranous enterocolitis, which has a high mortality. With newborn infants in whom dilatation of the bowel proximal to the aganglionic segment may not yet have developed, a barium enema may be normal. A definitive diagnosis is based on rectal biopsy, demonstrating absence of ganglion cells in the myenteric plexus and an abundance of acetylcholinesterase by histochemical techniques. Anal manometry demonstrates a characteristic failure of sphincter relaxation in response to rectal distension. Infants with Hirschsprung's disease usually are first treated by a colostomy with delayed repair after a period of growth. Older children with a dilated, hypertrophied proximal bowel require colostomy for initial decompression. Definitive treatment is by one of several pull-through operations featuring anastomosis of normally innervated colon to the anus.

Answer: A, B, C, D, E

23. A premature infant with respiratory distress at birth has been successfully weaned off the ventilator and now is being fed oral formula. The infant is noted to develop abdominal distension and passes blood-streaked stool. Appropriate management should include:

A. Anoscopy for probable neonatal fissure
B. Barium enema to exclude intussusception
C. Restriction of oral intake to clear fluids to prevent mucosal injury
D. Antibiotics only if specific pathogens are cultured from the stool
E. Cessation of all oral feedings

Sabiston: 1288
Schwartz: 1654

Comments: The most likely cause of the above clinical situation is necrotizing enterocolitis (NEC), a disease of premature infants and infants subjected to neonatal stress. The pathophysiology involves mucosal ischemia, bowel necrosis, perforation, peritonitis, and sepsis. It nearly always occurs in infants after the start of oral feedings. Clinical manifestations initially are formula intolerance, abdominal distension, blood-streaked stools with progression to frank peritonitis, and signs of systemic sepsis including acidosis, disseminated intravascular coagulation, and thrombocytopenia. Initial treatment is directed at the prevention of further mucosal injury and of septic complications. Oral feedings are stopped, tube decompression is instituted, broad-spectrum antibiotics are administered, and careful fluid and electrolyte support is provided. Close monitoring is mandatory, involving not only physical examination but also serial radiographs every 6 to 8 hours and serial biochemical assessment to detect signs of deterioration.

Answer: E

24. Which of the following are indications for operation in an infant with necrotizing enterocolitis?

A. Pneumatosis intestinalis
B. Portal vein gas
C. Pneumoperitoneum
D. Erythema and edema of the abdominal wall
E. Progressive thrombocytopenia

Sabiston: 1288
Schwartz: 1654

Comments: Pneumatosis intestinalis is a characteristic radiographic finding in necrotizing enterocolitis caused by invasion of the bowel wall by gas-forming organisms. Similarly, portal vein gas indicates the presence of gas-forming organisms that have been transported in the portal circulation to the liver. Neither of these radiographic findings alone, however, is an absolute indication for operation. Indications for surgical intervention are signs of perforation, peritonitis, or progressive clinical deterioration despite nonoperative therapeutic measures. These signs include pneumoperitoneum, an abdominal mass that may suggest abscess, tenderness, erythema and edema of the abdominal wall, and progressive acidosis or thrombocytopenia. When operation is performed, necrotic bowel is resected, abscesses are drained, and the ends of the retained bowel are brought out as enterostomies.

Answer: C, D, E

25. An infant recovers following resection and enterostomy for necrotizing enterocolitis. Prior to reestablishment of intestinal continuity, the work-up should include:

A. Sweat chloride test
B. Chromosomal studies
C. GI contrast studies
D. IVP

Sabiston: 1289
Schwartz: 1655

Comments: Following successful recovery from resection for NEC, bowel continuity can be re-established. It is important to visualize the distal bowel radiographically either by barium enema or by studies with contrast medium introduced through the distal enterostomy before reanastomosis, because stricture formation occurs in approximately 20% of infants. Stricture can occur after seemingly mild cases of NEC and can be a late cause of intestinal obstruction even in infants who did not require operation at the time of their acute illness. The other studies listed may be indicated depending on associated anomalies that the infant may have, but are not specific to the process of necrotizing enterocolitis. A sweat chloride test for cystic fibrosis should performed in any infant with meconium ileus, meconium plug syndrome, or hypoplastic left colon syndrome.

Answer: C

26. Contraindications to attempted barium enema reduction of an intussusception in a child include:

A. Pneumoperitoneum
B. Peritonitis
C. "Currant jelly" stool
D. Recurrence after previous hydrostatic reduction
E. Age over 5 years

Sabiston: 1282
Schwartz: 1655

Comments: Intussusception most commonly occurs in children under 3 years of age and usually as the result of hypertrophied lymphoid tissue in the terminal ileum. Barium enema can successfully reduce intussusception by hydrostatic pressure in approximately 60% of children and usually is the initial therapy. An attempt at hydrostatic reduction is contraindicated, however, in the presence of perforation or peritonitis. The passage of the characteristic "currant jelly" stool seen with intussusception may occur as the result of mucosal venous congestion and does not necessarily indicate necrosis. So, it does not contraindicate an attempt at nonoperative reduction. Recurrence no longer is considered an absolute indication for surgery, and a second attempt at hydrostatic reduction may be successful. Age alone does not mandate operation, although a leading point such as a polyp, Meckel's diverticulum, or tumor (lymphoma) is more likely to be found in older children and is more likely to require an operation. If an attempt at reduction by barium enema is unsuccessful, prompt operation is indicated.

Answer: A, B

27. Which of the following is/are true regarding the operative management of intussusception?

A. Resection should be performed without an attempt at intraoperative reduction, if reduction by barium enema has been unsuccessful
B. Primary ileocolic anastomosis may be performed if bowel resection is necessary
C. Following successful reduction by barium enema, delayed operation should be performed because of the risk of recurrence
D. Following successful reduction by barium enema in a child over 3 years old, exploration is indicated to exclude associated pathology

Sabiston: 1283
Schwartz: 1656

Comments: When nonviable bowel is encountered at the time of exploration for intussusception, resection is carried out without an attempt at reduction. Otherwise, reduction by gentle digital pressure is attempted; resection is performed if the intussusception is not reducible by this means. Primary anastomosis can generally be performed. Recurrent intussusception is unusual following successful reduction either by hydrostatic or by operative means. Contrast studies usually are sufficient to exclude significant associated pathology that would require operation in older children.

Answer: B

28. A mass located in the mesentery of the ileum adjacent to the bowel wall may be a(n):

A. Intestinal duplication
B. Meckel's diverticulum
C. Mesenteric cyst
D. Omphalomesenteric duct remnant

Schwartz: 1656

Comments: Intestinal duplications occur most commonly in the ileum; they present as cystic or tubular masses next to the bowel wall between the mesenteric leaves and contain elements of intestinal wall. Mesenteric cysts are also located within the mesentery but they do not contain any muscular wall. A Meckel's diverticulum is a type of omphalomesenteric duct remnant and, although found in the terminal ileum, is located on the antimesenteric side of the bowel.

Answer: A, C

29. Match each clinical characteristic in the left-hand column with the appropriate abdominal wall defects in the right-hand column.

A. Associated anomalies   a. Omphalocele
B. May close spontaneously   b. Gastroschisis
C. Require operation in the newborn   c. Umbilical hernia
D. Associated heat and fluid losses   d. None of the above
E. Closure may require prosthetic material

Sabiston: 1279, 1295
Schwartz: 1661

Comments: Each of these entities represents an abdominal wall defect at or near the umbilicus. **Omphalocele** results from failure of embryologic development of a portion of the anterior abdominal wall, presents as a truly midline sac-covered defect, and frequently is associated with other anomalies. In contradistinction, **gastroschisis** is thought to occur as the result of in-utero rupture of an umbilical hernia, and presents with eviscerated bowel through a defect without a sac and usually appears on the right side of the cord. The exposure of the extraperitoneal viscera to amnionic fluid and subsequently to the postnatal environment results in a burn-type physiology with significant fluid and heat losses that must be compensated for in the infant's resuscitation. **Umbilical hernias** result from failure of closure of the linea alba at the umbilical ring and may close spontaneously. Herniorrhaphy is done, usually at age 4 or 5, if spontaneous closure has not occurred. In the repair of both omphalocele and gastroschisis, when primary closure cannot be achieved because of the size of the defect and limited capacity of the abdomen, a Dacron sheet coated with Silastic (Silon) has been useful; a Gore-Tex sheet is now used more commonly.

Answer: A–a; B–c; C–a, b; D–b; E–a, b

30. Which of the following statements is/are true regarding imperforate anus?

A. Anomalies are defined as high or low according to the relationship of the rectum to the puborectalis mechanism
B. High anomalies are associated with a perineal fistula
C. Most female infants require initial colostomy
D. Imperforate anus may be associated with esophageal atresia and tracheoesophageal fistula
E. Pull-through techniques are highly successful in preserving continence

Sabiston: 1275
Schwartz: 1658

Comments: Imperforate anus is a type of anorectal agenesis in which the anus is absent and the rectum ends at varying levels in relation to the puborectalis mechanism. The blind rectum usually ends in a fistula which, in high lesions, usually opens into the prostatic urethra in males or the vagina in females. Low lesions present with a perineal fistula which often is seen in the median scrotal raphe of males or in the posterior vaginal fourchette of females. The level of the anomaly is the critical determinant of the type of correction required. Low lesions, which are suspected in the presence of a perineal fistula, can be corrected by a simple perineal approach. High lesions are initially treated by colostomy, followed by a definitive reconstructive procedure aimed at bringing the rectum through the puborectalis sling in order to achieve continence. Most cases of imperforate anus in females are of the low variety, whereas approximately one half of the lesions occurring in males are of the high variety. Historically, the various pull-through operations have not been too successful in achieving fecal continence. It appears, however, that the more recent approach of posterior sagittal anoplasty (described by Pena) may provide better long-term results. Imperforate anus may occur as part of the constellation of VATER anomalies (vertebral, anorectal, tracheoesophageal, renal/radial dystrophy). These, as well as associated genitourinary anomalies, must be excluded.

Answer: A, D

31. Parents of an infant with a unilateral undescended testicle should be advised that:

A. Correction of the problem should be carried out immediately
B. Spontaneous descent may occur, but if this has not happened by age 2 years, repair should be performed
C. Orchiopexy should be performed to prevent malignancy
D. Orchiopexy may prevent infertility

Sabiston: 1294
Schwartz: 1666

Comments: An undescended testicle must first be differentiated from a retractile testicle which, on careful examination, can be brought into the scrotum and does not require surgical treatment. In instances of bilateral undescended testes, serum gonadotropins and chromosomal studies may be helpful in establishing the presence of testicular tissue. Many infants with undescended testes will have spontaneous descent in the first year or so of life; if not, an orchiopexy should be carried out by the age of 2 years. There is evidence that in patients with undescended testes after the age of 2 years, spermatogenesis is impaired. Orchiopexy prior to this time may lessen the chance of infertility; however, patients with bilateral cryptorchidism in particular continue to have a high incidence of infertility. Cryptorchidism is associated with an increased risk of testicular cancer (predominantly seminoma); orchiopexy, however, does not diminish this risk, and these patients require periodic examination throughout their adolescent years. Additional reasons to perform orchiopexy include psychologic considerations, an increased incidence of testicular torsion, and the possibility of testicular trauma when the testicle is located at the pubic tubercle.

Answer: B, D

32. If at the time of orchiopexy, an undescended testicle cannot be brought down into the scrotum, appropriate treatment may include:

A. Orchiectomy
B. Attachment to the pubic tubercle and reoperation in 1 year
C. Division of the spermatic artery and vein to provide additional length
D. Termination of the procedure and treatment with chorionic gonadotropin

Sabiston: 1295
Schwartz: 1667

Comments: In most cases of cryptorchidism, particularly if the testicle is palpable, the testicle can be brought down into the scrotum without difficulty. The approach is through a herniorrhaphy incision; the cord is carefully dissected and an associated hernia sac, which is usually present, is dissected free and ligated at the internal ring.

The testicle is secured in a subcutaneous pouch in the scrotum after passage through the Dartos fascia. For the occasional instance when the testicle is in a higher retroperitoneal position and adequate length cannot be obtained for scrotal positioning, different approaches have been used including staged orchiopexy with reoperation in 6 to 18 months and division of the spermatic vessels, preserving the testicular blood supply along the vas deferens. Microvascular anastomosis has also been suggested. Human chorionic gonadotropin has been used as a nonoperative method of producing testicular descent. It is more successful in patients with bilateral undescended testes than in those with unilateral cases, but the success rate is not great.

Answer: B, C

33. Which of the following is/are true regarding the treatment of unilateral inguinal hernia in infants?

A. Operation should be delayed until 1 year of age since spontaneous obliteration of the processus vaginalis may occur
B. High ligation of an indirect hernia sac without formal floor repair is sufficient
C. A concerted attempt should be made to remove the distal hernia sac to prevent postoperative hydrocele
D. There is general agreement that contralateral exploration is indicated because of the high incidence of bilaterality

Sabiston: 1293
Schwartz: 1665

Comments: Inguinal hernias in children nearly always are due to failure of closure of the processus vaginalis. Repair is recommended at the time of diagnosis because there is a significant risk of incarceration. A patent processus vaginalis is not always associated with a clinical hernia, however, and some closure must occur during postnatal development since the patency rates are lower in adults. In infants with indirect inguinal hernia, simple high ligation and excision of the hernia sac at the internal ring is adequate treatment; routine repair of the inguinal floor should be avoided because it is unnecessary and risks injury to important fascial structures. It is not necessary to remove the entire distal hernia sac, and it should be left in place if its dissection might jeopardize cord structures. The role of exploration of clinically normal contralateral groins in infants is controversial. Although there is a high incidence of contralateral patent processus vaginalis, not all of these become clinically significant hernias.

Answer: B

34. A 3-month-old infant presents in the emergency room with a tender, firm right inguinal mass.

A. Reduction should be attempted after sedation
B. If reduction cannot be accomplished, herniorrhaphy should be performed promptly
C. Even if the hernia is reduced easily, emergency herniorrhaphy should be performed promptly
D. If the infant appears female, testicular feminization with torsion of an undescended testicle is likely

Sabiston: 1293
Schwartz: 1665

Comments: An incarcerated inguinal hernia in an infant can usually be reduced provided the infant is placed in a warm, calm environment and adequately sedated. Following successful reduction, repair should not be delayed unnecessarily. If the hernia cannot be reduced, then an emergency operation is obviously indicated. About 15% of hernias in children occur in females. Testicular feminization is present in only about 1% of female infants with inguinal hernias, and the presence of a hernia in a female infant, therefore, does not strongly suggest the diagnosis. Incarceration of an inguinal hernia risks not only intestinal ischemia, but testicular ischemia and subsequent atrophy as well. In females, the hernia sac may contain the ovary and tube, but ovarian ischemia is not common unless there is associated torsion.

Answer: A, B

35. Following elective repair of an inguinal hernia in a male infant, the child becomes anuric and edema of the abdominal wall is noted. The most likely diagnosis is:

A. Ischemic bowel
B. Synergistic bacterial infection
C. Iatrogenic urinary bladder injury
D. Iatrogenic ureteral injury

Sabiston: 1294

Comments: Complications are unusual following elective repair of groin hernias in children. Bladder injury may occur, however, if the incision is placed too far medially or if the bladder is involved as a sliding component and not recognized. In male infants, the bladder is the organ most frequently involved in sliding inguinal hernias, whereas in females the tube and ovary are more commonly involved.

Answer: C

36. Massive upper gastrointestinal bleeding in a child is most commonly caused by:

A. Gastritis
B. Peptic ulcer disease
C. Congenital arteriovenous malformations
D. Esophagogastric varices

Sabiston: 1289

Comments: Portal hypertension in children not uncommonly is first manifested by bleeding from esophagogastric varices. The portal hypertension frequently is the result of extrahepatic portal venous obstruction secondary to portal vein thrombosis and cavernomatous transformation of the portal vein. Gastritis and peptic ulcer disease may occur in children, but are not commonly the source of massive upper GI bleeding. The initial diagnostic approach to children with significant upper GI bleeding, as in adults, is by endoscopy. Bleeding varices may require endoscopic sclerotherapy or may require portal-systemic shunting.

Answer: D

37. Which of the following is/are true regarding hepato-portoenterostomy (Kasai procedure) in the treatment of biliary atresia?

A. Portoenterostomy is most successful when performed after 3 months of age, when the bile ducts are larger
B. When successful, portoenterostomy is rarely complicated by cholangitis
C. Portoenterostomy is no longer indicated as the initial surgical procedure if hepatic transplantation is available
D. Hepatic cirrhosis and portal hypertension remain problematic despite successful portoenterostomy

Sabiston: 1284
Schwartz: 1660

Comments: Biliary atresia occurs as part of a spectrum of anomalies known as infantile obstructive cholangiopathy. Although the etiology of these anomalies is unknown, it has been related to in-utero viral infection. Variable patterns of ductal involvement may occur, although commonly the extrahepatic bile ducts are obliterated and replaced by fibrous cords. Both the intrahepatic and extrahepatic biliary tree may be involved. The goal of treatment is to provide biliary drainage and to prevent late complications of biliary cirrhosis with secondary hepatic failure. Hepatoportoenterostomy is most successful in establishing bile drainage when performed in the first 2 months of life. The success rate falls dramatically after 3 months of age. Cholangitis, biliary cirrhosis, hepatic failure, and portal hypertension remain as late problems despite the fact that bile drainage is achieved. Hepatic transplantation has been successful in the treatment of this problem, but has not yet replaced an attempt at biliary enteric anastomosis as the initial procedure. An unsuccessful hepatoportoenterostomy does not preclude later hepatic transplantation. In order to minimize later cholangitic complications, long-term antibiotics, external venting of the Roux limb, and creation of a nipple valve in the Roux limb have been used.

Answer: D

38. The most common childhood malignancy is:

A. Lymphoma
B. Leukemia
C. Wilms' tumor
D. Neuroblastoma
E. Rhabdomyosarcoma

Sabiston: 1286
Schwartz: 1668

Comments: Malignancy is second only to trauma as the leading cause of death in childhood. In infants, malignant disease is the third most frequent cause of death following prematurity and congenital anomalies. Approximately 40% of childhood malignancies are leukemias. The most common solid tumor in children is neuroblastoma.

Answer: B

39. Match the characteristics in the left-hand column with the appropriate pediatric solid tumor(s) in the right-hand column.

A. Most common in first 3 years of life
B. Usually presents as an asymptomatic mass
C. Calyceal distortion on IVP
D. Elevated vanillylmandelic acid (VMA)
E. Primary treatment surgical
F. Overall 5-year survival over 75%

a. Wilms' tumor
b. Neuroblastoma

Sabiston: 1286
Schwartz: 1668

Comments: Neuroblastoma and nephroblastoma (Wilms' tumor) are the most common solid malignancies in children. The clinical presentation is often similar, presenting as an asymptomatic abdominal mass in children in the first years of life. Wilms' tumor, which is an embryonal sarcoma arising from the kidney, typically produces distortion of the renal collecting system on IVP. The lungs are the most common site of metastatic disease. Neuroblastoma arises from cells of neural crest origin, typically occurring in the adrenal medulla or posterior mediastinum. IVP differentiates adrenal neuroblastoma from Wilms' tumor by demonstrating renal displacement but no calyceal distortion. Because of continued catecholamine turnover, VMA levels are elevated in neuroblastoma and have been a useful biochemical marker. Neuroblastoma most commonly metastasizes to the liver and bone. The primary treatment of both of these lesions is by complete surgical excision, which is more often possible with Wilms' tumor. Both chemotherapy and radiotherapy are utilized but have been most useful in enhancing the survival of patients with Wilms' tumor, rather than neuroblastoma. The overall cure rate for Wilms' tumor is approximately 80% as compared with 30% for neuroblastoma. Younger children with neuroblastoma have a better prognosis, however, and infants under 1 year of age may attain a survival rate of 80%.

Answer: A–a, b; B–a, b; C–a; D–b; E–a, b; F–a

40. Which of the following is/are true regarding sacrococcygeal teratoma?

A. It is more common in males
B. When diagnosed after the neonatal period, it is usually benign
C. Excision should be performed in the newborn period
D. Malignant lesions should receive radiotherapy and chemotherapy prior to excision

Sabiston: 1288
Schwartz: 1670

Comments: Sacrococcygeal teratoma usually is identified by the presence of an external postsacral mass, although it may occur in the presacral space as a retrorectal lesion and not be noted until symptoms of rectal obstruction occur. When first noted in the neonatal period, most of these lesions are benign. Nonetheless, they should be excised promptly because of their marked potential for malignant degeneration. The incidence of malignancy and metastasis is high; the prognosis is worse when excision is delayed beyond the second month of life. There is a distinct female predominance of these lesions (80 to 85%). Malignant lesions do not respond well to radiotherapy or chemotherapy.

Answer: C

41. Match the characteristics in the left-hand column with the pediatric hepatic tumor(s) in the right-hand column.

A. More frequent
B. Better prognosis
C. Bimodal age distribution
D. Primary treatment surgical

a. Hepatoblastoma
b. Hepatocarcinoma

Sabiston: 1287
Schwartz: 1671

Comments: Hepatoblastoma and hepatocarcinoma are the two most common types of hepatic malignancies that occur in pediatric age groups. Hepatoblastoma is found most frequently in children under 3 years of age; hepatocarcinoma occurs in young infants and also in late childhood to early adolescence. Hepatoblastoma is the more frequent of the two lesions and also has the more favorable prognosis with an overall 5-year survival of 30 to 50%, whereas survival with hepatocarcinoma is approximately 15%. Alpha-fetoprotein is a useful biochemical marker for hepatic malignancies. The therapy of these tumors involves a multimodality approach, although surgical resection offers the best chance of cure.

Answer: A–a; B–a; C–b; D–a, b

CHAPTER 47

Transplantation

1. In which of the following clinical situations should organ or tissue donation be considered?

A. A 57-year-old man who dies of metastatic lung cancer
B. A 17-year-old man who is dead on arrival at the emergency room following a motorcycle accident
C. A 2-year-old child with irreversible brain death from bacterial meningitis, despite adequate treatment with appropriate antibiotics
D. A 24-year-old woman with irreversible brain injury following trauma who has a positive antibody to hepatitis surface antigen
E. A 35-year-old man who is brain dead after 2 weeks of hospitalization from ruptured intracerebral aneurysms and whose admission serum creatinine of 1.0 has risen to 3.0

Schwartz: 425, 427

Comments: The past or current presence of most common visceral malignancies is not a contraindication to corneal donation; the only contraindications are lymphoproliferative malignancies, lethal viral disease, or local ophthalmologic diseases. Because of the scarcity of pediatric donors, young children who have received appropriate antibiotic treatment for a septic disease, yet suffer brain death from septic or infectious causes, can be considered as liver donors. Bone donation should also be considered from every patient of age 18 to 40 years, especially if the tissues can be recovered within 6 hours of the time of death. In many cases, transient organ dysfunction is not a contraindication to organ donation. This is especially true of kidneys whose dysfunction almost certainly represents acute prerenal causes; upon reimplantation, eventual good restoration of organ function can be assumed.

Answer: A, B, C, D, E

2. The major reason for the shortage of cadaver organs available for transplantation is:

A. The result of laws relative to speed limits and to driving while intoxicated

B. Strong opposition by many religious denominations
C. The high frequency of refusal by the family
D. The high frequency of litigation against physicians who have declared patients brain dead
E. Inability or unwillingness of primary attending physicians to discuss the possibility of brain death with relatives and the possibility of organ donation

Schwartz: 425, 427

Comments: Despite the decreased death rate from highway accidents, it has been estimated that there are approximately 20,000 potential donors in the United States each year. Of these, fewer than 10 to 15% are utilized for organ donation. A minority of these refusals can be attributed to opposition on the part of the family. The overwhelming majority represent a failure or unwillingness of attending physicians to discuss with the families at the appropriate time the option of organ donation.

Answer: E

3. In evaluating a patient with end-stage renal failure, which of the following is/are absolute contraindications to consideration for renal transplantation?

A. Presence of cancer
B. History of pyelonephritis
C. Age greater than 50 years
D. Age less than 2 years
E. Long history of juvenile-onset diabetes mellitus

Sabiston: 408
Schwartz: 410

Comments: Because of the adverse effects of immunosuppressive drugs on infection or on cancer, transplantation is absolutely contraindicated in patients with uncontrollable infection or cancer. Pyelonephritis as an isolated event is not a contraindication to transplantation, and chronic infection is treated by bilateral nephrectomy. Patients who are considered cured from their cancer can be considered for transplantation, but not those with known existing cancer. With improvement in immunosuppression, the upper age limit for transplantation is being extended so that patients in their 50's, and even selected patients in their 60's with no other serious illnesses, can be considered as appropriate candidates for transplantation. Transplantation is the treatment of choice for children with end-stage renal disease, and many children less than 2 years of age have received transplants. Patients with serious systemic illnesses are at higher risk for complications following transplantation, but similarly are at higher risk with dialysis; almost certainly, they have a better chance of survival and rehabilitation with a successful renal transplant. For this reason, patients with diabetes are optimally treated with early transplantation.

Answer: A

4. A 40-year-old male has chronic glomerulonephritis; otherwise, his past history is unremarkable. Other than mild fatigue, his only abnormalities are a slowly rising BUN (90) and creatinine (7.0). No suitable living related donor is available, and the issue of access for dialysis has been raised. Which of the following operative procedures is/are appropriate for preparing this patient for dialysis and future cadaveric renal transplantation?

A. Scribner shunt
B. Arteriovenous (Brescia) fistula
C. Insertion of peritoneal dialysis catheter
D. Bilateral nephrectomy, splenectomy and dialysis access procedure
E. None of the above

Sabiston: 433
Schwartz: 412

Comments: Because of the shortage of cadaver organs, patients on dialysis may wait years for a kidney. There are advantages to peritoneal dialysis in some situations and the choice is determined by patient preference. The Scribner shunt with the plastic cannulae does not remain patent as long as the arteriovenous fistula. The immunologic advantages of splenectomy are countered by the long-term risk of infections and the advantages of apparent survival are not present at long-term analysis. Nephrectomy should be performed only for control of infection, symptomatic cystic disease, or uncontrollable hypertension.

Answer: B, C

5. With respect to organ donation by living relatives, which of the following statements is/are true?

A. Parents should preferentially be chosen, as their more advanced age allows less time for the acute and long-term adverse physiologic consequences of unilateral nephrectomy to become manifest
B. Children should preferentially be considered, as they present with the physiologically youngest organ
C. Siblings should be considered preferentially for immunologic reasons
D. None of the above

Sabiston: 410
Schwartz: 413

Comments: Long-term studies have shown no ill effects to living related donors who are adequately screened. It has also been shown that there is no advantage to having kidneys from a younger rather than an older donor, providing the renal function in any particular donor is normal. As histocompatibility antigens are inherited in mendelian fashion, 25% of siblings will be a perfect match, with a 95 to 98% long-term graft survival.

Answer: C

6. A cadaver kidney becomes available for a transplantation; which of the following is/are absolute contraindications to using this organ?

A. ABO incompatibility
B. Poor match based on HLA tissue typing
C. The presence of a current positive T-cell cross-match
D. A past, positive T-cell cross-match but a current negative T-cell cross-match
E. More than 36 hours of cold ischemia

Sabiston: 408
Schwartz: 411

Comments: ABO compatibility is an absolute requirement for renal transplantation. While there are rare instances in which ABO-incompatible kidney donors have been used successfully, this remains the exception to the standard rules of transplantation. • While there are many who feel there are advantages in emphasizing HLA-A, HLA-B, and HLA-D matching for transplantation of a cadaver kidney, the differences are relatively small; there are many transplant surgeons who believe that the longer waiting time for a kidney with these matching characteristics outweighs the advantages of a good HLA match. For this reason, they place minimal importance on tissue typing for cadaver recipients. • A currently positive T-cell cross-match indicates the presence of circulating antibodies against Class I antigens, and the certainty of hyperacute rejection. The current cross-match, therefore, must always be negative. It was believed that past sera with a positive T-cell cross-match would lead to an increased incidence of acute rejection and graft loss. Recent analysis of clinical studies has shown this not to be true and that many more transplants are performed across positive cross-matches with old or historical sera. Good renal function can be expected from kidneys that have been ischemic for 48 hours.

Answer: A, C

7. A patient receives a cadaver transplant without any operative incident; his initial immunosuppression does not include cyclosporine. During the first 24 hours postoperatively, the urine output averages 10 ml/hr. His vital signs have remained stable during the postoperative period. Regarding post-transplant oliguria, which of the following statements is/are true?

A. Surgical exploration should be performed, as oliguria in this situation is almost always due to technical problems
B. Anti-rejection treatment should be instituted, as the oliguria almost surely indicates acute rejection

C. The patient's drug regimen after transplantation should be closely evaluated, as the oliguria most typically indicates nephrotoxicity

D. Broad-spectrum antibiotics should be started, as infection is the most likely cause

E. None of the above

Sabiston: 414
Schwartz: 417

Comments: The most common cause of initial poor function or nonfunction of a cadaveric graft is preservation injury (acute tubular necrosis).

Answer: E

8. Which of the following is the single best method to evaluate early post-transplant oliguria when the patient is known to be well hydrated?

A. Immediate surgical exploration

B. Arteriogram

C. Biopsy

D. Intravenous urogram

E. Ultrasound with Doppler capability

Sabiston: 414
Schwartz: 417

Comments: Modern ultrasonographic techniques offer outstanding accuracy and precision in the ability to detect technical causes of allograft dysfunction. Doppler capability enables one to evaluate renal blood flow in both the artery and the vein. The parenchymal visualization is often so precise as to be able to differentiate rejection from other parenchymal processes. A diagnosis can almost always be made short of reoperation.

Answer: E

9. Regarding potential organ donors, which of the following statements is/are true?

A. A flat electroencephalogram is always necessary for the declaration of brain death

B. The presence of greater than 10^5 *Escherichia coli* organisms per milliliter in the urine is a contraindication to renal transplantation

C. Significant hypothermia is a contraindication to a declaration of brain death

D. A requirement for dopamine at a dose of 25 μg/kg/minute to maintain blood pressure constitutes a contraindication to using the kidney

E. None of the above

Sabiston: 410
Schwartz: 415

Comments: Brain death can be declared on the basis of clinical signs only. Although electroencephalograms were required in the past, the statutes in most states do not define the criteria for determining death. Reversible causes of profound cerebral dysfunction such as hypothermia and barbiturate therapy must be excluded. ● The coexistence of a urinary tract infection is not a contraindication to removal of kidneys, as this usually is a result of bladder catheterization and not pyelo-

nephritis. ● Although high-dose dopamine seriously affects the perfusion of the heart and liver, it does not cause serious long-term injury to the kidneys.

Answer: C

10. Regarding cyclosporine, which of the following statements is/are true?

A. Cyclosporine is a polysaccharide derived from *Pseudomonas* organisms; its major mechanism of action is based on its inability to block the synthesis of interleukin 1.

B. Clinical side effects of cyclosporine administration include nephrotoxicity, hepatotoxicity, and neurotoxicity

C. The major mechanism of action of cyclosporine is related to its ability to interfere with the synthesis of interleukin 1 by the macrophage

D. The major advantage for cyclosporine in renal transplantation is its ability to interfere with the immunologic memory so that patients with positive cross-matches can receive transplants to which they have performed antibodies

E. Renal biopsy is an ideal method by which to differentiate cyclosporine toxicity from rejection

Sabiston: 443
Schwartz: 386

Comments: Cyclosporine is a polypeptide derived from fungus; its mechanism of action is inhibition of synthesis of interleukin 2. ● Renal biopsies are very unreliable in differentiating nephrotoxicity from rejection. ● Cyclosporine has no effect on the immunologic memory; it does not allow patients with a positive cross-match to receive a transplant.

Answer: B

11. Which of the following statements is/are true regarding the effect of immunosuppression on the host immune system?

A. Immunosuppressive therapy accompanying transplantation contributes to a greatly increased incidence of visceral malignancies (e.g., of lung, colon, pancreas, and stomach)

B. Herpes-type viruses (CMV, EBV) remain the most serious infectious agent in the post-transplant period

C. The teratogenic effect of immunosuppressive drugs has resulted in strong advice to women not to have children following a successful organ transplant

D. Because of the patient's immunosuppressed state and generally increased susceptibility to infection, the ability to return to work in most cases is severely limited

E. None of the above

Sabiston: 446
Schwartz: 390

Comments: Herpes-type virus infections remain the most serious post-transplant infectious agent. Bacterial infections are not as proportionately increased, probably because the host defenses against them are humeral and the present immunosuppressive regimens affect primarily cellular immunity. The incidence of fetal anomalies associated with immunosuppression is not higher than non–immune-suppressed controls and in most cases, does not influence a successful pregnancy adversely. ● The incidence of cancer is indeed increased in transplant patients but appears confined to immunoproliferative malignancies, skin cancers, and malignancies with a possible viral etiology, such as cancer of the cervix.

Answer: B

12. Which of the following statements about current immunosuppressive medications is/are true?

A. The immunosuppressive mechanism of prednisone is based on its inability to interfere with secretion of interleukin 1 from the macrophages
B. Cyclosporine acts primarily to block the production of interleukin 2 from cytotoxic activated T cells
C. Azathioprine functions as an antimetabolite interfering with DNA synthesis and impedes the proliferation of lymphocytes
D. None of the above

Sabiston: 446
Schwartz: 386

Comments: These are straightforward explanations of the mechanisms of immunosuppressive activity of the primarily used immunosuppressive drugs. Prednisone and cyclosporine are now used mostly in combination as the protocol of choice in most centers for clinical immunosuppression in transplantation. Some centers have recommended triple therapy (azathioprine, prednisone, cyclosporine) to minimize the expense and nephrotoxic hazards of higher-dose cyclosporine.

Answer: A, B, C

13. A patient received a transplanted cadaver kidney that functioned immediately. He was sent home on the tenth post-transplant day receiving cyclosporine 10 mg/kg and with a creatinine of 1.5 and a BUN of 30. The blood pressure was elevated mildly. Three weeks after discharge, his creatinine rose to 2.5, his blood pressure and weight gradually increased, and his extremities became edematous. Which one or more of the following pathologic processes may explain this deterioration in renal function?

A. Renal artery stenosis
B. Rejection
C. Cyclosporine toxicity
D. Infection
E. Prerenal causes

Sabiston: 419
Schwartz: 418

Comments: The first four conditions are potential causes of early graft dysfunction. Oliguria and diminished renal function on the basis of a prerenal cause is very unlikely, as the patient is not clinically dehydrated. Although fever is absent, sepsis is a possible etiology.

Answer: A, B, C, D

14. The two best methods to determine the reason for the deterioration in renal allograft function in the patient described in Question 13 is:

A. Arteriogram
B. Biopsy
C. Ultrasound
D. Empiric reduction of cyclosporine dose
E. Renogram
F. Appropriate microbiologic culture

Sabiston: 419
Schwartz: 418

Comments: **Ultrasonography** is the presently preferred method of evaluating renal graft dysfunction for technical problems. Not only will the ultrasound demonstrate hydronephrosis or perirenal fluid accumulation, but the Doppler facilities will present an assessment of renal arterial and venous blood flow. Parenchymal visualization is not as exact. The Doppler information will give enough indications as to whether an arteriogram should subsequently be performed. It is difficult to differentiate between cyclosporine toxicity and rejection on the basis of **biopsy**. The pattern of interstitial nephritis is seen with both situations. **Arteriography** is almost certainly not indicated as an initial test, especially in a kidney where renal function is deteriorating; the arteriographic dye is most likely to exacerbate the deterioration in renal function. **Nuclide scanning** does not give the same kind of information regarding possible technical complications and is no better than ultrasound screening in evaluating renal blood flow.

Answer: C, D

15. The patient described in Question 13 had an IVP, which showed hydronephrosis and a distended ureter; some contrast material was seen in the bladder. The approach to management that should not be used is:

A. Antegrade (percutaneous) or retrograde (cystoscopic) examination of the ureter and passage of a stent
B. Surgical exploration to relieve the obstruction
C. Urgent surgical exploration to perform cutaneous ureterostomy
D. Observation for several weeks to allow edema of the ureter and bladder to resolve

Sabiston: 418

Comments: Surgical exploration of the transplant and correction of the stenosis was formerly the only available therapy. Cystoscopic examination and attempts at retrograde ureteral cannulation were not usually successful. Modern endourologic techniques are precise in that they permit delineation of the site of the obstruction and attempts at percutaneous dilatation to correct the obstruction and the antegrade placement of temporary stents. The stricture is not caused by edema, and delay of repair is dangerous.

Answer: D

16. A patient with deterioration of renal function similar to that described in Question 13 had an ultrasound

examination that suggested stenosis of the renal artery; an arteriogram showed a 90% renal artery stenosis. The treatment of choice is:

A. Reoperation with an attempt to repair the renal artery stenosis
B. Percutaneous balloon angioplasty
C. Medical management with antihypertensive therapy until the patient becomes more stable in 6 to 8 months
D. Intensive antirejection therapy

Sabiston: 419

Comments: Use of percutaneous balloon angioplasty has rapidly gained favor as an extremely effective form of therapy; it is safer than re-exploration of the operative site and has a higher rate of success.

Answer: B

17. With respect to cyclosporine, which of the following statements is/are true?

A. It is a peptide that is derived from fungi and that has immunosuppressive activity identical to that of azathioprine but is less toxic
B. It is more likely to produce malignancy than azathioprine
C. It is the most selective and specific drug currently available for maintenance immunosuppression
D. It can be toxic to the kidney and liver

Sabiston: 415, 443
Schwartz: 386

Comments: Cyclosporine is a peptide derived from fungi that has potent immunosuppressive activities. Originally, it was thought to inhibit the production of interleukin 1 and interleukin 2 and impair the expression of interleukin 2 receptors on T-lymphocyte cell surfaces. We now understand that cyclosporine inhibits messenger RNA that encodes for interleukin 2 production. Thus, this activity makes cyclosporine the most selective drug currently available for maintenance immunosuppression. Azathioprine (AZA) is immunosuppressive in a much different way. Specifically, AZA is a purine analog and is integrated into the DNA of actively dividing cells. Unfortunately, bone marrow cells as well as cells of the lymphoid system actively divide. As a result, one of the major side effects of AZA therapy is bone marrow toxicity. Cyclosporine does not have this undesirable side effect. Nonetheless, cyclosporine is not without risk: high blood levels of it are associated with both renal and hepatic toxicity. The risk of malignancy is no greater in cyclosporine-treated patients than in azathioprine-treated patients.

Answer: C, D

18. Matching for histocompatibility (HLA) antigens is:

A. Not important since the introduction of cyclosporine
B. More likely to occur with siblings of the patient than with cadaveric donors
C. Of no practical use in heart transplants
D. Common between spouses

Sabiston: 395
Schwartz: 368

Comments: The HLA complex encodes for a series of genes collectively referred to as major histocompatibility complex antigens. These antigens represent a major barrier to the success of allografts; recognition of HLA antigens by the host can result in graft rejection. The HLA antigens are found on the sixth chromosome in humans; since each individual has two such chromosomes (one maternal, one paternal), four different chromosomes can contribute to the HLA type of an individual. Thus, a father has chromosomes (a,b) and the mother (c,d). With rare exception, only four genetic combinations are possible in the offspring from such a union: ac, ad, bc, and bd. The probability that any two siblings will have identical HLA types is 25%; the probability that they will share one or the other chromosome is 50%; and the probability that they will not share any HLA antigens is 25%. Thus, within a family, there is a relatively high probability of finding individuals that share at least some HLA antigens. This is definitely not true when comparing random individuals within the population. One reason for this is that the HLA system encodes for more than 75 different antigens. Some investigators have felt that matching for HLA antigens is no longer important—that cyclosporine alone overcomes the barrier of the histoincompatibility. While this may be true with respect to 1-year survival of an allograft (50% prior to use of cyclosporine and 90% since the use of cyclosporine), recent data indicate that HLA matching is still beneficial, if one examines graft survival 5 years post-transplant. ● Generally, hearts are not cross-matched between donor and recipient; almost always, a negative cross-match will still allow for the transplant. In some cases, however, the recipient might be 100% sensitized to a random panel of cells; that is, serum from the potential recipient reacts with every cell on an HLA-typed panel. The only course if such an individual is to receive a heart is if the donor expresses the same HLA antigens and thus would not have antibodies directed to these antigens. In such circumstances, it is very important to pre-type the potential donor and recipient. ● In summary, matching for antigens of the HLA complex results in better prognosis for long-term allograft survival.

Answer: B

19. Relative to cross-matches between potential donors and recipients for solid organ transplants, which of the following statements is/are true?

A. A cross-match may be positive owing to autoreactive antibody unless a control is used
B. A positive cross-match is always a contraindication to solid organ transplantation
C. Cross-matches are positive when donor lymphocytes react with recipient serum
D. Cross-matches that are negative with current sera but positive in sera obtained 3 years previously should not preclude successful renal transplantation

Sabiston: 395
Schwartz: 370

Comments: By definition, a cross-match is positive when serum from a potential recipient binds to donor lymphocytes and, in the presence of complement, alters the membrane such that the cells are killed. Cytotoxic reactions that could be due to antibodies against HLA antigens are present on the donor cells; these antibodies could have developed as a result of blood transfusion, pregnancy, or a previous transplant. Another explanation for a positive cross-match is that the recipient may have circulating autoantibodies, which cross-react with donor lymphocytes. For this reason, an auto–cross-match is always performed. • Data now indicate that even if a serum test was positive in the past (>6 months old) against a donor, a transplant could still be performed if all current sera (<6 months old) had negative cross-matches. Although not all patients with past positive and current negative cross-matches have long-term survival (>1 year) of their allografts, none of them had hyperacute rejection.

Answer: B, C, D

20. Blood transfusions to potential kidney recipients:

A. Should be avoided at all costs
B. Enhance graft survival
C. Result in prolonged graft survival of HLA-mismatched grafts, especially if combined with azathioprine therapy
D. May sensitize the potential recipient
E. Promote extended graft survival via a clearly defined immunological network

Sabiston: 402, 408
Schwartz: 412

Comments: Pre-transplant blood transfusion to a kidney recipient treated with azathioprine and prednisone is beneficial in that it improves graft survival. Since the emergence of cyclosporine as the mainstay of immunosuppression, the benefits of transfusion have diminished. The risk of sensitizing patients to HLA antigens and thus producing a positive cross-match to potential donor tissue now appears to be a greater issue. Although blood should not be withheld if clinically necessary, widespread random transfusion is falling from favor. Donor-specific transfusion still offers an advantage, however. Many theories have been proposed to explain the mechanism of the blood transfusion effect, ranging from the removal of "high responders" from the recipient pool

to a complex network of idiotypic regulation of the immune response, but in essence the mechanism remains unknown.

Answer: B, C, D

21. Some believe that rejection of a transplanted kidney is initiated not by the parenchymal cells of the kidney, but rather by the "passenger cells." Which of the following statements about passenger cells is/are true?

A. They are composed of granulocytes and platelets
B. They express Class II HLA antigens
C. They can be eliminated by techniques such as high oxygen tension, in vitro culture, or antibodies directed against Class II antigens
D. They arise in the bone marrow
E. They are organ-specific

Sabiston: 416
Schwartz: 421

Comments: The concept that passenger cells initiate graft rejection has existed since the mid-1950's and continues to draw much attention. Currently, the passenger cell is thought to be a dendritic cell that originates in the bone marrow. Other candidates to become passenger cells include monocytes and B lymphocytes. The hallmark of these passenger cells is that they express Class II histocompatibility antigens. In contrast, the parenchymal cells of the kidney and of all other solid organs do not express these Class II antigens. This discrimination makes it possible to eliminate these potentially hazardous cells by methods including reagents directed against Class II antigens, culturing the allograft under high oxygen tension, or culturing the organ at 37° F or at ambient temperature. Passenger cells are not restricted to the kidney. In fact, they have been found in the heart, pancreas, liver, parathyroid, and islets of Langerhans. It does not appear that elimination of passenger cells by physical methods will in and of itself promote long-term graft survival in humans. However, a combination of passenger cell depletion plus short-term immunosuppression does promote graft survival in animals and may eventually be extended to humans.

Answer: B, C, D

CHAPTER 48

Lung, Chest Wall, and Mediastinum

1. Which of the following concerning surgical anatomy of the lungs is/are true?

A. The volumes of the right and left lung are approximately equal
B. The left mainstem bronchus is longer than the right
C. The trachea bifurcates at about the level of the 7th thoracic vertebra
D. The right pulmonary artery has a greater length than the left before giving off its first segmental branch

Sabiston: 1960
Schwartz: 605

Comments: The volume of the left lung is approximately 45% and the right 55% of the total pulmonary volume. The right mainstem bronchus is 1.2 cm in length. The left mainstem bronchus is 4 to 6 cm in length. The tracheal bifurcation lies at the level of the 4th or 5th thoracic vertebra. The right pulmonary artery passes from the left side of the mediastinum to the right pleural cavity before giving off a segmental branch.

Answer: B, D

2. Which of the following indicate(s) the patient is at high risk for respiratory failure following pulmonary resection?

A. $FEV_1 = 800$ ml
B. MVV = 150% predicted
C. $PaCO_2 = 29$ torr
D. V/Q scan shows 30% perfusion to operative side

Sabiston: 1973
Schwartz: 615

Comments: In evaluation of a patient for pulmonary resection, many aspects of pulmonary physiology must be considered. If the predicted postoperative FEV_1 will be less than 800 ml, the risk is prohibitive. The maximum voluntary ventilation (MVV) is an indicator of the status of the respiratory muscles, the compliance of the lung, and airway resistance. Studies have shown a 45% cardio-

pulmonary mortality rate after thoracotomy in patients with preoperative MVV less than 50% of the predicted value. ● Elevated $PaCO^2$ suggests serious abnormalities in alveolar ventilation. ● The ventilation-perfusion (V/Q) scan is a useful test to predict what the FEV_1 of the remaining lung will be after pneumonectomy.

Answer: A

3. Which of the following is the most sensitive diagnostic procedure for detecting a small pulmonary nodule?

A. PA and lateral x-rays of the chest
B. Whole-lung tomograms
C. CT scan of the thorax
D. Technetium perfusion scan

Sabiston: 178
Schwartz: 607

Comments: X-rays of the chest (PA and lateral views) are the least expensive but also the least sensitive. CT scans are quite sensitive and can identify approximately 50% more nodules than can whole lung tomograms. A technetium perfusion scan is the most sensitive for defects in pulmonary blood flow but does not display the detailed anatomy required to detect small pulmonary nodules.

Answer: C

4. In which one or more of the following is flexible fiberoptic bronchoscopy preferred to rigid bronchoscopy?

A. Patient comfort
B. Massive hemoptysis
C. Dilation of strictures
D. Segmental biopsies
E. Bedside aspiration

Sabiston: 1990

Comments: Introduction of the flexible bronchoscopy is much less uncomfortable to the patient, and can more

313

easily be used for bedside aspirations. In patients with massive hemoptysis the rigid bronchoscope accommodates the use of larger suction tubing and easier clearing of the airway. The lens of the flexible bronchoscope, on the other hand, frequently will be covered by fresh blood, preventing visualization of the tracheobronchial tree. The flexible bronchoscope is, in general, too flexible to dilate strictures. Segmental and subsegmental biopsies in the upper lobes can in general be done only with a flexible bronchoscope.

Answer: A, D, E

5. Which of the following complications is/are most common following pulmonary lobectomy?

A. Retained secretions and atelectasis
B. Bronchopleural fistula
C. Persistent air leak from the surface of the operated lung
D. Empyema
E. Persistent symptomatic air space

Sabiston: 331
Schwartz: 461

Comments: The most common postoperative complication is related to retained bronchial secretions and consequent atelectasis. This occurs in 10 to 20% of patients and is related to reflex splinting of the chest, shallow breathing, and an impaired cough. Air leaks, if they are not from the bronchial stump closure, usually close early. A small persistent air space may occur but usually causes no problems. An asymptomatic air space will gradually disappear with reabsorption of the air within the space. Bronchopleural fistula and empyema are uncommon following a lobectomy.

Answer: A

6. In patients who have sustained blunt trauma to the chest, which of the following would most likely be the cause of acute cardiopulmonary collapse?

A. Hemothorax
B. Pulmonary contusion
C. Acute adult respiratory distress syndrome (ARDS)
D. Pneumothorax
E. Rib fractures

Sabiston: 300
Schwartz: 621

Comments: Rib fractures are the most common injuries to the chest wall, but unless there is a flail segment, rib fractures usually do not cause respiratory insufficiency. Hemothorax can cause respiratory insufficiency but is less common than is pneumothorax. Pulmonary contusion causes a delayed ARDS due to increased alveolar edema. Pneumothorax can cause sudden cardiorespiratory collapse if not treated.

Answer: D

7. Of the following tumors of the chest wall, the most common is:

A. Osteogenic sarcoma
B. Fibrous dysplasia
C. Chondrosarcoma
D. Chondroma
E. Ewing's sarcoma

Sabiston: 2086
Schwartz: 646

Comments: Chest wall neoplasms are more often benign than malignant. **Chondrosarcoma** is the most common malignant neoplasm of the chest wall. It accounts for 45 to 60% of the malignant tumors, and is seen most often in patients between 30 and 50 years of age. **Fibrous dysplasia** is the most common benign tumor of the chest wall, accounting for 20 to 35% of these tumors. **Chondromas** represent 15 to 20% of benign tumors. **Osteogenic sarcoma** represents approximately 15% of malignant tumors of the chest wall. In general, benign tumors occur posteriorly and malignant tumors tend to occur anteriorly on the chest wall.

Answer: B

8. The most common tumor of the anterior mediastinal compartment is:

A. Thymoma
B. Neurofibroma
C. Enterogenous cyst
D. Pericardial cyst
E. Teratoma

Sabiston: 2093
Schwartz: 716

Comments: The common tumors of the anterior mediastinal compartment are thymoma, thyroid, and teratoma. Thymoma is the most common, accounting for about 20% in one series of over 2,000 cases. When all mediastinal compartments are considered, the most common tumor is the neurogenic tumor, accounting for about 22% of cases in the same series. Neurogenic tumors classically are located in the posterior compartments. Neurilemmoma is the most common neurogenic tumor. Pericardial cysts are the most common mediastinal cysts and usually occur at the right cardiophrenic angle.

Answer: A

9. Which of the following is the most common cause of acute mediastinitis?

A. Perforation of the esophagus secondary to instrumentation
B. Postoperative infection following median sternotomy for open heart surgery
C. Traumatic injury to the mediastinum and mediastinal structures
D. Intrathoracic leak of an anastomotic suture line
E. Erosion of foreign body from the tracheobronchial tree or esophagus

Sabiston: 2091
Schwartz: 725

Comments: Currently the most common setting of mediastinitis is cardiac surgery through median sternotomy incision. Prolonged perfusion time, poor cardiac output postoperatively, and postoperative bleeding of sufficient magnitude to require re-exploration are common predisposing factors. Perforation of the esophagus, anastomotic leaks, and traumatic injuries can rapidly lead to a fulminating illness. The standard treatment is appropriate antibiotic therapy, drainage of the contaminated area, and either repair or exclusion of the esophagus.

Answer: B

10. Which of the following tumors has/have a higher incidence and death rate in asbestos workers?

A. Cancer of the lung
B. Pleural mesothelioma
C. Cancer of the esophagus
D. Cancer of the stomach

Sabiston: 2030
Schwartz: 658

Comments: All of the above neoplasms occur more commonly in asbestos workers. Usually there is a long latent period (15 to 35 years) between exposure to asbestos and the development of tumors. Among asbestos workers, 6 to 7% of all deaths are due to mesothelioma and 20% are due to carcinoma of the lung. Deaths from carcinoma of the esophagus are 2.5 times higher than expected; deaths from stomach cancer are 1.5 times higher.

Answer: A, B, C, D

11. In a patient with a malignant pleural effusion, which of the following is/are considered definitive therapy?

A. Thoracentesis
B. Closed tube thoracostomy
C. Closed tube thoracostomy with instillation of a sclerosing agent
D. Pleurectomy
E. Pleuroperitoneal shunt

Sabiston: 2022
Schwartz: 653

Comments: Thoracentesis alone, in the treatment of a malignant effusion, has a 97 to 99% failure rate. Closed tube thoracostomy alone has a high failure rate. The principle of total removal of the fluid (generally with chest tube drainage) and obliteration of the space between the pleura and the lung will effectively control the effusion. Obliteration of the pleural space usually can be accomplished by injection of a sclerosing agent such as tetracycline or nitrogen mustard into the pleural space through the chest tube. Occasionally parietal pleurectomy may be necessary to obliterate the space. Complications are frequent and mortality rates are significant with pleurectomy. Pleuroperitoneal shunt is a recent technique that can be effective for unresolving benign pleural effusions.

Answer: C, D

12. Empyema thoracis can be caused by which of the following?

A. Pneumonia with subsequent pyogenic infection of the associated effusion
B. Infections associated with a surgical procedure on the lung
C. Penetration of the pleural space by a foreign body
D. Nonsterile technique when performing a thoracentesis

Sabiston: 2028
Schwartz: 655

Comments: Empyema is most commonly secondary to a parapneumonic effusion becoming infected. This is becoming less frequent with the early use of antibiotics for pneumonia. Any trauma, especially penetration of the chest with a nonsterile foreign body, can lead to an empyema.

Answer: A, B, C, D

13. Which of the following methods is/are useful in the treatment of empyema thoracis?

A. Antibiotic therapy alone
B. Thoracentesis
C. Dependent open drainage of the empyema cavity
D. Decortication and pulmonary resection

Sabiston: 2028
Schwartz: 655

Comments: Antibiotic therapy alone without additional management of the empyema cavity is ineffective. If the effusion is still very fluid rather than viscid, thoracentesis with aggressive antibiotic therapy may abort the process. However, frequently it is not possible to remove all the fluid from the pleural space; this will lead to progression of the empyema. In a well-established empyema, initial drainage is established by closed tube thoracostomy, followed by dependent open drainage achieved by a rib resection and possibly an Eloesser flap. Decortication and pulmonary resection may be necessary for the cavity of a chronic empyema in which the lung does not re-expand after 4 to 6 weeks of the standard treatment outlined above, or for the acute empyema that has not responded to nonoperative therapy.

Answer: B, C, D

14. The most common tumor involving the trachea is:

A. Adenoid cystic carcinoma
B. Squamous cell carcinoma
C. Carcinoid
D. Mucoepidermoid carcinoma

Schwartz: 715

Comments: Squamous cell carcinoma remains the most common primary tumor of the trachea, accounting for approximately two thirds of primary tracheal tumors. Adenoid cystic carcinoma (formerly called cylindroma) accounts for one fourth of primary tracheal tumors. Secondary involvement of the trachea by carcinoma of the esophagus, lung, thyroid gland, or larynx is far more common than are primary tumors of the trachea.

Answer: B

15. Which of the following can cause lung abscesses?

A. Aspiration in an alcoholic or in a debilitated patient
B. Aspiration secondary to esophageal disease
C. Infection of a structural abnormality in the lung
D. Hematogenous spread of bacteremia

Sabiston: 2007
Schwartz: 678

Comments: Aspiration from any cause, but especially in alcoholics and in debilitated patients, is a frequent cause of lung abscess. Anaerobic bacterial organisms are most commonly responsible. Hematogenous spread of bacteria tends to cause multiple abscesses and has a much higher rate of morbidity and mortality. Achalasia, esophageal reflux, and cricopharyngeal diverticula may lead to pulmonary infection as a consequence of aspiration of esophageal contents. Pulmonary sequestration often presents as an abscess.

Answer: A, B, C, D

16. The standard therapy for pulmonary abscess includes:

A. Antibiotics
B. Bronchoscopy
C. Early surgical resection of the involved area of the lung
D. Tube drainage of the abscess cavity

Sabiston: 2009
Schwartz: 678

Comments: Treatment of pulmonary abscesses consists of diagnostic bronchoscopy to remove any foreign bodies, to evaluate for bronchial stenosis or obstruction, and to collect secretions for culture and cytology, and administration of the appropriate antibiotics. With adequate therapy, complete collapse of the abscess cavity wall and complete healing generally take place in 10 to 14 weeks. Failure of an abscess cavity to heal should alert the physician to a possible underlying carcinoma. Patients who have persistent cavities or cavities that are initially 6 cm or larger are candidates for an operation. Massive bleeding or empyema also requires surgery, which should include resection of the entire lobe. Tube drainage should be done only if the abscess cavity is adherent to the pleura.

Answer: A, B

17. Which of the following is/are considered atypical forms of mycobacteria?

A. *M. kansasii*
B. *M. tuberculosis*
C. *M. intracellularis*
D. *M. scrofulaceum*

Sabiston: 2037
Schwartz: 681

Comments: *M. tuberculosis* is the common species involved in *Mycobacterium* infection and accounts for 85 to 97% of *Mycobacterium* infections. It is estimated that approximately 7% of the population is infected with the bacillus. All other forms of *Mycobacterium* are called atypical forms. Note that all of these stain positive as acid-fast organisms on smears, and therefore the atypical organism can be detected only by cultures, which require 4 to 6 weeks.

Answer: A, C, D

18. Which of the following is/are considered first-line drugs for the treatment of infection with *M. tuberculosis*?

A. Isoniazid
B. Ethambutol
C. Rifampin
D. Streptomycin
E. Para-aminosalicylic acid

Sabiston: 2039
Schwartz: 683

Comments: Isoniazid, ethambutol, and rifampin are considered first-line drugs in the treatment of *Mycobacterium tuberculosis*. Single-drug treatment is discouraged since there occurs early development of bacterial resistance. Resistance is frequently prevented when two or more drugs are used in combination. Streptomycin is less frequently used since it needs to be administered by injection. All other drugs are second-line drugs and are used when resistance to the first-line drugs develops.

Answer: A, B, C

19. Which of the following characterize(s) extralobar pulmonary sequestration?

A. Venous drainage to pulmonary vein
B. Venous drainage to azygos vein
C. Arterial supply from aorta
D. Associated with congenital diaphragmatic hernia

Schwartz: 1642

Comments: Extralobar sequestration receives its arterial supply via small vessels from various adjacent systemic vessels including the aorta. Its venous drainage is into the azygos system. Intralobar sequestration receives its arterial supply from a large artery off the aorta; often this branch may originate from below the diaphragm. The venous drainage is into the pulmonary veins. Extralobar sequestration is often associated with congenital diaphragmatic hernia.

Answer: B, C, D

20. The most common cause of spontaneous pneumothorax is:

A. Tuberculosis
B. Rupture of small blebs
C. Emphysema

D. Various types of pulmonary neoplasms
E. Endometriosis

Sabiston: 2023
Schwartz: 675

Comments: The most common cause of spontaneous pneumothorax is rupture of small blebs generally located in the apex of the lung in persons without underlying lung disease. The highest incidence is in tall, thin individuals 20 to 40 years of age. Men are affected 5 to 6 times more frequently than are women. Chronic bronchitis and emphysema account for 10% of spontaneous pneumothorax. Prior to effective drug therapy for this disease, tuberculosis was thought to be the most common cause of spontaneous pneumothorax. Metastatic sarcoma is known to erode through the visceral pleura, causing a spontaneous pneumothorax. Endometriosis may cause pneumothorax with menses (catamenial pneumothorax).

Answer: B

21. Which of the following is/are indication(s) for surgical intervention in a patient with a pneumothorax?

A. Recurrent spontaneous pneumothorax
B. At the end of a 3-day trial of closed drainage of a spontaneous pneumothorax with a persistent air leak
C. Complete collapse of the lung in a patient with an initial spontaneous pneumothorax
D. Initial pneumothorax in a commercial airline pilot

Sabiston: 2023
Schwartz: 675

Comments: Recurrence of a spontaneous pneumothorax is generally considered an indication for its operative repair. The incidence of a recurrence after an initial pneumothorax is 15 to 20%. However, the incidence of a subsequent spontaneous pneumothorax following recurrence is 70 to 80%. Operative repair may be suggested for a patient with an initial spontaneous pneumothorax when that individual's occupation entails immediate responsibility for other persons' safety (e.g., an airplane pilot) or for those who live in remote areas. Operative repair of persistent air leaks from spontaneous pneumothorax is not considered until at least 7 to 10 days of closed therapy. Other indications for early operation are massive air leak preventing lung re-expansion, hemopneumothorax, or a large solitary bulla.

Answer: A, D

22. Which of the following disease processes can lead to massive hemoptysis?

A. Bronchogenic carcinoma
B. Bronchiectasis
C. Broncholith
D. Tuberculosis
E. Lung abscess

Sabiston: 2023, 2038, 2060
Schwartz: 678

Comments: Lung abscess, tuberculosis, and bronchiectasis frequently can lead to massive hemorrhage, this being considered as more than 600 ml in 24 hours. Both active tuberculosis and chronic cavitary tuberculosis can present with massive exsanguinating hemorrhage. While bronchogenic carcinoma can present with major hemorrhage if the tumor erodes into a major pulmonary artery or vein, this is a less frequent occurrence. Broncholiths almost never cause massive hemorrhage. The quantity of blood may vary from 1 to 50 ml.

Answer: A, B, D, E

23. True or False: Bronchial adenomas are considered benign tumors of the lung.

Sabiston: 2054
Schwartz: 707

Comments: The term "adenoma" suggests a benign process. The term "bronchial adenoma" is of historical interest only. Today, these tumors are identified as bronchial carcinoids, adenoid cystic carcinomas, and mucoepidermoid carcinomas. These tumors are frankly malignant, although the natural history is prolonged. Approximately 10 to 15% of patients will have metastases. The survival rates are between 75 and 90%.

Answer: False

24. Which of the following is the most common type of "bronchial adenoma"?

A. Cylindroma
B. Carcinoid adenoma
C. Mucoepidermoid tumor
D. Hamartoma
E. Mixed tumor of salivary gland type

Sabiston: 2054
Schwartz: 707

Comments: Carcinoid adenomas account for approximately 85% of all "bronchial adenomas." Adenoid cystic carcinomas, which in the past were called cylindromas, account for 10 to 15% of "adenomas." These tumors are more malignant than carcinoid adenomas and have a poorer prognosis. All other "adenomas" are rare. Hamartoma is not a bronchial adenoma but rather a tumor consisting of a disorganized arrangement of tissues normally present in the lung.

Answer: B

25. Which of the following affect(s) the TNM stage of a lung cancer?

A. Cell type
B. Location of tumor
C. Spread of tumor to mediastinal lymph nodes
D. Hypercalcemia
E. Ten pound weight loss

Sabiston: 2068
Schwartz: 707

Comments: TNM staging is based on the characteristics of the primary **T**umor, the **N**odal status, and the presence or absence of distant **M**etastases. The location of the primary tumor in relation to visceral pleura, chest wall, mediastinal structures, and carina, as well as its size, determine the T classification. Spread of tumor to mediastinal nodes is considered N2 and therefore Stage III disease. Cell type and systemic manifestations do not enter into staging of lung cancer.

Answer: B, C

26. Which of the following is/are absolute contraindication(s) to surgical resection of a lung tumor?

A. Vagus nerve involvement as evidenced by ipsilateral cord paralysis
B. Pleural effusion
C. Chest wall invasion of the tumor
D. Liver metastases
E. Mediastinal node involvement on the ipsilateral side

Sabiston: 2064
Schwartz: 689

Comments: **Vagus nerve involvement** is usually betrayed by left vocal cord paralysis and indicates invasion of the left recurrent nerve in the aorticopulmonary window; tumor in this area generally is considered nonresectable. Occasionally, however, the left vagus nerve can be involved above the aortic arch by direct invasion of the mediastinum. Although this is classified as Stage III disease, it is not an absolute contraindication to resection. **Pleural effusion** that contains malignant cells makes the disease noncurable by operation. Such an effusion, however, must be shown cytologically to be malignant before such a patient is denied an operation. **Chest wall invasion,** although constituting Stage III disease, can be resected for cure; there are reasonable survival rates in those instances in which it is part of a superior sulcus tumor. **Mediastinal lymph node involvement** on the ipsilateral side, particularly with squamous cell carcinomas, can likewise be resected for cure and with the expectation of reasonable survival rates. **Liver metastases** constitute an absolute contraindication to pulmonary resection since, under these conditions, the lung cancer is categorically noncurable.

Answer: D

27. Which of the following extrapulmonary manifestations of carcinoma of the lung is/are associated with small cell (oat cell) carcinoma?

A. Cushing's syndrome
B. Excessive production of antidiuretic hormone
C. Carcinoid syndrome
D. Hypercalcemia

Sabiston: 2061
Schwartz: 694

Comments: Hypercalcemia is most frequently associated with squamous cell carcinoma. Cushing's syndrome, excessive production of antidiuretic hormone, and the carcinoid syndrome generally are associated with small cell

(oat cell) carcinoma. All the listed manifestations, however, are not secondary to metastasis but presumably are the result of secretion of endocrine-like substances by the tumor.

Answer: A, B, C

28. List the following lung tumors in decreasing order of frequency.

A. Small cell
B. Squamous cell
C. Large cell
D. Adenocarcinoma

Sabiston: 2058
Schwartz: 690

Comments: Squamous cell carcinoma remains the most common carcinoma of the lung accounting for 35 to 60% (average 45%) of all lung carcinomas. Small cell carcinoma accounts for approximately 35% of lung carcinomas. Both of these tumors tend to occur in the central zone of the lung. Adenocarcinoma accounts for 15 to 20% of lung carcinomas but seems to be increasing in frequency, particularly in women who are cigarette smokers. Bronchioloalveolar-type carcinoma is included in the adenocarcinoma group. Large cell carcinoma accounts for 5 to 15% of all lung carcinomas.

Answer: B, A, D, C

29. In the general population, what percentage of non–symptom-producing solitary pulmonary nodules are carcinoma?

A. 5%
B. 20%
C. 35%
D. 50%

Sabiston: 2072
Schwartz: 686

Comments: In the general population only 5% of "coin" lesions discovered on routine screening chest x-ray are carcinomas, the majority being granulomas. In patients over 50 years who have had resection of such a "coin" lesion, however, the incidence of cancer is 50%. In those aged 80 years or older, the rate of malignancy of these lesions increases to almost 100%.

Answer: A

30. A "coin" lesion is found during a periodic health check-up of a 60-year-old white man who is a heavy cigarette smoker. Which of the following should routinely be done in the evaluation of this lesion?

A. Bronchoscopy
B. PPD skin test
C. Serial x-rays to evaluate doubling time
D. Percutaneous needle biopsy
E. Laminograms of the lesion
F. CT scan of the chest

Sabiston: 2072
Schwartz: 686

Comments: **Laminograms** of the lesion should be done to determine if calcification is present. Laminar layers, large central core, or "popcorn" distribution of the calcium generally indicates that the lesion is benign. A **PPD skin test**, if positive, indicates that the lesion may be a granulomatous process. **CT scan** is useful as a means to determine if there are any other nodules, possibly indicating metastatic disease from a primary tumor elsewhere. By extending the scan to the upper abdomen, the liver and adrenals may be checked for metastasis. In the event that this is a primary lung carcinoma, it also identifies enlarged mediastinal nodes. **Bronchoscopy** should be performed since, with radiologic guidance, a diagnosis can be established in some cases with very little morbidity. **Serial x-rays** observed for change can be most useful if x-rays are available from earlier dates showing the tumor when it was smaller. Choosing to only observe the tumor while waiting for later x-rays to determine doubling time generally is not advisable. **Percutaneous needle biopsy** is a means of obtaining a positive diagnosis of carcinoma, if it cannot be obtained by bronchoscopic biopsy. However, it serves only to confirm the need for surgical resection. A negative biopsy may indicate only that the lesion was not adequately sampled, and in general operation would still be indicated.

Answer: A, B, E, F

31. The overall 5-year survival rate of patients with carcinoma of the lung is:

A. 10%
B. 20%
C. 30%
D. 40%
E. 50%

Sabiston: 2057, 2071

Comments: The 5-year survival rate of all patients who develop carcinoma of the lung is 8 to 10%. The 5-year salvage rate after surgical resection is 20 to 35%. However, for patients who have T1 lesions without nodal involvement and no distant metastasis, the survival rate can be as high as 80%.

Answer: A

32. Which of the following factors is/are suspected to contribute to the development of lung cancer?

A. Cigarette smoking
B. Asbestos mining and use
C. Exposure to hydrocarbons
D. Radioactive ore mining
E. Polluted urban air

Sabiston: 2057
Schwartz: 690

Comments: All of the listed agents are reported to increase the incidence of carcinoma of the lung. Cigarette smoking appears to be the major contributing factor in the development of lung carcinoma. Cessation of smoking appears to reduce the risk of developing carcinoma

of the lung, but the risk may never be reduced to the level of a person who has never smoked.

Answer: A, B, C, D, E

33. List in decreasing order of frequency the organs involved with metastases from bronchogenic carcinoma.

A. Adrenals
B. Liver
C. Bone
D. Brain
E. Kidneys

Sabiston: 2059

Comments: The liver is the most common site of metastasis outside the thoracic cavity, accounting for approximately 33% of the incidence of organ involvement in several series. The adrenals are the second most common (20 to 33%), followed by bone (15 to 20%), as found in the same series; the brain and kidneys follow in that order. This information can be of value in determining whether a patient should be evaluated for metastases.

Answer: B, A, C, D, E

34. The most common benign tumor of the lung is:

A. Neuroma
B. Fibroma
C. Hamartoma
D. Plasmacytoma
E. Lipoma

Sabiston: 2049
Schwartz: 710

Comments: Hamartoma is the most common benign tumor in the lung. Its major component is cartilage; it is pathologically designated a chondroma or chondromyxoid hamartoma. These tumors average 2 to 3 cm in size and occur more commonly in the fifth and sixth decade of life. Operation is necessary, as one cannot differentiate these from malignant neoplastic pulmonary lesions. The other types of benign tumors of the lung are rarely encountered.

Answer: C

35. A patient being followed after apparently successful treatment of a squamous cell cancer of the head and neck is found to have a new solitary pulmonary nodule. The most likely diagnosis of this lesion is a:

A. Solitary metastasis
B. Granuloma
C. New lung primary carcinoma
D. Benign lung tumor

Sabiston: 2072
Schwartz: 710

Comments: When evaluating chest x-rays for new lung lesions, this should be done in the context of the time frame in which a patient is at risk from a previous malignancy. Generally, a new lung lesion in a patient who previously had a known primary head and neck tumor, especially a squamous cell carcinoma, is most likely a new primary cancer rather than a solitary metastasis. In a patient who previously had a melanoma or sarcoma, however, a solitary lesion in the lung is more likely to be a metastasis. In patients with known cancers of the gastrointestinal tract, genitourinary tract, or breast, a solitary pulmonary nodule has an equal chance of being a metastasis or a new primary lung cancer.

Answer: C

36. A metastasis to the lung from a known malignant tumor elsewhere should not be resected if:

A. The primary tumor is not controlled
B. There are bilateral metastases
C. There is metastatic disease in other organs besides the lung
D. There are multiple unilateral metastases
E. The cell type is unfavorable

Sabiston: 2072
Schwartz: 710

Comments: Before resection of a metastatic neoplasm to the lung, the primary tumor must be under control and there must be assurance that no other organ is involved with metastasis. The planned operation must be able to remove all known tumor, and the patient must be able to tolerate removal of involved lung tissue. Therefore, whether the lesions are multiple or bilateral, these lesions should be resected if the lung tissue that remains permits adequate pulmonary function. Several other factors may influence the decision to operate, including histologic type, disease-free interval, tumor doubling time, or the presence of secondary nodal metastasis. Each of these factors has been shown to influence survival, but none of these unfavorable situations is an absolute contraindication to resection.

Answer: A, C

Cardiac Surgery—Congenital Diseases

CHAPTER 49

1. True statements regarding the epidemiology and etiology of congenital heart disease include:

A. The frequency is 3 to 4 cases per 100,000 live births
B. The risk in siblings of children with congenital heart disease is 2%
C. The heart is formed between the eighth and twelfth weeks of intrauterine life
D. Many infectious diseases are known to cause congenital heart disease
E. Congenital heart malformations commonly occur in association with noncardiac developmental defects

Schwartz: 733

Comments: The heart develops between the third and eighth weeks of intrauterine life. Usually, congenital heart disease is an isolated malformation without known cause. Maternal rubella in the first trimester is one of the few infectious diseases known to cause congenital heart disease. It can produce mental deficiency, deafness, cataracts, and patent ductus arteriosus. Down's syndrome is another abnormality associated with a high incidence of congenital heart disease (atrioventricular canal, partial or complete).

Answer: A, B

2. Features of fetal circulation and heart anatomy include:

A. Of the six branchial aortic arches present in the fetus, only the fourth and sixth persist, as the aorta and ductus arteriosus, respectively
B. Transposition of the great vessels and aortic defects arise from abnormal development of primitive bulbus cordis
C. Fetal pulmonary vascular resistance is high, causing a right-to-left atrial shunt via the patent foramen ovale and from the pulmonary artery to the descending aorta via the patent ductus arteriosus

D. Fetal pulmonary artery anatomy features an abundance of smooth muscle in the media of the arterial wall
E. Fetal pulmonary vascular resistance falls to that seen in normal adults within the first month of life

Schwartz: 733

Comments: Fetal circulation is characterized by several distinct features (A to D above). The increased vascular resistance of the fetal pulmonary circulation falls to levels found in adults between the first and third years of life. Persistence of fetal histology in the pulmonary arteries in children is associated with pulmonary hypertension. The normal decrease in fetal pulmonary vascular resistance after birth allows closure of the foramen ovale. In 10 to 20% of adults, the foramen ovale remains patent. This usually is of no clinical significance; however, in the presence of increasing pulmonary vascular resistance in adulthood, this opening allows shunting of unoxygenated blood to the left side of the heart, leading to cyanosis. Although in most individuals the patent ductus arteriosus closes by 3 months, in a small percentage it remains patent, allowing left-to-right shunting of blood as systemic vascular pressures rise and pulmonary vascular resistance falls.

Answer: A, B, C, D

3. Match the items in the two columns.

Defect	Pathophysiologic Effect
A. Obstructive lesions	a. Cyanotic shunt
B. Right-to-left shunt	b. Acyanotic shunt
C. Left-to-right shunt	c. Increased ventricular work

Sabiston: 2173
Schwartz: 734

Comments: Congenital heart defects can be divided into four categories, each associated with distinct physiologic

321

abnormalities. **Obstructive lesions** (pulmonic stenosis, aortic stenosis, coarctation) restrict the flow of blood and increase the workload of the obstructed ventricle. **Left-to-right shunts** (atrial septal defect, ventricular septal defect, and patent ductus arteriosus) allow mixing of oxygenated blood with unoxygenated blood and create problems associated with increased volume of flow. **Right-to-left shunts** (tetralogy of Fallot) result from a combination of septal defects associated with obstruction of ventricular emptying, leading to cyanosis. **Complex malformations** (transposition of the great vessels, tricuspid atresia) result from gross errors in development and lead to varying degrees of heart failure and cyanosis.

Answer: A–c, B–a, C–b

4. True or False: Surgical therapy of congenital heart defects should be delayed until cardiac enlargement occurs unless heart failure develops.

Sabiston: 2173
Schwartz: 734

Comments: Congenital heart disease generally progresses through four stages. **First Stage:** Abnormal physical findings such as the systolic murmur of pulmonary valvular stenosis may be evident. **Second Stage:** Physiologic disturbances, such as pressure gradients across stenotic valves, increased blood flow through shunts, or the elevation of pulmonary artery pressure, may be detectable. **Third Stage:** Ventricular enlargement due to outflow stenosis or pulmonary hypertension may be evident. **Fourth Stage:** Cardiac failure occurs, resulting from chronic increased workload placed on the heart because of the underlying defect. Diagnosis and therapy should be undertaken before the later stages are reached because severe ventricular hypertrophy and elevated pulmonary vascular resistance can progress to a point of irreversibility. In all forms of congenital heart disease, susceptibility to bacterial endocarditis increases because the localized turbulence of blood flow predisposes to deposition of bacteria during transient bacteremia.

Answer: False

5. Which of the following statements regarding obstructive congenital heart lesions is/are true?

A. The most common obstructive lesions are pulmonic valvular stenosis, aortic valvular stenosis, and coarctation of the aorta
B. Obstructive congenital heart lesions produce "systolic" overloading and concentric hypertrophy
C. Concentric hypertrophy produces marked cardiac enlargement detected by physical examination and routine chest x-ray
D. Electrocardiographic changes occur only after there is marked enlargement of the cardiac silhouette
E. Angina pectoris, arrhythmia, a predisposition to sudden death, and end-stage cardiac failure result from progressive obstruction

Sabiston: 2173, 2261
Schwartz: 735

Comments: The concentric hypertrophy of obstructive congenital heart lesions is not easily detected by clinical means or by chest x-ray. Electrocardiographic changes are the most useful in making the diagnosis and can indicate the degree of ventricular hypertrophy present. Echocardiogram and Doppler examination are additional noninvasive tests useful in assessing chamber size and degree of obstruction.

Answer: A, B, E

6. Which statement(s) regarding left-to-right shunts is(are) true?

A. The most common causes are atrial septal defect, ventricular septal defect, and patent ductus arteriosus
B. Recirculation of blood through the pulmonary circuit produces marked cyanosis, pulmonary congestion, and the tendency to develop pulmonary hypertension
C. Left-to-right shunts lead to diastolic overloading and cardiac dilatation manifested on chest x-ray as ventricular enlargement.
D. The shunt becomes physiologically significant when pulmonary blood flow is 1.5 to 2 times as great as systemic blood flow

Sabiston: 2173, 2191, 2212
Schwartz: 735

Comments: Persistent patency of the ductus arteriosus or defects in the atrial or ventricular septa permit flow of blood from left to right as a consequence of the higher pressures in the left side of the heart compared with the greater compliance and lower pressure in the right side. Because the shunt carries oxygenated blood, cyanosis does not occur. Pulmonary congestion and a tendency to develop pulmonary hypertension does occur. Unlike obstructive lesions, these lesions produce diastolic overloading and cardiac dilatation seen as ventricular enlargement on chest x-ray. Electrocardiographic changes are less prominent than those seen with concentric hypertrophy. Cardiac failure tends to occur earlier than it does with obstructive lesions. Pulmonary flow may reach levels 3 to 4 times that of systemic blood flow. The resultant congestion produces a susceptibility to bacterial infection, which in turn leads to recurrent bouts of pneumonia.

Answer: A, C, D

7. True or False: The gracile habitus often seen in association with patent ductus arteriosus results from a genetic metabolic defect.

Sabiston: 2174
Schwartz: 736

Comments: Large left-to-right shunts are associated not only with increased pulmonary blood flow but also with decreased systemic blood flow. This decrease is associated with retardation of normal growth and development and is most evident in children with patent ductus arteriosus or atrial septal defects. The gracile habitus describes children who appear frail and underweight. Increases in growth and weight occur when the cardiac defect is corrected. Mental retardation is more common in children with congenital heart disease; this, however, does not improve after surgical correction.

Answer: False

8. True statements regarding pulmonary hypertension include:

A. The most important parameter in evaluation of pulmonary hypertension is the systolic pressure of the pulmonary artery
B. Pulmonary hypertension becomes irreversible by the age of 1 year in patients with increased pulmonary artery blood flow
C. Susceptibility to development of pulmonary hypertension varies with individuals
D. An atrial septal defect should be surgically corrected before 1 year of age to avoid pulmonary hypertension

Sabiston: 2214
Schwartz: 735

Comments: Pulmonary hypertension may result from an increase in pulmonary blood flow, histologic changes in pulmonary arterioles, and from pulmonary venous obstruction. The most important physiologic measurement is the pulmonary vascular resistance, not the absolute level of pulmonary arterial pressure. Although in the fetus and in young infants there is smooth muscle hypertrophy of the media, in older children and adults, there occurs thickening of the intima with an associated fibrosis; this leads to decreased arteriolar distensibility and, consequently, increased pulmonary vascular resistance. The pressure under which blood enters the pulmonary artery seems to be more important than the volume of blood flow. The incidence of pulmonary hypertension is higher with ventricular septal defect than it is with atrial septal defect, which produces a similar increase in blood flow, but at a lower pressure. There is variability in the age at which various lesions produce pulmonary hypertension. Children with ventricular septal defect, patent ductus arteriosus, or aortopulmonary windows should be corrected in the first 1 to 2 years of life. Transposition of the great vessels or truncus arteriosus may require correction during the first few weeks or months of life. Simple atrial septal defects rarely require surgical correction at an early age.

Answer: C

9. True statements regarding right-to-left shunts include:

A. Venous blood is shunted into the systemic circulation, producing arterial hypoxemia and cyanosis
B. A right-to-left shunt usually occurs in the face of a septal defect associated with obstruction of flow into the pulmonary artery
C. There is an increase in cardiac output
D. As is the case with left-to-right shunts, congestive heart failure develops ultimately
E. The most common lesion producing a right-to-left shunt is the tetralogy of Fallot

Sabiston: 2223
Schwartz: 736

Comments: The classic congenital abnormality producing a right-to-left shunt is the tetralogy of Fallot, a combination of ventricular septal defect and pulmonary stenosis.

Other lesions include transposition of the great vessels, tricuspid atresia, truncus arteriosus, and total anomalous drainage of the pulmonary veins. Right-to-left shunts do not produce an increase in cardiac output, and blood flow is often less than normal. Heart failure, therefore, is rare with an uncomplicated right-to-left shunt.

Answer: A, B, E

10. True statements regarding the cyanosis of right-to-left shunts include:

A. The degree of cyanosis depends on the degree of anoxia and on the hemoglobin concentration
B. Peripheral cyanosis results simply from a decrease in cardiac output. Central cyanosis is caused by a defect in oxygenation or by an intracardiac shunt
C. Clubbing and polycythemia are irreversible sequelae of chronic cyanosis
D. Increasing blood flow through the pulmonary circuit can reduce cyanosis and improve oxygen transport
E. Squatting increases peripheral vascular resistance, which increases pulmonary blood flow and thus relieves exertional dyspnea in cyanotic children

Sabiston: 2224
Schwartz: 736

Comments: The degree of cyanosis depends on the ratio between oxygenated and unoxygenated blood in the arterial circulation. About 5 gm of reduced hemoglobin is required to produce visible cyanosis. Surgical creation of a systemic-pulmonary shunt increases pulmonary blood flow and can help compensate for cyanosis. Polycythemia is a physiologic response to cyanosis and can lead to levels of hematocrit as high as 80%. High levels of hematocrit increase blood viscosity and, should dehydration occur, predispose individuals to venous thrombosis. Clubbing of the digits is usually not prominent until a cyanotic child is 1 to 2 years of age. If the anoxia is severe, however, clubbing may occur within several weeks. It subsides gradually following correction of the shunt.

Answer: A, B, D, E

11. True or False: In children with severe anoxia, cyanotic spells are common up to 10 years of age.

Sabiston: 2195, 2224
Schwartz: 737

Comments: Cyanotic spells are periodic episodes of unconsciousness related to cerebral anoxia. They often appear in the third to fourth month of life, but, with extreme anoxia, may appear in the first few weeks; they are rare after the fifth to sixth year. Because they may result in permanent neurologic injury or even death, emergency surgical treatment to improve oxygen content is indicated. Cyanotic children often may suffer from neurologic injury caused by brain abscesses that result from endocarditis (especially in tetralogy of Fallot) or paradoxic embolism through an intracardiac defect. The occurrence of CNS symptoms caused by any of these sources is a strong indication for early surgical therapy.

Answer: False

12. True or False: In children with congenital heart disease, the increased bronchial circulation due to cyanosis often leads to hemoptysis.

Schwartz: 737

Comments: Pulmonary blood flow usually is less than normal in cyanotic children. Hemoptysis is rare even though the bronchial circulation may be greatly increased. Extrapulmonary collaterals may lead to epistaxis in some children.

Answer: False

13. Match the items in the two columns.

Congenital Defect	Radiographic Change
A. Tetralogy of Fallot	a. Egg-shaped heart
B. Transposition of great vessels	b. Sabot-shaped heart
C. Total anomalous pulmonary venous return	c. Figure-of-8 abnormality
D. Aortic stenosis, mitral insufficiency, coarctation, patent ductus arteriosus, ventricular septal defect, and tricuspid atresia	d. Left atrial enlargement
E. Mitral insufficiency, ventricular septal defect, patent ductus arteriosus, and left ventricular failure	e. Right atrial enlargement
F. Ebstein's malformation, atrial septal defect, pulmonic stenosis	f. Left ventricular enlargement
G. Pulmonic stenosis, pulmonary hypertension, atrial septal defect, ventricular septal defect	g. Right ventricular enlargement

Sabiston: 2196, 2208, 2216, 2224, 2242, 2251, 2263
Schwartz: 738

Comments: The chest x-ray plays an important role in the evaluation of congenital heart disease. Certain lesions (choices A–C) produce characteristic changes in cardiac contour, whereas others (choices D–G) produce enlargement of the various heart chambers (there is some overlap). The electrocardiogram enables one to detect selective right vs. left ventricular hypertrophy and is, therefore, an important adjunct to the noninvasive evaluation of congenital heart disease.

Answer: A–b; B–a; C–c; D–f; E–d; F–e; G–g

14. True or False: The appearance of rales is the first sign of congestive heart failure in children.

Schwartz: 738

Comments: Unlike congestive heart failure in adults, the hallmark of congestive heart failure in children is hepatic enlargement, which precedes the appearance of rales.

Answer: False

15. Match the items in the two columns.

Comment/Pathology	Auscultatory Findings
A. Common, but of little diagnostic significance	a. Systolic murmurs
B. Infrequent, but when present is a significant finding	b. Increased second heart sound
C. Pulmonary hypertension	c. Diastolic murmurs
D. Pulmonary stenosis or atresia	d. Variable splitting of second heart sound
E. Atrial septal defect	e. Decreased second heart sound

Schwartz: 738

Comments: Proper auscultation of the heart can often lead to the correct diagnosis of a congenital cardiac abnormality.

Answer: A–a; B–c; C–b; D–e; E–d

16. True statements regarding cardiac catheterization for the evaluation of congenital heart disease include:

A. All the needed information can be obtained by catheterization of the left side
B. Cardiac catheterization provides the information necessary to calculate the pulmonary vascular resistance
C. A difference of oxygen saturation between chambers as small as 1 volume % is usually sufficient to diagnose intracardiac left-to-right shunts
D. Cardiac catheterization provides the information needed to calculate the functional cross-sectional area of stenotic valves

Sabiston: 2139
Schwartz: 740

Comments: Cardiac catheterization is essential to the complete evaluation of congenital heart defects. A complete study requires catheterization of the right and left sides. Pulmonary vascular resistance is calculated from pulmonary blood flow and pulmonary artery pressure. Functionally significant stenosis exists in the following circumstances: mitral valve—an area smaller than 1.5 cm²; aortic valve—an area smaller than 0.8 cm²; pulmonary valve—an area smaller than 0.8 cm².

Answer: B, C, D

17. True statements regarding pulmonic stenosis include:

A. The most common cause is hypoplasia of the pulmonic valve annulus
B. The physiologic abnormality is obstruction of flow from the right ventricle, with secondary concentric hypertrophy
C. Right atrial enlargement can occur, leading to stretching of the foramen ovale
D. The most common symptom is dyspnea on exertion
E. Electrocardiographic abnormalities provide an accurate guide to the severity of obstruction

Sabiston: 2226, 2230
Schwartz: 741

Comments: Pulmonic stenosis accounts for 10% of congenital abnormalities. It is a spectrum of disorders involving fusion of the cusps of the pulmonary valve (the most common cause), hypoplasia of the valvular annulus, poststenotic dilatation of the main pulmonary artery, and concentric hypertrophy of the right ventricle. Uncommonly, there is stenosis of the distal pulmonary arteries. Five to 10% of these patients have an isolated infundibular stenosis. The occurrence of pulmonary stenosis with other abnormalities is rare. Elevated right ventriclar pressures are eventually transmitted to the right atrium at levels capable of stretching open the foramen ovale. This produces a right-to-left shunt with its attendant triad of cyanosis, polycythemia, and clubbing. Right ventricular pressures raised above those of the left ventricle exclude the diagnosis of ventricular septal defect. Mild cases without electrocardiographic changes may follow a benign course and do not require surgical treatment. Goals of surgical therapy are to perform valvulotomy, to patch repair a hypoplastic annulus or outflow tract abnormalities, and to close the patent foramen ovale, if present.

Answer: B, C, D, E

18. True statements regarding congenital aortic stenosis include:

A. When caused by rheumatic fever, there usually is concomitant mitral valve disease
B. As in pulmonic stenosis, valvular calcification is common
C. The degree of stenosis alone determines the severity of obstruction and the resultant ventricular hypertrophy
D. Unlike pulmonic stenosis, ventricular enlargement is rarely seen on chest x-ray
E. Congenital aortic stenosis may be the result of cusp fusion, severe hypoplasia of the valve, or subvalvular stenosis

Sabiston: 2261
Schwartz: 745

Comments: Congenital aortic stenosis accounts for 10% of congenital heart abnormalities, is 3 to 4 times more common in males, and in 20% of cases is associated with other cardiac defects (patent ductus arteriosus, ventricular septal defect, coarctation of the aorta). The most common abnormality is fusion of the commissure between the right and left coronary cusps, producing the classic bicuspid valve. Unlike pulmonary stenosis, valvular calcification is very common by the third decade. Its appearance often heralds the onset of severe symptoms in previously asymptomatic patients. An electrocardiogram enables one to detect the hypertrophy of aortic stenosis, but severe obstruction may exist without significant electrocardiographic changes. Measurement of peak systolic gradients provides a reliable assessment of the severity of the stenosis. Although often slow to develop, the symptoms of fatigue, dyspnea, angina, and syncope appear at gradients greater than 50 mm Hg. Overt congestive heart failure is rare; however, sudden death may occur secondary to ventricular fibrillation. The four most common physical findings are systolic murmur, slow carotid upstrokes, forceful left ventricular impulse, and a narrow pulse pressure. A gradient greater than 50 mm Hg and a cross-sectional area smaller than 0.5 cm^2 are considered indications for operation. Valvulotomy or re-

section of subaortic stenosis is the usual initial operation. As many as 20 to 30% of patients return for a second operation for valve replacement.

Answer: A, C, D, E

19. Match the items in the two columns.

Clinical Comment	Type of Stenosis
A. Diagnosis requires cardiac catheterization and angiography	a. Supravalvular aortic stenosis
B. Pressure gradient increases with isoproterenol	b. Idiopathic hypertrophic subaortic stenosis (IHSS)
C. Broad forehead, heavy cheeks, protuberant lips, pointed chin, mental retardation	c. Both
D. Associated cardiac abnormalities are frequent	d. Neither
E. Family history of heart disease, with reports of sudden death, is common	
F. Syncope, dyspnea, angina, and sudden death are common symptoms	

Sabiston: 2261
Schwartz: 749

Comments: As with other forms of aortic stenosis, supravalvular stenosis and idiopathic hypertrophic subaortic stenosis (IHSS) have the potential to produce syncope, dyspnea, angina, and sudden death. Patients with IHSS, however, are often symptom-free as children. Supravalvular stenosis is the rarest form of aortic stenosis and presents as an hourglass, a diffuse hypoplastic, or a membranous form. One fifth of these patients have the typical facies previously described; one third have associated aortic cusp abnormalities; and one half have coronary artery abnormalities. In the absence of the typical facies, angiography is needed to make a diagnosis. IHSS is caused by a hypertrophic myopathy of the left ventricular outflow tract. Angiography is needed to differentiate this lesion from other forms of aortic stenosis. Patients may be treated medically by reduction of after-load. Resection of the hypertrophied area in those who fail to respond to medical care does not alter the underlying progressive ventricular hypertrophy.

Answer: A–c; B–b; C–a; D–a; E–b; F–c

20. True statements regarding coarctation of the aorta include:

A. The lesion occurs usually 2 to 4 cm distal to the left subclavian artery
B. Early left ventricular failure requiring surgical correction in infants is common
C. Leg claudication and poststenotic aortic aneurysms are common
D. Arm hypertension, decreased or absent leg pulses, and a systolic murmur over the left hemithorax are the classic physical findings
E. Operative complications include paraplegia and paradoxical postoperative hypertension

Sabiston: 2178
Schwartz: 751

Comments: Coarctation of the aorta accounts for 10 to 15% of congenital heart defects and occurs twice as frequently in males. It usually occurs distal to the left subclavian artery in association with the ligamentum arteriosum. Occasionally, in infants, severe left ventricular failure will develop, requiring immediate surgical correction. The majority of patients are without symptoms but have severe arm hypertension. Collateral flow via the intercostal arteries is sufficient, so that claudication is unusual and heart failure is delayed until early adult life. These intercostal collateral arteries produce the classic rib-notching seen on chest x-ray. The findings on physical examination, and on chest x-ray as described above, and an electrocardiogram showing left ventricular hypertrophy establish the diagnosis. In the past, operation has been postponed until ages 5 to 7 years because of the high rate of recurrence of coarctations repaired in infants by end-to-end anastomosis. The use of subclavian flaps rather than end-to-end anastomosis makes repair by age 2 years possible in most cases. During operation, cross-clamping the aorta is generally well tolerated for up to 20 minutes in patients with good collateral flow. Aortic shunts may be considered when distal aortic pressures are less than 60 mm Hg (usually the result of poor collateralization). Paradoxical postoperative hypertension requires medical treatment to avoid abdominal complications such as intestinal necrosis or pancreatitis.

Answer: A, D, E

21. Match the items in the two columns:

Anomaly	Comment
A. Persistent atrioventricular canal	a. Patent atrial septal defect required for survival
B. Secundum atrial septal defect	b. Often associated with anomalous pulmonary veins
C. Ostium primum	c. Associated with anterior mitral valve cleft
D. Total anomalous pulmonary venous drainage	d. Atrial septal, ventricular septal, mitral, and tricuspid defects
E. Partial anomalous pulmonary venous drainage	e. Physiologic derangement like that of atrial septal defect

Sabiston: 2191
Schwartz: 759, 761, 763

Comments: All the listed anomalies produce left-to-right shunting. While secundum defects and anomalous pulmonary veins cause simple left-to-right shunts, ostium primum and atrioventricular (AV) canal defects produce varying degrees of mitral (primum) or mitral and tricuspid (AV canal) insufficiency as well. The common AV canal is a severe defect characterized by a clinical course of severe cardiac failure and cardiac enlargement during the first few years of life. Early operative repair should be attempted; AV canal has a 15 to 20% mortality rate.

Answer: A–d; B–b; C–c; D–a; E–e

22. Match the items in the two columns.

Clinical Comment	Heart Defect
A. Associated with Down's syndrome	a. Secundum atrial septal defect
B. Patients may be without symptoms into adult life	b. Ostium primum
C. Arrhythmias secondary to atrial hypertrophy	c. Both
D. Conduction defects due to bundle fibrosis	d. Neither
E. Twice as frequent in females	

Sabiston: 2191
Schwartz: 759, 763

Comments: The secundum atrial septal defect occurs twice as frequently in females, accounting for 10 to 15% of congenital heart defects, whereas ostium primum defects (also known as partial endocardial cushion defects) are relatively rare. Secundum defects can be high (sinus venosus defect), low, or in the middle of the atrial septum; 15% are associated with anomalous pulmonary veins. Most infants are symptom-free and remain so until left atrial pressures rise above those in the right atrium. Pulmonary congestion, pulmonary hypertension, and congestive heart failure may then result and often are not noticed until the third to fourth decade of life. Arrhythmias due to chronic right atrial enlargement are not unusual. Primum defects allow shunting via a low atrial septal defect and regurgitation through a cleft in the anterior leaf of the mitral valve. When regurgitation is severe, left ventricular failure and pulmonary hypertension appear early, and cardiac function is more severely impaired than with secundum defects. The electrocardiogram in secundum defects shows mild right ventricular hypertrophy, right axis deviation, and occasional right bundle branch block; in primum defects, it shows right and left ventricular hypertrophy and left axis deviation. A counterclockwise loop in the frontal plane of the vectorcardiogram is almost pathognomonic of ostium primum defects.

Answer: A–b; B–c; C–a; D–b; E–a

23. Which of the following statements is/are true regarding partial and total anomalous pulmonary venous drainage?

A. All patterns of partial anomalous pulmonary venous drainage require surgical correction
B. The scimitar syndrome is the association of partial pulmonary venous drainage with syphilitic bone changes
C. Fifty percent of partial anomalous pulmonary veins are found with an intact atrial septum
D. Partial anomalous pulmonary veins arise more commonly from the right lung
E. Balloon septostomy is used to palliate infants with partial anomalous pulmonary venous drainage

Sabiston: 2206
Schwartz: 761

Comments: Only rarely are partial anomalous pulmonary veins found with an intact atrial septum; usually they arise from a single lung, most commonly the right. Right anomalous pulmonary veins entering the superior vena cava usually are associated with a high secundum atrial septal defect known as sinus venosus defect. Right anomalous pulmonary veins may also enter the right atrium or the inferior vena cava. Anomalous left pulmonary veins usually enter a persistent left superior vena cava, the innominate vein, or rarely the coronary sinus. Single anomalous pulmonary veins may be physiologically harmless and require no treatment. Total anomalous pulmonary venous drainage is a far more serious defect, causing complete shunting of pulmonary venous return to the right side of the heart. The three types of total anomalous pulmonary venous drainage are (1) supracardiac, (2) intracardiac, and (3) infracardiac. The usual pattern is emptying of the veins into a persistent left superior vena cava that reaches the right side of the heart via the innominate vein and right superior vena cava. In this situation, life is possible only if a patent atrial septal defect allows oxygenated blood to reach the left side of the heart. Infants with this defect are critically ill and may be palliated by balloon septostomy until definitive surgical procedures can be undertaken. The scimitar syndrome describes the radiologic appearance created by the shadow of an anomalous right pulmonary vein arising parallel to the right border of the heart. It is often associated with defective development of the right lung and the anomalous origin of its pulmonary arteries from the aorta.

Answer: D

24. True statements regarding ventricular septal defects include:

A. There are two general anatomic types of ventricular septal defect—membranous and muscular
B. Defects less than 2 cm in diameter are generally well tolerated
C. Ventricular septal defect commonly occurs in association with other congenital cardiac anomalies
D. Banding of the pulmonary artery is the operation of choice in infants younger than 2 years
E. Operation between ages 4 and 6 years is recommended in symptomatic children if the pulmonary blood flow is 1.5 to 2 times the normal flow

Sabiston: 2212
Schwartz: 767

Comments: Ventricular septal defects account for 20 to 30% of congenital heart defects. Associated anomalies are common (patent ductus arteriosus, coarctation, atrial septal defect, aortic insufficiency). Four general anatomic types of ventricular septal defect have been recognized: perimembranous, subarterial, atrioventricular canal, and muscular. Defects in the membranous septum are the most frequent (85 to 90%). Of the four types, the muscular defects are often multiple. Defects less than 1 cm in diameter are associated with pulmonary blood flow less than 2 times the systemic flow, with few adverse physiologic consequences. Larger defects can produce cardiac failure, pulmonary hypertension, and death. In symptomatic infants with large lesions, surgical correction is indicated. If such infants are left untreated, increased pulmonary vascular resistance may become irreversible by the age of 2 years. Up to 25% of small ventricular septal

defects will spontaneously close. In the absence of symptoms, and since spontaneous closure rarely occurs beyond this point, repair is delayed until the age of 5 to 6 years. If at this age there is evidence of increased heart size or the pulmonary artery flow is demonstrated to be greater than 1.5 to 2 times the normal flow, repair should be undertaken. Bacterial endocarditis is the only known risk from small ventricular septal defects and requires prophylactic antibiotics in asymptomatic patients.

Answer: C

25. True or False: The major reason for transatrial repair of ventricular septal defects is to avoid injury to the coronary arteries.

Sabiston: 2220
Schwartz: 769

Comments: Repair of a ventricular septal defect usually occurs through a ventriculotomy. Care must be taken to avoid injuring underlying significant coronary arteries. Anomalous coronary arteries are often found in association with ventricular septal defects. The most common is origin of the left anterior descending artery from the right coronary artery. For this reason, transatrial repair or the use of transverse ventriculotomy is the preferred operative approach. The other major consideration is avoidance of heart block. Because cardioplegia is used during repair, dependence on the electrocardiogram is not adequate protection. The conduction bundle is identified using anatomic landmarks, and sutures are placed carefully to avoid injuring it.

Answer: True

26. True or False: Eisenmenger's syndrome is a classic conduction defect resulting from inappropriate repair of a ventricular septal defect.

Sabiston: 2215
Schwartz: 768

Comments: Eisenmenger's syndrome is the end stage of progressive pulmonary hypertension that results from a large left-to-right shunt. Most commonly occurring with uncorrected ventricular septal defects, it can also occur from patent ductus arteriosus, transposition, and truncus arteriosus and rarely can occur in association with a persistent atrial septal defect. It is characterized by pulmonary vascular resistance ultimately rising to levels above systemic vascular resistance, causing reversal of the original left-to-right shunt and producing cyanosis.

Answer: False

27. Which of the following statements is/are true regarding patent ductus arteriosus?

A. It is more common in males
B. It almost always is an isolated defect
C. Because of its small diameter, a patent ductus arteriosus cannot shunt more than 20% of the left ventricular output
D. Bacterial endocarditis is a rare complication of a patent ductus arteriosus

E. The presence of cyanosis is a contraindication to closure

Sabiston: 2173
Schwartz: 771

Comments: Patent ductus arteriosus accounts for 15% of congenital heart defects, occurs 2 to 3 times more frequently in females, and is found in association with other cardiac defects in 15% of cases. It originates from the 6th left aortic arch, runs from the pulmonary artery to the aorta distal to the left subclavian artery, and usually closes after birth, probably in response to rising arterial oxygen tension. As much as 70% of the left ventricular output may be shunted by a large patent ductus arteriosus. Occasionally, a patent ductus arteriosus can produce severe congestive heart failure in infants up to age 2 years; after that, it is rare until adulthood. As with any lesion that increases pulmonary artery flow, the potential for pulmonary hypertension exists. There is an unusual propensity for bacterial endocarditis involving *Streptococcus viridans*, which develops in 20 to 25% of these patients. The hallmark of a patent ductus arteriosus is a continuous machinery murmur associated with a widened pulse pressure. Chest x-ray may show left ventricular hypertrophy (LVH), increased pulmonary vascular markings, and an enlarged pulmonary conus. The electrocardiogram varies from possibly being normal, with a small patent ductus arteriosus, to showing left ventricular hypertrophy with large lesions. Although physical examination and echocardiogram are sufficient in many cases, aortography provides the definitive anatomic diagnosis. Cyanosis is considered a contraindication to surgical closure, since its presence implies the presence of either an associated cyanosis-producing lesion, such as tetralogy, or Eisenmenger's syndrome. In the first instance, the patent ductus arteriosus is an important ancillary source of blood flow to the lungs; in the second, it helps decrease pulmonary hypertension by shunting blood away from the pulmonary circuit.

Answer: E

28. True or False: Indomethacin has replaced surgery as the initial treatment of choice for patent ductus arteriosus in a premature infant.

Sabiston: 2174
Schwartz: 776

Comments: The incidence of patent ductus arteriosus in premature infants varies inversely with the birth weight and gestational age and is as high as 80%. Indomethacin, by blocking the synthesis of prostaglandins, hastens the closure of a patent ductus arteriosus. Indomethacin is effective in closing a patent ductus arteriosus but is associated with impairment of renal function, coagulation, and occasionally gastrointestinal bleeding. Surgical division or ligation is very safe and is associated with significantly less enterocolitis. Once a patent ductus arteriosus is diagnosed, a trial of indomethacin is indicated. Surgery is reserved for cases of indomethacin intolerance or failure to produce closure.

Answer: True

29. Which of the following statements regarding tetralogy of Fallot is/are correct?

A. It consists of right ventricular outflow obstruction, ventricular septal defect, dextroposition of the aorta, and right ventricular hypertrophy
B. It is the dextroposition of the aorta that allows right-to-left shunting of blood through an otherwise uncomplicated ventricular septal defect
C. Cardiac enlargement and heart failure are common because of the right ventricular outflow obstruction
D. The clinical course of the disease may be grouped according to the time of appearance of cyanosis
E. The long-term surgical results are poor

Sabiston: 2223
Schwartz: 776

Comments: Tetralogy of Fallot is the most common cyanotic heart malformation (50%). The right ventricular outflow obstruction is severe enough to limit blood flow to the lungs and to raise right ventricular pressures to those seen in the left ventricle, thereby causing right-to-left shunting of blood through the ventricular septal defect. Since the ventricular septal defect decompresses the obstructed right ventricle, cardiac enlargement and failure are rare. The hallmarks of the disease are cyanosis and dyspnea on exertion. Also frequently seen are cyanotic spells and squatting. One third of the patients are cyanotic at birth and do not survive unless an operation is performed. These patients often are palliated by a subclavian artery to pulmonary artery (Blalock-Taussig) shunt or a right pulmonary artery to aorta (Waterston) shunt. The definitive operation is then postponed until the patient is 6 to 12 months of age. One third of the patients become cyanotic in the first year of life and are also severely disabled. One third of patients develop cyanosis in later years and may have minimal disability and mild polycythemia—the so-called pink tetralogies. A chest x-ray in such an individual demonstrates a normal-sized heart of unusual contour (sabot-shaped heart) due to right ventricular enlargement and a small pulmonary artery. The electrocardiogram demonstrates right ventricular hypertrophy with right axis deviation. Cardiac catheterization is required to plan the proper operation; the long-term prognosis after definitive repair is good. Lesions to be distinguished from tetralogy include truncus arteriosus, transposition of the great vessels, and pulmonary valvular stenosis with a patent foramen ovale.

Answer: A, D

30. Which statement(s) is(are) true regarding transposition of the great vessels?

A. The aorta arises from the right ventricle and carries unoxygenated blood to the body
B. The pulmonary artery arises from the left ventricle and carries unoxygenated blood to the lung
C. A patent ductus arteriosus, ventricular septal defect, or an atrial septal defect is necessary for survival
D. In those individuals with a large ventricular septal defect, survival to the second or third decade is not uncommon
E. As in tetralogy of Fallot, congestive heart failure is rare

Sabiston: 2249
Schwartz: 782

Comments: Transposition of the great vessels accounts for 30 to 40% of cyanotic heart disease in the neonate. Blood flows in two noncommunicating parallel circuits; some type of left-to-right shunt allowing admixture is necessary for survival. Fifty percent of these infants are born with a patent ductus arteriosus; a patent foramen ovale is common, and 50 to 70% have a ventricular septal defect. Severe anoxia and progressive heart failure (due to high cardiac output and desaturation of coronary blood flow) are the major physiologic handicaps. Infants with an intact ventricular septum and patent foramen ovale are the most severely affected. Those with a ventricular septal defect and pulmonary artery stenosis have the most favorable outlook because the stenosis protects against the effects of increased pulmonary blood flow. The lesion is highly lethal; 90% of patients die in the first 6 months of life if they are not treated. A chest x-ray reveals an egg-shaped heart caused by a prominence of the right ventricle and dilatation of the right atrium. The electrocardiogram demonstrates right ventricular hypertrophy. Left ventricular hypertrophy may develop in the face of pulmonary stenosis. At birth, infants require enlargement of the pulmonary-systemic communication, usually by balloon septostomy, if they are to survive. Those with large ventricular septal defects should undergo pulmonary artery banding or definitive surgical repair to avoid the development of irreversible pulmonary hypertension. Occasionally, infants with pulmonary artery stenosis require a palliative systemic-pulmonary shunt to increase pulmonary blood flow. With appropriate palliation, definitive surgery can be delayed for 2 to 3 years.

Answer: A, C

31. Which statement(s) is(are) true regarding tricuspid atresia?

A. The basic defect is atresia of the aortic and pulmonary tricuspid valves
B. Absence of a murmur is a good prognostic sign
C. The electrocardiogram uniformly demonstrates left ventricular hypertrophy and left axis deviation
D. Ligation of a patent ductus arteriosus, if present, is indicated to prevent irreversible pulmonary hypertension
E. The Fontan procedure is performed as soon as the diagnosis is made

Sabiston: 2241
Schwartz: 785

Comments: Three to 8% of cyanotic heart lesions are caused by tricuspid atresia, which consists of underdevelopment of the right ventricle, tricuspid valve, and pulmonary valve, severely limiting pulmonary blood flow. If life is to continue, an atrial septal defect must be present to allow decompression into the left atrium. The degree of impairment to pulmonary flow determines the severity of the right ventricular hypoplasia. Initially, a patent ductus arteriosus provides natural relief, but decompensation occurs after it closes. The absence of a murmur implies a very low blood flow and thus a poor

prognosis. The electrocardiogram is important diagnostically: it demonstrates left ventricular hypertrophy and left axis deviation in contrast to the right ventricular hypertrophy seen with most other forms of cyanotic heart disease (i.e., tetralogy and transposition). A palliative systemic-pulmonary shunt is indicated once the diagnosis is made. Other options include the Potts type of aortic-pulmonary shunt in infants and the Blalock-Taussig subclavian-pulmonary shunt or the Glenn caval-pulmonary shunt in older children. The Fontan procedure, usually performed in older children after initial palliation, is the creation of a right atrium–pulmonary artery communication using a valved conduit.

Answer: C

32. Match the items in the two columns.

Congenital Defects	Characteristics
A. Ruptured aneurysm of sinus of Valsalva	a. Pulmonary congestion, pulmonary hypertension, and cardiac failure
B. Truncus arteriosus, aortopulmonary window	b. Defective separation of aorta and pulmonary artery
C. Cor triatriatum, congenital mitral stenosis	c. Atrialized right ventricle
D. Ebstein's anomaly	d. Congenital or syphilitic in origin
E. Anomalous origin of left coronary artery from pulmonary artery	e. Multiple left ventricular infarctions
F. Anomalous origin of right coronary artery from pulmonary artery	f. Innocuous; compatible with normal longevity

Sabiston: 1794, 2177, 2243, 2316, 2321, 2347, 2373
Schwartz: 787, 795

Comments: There are a number of rare but interesting congenital heart defects. **Cor triatriatum**—the presence of an abnormal chamber superior and posterior to the left atrium—and congenital mitral stenosis both produce elevation of left atrial pressure with accompanying pulmonary congestion, pulmonary hypertension, and heart failure. **Aortopulmonary window** results from an abnormal separation of the primitive truncus arteriosus into the aorta and pulmonary artery. The aortic and pulmonary valves are normal, and the defect produces a large left-to-right shunt similar to that of a patent ductus arteriosus. **Truncus arteriosus** is a more profound abnormality in the division of the truncus arteriosus into aorta and pulmonary artery and consists of a common arterial trunk from which the entire circulation arises. There is always an associated ventricular septal defect. The physiologic derangement is severe, and surgical correction is difficult. **Ebstein's anomaly** results from downward displacement of a portion of the tricuspid valve, producing atrialization of a portion of the right ventricle. The physiologic result is inadequate cardiac output from the right ventricle. The right atrium becomes dilated, and cyanosis develops owing to right-to-left shunting of blood through the foramen ovale. In congenital **aneurysms of the sinus of Valsalva,** the media of the aortic wall do not extend to the annulus of the aortic valve ring. These aneurysms can also result from syphilis or other infections. Seventy percent of cases involve the right coronary sinus, with rupture occurring into the right ventricle. The average age of rupture is 31 years, and the rupture, unless corrected, is usually followed by fatal heart failure within 1 year. Multiple **anomalies of the coronary arteries** exist. Anomalous origin of the left coronary artery from the pulmonary artery is a severe lesion causing death in most patients within the first year of life. Reimplantation or grafting into the aorta can correct the defect. Anomalous origin of the right coronary artery from the pulmonary artery is innocuous and compatible with normal longevity. Coronary arteriovenous fistula is an abnormal direct communication between a coronary artery and a cardiac chamber. Usually, the abnormal opening is into the right atrium or right ventricle, constituting a left-to-right shunt. Ligation of the fistula is curative.

Answer: A–d; B–b; C–a; D–c; E–e; F–f

CHAPTER 50

Cardiac Surgery—Acquired Diseases

1. The standard technique of perfusion during extracorporeal circulation involves which of the following?

A. Cannulation of the right atrium for aspiration of venous blood
B. Femoral artery cannulation for retrograde perfusion
C. Cannulation of the ascending aorta for return of oxygennated blood
D. Discarding of intracardiac blood

Schwartz: 811

Comments: The development of extracorporeal circulation has made possible the scope of cardiac surgery performed today. Perfusion technique involves aspiration of venous blood through large cannulas inserted into the right atrium and advanced into the venae cavae, followed by oxygenation and subsequent return through a cannula in the ascending aorta. ● Femoral arterial cannulation is associated with a small but definite risk of retrograde dissection of the aorta. ● Most heart-lung machines use a roller pump with either a bubble or a membrane oxygenator and a heat exchanger in the circuit for temperature control. Specifics of perfusion rates must be tailored to the individual circumstance; general guidelines suggest flow rates of approximately 2.5 l per m per minute or 50 to 70 ml per kg per minute for normal-sized adults. Shed blood is aspirated, filtered, and returned to the oxygenator.

Answer: A, C

2. The maximum amount of time extracorporeal circulation can be tolerated before significant risk of physiologic injury and metabolic defects occur is:

A. 2 to 4 hours
B. 6 to 8 hours
C. 10 to 12 hours
D. 14 to 16 hours
E. 18 to 20 hours

Schwartz: 813

Comments: Tolerance of extracorporeal circulation is variable. Six to 8 hours is an accepted range, although physiologic injury may occur earlier, and occasionally patients may undergo longer perfusion with relatively few consequences. Physiologic defects observed with extracorporeal circulation include progressive sludging of blood elements in the capillary microcirculation, red cell hemolysis, coagulation defects, denaturation of plasma proteins, and occasional fat embolism.

Answer: B

3. Complications of prolonged extracorporeal circulation include:

A. Postoperative bleeding
B. Renal insufficiency
C. Respiratory insufficiency
D. Psychosis
E. Pancreatitis

Schwartz: 813

Comments: The physiologic and metabolic injuries resulting from prolonged extracorporeal circulation are exhibited in several ways. Postoperative bleeding may occur owing to destruction of clotting factors, destruction of platelets, impairment of platelet function, and improper titration of protamine to reverse systemic heparinization. The coagulation defect may be transient and occasionally may resolve within the first 12 hours following perfusion. The importance of meticulous surgical hemostasis is apparent. Both renal and respiratory insufficiency are usually transient and often require prolonged supportive treatment. A variety of CNS changes may occur. These changes have both metabolic and organic causes, which may be manifest by localized or generalized deficit of variable severity and duration. Infrequently, pancreatitis occurs, likely secondary to hypoperfusion.

Answer: A, B, C, D, E

4. Following aortic valve replacement for calcific aortic stenosis, a patient develops seizures. The most likely causes include:

A. Air embolism
B. Calcium emboli
C. Emboli from a left atrial thrombus
D. Emboli from aortic atherosclerosis
E. Extracorporeal circulation

Schwartz: 816

Comments: Seizures occur not infrequently as a manifestation of focal injury to the central nervous system. Air embolism is a result of incomplete evacuation of air from the cardiac chambers following open heart surgery. Evacuation may be facilitated by the use of a left ventricular vent or an aortic vent or both, which are left in place until after the heart is beating. During this time cardiopulmonary bypass is gradually reduced, the patient is rotated, and the heart is manipulated to assist in removal of air from within the cardiac chambers. ● Calcium fragments may embolize after removal of calcific debris from a diseased aortic valve. Cannulation and/or clamping of a diseased aorta may result in dislodgement of arteriosclerotic debris. ● Left atrial thrombi are another potential source of cerebral emboli. This is usually seen in patients with mitral stenosis. ● The usual neurologic deficit observed following prolonged extracorporeal circulation is a transient generalized depression of cerebral function related to hypoperfusion of the microcirculation.

Answer: A, B, D

5. Indications for coronary artery bypass may include:

A. Unstable angina
B. Left main coronary artery disease
C. Three-vessel disease
D. Two-vessel disease
E. Single-vessel disease

Sabiston: 2292
Schwartz: 853

Comments: Coronary revascularization not only relieves angina, which is the most common symptom of ischemic heart disease, but in selected groups of patients, results have indicated that it improves longevity. In patients with single-vessel disease, the results of surgical and medical treatment have shown similar survival rates. A usual indication for coronary bypass in patients with single-vessel disease is angina refractory to maximum medical treatment. It has been shown that patients with multivessel disease and compromised left ventricular function have exhibited an improved survival rate, even in the face of mild or moderate angina pectoris. Significant improvement in survival rate has been noted in patients with greater than 50 percent narrowing of the left main coronary artery and triple-vessel disease with impaired left ventricular function. Surgical treatment of patients with unstable angina pectoris offers significant benefit if the patient is unresponsive to intensive medical therapy.

Answer: A, B, C, D, E

6. Contraindications to coronary artery bypass include:

A. Refractory congestive heart failure
B. Severely depressed left ventricular ejection fraction (less than 0.20)
C. Age over 70 years
D. Angiographic inability to visualize a patent distal vessel
E. Acute myocardial infarction

Sabiston: 2293
Schwart: 855

Comments: Most authorities would consider congestive heart failure with pulmonary hypertension (in the absence of mechanical defects such as LVA, MR, VSD) the only cardiac contraindication to bypass grafting. With current techniques of myocardial preservation and revascularization, bypass can be successfully performed in patients who, for various reasons, were once considered excessive risk candidates for bypass. Angiographic visualization depends upon technique and collateral circulation and is not a reliable criterion of operability. Revascularization may be beneficial in the face of an acute, evolving myocardial infarction if the patient can be operated on within the first 3 to 6 hours. The role of surgery in relation to balloon angioplasty and thrombolytic therapy in this setting has not yet been fully defined.

Answer: A

7. The operative mortality of coronary artery bypass approximates 10% in which of the following situations?

A. Elective operation
B. Revision of failed coronary artery bypass surgery
C. Emergency coronary artery bypass
D. Severely impaired left ventricular function
E. None of the above

Sabiston: 2293
Schwartz: 856

Comments: Improvement in anesthetic and surgical techniques and methods of myocardial protection have reduced the mortality of elective coronary artery bypass to approximately 1 to 2%. The risk is somewhat higher in certain groups of patients, but even in higher risk categories or in situations of emergency coronary artery bypass or revision of failed bypass surgery, the risk rarely exceeds 3 to 5%.

Answer: E

8. Which of the following statements is/are true regarding the prognosis of coronary artery disease?

A. Most patients die within 1 to 2 years of onset of congestive heart failure
B. Ventricular function influences survival more than does the extent of vessel involvement
C. Mortality of an acute myocardial infarction is approximately 50%
D. Acute myocardial infarction is the most common cause of sudden cardiac death

Schwartz: 853

Comments: Manifestations of coronary occlusive disease include angina pectoris, myocardial infarction, congestive heart failure, arrhythmias, and sudden death. Sudden death is often the result of ventricular fibrillation without demonstrable infarction. The current mortality of an acute myocardial infarction is approximately 10%. With destruction of significant left ventricular muscle mass, chronic congestive heart failure occurs, and the prognosis is poor. Data suggest that while both the extent of coronary vessel involvement and the status of the left ventricle are important prognostically, it is left ventricular function that allows the most accurate prediction of long-term survival.

Answer: A, B

9. Results of coronary artery bypass grafting include:

A. Complete pain relief in the majority of patients
B. Improvement in left ventricular function
C. Prolonged life in patients with two- and three-vessel disease or left main vessel disease
D. 5-year survival rate of 85 to 95%
E. Diminished risk of sudden death

Sabiston: 2302
Schwartz: 855

Comments: Coronary artery bypass grafting decreases angina in 90% of patients and completely relieves pain in approximately two thirds. There is both hemodynamic and clinical evidence of improved left ventricular function. The overall 5-year survival rate following myocardial revascularization is generally in the 85 to 95% range. Improvement in survival rate has been documented only in patients with triple-vessel and left main coronary disease. The survival rate has been shown to be significantly better than with medical therapy for patients with left main lesions or with three-vessel disease. It appears that the risk of sudden cardiac death is decreased by coronary artery bypass grafting, and there is evidence that the incidence of myocardial infarction is also reduced following successful revascularization.

Answer: A, B, D, E

10. A 55-year-old patient in the coronary care unit develops refractory angina 2 days after being hospitalized for an acute myocardial infarction. Which of the following statements is/are true regarding coronary artery bypass in this situation?

A. It should be performed only if there is left main coronary disease
B. Operative mortality and long-term survival are poor compared with patients who have unstable angina not precipitated by myocardial infarction
C. It should be preceded by streptokinase therapy if multivessel disease is also present
D. The operative mortality is under 5%

Sabiston: 2293

Comments: Unstable angina is preceded by myocardial infarction in approximately one half of patients. The initial treatment of patients with unstable angina involves intensive medical therapy with beta-blocking agents, nitrates, and calcium channel–blocking drugs. Patients who fail to respond to medical treatment should have an operation on an emergency basis if they have reconstructible vessels. The operative mortality is approximately 4%. Among patients who respond to initial medical management, approximately 15% per year require later myocardial revascularization, with results that are comparable to those seen in patients with stable angina. Prognosis does not seem to differ between patients with unstable angina preceded by an acute myocardial infarction and those without infarction.

Answer: D

11. A patient develops angina 3 years after coronary artery bypass. Angiography is most likely to reveal:

A. A dominant right coronary system
B. Progressive atherosclerosis in the coronary arteries
C. Progressive atherosclerosis in vein graft
D. Vein graft thrombosis

Sabiston: 2303
Schwartz: 856

Comments: The rate of recurrence of angina following coronary artery bypass grafting is approximately 5 to 7% per year. Surgery, unfortunately, does not slow the progression of atherosclerosis, which is the primary cause of recurrent symptoms. Graft occlusion may also occur as a result of thrombosis, intimal fibrosis, or fibrous endarteritis. Vein grafts may also be involved with atherosclerosis; this usually occurs later in the postoperative course. Overall vein graft patency is approximately 80% after 5 years. There is evidence that internal mammary artery grafts have a lower rate of late atherosclerotic involvement and better rates of patency than vein grafts.

Answer: B

12. A patient is in ventribular fibrillation with a PaO_2 of 100 mm Hg and a pH of 7.20. An initial attempt at defibrillation with DC current at a charge of 300 watt-seconds is unsuccessful. Appropriate treatment includes:

A. Increasing charge to 800 watt-seconds
B. Administration of sodium bicarbonate
C. Administration of epinephrine
D. Confirmation of electrode placement
E. Repeat defibrillation using AC current

Sabiston: 2170
Schwartz: 819

Comments: Unless coronary thrombosis has occurred, it is usually possible to defibrillate most fibrillating hearts. Acidosis, hypoxia, and inadequate delivery of current are causes of failure of defibrillation. Direct current defibrillation with 300 watt-seconds is preferred to alternating current. Epinephrine stimulates myocardial tone and may facilitate defibrillation.

Answer: B, C, D

13. Ventricular aneurysms usually have which of the following characteristics?

A. Result from myocardial infarction
B. Involve the posterior left ventricle
C. Present with peripheral emboli from a mural thrombosis
D. Cause death because of rupture

Sabiston: 2310
Schwartz: 858

Comments: The great majority of ventricular aneurysms result from transmural infarction. They most frequently involve the anterior left ventricle in the distribution of the left anterior descending artery. The most common complication is congestive heart failure, followed by arrhythmias and angina. Peripheral emboli may occur but are infrequent. Death due to rupture of a ventricular aneurysm is also an unusual event.

Answer: A

14. Which of the following statements is/are true regarding surgical treatment of ventricular aneurysm?

A. Aneurysms smaller than 5 cm are usually insignificant
B. Indications include congestive heart failure and malignant arrhythmias
C. Preservation of the left anterior descending artery is mandatory
D. Complete aneurysmectomy is preferred
E. Concomitant coronary artery bypass is usually performed

Sabiston: 2311
Schwartz: 859

Comments: Resection of ventricular aneurysms is indicated for the treatment of congestive heart failure and, in some instances, for treatment of recurrent malignant ventricular arrhythmias. Concomitant coronary artery bypass is performed as indicated in association with left ventricular aneurysm resection. Rather than performing complete excision of all scar tissue, the surgeon leaves a rim of scar in order to avoid compromise of collateral circulation and possible narrowing of the left ventricular chamber. An effort is made to preserve and/or bypass the left anterior descending artery if significant flow to the ventricular septum can be affected via this channel but preservation is not mandatory since it is often the vessel that has been involved in the infarction precipitating the aneurysm.

Answer: A, B, E

15. Treatment of acute pyogenic pericarditis may require:

A. Parenteral antibiotics that are active against *Staphylococcus, Streptococcus,* and *Haemophilus* species
B. Serial pericardial aspirations
C. Subxiphoid pericardiotomy
D. Radical pericardiectomy

Sabiston: 2130
Schwartz: 860

Comments: Pyogenic pericarditis is rare. Today it is usually seen in infants or young children, in whom it is associated with a high mortality rate. *Staphylococcus aureus* and *Streptococcus* species are the most common organisms in adults, whereas *Haemophilus influenzae* and *Neisseria meningitidis* predominate in infants and children. Parenteral antibiotics combined with serial pericardial aspirations and occasional intrapericardial instillation of antibiotics are usually adequate treatment. Surgical drainage may be necessary, but radical pericardiectomy is not indicated.

Answer: A, B, C

16. Which of the following statements is/are true concerning chronic constrictive pericarditis?

A. It is usually caused by mycobacterium
B. It is best treated with a combination of diuretics and inotropic agents
C. Pericardiectomy is successful in 50% of patients with chronic constrictive pericarditis
D. It is characterized by equalization of right- and left-sided pressures

Sabiston: 2126
Schwartz: 861

Comments: Chronic constrictive pericarditis most often occurs secondary to a viral process, although in most cases the true etiology is unknown. Tuberculosis was once thought to be the most frequent cause. The disease is marked by progressive edema, ascites, hepatic enlargement, and dyspnea on exertion. Hemodynamic findings include evaluation of the right ventricular end-diastolic, right atrial, and central venous pressures to levels equal to those of the pulmonary artery wedge and left ventricular end-diastolic pressures. Pericardiectomy is the treatment of choice and is successful in 90% of cases if adequate resection is performed.

Answer: D

17. Accepted indications for transluminal coronary balloon angioplasty include:

A. Isolated left main artery disease
B. Acute evolving myocardial infarction with critical coronary stenosis
C. Stenotic vein bypass grafts
D. Intraoperative dilatation distal to bypass grafts
E. Distal segmental lesions

Sabiston: 2302

Comments: The treatment of occlusive peripheral arterial disease, renal arterial disease, and coronary disease with balloon angioplasty has been increasing. Its role in relation to that of operation for coronary artery disease is not yet fully defined. It has been used in several settings, however, and usually is applied to distal segmental lesions in which a bypass graft is not possible. Approximately 5% of patients require emergency coronary artery bypass following balloon angioplasty because of complications; approximately one third of patients ultimately fail. Isolated left main artery disease is not an indication for balloon angioplasty but should be managed by operation.

Answer: B, C, D, E

18. Following open heart surgery, a patient develops chest pain, fever, tachycardia, and a pericardial friction rub. Which of the following statements is/are true regarding this situation?

A. This picture usually is accompanied by pleural effusion and evidence of congestive heart failure
B. The most likely diagnosis is pulmonary embolism
C. Usually there will be an associated leukocytosis or eosinophilia
D. Primary treatment should include antibiotics
E. The patient likely will respond well to anti-inflammatory agents.

Sabiston: 2131, 2301
Schwartz: 816, 856

Comments: Following procedures in which the pericardium is entered, transient pericardial inflammation known as the postpericardiotomy syndrome may occur. Clinical manifestations include pain, fever, tachycardia, arrhythmias, and sometimes a pericardial friction rub. Usually there is no leukocytosis or eosinophilia. Patients usually respond well to a short course of indomethacin or steroids.

Answer: E

19. Five hours following coronary artery bypass, a patient suddenly becomes hypotensive. Cardiac index is less than 2 L per minute. Central venous pressure is 22 mm Hg. Left atrial pressure is 25 mm Hg. Immediate treatment should include:

A. Angiography for probable graft occlusion
B. Intra-aortic balloon counterpulsation
C. Ntiroprusside for afterload reduction
D. Mediastinotomy
E. Inotropic agent

Sabiston: 2299
Schwartz: 814

Comments: Hypotension and low cardiac output following open heart surgery require prompt and careful evaluation. Specific causes include inadequate blood volume, occult bleeding, cardiac tamponade, arrhythmias, myocardial insufficiency, and acidosis. The finding of elevated filling pressures with equalization of right- and left-sided pressures, particularly with increased early postoperative bleeding, suggests the diagnosis of cardiac tamponade, in which case immediate reoperation is mandatory. Significant elevation of filling pressures in association with low cardiac output may also be indicative of cardiac failure, which may be treated with inotropic agents, digitalis, and counterpulsation. Chest x-ray is of variable diagnostic value, occasionally revealing widening of the mediastinum and occasionally allowing detection of occult accumulation of blood in a pleural space.

Answer: D

20. Aortic stenosis presenting in an adult may result from:

A. Bacterial endocarditis
B. Marfan's syndrome
C. Rheumatic fever
D. Congenital bicuspid valve
E. Syphilis

Sabiston: 2336
Schwartz: 835

Comments: Aortic stenosis presenting in an adult may result from rheumatic fever or from a congenital valvular deformity. A congenital biscuspid valve may remain asymptomatic for many years, but the deformed valve is susceptible to endocarditis and eventually develops calcification and symptomatic stenosis. Aortic insufficiency commonly follows bacterial endocarditis. Aortic insufficiency may also result from dilatation of the aortic annulus due to an ascending aortic aneurysm, as seen with Marfan's syndrome or, more rarely, syphilis.

Answer: C, D

21. The most common clinical manifestation of aortic stenosis is:

A. Syncope
B. Angina pectoris
C. Dyspnea on exertion
D. Atrial fibrillation

Sabiston: 2338
Schwartz: 836

Comments: Characteristically, patients with aortic stenosis remain asymptomatic for many years but deteriorate rapidly once symptoms begin. About two thirds of patients develop angina pectoris. This coronary insufficiency is secondary to inadequate cardiac output or results from compromised coronary arterial blood flow caused by elevated left ventricular end-diastolic pressure. Syncope, present in one third of patients, also reflects impaired cardiac output but in some patients may be related to a conduction abnormality due to calcification of the atrioventricular node. Signs of left ventricular failure and atrial fibrillation resulting in elevated left atrial pressures are evidence of more advanced disease.

Answer: B

22. Which of the following statements is/are true regarding the prognosis of adults with aortic stenosis?

A. Sudden death accounts for most fatalities
B. Left ventricular failure signifies a worse prognosis than does syncope or chest pain
C. Symptomatic patients have a greater risk of sudden death than do asymptomatic patients
D. Intensity of the murmur correlates with severity of disease

Sabiston: 2338
Schwartz: 836

Comments: Once patients with aortic stenosis develop symptoms, prognosis is poor. With angina or syncope, the average life expectancy of untreated patients is 3 to 4 years; death occurs 1 to 2 years after left ventricular failure. Sudden death occurs more frequently with aortic stenosis than with any other valvular lesion. It accounts for approximately 20% of deaths from aortic stenosis and is always a risk, but it occurs more frequently in symptomatic patients. The loudness of the classic systolic diamond-shaped ejection murmur reported over the aortic area and the apex does not have prognostic significance.

Answer: B, C

23. Indications for operation in patients with aortic stenosis include:

A. All symptomatic patients
B. Systolic pressure gradient greater than 50 mm Hg in asymptomatic patients
C. Valvular cross-sectional area smaller than 1 cm^2
D. Concomitant coronary artery disease

Sabiston: 2338
Schwartz: 836, 841

Comments: All symptomatic patients require prompt valve replacement because of the high risk of sudden death and deterioration. Peak systolic gradients across the valve of greater than 50 to 60 mm Hg and cross-sectional areas of 0.8 to 1 cm^2 generally are found with moderately severe aortic stenosis and are indications for valve replacement, even if symptoms are absent. Patients with aortic stenosis may have associated coronary artery disease; bypass of critical lesions does not add significantly to operative risk. Five-year survival rate following aortic valve replacement is approximately 80%.

Answer: A, B, C, D

24. Select the type of prosthetic heart valve most appropriate for each given clinical situation.

Patient	Valve
A. Child with congenital aortic stenosis	a. Bioprosthetic
B. Patient with hereditary coagulopathy	b. Mechanical
C. 24-year-old with mitral stenosis	c. Neither
D. Patient with chronic renal failure	
E. 24-year-old woman with mitral stenosis who desires children	

Sabiston: 2366

Comments: The ideal prosthetic heart valve has not yet been developed; selection is based on patient characteristics, operative findings, and surgeons' preference. Bioprosthetic valves (glutaraldehyde-fixed porcine heterografts or bovine pericardium) have a low rate of thromboembolism and therefore do not require long-term anticoagulation. The problem with bioprosthetic valves, however, is long-term durability; the rate of valve

failure is 2 to 5% yearly, and this rate increases after the first 6 years. These valves are contraindicated in children, in those under 20 to 30 years of age, and in patients with chronic renal failure who require hemodialysis. Mechanical heart valves are durable, but their usefulness is limited by the need of permanent anticoagulation, which is contraindicated in certain clinical states (e.g., pregnancy, coagulopathy, ulcer disease). Thromboembolic complications occur at a 2 to 5% annual rate even in patients who are adequately anticoagulated. Adults with mechanical valves require permanent anticoagulation therapy, which carries a mortality of approximately 1% per year. The risk of prosthetic valve endocarditis is about 1 to 2% per year for both bioprosthetic and mechanical valves; it has been suggested that infection of tissue valves may respond better to antibiotic therapy alone.

Answer: A–b; B–a; C–c; D–b; E–a

25. Cardiac catheterization of a 40-year-old woman with a recent history of dyspnea on exertion, hemoptysis, and paroxysmal nocturnal dyspnea demonstrates a left atrial pressure of 28 mm Hg. The primary determinants of this pressure include:

A. Size of the left atrium
B. Cross-sectional area of the mitral opening
C. Cardiac output
D. Cardiac rate
E. Pulmonary artery pressure

Sabiston: 2350
Schwartz: 821

Comments: The primary physiologic consequences of mitral stenosis are increased left atrial pressure, decreased cardiac output, and increased pulmonary vascular resistance. The clinical manifestations of these changes include the typical symptoms of congestive heart failure, pulmonary edema, and right-sided heart failure, as well as atrial fibrillation and arterial embolism. Actual left atrial pressure is determined by the size of the mitral orifice, cardiac output, and heart rate. Severity of disease is best classified by calculation of the cross-sectional area of the valve, which takes into consideration both pressure gradient and cardiac output. Mitral valve area (MVA) of approximately 1 cm^2 or less is indicative of significant stenosis, although low flow rates and the presence of mitral regurgitation may influence calculations. When left atrial pressures exceed plasma oncotic pressure (24 to 30 mm Hg), pulmonary edema develops.

Answer: B, C, D

26. Indications for valvulotomy or valve replacement in patients with significant mitral stenosis include:

A. Asymptomatic patients
B. Atrial fibrillation
C. Congestive heart failure
D. Pulmonary hypertension
E. Systemic embolization

Sabiston: 2351

Comments: The natural history of mitral stenosis is one of progressive symptomatology. Most asymptomatic patients are treated medically and observed. Symptomatic patients whose treatment is only medical eventually die from their cardiac disease. Indications for operative intervention include congestive heart failure (with New York Heart Association class III or IV symptoms), onset of atrial fibrillation with significant mitral stenosis, pulmonary hypertension, systemic embolization, and infective endocarditis. Surgical therapy is also recommended for patients who have mild symptoms and a severe reduction in valvular area.

Answer: B, C, D, E

27. The treatment of mitral stenosis is by a judicious combination of medical and surgical therapy. Which of the following statements is/are true regarding results of surgical treatment for symptomatic mitral stenosis?

A. Survival rate is increased compared with that of medical therapy
B. Surgical treatment is usually curative
C. Commissurotomy decreases the risk of systemic embolization and endocarditis
D. Pulmonary vascular resistance usually diminishes following valve replacement or commissurotomy
E. Ten-year survival rate exceeds 90%

Sabiston: 2352

Comments: Surgical treatment of mitral stenosis by commissurotomy or valve replacement produces physiologic and clinical improvement, although results tend to deteriorate over time. Patients require continued follow-up, and if symptoms reappear, the patient should be evaluated for reoperation. A second commissurotomy is occasionally possible, but often valve replacement is required.

Answer: A, C, D, E

28. The most common cause of mitral insufficiency is:

A. Bacterial endocarditis
B. Rheumatic fever
C. Mitral valve prolapse
D. Papillary muscle dysfunction
E. Rupture of chordae tendineae

Sabiston: 2353
Schwartz: 831

Comments: Rheumatic fever is the most common cause of both mitral regurgitation and mitral stenosis. Although mitral stenosis almost exclusively results from rheumatic fever, mitral regurgitation may have other causes, including mitral valve prolapse, idiopathic calcification, bacterial endocarditis, chordal rupture, and ischemic heart disease. An etiology other than rheumatic fever can often be suspected on the basis of the history and clinical presentation.

Answer: B

29. Which of the following statements is/are true regarding patients with mitral regurgitation compared with those who have mitral stenosis?

A. They more often develop left ventricular failure
B. They rarely develop atrial fibrillation
C. They less commonly develop systemic emboli
D. In general, they have a poorer prognosis postoperatively
E. Pulmonary hypertension usually fails to resolve following valve replacement

Sabiston: 2353

Comments: The physical signs of pulmonary hypertension and right heart failure produced by mitral regurgitation are similar to those seen in mitral stenosis. Unlike patients with mitral stenosis, however, patients with mitral regurgitation ultimately develop left ventricular failure owing to chronic overload. Atrial fibrillation is a common manifestation of mitral regurgitation; embolization does occur, but it is less common than in mitral stenosis. The natural history of mitral regurgitation and the results of operative correction are somewhat more variable than those with mitral stenosis because of the different etiologic factors that may produce mitral incompetence. Pulmonary hypertension will usually resolve after successful valve replacement. In most studies, success of valve replacement for mitral insufficiency is less long-term than that for isolated mitral stenosis.

Answer: A, C, D

30. A 60-year-old man with a history of dyspnea on exertion, angina, palpitations, and episodes of severe diaphoresis has a high-pitched diastolic murmur along the left sternal border. Expected findings include:

A. Enlargement of both the left atrium and the left ventricle on chest x-ray
B. Systolic ejection murmur
C. Bounding peripheral pulses
D. Atrial fibrillation
E. Elevated thyroid function tests

Schwartz: 842

Comments: Common symptoms of aortic insufficiency include angina, progressive dyspnea, palpitations, and peripheral vasomotor changes. Signs of pulmonary congestion occur later as left ventricular failure develops. Findings on physical examination include a normal cardiac rhythm and bounding peripheral pulses due to the widened pulse pressure. The classic decrescendo diastolic murmur is present and is accentuated by leaning forward. A systolic ejection murmur may also be heard but does not usually represent aortic stenosis. Enlargement of the left ventricle is seen on chest x-ray.

Answer: B, C

31. The best indications for operative intervention in aortic insufficiency are:

A. Progressive symptoms
B. Loudness and length of diastolic murmur

C. Increasing left ventricular size
D. Magnitude of reflux as measured during catheterization

Sabiston: 2338
Schwartz: 842

Comments: Patients with aortic insufficiency generally remain asymptomatic for many years, although there is significant variability among patients. Progressive symptoms of heart failure or ischemia and increasing left ventricular size on chest x-ray or echocardiography are generally considered indications for operation. The loudness of the diastolic murmur does not correlate with severity of disease. The length of the murmur reflects to some extent the patient's physiologic status in that a longer murmur reflects a greater degree of regurgitation. Short murmurs may be heard, however, both in patients with early disease and minimal regurgitation and in patients with end-stage disease and elevated left ventricular end-diastolic pressures. Measurement of reflux is possible during cardiac catheterization, but this has not yet proved to be useful in the selection of patients for operation.

Answer: A, C

32. Tricuspid valvular disease most commonly is:

A. Functional rather than organic
B. The end result of rheumatic fever
C. Tricuspid stenosis
D. Treated by valve excision without replacement

Sabiston: 2357, 2364
Schwartz: 844

Comments: Insufficiency is the most common hemodynamic abnormality of the tricuspid valve. Most often this is a functional disorder secondary to right ventricular dilatation, which is due to mitral disease, pulmonary hypertension, or other causes of right ventricular failure. Organic causes of tricuspid insufficiency, such as rheumatic fever, endocarditis, or carcinoid syndrome, are less common. Tricuspid stenosis is infrequent and usually of rheumatic origin. Treatment of significant tricuspid insufficiency or stenosis generally involves valve repair or replacement. Isolated organic disease of the tricuspid valve is most commonly seen as a result of endocarditis secondary to intravenous drug abuse. Total valve excision without replacement has been an occasional alternative in this difficult situation.

Answer: A, B

33. Match the items in the two columns.

Valvular Lesion	Clinical Effect
A. Aortic insufficiency	a. Masking of mitral stenosis
B. Mitral insufficiency	b. Masking of tricuspid valve disease
C. Mitral stenosis	c. Masking of aortic stenosis

Sabiston: 2337, 2347
Schwartz: 846

Comments: Rheumatic heart disease frequently involves more than one cardiac valve, but multivalvular involvement may not always be clinically apparent. Cardiac catheterization is, therefore, critical to the evaluation of patients preoperatively, since failure to correct all significant valvular lesions is associated with higher morbidity and mortality. With mitral stenosis, the restricted volume of blood entering the left ventricle may mask an associated aortic stenosis. Similarly, the findings of tricuspid disease are frequently overshadowed by concomitant auscultatory findings and right ventricular failure secondary to mitral regurgitation. Prominent aortic insufficiency may obscure the murmur of mitral stenosis; conversely, severe mitral stenosis may limit the physiologic consequences of aortic insufficiency. When cardiac failure results from aortic insufficiency, the subsequent left ventricular dilatation that occurs may produce a functional mitral insufficiency in an otherwise normal valve.

Answer: A–a; B–b; C–c

34. The cardiac chamber most frequently injured by penetrating trauma is the:

A. Left ventricle
B. Right ventricle
C. Left atrium
D. Right atrium

Schwartz: 847

Comments: The right ventricle is the most anterior chamber of the heart and consequently is the structure most susceptible to penetrating injury. Cardiac injury may produce exsanguination, cardiac tamponade, and, rarely, cardiac failure secondary to damage to a major coronary artery, a valve, or the conduction system. The key to saving patients who arrive in the emergency room with cardiac injury is prompt recognition and treatment of tamponade while other resuscitative measures are instituted. Nonpenetrating cardiac trauma usually produces diffuse contusion, which warrants cardiac monitoring in an intensive care setting.

Answer: B

35. The most common primary malignant cardiac neoplasm is:

A. Myxoma
B. Rhabdomyoma
C. Sarcoma
D. Lymphoma

Sabiston: 2405
Schwartz: 849

Comments: The most common cardiac neoplasms are metastatic. Most primary cardiac neoplasms are benign, and, of these, myxoma is the most common, followed by rhabdomyoma. Approximately 20% of primary tumors are malignant; these are almost always rhabdomyosarcoma and angiosarcoma, and they will generally have systemic metastases at the time of diagnosis.

Answer: C

36. Which of the following statements is/are true regarding metastatic cardiac neoplasms?

A. Most lesions are asymptomatic
B. Metastatic tumors usually involve cardiac valves and produce typical murmurs
C. Excision of solitary lesions produces survival comparable to that seen with solitary liver metastases
D. Generally lesions are multiple and not amenable to surgical treatment

Sabiston: 2409
Schwartz: 851

Comments: Leukemia, lymphoma, lung and breast cancer, and melanoma are among the more common neoplasms that can involve the heart. It is extremely unusual for the heart to be the only site of metastasis or for there to be only a solitary metastasis to the heart. From a cardiac standpoint, most patients with such metastases are asymptomatic. Among those with symptoms, bloody pericardial effusion is the most common manifestation. Valvular involvement is rare. Treatment, therefore, is palliative and aimed at the primary disease process and relief of symptomatic pericardial effusion. In rare selected patients with solitary metastases to the overflow tract, resection may be indicated. For the most part, however, the role of cardiac surgery is limited to resection of renal tumors that have extended through the cava to the atrium and decompression of symptomatic pericardial effusions.

Answer: A, D

37. Physiologic effects of intra-aortic balloon pumping include:

A. Decreased cardiac afterload
B. Increased coronary blood flow
C. Decreased left ventricular end-diastolic pressure
D. Decreased left ventricular preload

Sabiston: 2468
Schwartz: 866

Comments: An electronically synchronized intra-aortic balloon pump, which inflates during diastole and deflates with systole, has physiologic effects that both decrease myocardial oxygen consumption and increase coronary blood flow. Deflation of the balloon reduces impedance to aortic flow, thereby reducing afterload and improving cardiac output. Left ventricular end-diastolic volume and pressure are reduced, and diastolic coronary blood flow is enhanced, particularly in failing hearts. Pulmonary artery diastolic pressure is decreased, thus reducing left ventricular preload.

Answer: A, B, C, D

38. Which of the following statements appropriately describe(s) indications for and effects of intra-aortic balloon pumping (IABP)?

A. IABP is indicated in myocardial infarction with cardiogenic shock to decrease infarct size
B. In patients with refractory unstable angina, IABP effectively relieves pain

C. IABP is indicated for support of cardiac failure following cardiopulmonary bypass, even though most patients cannot be successfully weaned from it
D. IABP is indicated in severe aortic insufficiency to decrease peripheral resistance

Sabiston: 2471

Comments: Indications for intra-aortic balloon pumping include the following: cardiac failure after cardiopulmonary bypass; refractory unstable angina; preoperative treatment of septal defects, mitral regurgitation, arrhythmias, ventricular aneurysms, and occasionally cardiogenic shock. IABP no longer is commonly used for the treatment of cardiogenic shock that is associated with myocardial infarction because most patients cannot be successfully weaned from it and there is no conclusive evidence that IABP decreases infarct size. IABP is particularly effective for controlling pain in patients with angina refractory to pharmacologic manipulation. IABP has also been successful in the support of patients with cardiac failure following cardiopulmonary bypass; most such patients can be weaned successfully, and with long-term survival. Severe aortic insufficiency is a contraindication to balloon counterpulsation because regurgitation and cardiac failure are exacerbated.

Answer: B

39. Which of the following are indications for placement of a permanent cardiac pacemaker?

A. Sick sinus syndrome
B. Complete AV block
C. Mobitz Type II AV block
D. Stokes-Adams attacks
E. Mobitz Type I AV block

Sabiston: 2418

Comments: There is some disagreement regarding the total list of indications for either temporary or permanent cardiac pacing. Most would agree that indications for permanent pacing include the following: sick sinus syndrome or bradytachycardia syndrome; Mobitz Type II AV block (since it frequently leads to complete AV block); complete AV block; symptomatic bilateral bundle branch block and bifascicular or incomplete trifascicular block with intermittent complete AV block following myocardial infarction. Stokes-Adams attacks consisting of intermittent syncopal episodes and sometimes convulsions are manifestations of complete heart block. Mobitz Type I AV block (Wenckebach) rarely requires pacing.

Answer: A, B, C, D

40. Open-chest cardiac massage may be indicated in patients with which of the following?

A. Blunt thoracic trauma
B. Penetrating thoracic trauma
C. Barrel chest
D. Spinal deformities

Sabiston: 2170
Schwartz: 819

Comments: Open-chest cardiac compression may be life-saving in certain circumstances. It is particularly indicated in cases of blunt or penetrating thoracic injury when there is suspected cardiac tamponade, massive intrathoracic hemorrhage, penetrating cardiac injury, or an open pericardium. It may be necessary in patients in whom external compression is unsuccessful; this some-times occurs in patients with a barrel chest and emphysema or in those with spinal deformities. To perform open cardiac massage, the chest is opened through the left 5th intercostal space. On opening the pericardial sac, care should be taken not to injure the phrenic nerve.

Answer: A, B, C, D

CHAPTER 51

Urology

1. Which of the following statements is/are true regarding renal vascular anatomy?

A. Renal arteries are end-arteries
B. The right renal artery crosses ventral to the vena cava
C. The left renal vein crosses ventral to the aorta
D. The right adrenal and gonadal veins empty into the right renal vein

Schwartz: 1679

Comments: Approximately two thirds of normal kidneys are supplied by a single renal artery arising from the aorta, near the upper aspect of the 2nd lumbar vertebra. Each renal artery has approximately five segmental branches that are end-arteries; occlusion of the segmental vessels therefore causes infarction. Renal arterial anomalies are more often present in abnormally located kidneys. Venous drainage of the kidney often involves collateral vessels, particularly on the left side via the gonadal, adrenal, and lumbar veins. The renal vein itself is usually singular on the left and, approximately 10% of the time, is multiple on the right. Since the aorta in normal individuals lies to the left side of the vena cava, the right renal artery crosses behind the vena cava and the left renal vein crosses anterior to the aorta. This is consistent with the general anatomic principle that major systemic veins pass ventral to their associated arteries. The longer length of the left renal vein is advantageous when the left kidney is used as a donor organ during renal transplantation.

Answer: A, C

2. Which of the following statements is/are true regarding the course of the normal ureter?

A. It is anterior to the uterine artery in the female
B. It is anterior to gonadal vessels
C. It crosses the iliac vessels near their bifurcation
D. It is anterior to the vas deferens in the male

Sabiston: 1653
Schwartz: 1680

Comments: Understanding the normal location of the ureters and the displacement possible in certain disease states is a prerequisite of performing operations in the abdominal or pelvic areas. The ureters are retroperitoneal, originating at the renal pelvis and running a linear cephalocaudad course lateral to the transverse processes of the lumbar vertebrae, crossing the iliac arteries near their bifurcation, and then entering the true pelvis. In the course of descent, the right ureter lies behind the root of the small bowel mesentery, and the left ureter lies behind the sigmoid mesocolon. Both of them lie medial and posterior to the gonadal vessels; they course dorsal to the uterine arteries in the female and to the vas deferens in the male.

Answer: C

3. Match the illustration with the pathology.

A. Testicular tumor
B. Spermatocele
C. Chronic epididymitis
D. Acute/subacute epididymitis
E. Hydrocele

Sabiston: 1679
Schwartz: 1684

Comments: **Hydrocele** can be idiopathic or secondary to a disease process such as epididymitis, trauma, mumps, and tuberculosis. Typically, it is a nontender mass that is translucent. It can obscure palpation of the testis; it is important to be aware of this in younger men, because as many as 20% of acute hydroceles in such individuals are secondary to testicular tumors. If the mass with all the characteristics of a hydrocele empties when the patient is in the supine position, then very likely there is a patent processus vaginalis. • **Spermatocele** is a simple or multiloculated cyst at the head of the epididymis and usually requires no treatment unless it is symptomatic. It transilluminates and can be palpated as being discrete from the testes. • **Epididymitis**, if acute, leaves the patient with an exquisitely tender scrotum whose skin may be red and edematous. There may be a mass, but often

341

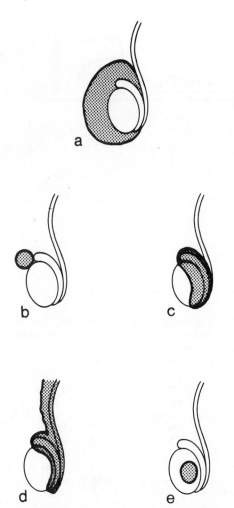

From Frank IN: Chapter 40 in Schwartz SI, et al. (eds.): Principles of Surgery. 4th ed. Copyright © 1984 by McGraw-Hill, Inc. Used by permission of McGraw-Hill Book Company.

this is difficult to appreciate because the patient will not permit a deliberate examination. In **chronic epididymitis** the mass is nontender and firm to hard, and can have beading of the entire vas deferens. If, in addition, a fistula is present, the most likely cause is tuberculosis. ● **Testicular cancer** is the most serious condition that can be present in the scrotum, and a mass therein must be so viewed until proved otherwise. The mass usually is firm, cannot be transilluminated, and is not tender; if it is tender, this may have a sudden onset and follow a seemingly trivial injury that causes bleeding in the tumorous testicle. Ultrasonographic examination of such a mass has greatly facilitated making the diagnosis within such a clinical setting.

Answer: A–e; B–b; C–d; D–c; E–a

4. Complete the following statement: The new onset of a left varicocele or the presence of a right varicocele in a patient over the age of 40 years

A. Most often is seen in association with an indirect inguinal hernia
B. Suggests testicular tumor

C. Suggests renal tumor
D. Suggests infertility

Sabiston: 1680
Schwartz: 1685

Comments: Most varicoceles occur on the left side and are idiopathic; the longer course of the left spermatic vein and abnormalities of venous valves have been suggested as etiologic factors. Obstruction of the vena cava or left renal vein also leads to varicocele formation. The presence of a right varicocele, which is uncommon, or the new onset of a left varicocele should alert the clinician to possible malignant venous obstruction. Failure of a varicocele to drain with the patient in the supine position also suggests venous obstruction as the etiologic mechanism. Varicoceles have been associated with infertility, although the clinical situation described above does not itself suggest that the patient is infertile.

Answer: C

5. While lifting a spare tire, a 40-year-old develops sudden left testicular pain. Examination reveals a tender scrotal mass. Differential diagnosis includes:

A. Epididymitis
B. Inguinal hernia
C. Testicular torsion
D. Renal calculus
E. Testicular tumor

Sabiston: 1679
Schwartz: 1684, 1696

Comments: The differential diagnosis of a tender scrotal mass includes testicular torsion, epididymitis, orchitis, tumor, acute hydrocele, and inguinal hernia. The onset of any of these may be fairly acute and demands prompt attention. Acute epididymitis is most commonly caused by retrograde extension of infection from the prostate, seminal vesicles, or bladder. Traumatic, sterile epididymitis may occur when there is a sudden increase of intra-abdominal pressure and retrograde extravasation of urine into the epididymis. Ureteral obstruction due to calculus disease may produce pain radiating to the scrotum but is not associated with tender scrotal mass. Testicular tumors, although often nontender, may present acutely as the result of hemorrhage within them. Testicular cancer should always be considered in the differential diagnosis of a scrotal mass, whether tender or nontender.

Answer: A, B, C, E

6. In which of the following patients does a first-time, uncomplicated urinary tract infection (cystitis) require further evaluation?

A. Adult male
B. Female child
C. Adult female
D. Male child
E. None of the above

Sabiston: 1644
Schwartz: 1693

Comments: Urinary tract infections include both uncomplicated lower urinary tract infections, such as cystitis, as well as more serious infections such as pyelonephritis, which may be associated with systemic sepsis. Most urinary tract infection is the result of ascending contamination, although infection may occasionally be caused by hematogenous dissemination. Urinary tract infections are more common in females than males because of the shorter urethra. Uncomplicated lower urinary tract infection in an adult female does not require further evaluation. In male patients or children, however, anatomic or functional obstructive uropathy should be excluded as a predisposing factor; evaluation may include cystoscopy as well as radiologic and manometric studies. Correctable anatomic abnormalities should also be sought in adult females with recurrent urinary tract infection.

Answer: A, B, D

7. Match the characteristics in the left column with the appropriate response(s) in the right column.

A. Usually caused by gonococcus
B. Pyuria is characteristic
C. Usually results from venereal transmission
D. Urethral discharge is characteristic
E. Result of ascending infection

a. Acute urethritis
b. Acute prostatitis
c. Both
d. Neither

Sabiston: 1682, 1689
Schwartz: 1694

Comments: Acute urethritis and prostatitis are both usually the result of ascending infection. Acute urethritis usually is venereally acquired but nongonococcal in origin. Chlamydial organisms are commonly implicated, although *Trichomonas* and bacterial, viral, or fungal infection may also be responsible. Dysuria, frequency, and urethral discharge are common manifestations. Acute prostatitis usually is caused by the same organisms responsible for cystitis (gram-negative bacteria) but may also be due to the organisms producing acute urethritis. Dysuria, frequency, urgency, perineal discomfort, urinary retention, and fever and chills are common symptoms. The prostate is markedly tender on examination. Although pyuria will be present with both acute gonococcal urethritis and acute prostatitis, the two might be differentiated by obtaining a split urine sample and looking at the first voided specimen (urethral urine) and at a midstream specimen (bladder urine). In acute prostatitis, the two samples will both contain essentially the same degree of pyuria. In acute urethritis, marked pyuria will be present only in the first specimen.

Answer: A–d; B–c; C–a; D–a; E–c

8. Which of the following statements is/are true regarding chronic prostatitis?

A. It is most often the result of inadequately treated gonococcal infection
B. Prostate may be nontender, and urinalysis may be normal

C. Prostatic massage is contraindicated because of the risk of dissemination
D. Chronic prostatitis is best treated with prostatic resection, even in the absence of obstructive symptoms

Sabiston: 1682
Schwartz: 1696

Comments: Chronic prostatitis is manifested by symptoms of recurrent lower urinary tract infection and perineal discomfort. Several features differentiate it from acute prostatitis. The prostate itself usually is not tender, and urinalysis may be normal, although prostatic massage may yield a urethral discharge that can be examined and cultured. Identification of the specific offending pathogen and successful treatment can be difficult. Treatment includes antimicrobial agents, treatment of symptoms as with sitz baths and anti-inflammatory agents, and measures to facilitate prostatic drainage, such as prostatic massage. (Note that prostatic massage is avoided in acute prostatitis to avoid dissemination.) If chronic prostatitis has been precipitated by obstructive uropathy, prostatectomy may be beneficial, but it is not generally indicated or curative in situations of chronic prostatitis without obstruction.

Answer: B

9. Indications for prostatic resection in a patient with benign prostatic hypertrophy include:

A. Associated symptoms of prostatitis
B. Obstructive symptoms with normal rectal examination
C. Increased risk of prostatic cancer
D. Recurrent urinary tract infection and residual urine of 100 ml
E. Acute urinary retention

Sabiston: 1684
Schwartz: 1716

Comments: The indications for operation to remove prostatic tissue in patients with benign prostatic hypertrophy (BPH) include the presence of significant residual urine (greater than 100 ml) and troublesome symptoms of obstructive uropathy (frequency, nocturia, hesitancy, sexual dysfunction) or the secondary effects of obstruction, which may include persistent infection, vesicle diverticuli or calculi, and renal dysfunction. Acute urinary retention occurs when there is decompensation of the detrusor muscle due to long-standing obstruction; this also constitutes an indication for operation. The presence on rectal examination of a normal-sized prostate does not exclude obstruction by benign prostatic hypertrophy, since an enlarged median bar and a normal posterior component can produce significant bladder neck obstruction yet a negative rectal examination for prostatic enlargement. Symptoms of chronic prostatitis without obstruction are not alone an indication for operation. Benign prostatic hypertrophy occurs in most males with increasing age and is not a risk factor for prostatic cancer. It should be noted, however, that operations for BPH do not effect a total prostatectomy, so that prostate cancer can still occur following resections for a benign disease.

Answer: B, D, E

10. Match the surgical approach to the prostate in the left column with the appropriate responses in the right column when operating for benign prostatic hyperplasia (BPH).

A. Suprapubic
B. Retropubic
C. Perineal
D. Transurethral

a. Higher risk of recurrent prostatic obstruction
b. Treatment of associated bladder calculi
c. Treatment of associated inguinal hernia
d. Large prostate in elderly, debilitated patient

Sabiston: 1684
Schwartz: 1716

Comments: Prostatic resection for BPH can be accomplished via a transurethral approach or by one of several open techniques. All of these approaches involve removal of the central adenomatous hyperplastic part of the prostate and are not meant to accomplish total prostatectomy. Transurethral resection (TUR) is the most commonly performed and is particularly suitable for adenomas that can be resected within 1 hour. Size, therefore, is the predominant factor in selection of the transurethral approach. TUR does, however, carry a higher risk of recurrent obstruction than do open techniques. Suprapubic prostatectomy involves a transvesical approach, which is useful in the treatment of associated bladder diverticulum or calculi or when there is significant intrusion of the prostate into the bladder or a large middle lobe. A retropubic prostatectomy is similar to a suprapubic prostatectomy, except the incision is made in the prostatic capsule, and a bladder incision is avoided. Both the suprapubic and retropubic approaches permit repair of an associated inguinal hernia, and the morbidity and mortality of both approaches are equivalent. The perineal approach, performed through an incision anterior to the rectum, is primarily for very large prostates that cannot be resected transurethrally in elderly patients who cannot tolerate a low abdominal incision. The small perineal incision has a lower incidence of abdominal ileus and respiratory complications. Radical prostatectomy for prostate cancer can be performed via a retropubic or perineal approach.

Answer: A–b, c; B–c; C–d; D–a

11. Which of the following statements is/are true regarding prostate cancer?

A. Most lesions arise from the central portion of the gland
B. Ten percent of prostate nodules detected on rectal examination are malignant
C. Most lesions are adenocarcinomas
D. Bony metastases are usually osteolytic

Sabiston: 1686
Schwartz: 1717

Comments: Carcinoma of the prostate is the most common non-skin cancer in men over the age of 65 years and is the third leading cause of cancer deaths in the male population. Histologically, most of these lesions are adenocarcinomas; squamous cell carcinoma and sarcoma of the prostate occur rarely. No definite etiologic factors have been established, although there is a relationship to androgen stimulation. Most prostate cancers arise in the periphery of the gland and are asymptomatic until urinary obstruction or symptoms of metastatic disease develop. Annual rectal examination in all men over age 50 is the most important means of early detection; over one half of prostate nodules detected on examination are malignant. Prostate cancer has a characteristic pattern of distant metastases. Bony lesions are particularly common in the pelvis and lumbosacral spine, and in most cases combined osteoblastic and osteolytic lesions occur. Pulmonary metastases are characterized by a miliary, interstitial pattern. In advanced stages, adenocarcinoma of the prostate may metastasize to almost any site.

Answer: C

12. Which of the following statements is/are true regarding serum acid phosphatase in prostatic disease?

A. Acid phosphatase is the most sensitive method of screening for prostatic carcinoma
B. Acid phosphatase has been useful as a tumor marker in assessing treatment results for prostatic cancer
C. Acid phosphatase may be elevated after rectal examination of a normal prostate
D. Acid phosphatase elevations are specific to prostatic cancer
E. Acid phosphatase that is elevated in a patient with prostatic cancer usually precludes a surgical cure

Sabiston: 1686
Schwartz: 1718

Comments: Serum acid phosphatase originates from many sources, including the prostate. The prostatic fraction can be determined by addition of tartrate to serum, and this allows differentiation of elevations due to prostatic cancer from other causes of elevations in total acid phosphatase, such as myeloma or bony tumors. The normal prostate contains acid phosphatase, and mild serum elevations may be detected up to 36 hours following rectal examination of the prostate. Elevations may also occur in patients with benign prostatic disease and acute urinary retention or infarction of the prostate. The presence of an elevated acid phosphatase in prostatic carcinoma usually signifies metastatic disease or extensive local disease, thus diminishing the possibility of successful surgical extirpation for cure. Serum acid phosphatase is not useful as a screening method, because it is not generally elevated with early disease. Rectal examination of the prostate is the most important method of detecting asymptomatic prostate cancer.

Answer: B, C, E

13. A patient in good general health presents with an asymptomatic prostate nodule. Biopsy reveals adenocarcinoma. Metastatic work-up is negative. Which one or more of the following therapies may be appropriate?

A. Transurethral prostate resection
B. Radical prostatectomy

C. Orchiectomy
D. Administration of diethylstilbestrol
E. Local radiotherapy alone

Sabiston: 1687
Schwartz: 1717

Comments: When a prostate nodule is detected, transperineal or transrectal biopsy should be performed to confirm the diagnosis. Then a thorough metastatic evaluation is performed to stage the extent of disease so as to determine the most appropriate therapy. Basic evaluation for metastases includes chest x-ray, bone scan, and serum acid phosphatase. Computed tomography of the pelvis may be useful in determining the extent of local disease and the presence of pelvic lymphadenopathy. Lymph nodes may also be assessed by lymphangiography. The best results of therapy for early prostate cancer are obtained with radical prostatectomy involving removal of the entire prostate and seminal vesicles. If staging pelvic lymphadenopathy is performed, and if, on frozen section, the lymph nodes are positive, the operation usually is terminated; if the lymph nodes are negative, the operation is continued as a radical prostatectomy. Early lesions have also been treated with external beam radiotherapy and interstitial I-125 seed implants, but radiotherapy has not yet been proved to be as effective as surgical treatment.

Answer: B, E

14. A patient presents with a hard, irregular prostate, elevated acid phosphatase, and multiple osteoblastic lesions in the sacrum and lumbar spine. Biopsy of the prostate reveals well-differentiated adenocarcinoma. Which one or more of the following therapies is/are indicated?

A. Transurethral prostate resection
B. Radical prostatectomy
C. Hormonal therapy
D. Radiation therapy
E. Cytotoxic chemotherapy

Sabiston: 1687
Schwartz: 1718

Comments: The treatment of locally advanced or metastatic prostate cancer is palliative. The primary method of therapy is by hormonal manipulation consisting of bilateral orchiectomy or the administration of exogenous estrogens such as diethylstilbestrol. Hormonal therapy is the primary means of palliating bone pain, obstructive uropathy, and the general debility of metastatic disease. When hormonal treatment fails to palliate, then transurethral resection of the prostate, local radiation to painful metastases, and chemotherapy are employed. Radical surgical resection is not indicated.

Answer: C

15. Urinary tract calculi are most commonly composed of:

A. Cystine
B. Uric acid
C. Ammonium magnesium phosphate
D. Calcium oxalate
E. Pure calcium phosphate

Sabiston: 1647
Schwartz: 1697

Comments: See Question 16.

16. For which of the following types of renal calculi is growth not affected by manipulation of urinary pH?

A. Cystine
B. Uric acid
C. Ammonium magnesium phosphate
D. Calcium oxalate
E. Calcium phosphate

Schwartz: 1701

Comments: Renal calculi result from a variety of metabolic conditions; determination of stone composition is important for both the recognition of the underlying abnormality and the institution of appropriate therapy aimed at removing the stone and preventing recurrence. Most urinary calculi (up to 75%) are calcium oxalate stones; approximately one half of these are mixtures of calcium oxalate and phosphate. Ammonium magnesium phosphate stones are the next in frequency and are usually associated with infection. Urinary calculi can sometimes be dissolved by appropriate manipulation of urinary pH. Uric acid and cystine stones form in acid urine, and solubility is increased by alkalinization. Ammonia magnesium phosphate calculi form in alkaline urine, and solubility is increased by acid urine. The problem, however, is that in the presence of infection, urea-splitting organisms form ammonias and thence an alkaline urine, and adequate pH manipulation cannot be obtained without control of infection. Calcium phosphate and calcium oxalate stones are not generally altered by variations of urinary pH within the normal range. Stone composition also is related to ability to visualize stones on plain x-rays. Calcium-containing stones in particular are radiopaque; however, ammonium magnesium phosphate and cystine stones can also be visualized. Uric acid stones are typically radiolucent.

Answer: Question 15: D
Question 16: D, E

17. Which of the following is/are indication(s) for endoscopic, percutaneous, or open surgical removal of renal calculi?

A. Impaired renal function
B. Any oxalate stone
C. Intractable pain
D. Persistent obstruction

Sabiston: 1647
Schwartz: 1699

Comments: The simple presence of a renal or ureteral calculus is not alone an indication for intervention by invasive techniques. Medical management involving analgesics, hydration, diuretics, appropriate urinary pH adjustment, and antibiotics will often result in spontaneous passage. Invasive attempts at removal are indicated when calculi produce persistent obstruction, intractable pain, or refractory infection, or when they are associated with impaired renal function. Approaches to stone removal include transurethral manipulation, percutaneous nephrostomy, extracorporeal shock wave lithotripsy, and open surgical techniques.

Answer: A, C, D

18. The anatomic abnormality found in torsion of the testicle in adolescence most commonly involves which one of the following?

A. Intravaginal torsion of the spermatic cord
B. Extravaginal torsion of the spermatic cord
C. Torsion of the appendix testis
D. Torsion of the appendix epididymis

Sabiston: 1677
Schwartz: 1685

Comments: There are two main types of torsion of the testicle. In the neonate, torsion of the spermatic cord occurs before attachment of the gubernaculum, allowing torsion of the entire testicle and tunica vaginalis. This is called extravaginal torsion. The second type of torsion occurs in adolescents and older men and is called intravaginal torsion of the spermatic cord. The tunica vaginalis, at this time, is fixed to the dartos fascia by the gubernaculum and cannot turn. This type of torsion is most commonly associated with a short mesenteric attachment between the cord and the testicle and epididymis. This allows the testicle to fall forward (producing the "bell clapper" deformity), and torsion can therefore occur within the tunica vaginalis. Since this deformity is often bilateral, fixation of the contralateral testes should be performed at the time of correction of testicular torsion. The appendix testis and appendix epididymidis are small, cystic, embryologic remnants attached to the superior pole of the testis and head of the epididymis, respectively. Torsion of these appendages can produce acute pain and swelling similar to torsion of the spermatic cord but does not result in testicular infarction. Transillumination may reveal the "black dot" sign representing the infarcted structure. Exploration may be required to exclude testicular ischemia.

Answer: A

19. An adolescent male presents with a 3-hour history of acute, severe scrotal pain. Examination reveals scrotal swelling and tenderness that does not permit discrete palpation of the epididymis. Best treatment at this point is:

A. Heat, scrotal elevation, and antibiotics
B. Manual attempt at detorsion
C. Analgesics and re-examination
D. Radioisotope scan to assess testicular blood flow
E. Surgical exploration

Sabiston: 1677
Schwartz: 1685

Comments: When examining the acutely painful scrotum, one should attempt to differentiate epididymitis from testicular torsion, but this may not be possible. Doubtful cases should be treated as testicular torsion until proved otherwise. Since irreversible testicular ischemia occurs within 4 hours when there is complete torsion, prompt surgical exploration is indicated, even if there is diagnostic uncertainty. Use of the Doppler and nuclear medicine scans may be helpful in the assessment of testicular blood flow, but normal studies do not exclude torsion, and in questionable cases, additional diagnostic studies should not be performed if they will cause unnecessary delay in operative intervention and potentially jeopardize the opportunity for testicular salvage.

Answer: E

20. Which one or more of the following are principles of repair of an intraoperative ureteral injury?

A. Use of nonabsorbable suture material
B. Use of absorbable suture material
C. Extensive ureteral dissection to minimize tension
D. Drainage
E. Intraureteral stent

Sabiston: 322, 1654
Schwartz: 1722

Comments: Ureteral injuries are usually iatrogenic and occur during the course of retroperitoneal dissection of various abdominal and pelvic operations. In cases of transection, repair should be carried out using absorbable suture material and a Silastic stent. Nonabsorbable suture should be avoided because it may serve as a nidus for calculus formation. Extensive ureteral dissection should be avoided in order to preserve the segmental blood supply. Drains should be placed to accommodate any anastomotic leak. When injury involves the low ureteral segment, ureteroneocystostomy is recommended.

Answer: B, D, E

21. A 32-year-old man presents with a nontender, hard testicular lump. Appropriate treatment includes which one or more of the following?

A. Determination of serum alpha-fetoprotein and human chorionic gonadotropin levels
B. Incisional biopsy via a scrotal incision
C. Incisional biopsy via an inguinal incision
D. Orchiectomy via a scrotal incision
E. Orchiectomy via an inguinal incision

Sabiston: 1676
Schwartz: 1719

Comments: Malignancy should be suspected whenever a testicular mass is detected. Serum should be obtained for determination of alpha-fetoprotein level and for the beta subunit of human chorionic gonadotropin, as these are useful tumor markers in many testicular cancers. The primary diagnostic maneuver is orchiectomy, and this should be carried out promptly via an inguinal incision. The testicular vessels are controlled at the internal ring; the testicle is then inspected. If a testicular mass is confirmed, orchiectomy is usually performed. Since these tumors are heterogeneous, examination of only a portion of the mass can lead to an erroneous diagnosis. Incisional biopsy, therefore, has no role in this setting. Additionally, it can lead to implantation of tumor in the incision. It is very uncommon for an experienced urologist to make an error in diagnosis. The testicle could be affected by a noncancerous condition, which is also usually best treated by orchiectomy. A scrotal approach is contraindicated; it does not permit control of vessels prior to manipulation of the testicle in a maneuver that may dislodge cells into the venous drainage.

Answer: A, E

22. A testicular mass in a 30-year-old would most likely be which one of the following?

A. Benign tumor
B. Seminoma
C. Teratocarcinoma
D. Choriocarcinoma
E. Embryonal cell carcinoma

Sabiston: 1676
Schwartz: 1719

Comments: The overwhelming majority of testicular masses are found in patients in the 20- to 35-year age group and are malignant tumors. Benign fibromas of the tunica vaginalis may occur but are rare. Malignant tumors may be of germinal cell or nongerminal cell origin. Germinal cell tumors are by far the most common and include seminoma, embryonal cell carcinoma, teratocarcinoma, choriocarcinoma, and combinations of these. Seminomas account for approximately 40% of all malignant testicular lesions. Embryonal carcinoma is the most common testicular tumor of childhood. Tumors of nongerminal cell origin, such as Leydig cell tumors and androblastomas, are unusual but are notable in that they may produce excess androgens.

Answer: B

23. Match the statement in the column on the left with the appropriate type(s) of testicular cancer in the column on the right.

A. Radiotherapy is the primary treatment modality
B. Retroperitoneal node dissection is initial therapy if there are no pulmonary metastases
C. Combination chemotherapy is the primary treatment modality
D. Pulmonary metastases are usually present at the time of diagnosis
E. Five-year survival rates approximate 90%

a. Seminoma
b. Choriocarcinoma
c. Embryonal cell carcinoma
d. None of the above

Sabiston: 1676
Schwartz: 1720

Comments: When the diagnosis of testicular cancer has been established, further treatment depends upon the histologic diagnosis and the stage of disease. **Seminoma** tends to be a slower growing tumor, which spreads predominantly by lymphatic routes. It is extremely radiosensitive, even when metastatic. For this reason, radiotherapy is generally preferred and retroperitoneal node dissection not performed. Seminoma has the best prognosis of any testicular cancers, with a 5-year survival rate of about 90%. **Choriocarcinoma**, in contradistinction, is an extremely malignant tumor, with rapid hematogenous spread to the lungs. Initial treatment, therefore, involves multiagent chemotherapy if pulmonary metastases are present, although response rates are not as good as for other resectable germ cell tumors. **Embryonal carcinoma** has a more intermediate course. In the absence of pulmonary metastases, retroperitoneal node dissection is performed. If findings are positive, then adjuvant chemotherapy is instituted. In patients with pulmonary metastases or extensive retroperitoneal disease, initial chemotherapy may be followed by retroperitoneal node dissection if there is good response but a retroperitoneal mass persists. Tumors of combined histologies are treated according to the more malignant element.

Answer: A–a; B–c; C–b; D–b; E–a

24. In a male with pelvic fracture due to blunt trauma, retrograde urethrography demonstrates disruption of the membranous urethra. Which one or more of the following constitute(s) appropriate initial treatment?

A. Passage of a transurethral catheter
B. Suprapubic cystostomy
C. Perineal repair
D. Retropubic repair
E. Transabdominal repair

Sabiston: 1689
Schwartz: 1722

Comments: Blunt pelvic trauma is the most common cause of urethral injury. Disruption usually occurs at the membranous portion of the urethra, since the posterior prostatic and membranous portions are relatively fixed by puboprostatic ligaments and the urogenital diaphragm. Urethral injury should be suspected if blood is noted at the meatus or if the patient is unable to void clear urine normally. Passage of a catheter should not be attempted under these circumstances; retrograde urethrography should be obtained. If urethral injury is confirmed, treatment depends upon the extent of the patient's injuries but can initially be accomplished safely with suprapubic cystostomy. Untreated urethral injuries can result in stricture and incontinence. Penetrating urethral injuries can often be treated by initial repair and urinary diversion.

Answer: B

25. Which of the following statements is/are true regarding bladder trauma?

A. Injury is usually intraperitoneal when associated with pelvic fracture
B. Single-view retrograde cystogram in the emergency room demonstrates most significant bladder injuries
C. Primary multiple-layer closure is indicated

D. Iatrogenic injury usually requires repair and supra-pubic cystostomy

Sabiston: 1663
Schwartz: 1722

Comments: Bladder injury may occur as the result of blunt or penetrating trauma or may be incurred accidentally during pelvic operations. When associated with pelvic fracture, the site of injury is usually extraperitoneal, having been caused by bony perforation. Blunt injury without fracture is associated with intraperitoneal rupture, particularly if the bladder was full at the time of injury. Bladder injury should be suspected in any patient with lower abdominal trauma if there is any hematuria, or if the patient is unable to void. Cystography may miss significant injury if anteroposterior as well as lateral drainage films in particular are not obtained. The usual treatment involves a 2- or 3-layer closure, with transurethral or suprapubic drainage. Iatrogenic injury recognized at the time of operation does not generally warrant suprapubic cystostomy but does require repair and urethral catheter drainage for 4 to 5 days. It is necessary also to be vigilant that the Foley catheter does not become clogged, as with blood.

Answer: C

26. Which of the following statements is/are true regarding vesicointestinal fistulas?

A. They are most commonly caused by Crohn's disease
B. They are the only cause of pneumaturia
C. Cystoscopy is useful diagnostically
D. Successful repair requires a two-stage procedure

Sabiston: 1660

Comments: Vesicoenteric fistulas most commonly involve the sigmoid colon and result from diverticulitis. Other causes of these fistulas include Crohn's disease, colorectal malignancy, and, rarely, primary bladder malignancy. Pneumaturia is a classic symptom, but it can also be caused by infection with gas-producing bacterial organisms and fermentation of carbohydrates in diabetic urine. The diagnosis can often be established on the basis of cystoscopic findings, although anatomic visualization of the fistula itself may require gastrointestinal contrast studies. Resection of the fistula and abnormal bowel with primary repair of the bladder can usually be carried out as a single procedure unless there is an accompanying abscess. In such a case, a two-stage procedure with later re-establishment of intestinal continuity may be required.

Answer: C

27. Which of the following statements is/are true regarding bladder cancer?

A. Adenocarcinoma is the most common histologic type
B. Prognosis is related to histologic grade of the tumor
C. Painless hematuria is the most common presenting symptom
D. Early pulmonary metastases are characteristic

Sabiston: 1665
Schwartz: 1714

Comments: Cancer of the urinary bladder has a peak incidence in the 50 to 70 year age group and is more common in men than women. Ninety percent of these tumors are transitional cell in type; squamous cell cancer and adenocarcinoma occur infrequently. Painless hematuria, either gross or microscopic, is the most common initial manifestation. Approximately 30% of patients present with symptoms of bladder irritability; 30% may have an associated urinary tract infection. The prognosis of bladder cancer is directly related to both stage and histologic grade. Bladder malignancies metastasize via both pelvic lymphatic and hematogenous routes to lung, liver, and bone as well as to other distant sites.

Answer: B, C

28. Appropriate treatment of locally invasive bladder cancer involving the muscular wall includes which one or more of the following?

A. Radical cystectomy alone
B. Preoperative radiotherapy and radical cystectomy
C. Preoperative chemotherapy and radical cystectomy
D. Radiotherapy alone
E. Intravesical chemotherapy

Sabiston: 1666
Schwartz: 1714

Comments: The appropriate local treatment of bladder cancer is dependent upon tumor stage. Lesions confined to the mucosa can be treated with transurethral resection, fulguration, or intravesical chemotherapeutic agents; then a careful surveillance program must be maintained. The treatment of lesions with submucosal invasion has been controversial as to whether intravesical chemotherapy is appropriate and as to the necessary extent of surgical resection. Lesions invading the muscular wall of the bladder are best treated by radical cystectomy. In men this includes removal of the bladder, prostate, seminal vesicles, and adjacent perivesical tissues; in women this includes the bladder, uterus, fallopian tubes, ovaries, anterior vagina, and urethra. The role of segmental cystectomy with muscular invasion is controversial. The need to remove the entire urethra in the male also requires consideration because of a significant incidence of recurrence in the retained urethra. Preoperative radiation has been favored in the treatment of locally invasive lesions, although its benefit is still being evaluated. Combined clinical studies suggest that preoperative radiotherapy may confer survival advantage on patients with deep muscular or perivesical invasion. Because the 5-year survival rate of patients with muscle invasion following cystectomy (with or without radiotherapy) is only 50%, and the major cause of death is metastatic disease, there is currently considerable interest in the use of adjuvant chemotherapy (either pre- or postcystectomy). With recent studies showing combination chemotherapy (with *cis*-platinum, doxorubicin [Adriamycin], vinblastine, and methotrexate) in patients with advanced disease giving response rates of from 50 to 70%, these agents now are being used (in numerous studies) prior to cystectomy when muscle invasion is present.

Answer: A, B, C

29. Complications of ureterosigmoidostomy include:

A. Retrograde urinary tract infection
B. Hyperchloremic acidosis
C. Hypochloremic alkalosis
D. Colon malignancy

Sabiston: 1668

Comments: Following cystectomy, some method of urinary diversion must be provided. This can take the form of cutaneous ureterostomy or anastomosis of the ureters to a segment of small bowel or colon that serves as a conduit. Formerly, ureterosigmoidostomy was used, but it has been abandoned in most situations, because of the associated complications and the development of newer methods of diversion. Complications of ureterosigmoidostomy include retrograde infection from reflux of colonic contents, electrolyte abnormalities due to absorption of urinary components by the colon, and an increased incidence of colon malignancy that has been related to mixing of fecal and urinary streams.

Answer: A, B, D

30. A properly constructed cutaneous ureteroileostomy (ileal conduit) should:

A. Provide an adequate reservoir for urine storage
B. Prevent ureteral reflux
C. Require catheterization for emptying
D. Separate the urinary and fecal streams

Sabiston: 1668
Schwartz: 1723

Comments: The use of an isolated segment of ileum to serve as a conduit between the ureters and the skin has become the most common form of urinary diversion. It is used for patients with cystectomy as well as those with renal dysfunction secondary to chronic lower urinary tract dysfunction (for example, neurogenic bladder). Recently, there has been increased use of the sigmoid as a conduit as well as interest in attempts to create a continent urinary reservoir that would require catheterization for emptying and, therefore, offer the patient greater control over this function. The purpose of creating an ileal conduit is to create a route (unidirectionally within the conduit) for transport of urine; it is not a reservoir for storage. Stasis in the bowel segment predisposes to infection, stone formation, and ureteral reflux. Some degree of ureteral reflux can be expected normally with an ileal conduit.

Answer: D

31. A patient is stable following resuscitation for blunt abdominal trauma. Gross hematuria is noted, and an IVP fails to visualize one kidney. Which one of the following procedures should be performed next?

A. Operative exploration
B. Arteriography
C. Retrograde pyelography
D. Renal scan

Sabiston: 1652
Schwartz: 1720

Comments: Renal injury should be suspected whenever a traumatized patient is found to have hematuria or when the nature of the injury or associated findings suggest this possibility (for example, penetrating retroperitoneal trauma, radiographic obliteration of the psoas shadow or renal outline, fractures of the lower ribs or transverse vertebral processes). Initial imaging of the kidney can be obtained by intravenous pyelography or a CT scan with infusion. If the patient is hemodynamically unstable with evidence of ongoing hemorrhage, laparotomy is performed without further diagnostic studies. However, if the patient is stable and an IVP fails to visualize the kidney, arteriography should be performed next because of the possibility of renal vascular injury, which typically occurs in acceleration-deceleration injuries resulting in intimal disruption and renal artery thrombosis. This entity requires prompt recognition and treatment if one is to salvage the kidney. Radioisotope scans also reflect renal blood flow and function but do not provide precise anatomic detail. Retrograde pyelography may be useful in evaluating ureteral injuries and urinary extravasation. If the kidney fails to visualize on the arteriographic image, exploration is indicated.

Answer: B

32. Which of the following statements is/are true regarding the management of renal trauma?

A. Contusions are treated by observation until the hematuria subsides
B. Parenchymal lacerations require routine exploration because of the risk of secondary hemorrhage or infection
C. Retroperitoneal flank hematomas encountered during laparotomy require exploration
D. On exploring a perinephric hematoma, Gerota's fascia is first opened and vascular control obtained

Sabiston: 1652
Schwartz: 1720

Comments: As with any visceral organ, a spectrum of renal injuries may occur following blunt or penetrating trauma. Renal contusions are managed conservatively and require no specific therapy, other than rest. Parenchymal lacerations confined to the renal cortex may also be treated nonoperatively if the patient is stable. Deeper lacerations extending into the calyceal system usually require primary surgical repair. It is generally recommended that lateral retroperitoneal hematomas be explored because of the possibility of significant renal parenchymal or vascular injury, even if the hematoma is not expanding. The key surgical principle in the approach to the injured kidney is to obtain control of the vascular pedicle first. If Gerota's fascia is incised first, tamponade effect may be released, and significant hemorrhage can result. Initial vascular control allows accurate assessment of the extent of injury and may permit primary repair or partial nephrectomy rather than removal of the entire organ. Before a kidney is removed, the presence of a functioning kidney on the contralateral side should be verified.

Answer: A, C

33. Which one of the following is the most common asymptomatic solid renal mass?

A. Wilms' tumor
B. Renal cell carcinoma
C. Renal sarcoma
D. Transitional cell carcinoma
E. Metastatic tumor

Sabiston: 1651, 1656
Schwartz: 1706

Comment: Occasionally, asymptomatic mass lesions of the kidney are identified on IVP or ultrasonogram; the great majority of them are benign renal cysts. Among malignant lesions detected as asymptomatic renal masses, metastatic tumor is the most common, and the breast is the most frequent primary site. Although renal adenocarcinoma is the most common primary renal malignancy, usually it is detected because of symptoms. Most cancers arising from the renal pelvis are transitional cell in type and present with hematuria. Renal sarcoma is uncommon. Wilms' tumor is one of the most common solid tumors of childhood and often presents as an asymptomatic abdominal mass.

Answer: E

34. Which one of the following is seen most commonly with renal cell carcinoma?

A. Hypertension
B. Erythrocytosis
C. Hematuria
D. Acute varicocele
E. Fever

Sabiston: 1650
Schwartz: 1706

Comments: Among the many symptoms that have been associated with renal cell carcinoma, hematuria, pain, and abdominal mass are the most common. Most patients, however, do not present with the classic triad involving all three of these symptoms. Hypertension may result from renal vascular compression but is more commonly seen in Wilms' tumor. Fever is thought to result from tumor necrosis. A small percentage of patients exhibit erythrocytosis, which has been related to the production of erythropoietin by the tumor. It is more common, however, for patients with renal carcinoma to present with anemia than with erythrocythemia. A small percentage of patients with renal tumors develop renal vein thrombosis and a subsequent acute varicocele.

Answer: C

35. Which of the following statements is/are true regarding treatment of renal cell carcinoma?

A. Induction chemotherapy followed by nephrectomy yields best overall results
B. Radical nephrectomy involves removal of the kidney, adrenal gland, perinephric fat, and regional lymph nodes
C. Regional lymphadenectomy for lesions extending outside the kidney is the most important prognostic determinant
D. Nephrectomy is indicated even in the presence of distant metastases so as to improve chemotherapeutic effectiveness

Sabiston: 1651
Schwartz: 1707

Comments: The treatment of renal cell carcinoma and the subsequent prognosis is determined by the anatomic extent of disease. Treatment of local disease focuses on tumor removal by radical nephrectomy. Operation alone offers an excellent prognosis in patients with early lesions confined within the renal cortex. A survival advantage for those having regional lymphadenectomy has not been definitively established. Metastases frequently occur by hematogenous routes as well and may negate any theoretic advantage of even more radical local surgery. Postoperative radiotherapy may have value in patients with large tumors and extensive local invasion. In the presence of distant metastases, nephrectomy may still be appropriate to control bleeding, pain, or infection. Nephrectomy has not been shown to enhance the response to adjuvant chemotherapy. Chemotherapy for renal adenocarcinoma in general has not been satisfactory. In selected circumstances, patients with isolated metastases have benefited from resection of their metastatic disease.

Answer: B

36. Transitional cell cancers of the renal pelvis are best treated by which one of the following?

A. Nephrectomy
B. Nephroureterectomy with excision of ureter to the level of the bladder
C. Nephroureterectomy with excision of bladder cuff
D. Nephroureterectomy and total cystectomy
E. Radiotherapy

Sabiston: 1656
Schwartz: 1709

Comments: Transitional cell cancers of the renal pelvis and ureter are notable for their multicentricity and their tendency to spread by direct extension to other parts of the uroepithelium. Approximately 25% of patients develop recurrence of the cancer in any ureteral remnant. For this reason, nephroureterectomy with excision of a cuff of bladder at the ureteral orifice has been the standard treatment. There is no specific role for radiotherapy in the primary treatment of these lesions.

Answer: C

37. Which of the following statements is/are true regarding vasectomy?

A. It produces prompt sterility
B. Duplication of the vas deferens is a common cause of failure

C. It is a safe outpatient procedure
D. The pregnancy rate after vasovasostomy approaches 50%

Sabiston: 1678
Schwartz: 1729

Comments: Vasectomy for the purpose of sterilization has become a commonplace procedure that is safely performed in the outpatient setting. Careful attention must be given to appropriate patient screening, preoperative patient education, and informing patients of the risks, chance of failure of the procedure, and alternative methods of birth control. Patients also must be instructed that viable spermatozoa remain in the seminal tract distal to the site of vasectomy for several weeks after the operation; careful follow-up examination of semen must be performed at 6 to 8 weeks to confirm whether the patient is, in fact, sterile. The procedure should be considered a permanent form of sterilization, although with microsurgical techniques, reanastomosis of the vas deferens can be performed in over 90% of cases, with a success rate (as attested to by subsequent pregnancy) approaching 50%.

Answer: C, D

CHAPTER 52

Gynecology

1. Which of the following statements is/are true regarding embryologic development of the female genital tract?

A. The uterus represents fusion of the müllerian ducts
B. The internal genitalia are partially derived from the ectoderm
C. The development of the female genitalia occurs independently of androgenic influence
D. Urologic and gynecologic developmental anomalies rarely coexist

Sabiston: 1601
Schwartz: 1733

Comments: Urogenital development in the male and female results from the appropriate migration and/or fusion of the müllerian and wolffian ducts. Prior to the eighth week of development, there is no evident sexual differentiation morphologically. Subsequently, müllerian development and fusion result in the formation of the uterus and vagina. Normal müllerian development is inhibited by testicular androgens, as has been proved by studies that showed that castrated male rabbit fetuses uniformly undergo normal müllerian development. As fetal development proceeds, the müllerian structures join with the endodermally derived structures of the urogenital sinus to complete the development of the internal genitalia. The external genitalia are derived from the ectoderm and include the vulva, major and minor labia, and clitoris. Embryologically, müllerian and wolffian abnormalities frequently coexist, and therefore one must be alert to the possibility of urologic abnormalities in patients with developmental gynecologic abnormalities.

Answer: A

2. Which of the following anomalies of uterine development have been described?

A. Normal appearance of uterus externally; septum reaching the cervix internally
B. Separate uteri, each with a separate vagina
C. Complete atresia at level of cervix

D. Complete separation of one uterine horn from an otherwise normal opposite horn and vagina

Sabiston: 1601, 1612
Schwartz: 1735

Comments: Since normal development of the uterus and vagina depends upon proper fusion of the müllerian ducts, anomalies of fusion may result in a number of partial or complete uterine and/or vaginal separations. The uterus may appear normal externally but have a midline septum that may vary in prominence from barely noticeable to completely separating the genitalia into two uterine and vaginal cavities. When external fusion is incomplete, the uterus is considered to be bicornuate, and this anomaly can vary in its severity. Failure of fusion may result in one of the horns of the uterus remaining unconnected to the normally developing opposite side. Occasionally, partial atresia of the otherwise normally fused müllerian ducts may occur, often at the level of the cervix. Since ovarian development is usually normal in these circumstances, these anomalies usually do not become apparent until childbearing years. Although normal pregnancies may occur in some patients with müllerian fusion anomalies, the smaller capacity of the uterus resulting from these anomalies frequently leads to habitual abortion.

Answer: A, B, C, D

3. Match the following anatomic structures with their appropriate description:

Structure	Description
A. Skene's glands	a. Labial glands
B. Bartholin's glands	b. Supports uterus at apex of vagina
C. Round ligament	c. Uterine blood supply
D. Broad ligament	d. Periurethral glands
E. Infundibulopelvic ligament	e. Ovarian blood supply
F. Cardinal ligament	f. Equivalent of vas deferens

Sabiston: 1602
Schwartz: 1735

Comments: Understanding the anatomic relationships of the female pelvis and perineum is crucial to proper diagnosis and safe operations in these areas. The surgeon operating on the pelvis must be cognizant of the structures that support and provide blood to the ovaries and uterus in order to avoid their inadvertent devascularization or hemorrhage. Awareness of the normal course of the ureter is fundamental to safe pelvic dissection. The ureter passes deep to the infundibulopelvic ligament over the bifurcation of the iliac vessels at the pelvic brim and deep to the uterine artery at the level of the cervix.

Answer: A–d; B–a; C–f; D–c; E–e; F–b

4. Match the following:

Anatomic Abnormality	Predisposing Factor
A. Urethrocele	a. Weakness in the area of the cul-de-sac
B. Rectocele	b. Weakness in the distal anterior vaginal wall
C. Enterocele	c. Weakness in the ligamentous support of the uterus
D. Uterine prolapse	d. Protrusion of the posterior wall of the vagina
E. Cystocele	e. Protrusion of the anterior wall of the vagina

Sabiston: 1617
Schwartz: 1736

Comments: Anatomic support for the uterus and vagina is provided by a number of ligaments, fascial thickenings, and muscular slings. Weakness in one or more of these structures may result in the abnormalities listed above. Pelvic relaxations of varying types and degrees are found in all women who have delivered children vaginally. Although symptom-producing pelvic relaxations may occur in any age group, they are most common after the climacteric. When they are symptomatic, they should always be treated surgically unless there are strong medical contraindications to anesthesia. The natural history of mild to moderate relaxation is progression to more severe forms, with resulting repair of tissues less favorable than when tissues are stronger.

Answer: A–b; B–d; C–a; D–c; E–e

5. Which of the following statements regarding gonadotropic hormones is/are correct?

A. Follicle stimulating hormone (FSH) facilitates granulosa cell proliferation and maturation of the oocyte
B. Luteinizing hormone (LH) has no significant role in progesterone and estrogen production
C. Human chorionic gonadotropin (HCG) is produced by the corpus luteum and helps maintain pregnancy during the first 6 weeks following fertilization
D. Beta HCG assay makes detection of pregnancy possible within 72 hours of implantation
E. HCG may be a marker for nongynecologic malignancies

Sabiston: 1606
Schwartz: 1737

Comments: The endrocrinologic relationships between the hypothalamus, pituitary, ovary, and placenta are complex and depend on a number of interrelated feedback mechanisms. FSH has its principal role in the early portion of the menstrual cycle, during which it facilitates follicular development, granulosa cell proliferation, and maturation of the oocyte. Following ovulation, LH is responsible for transformation of the ovarian follicle to a corpus luteum and supports the production by the corpus luteum of progesterone and estrogen. HCG is a glycoprotein normally secreted by the placenta during pregnancy. Whereas its alpha subunit is chemically similar to that of FSH, LH, and TSH (thyroid stimulating hormone), its beta subunit is highly specific and is elevated to detectable serum levels within 72 hours after implantation of a fertilized ovum. HCG also supports the production of estrogen and progesterone by the corpus luteum during early pregnancy. In addition, HCG has been used as a specific tumor marker for trophoblastic tumors and for germ cell tumors of the ovary and testis, as well as for some nongynecologic tumors, including hepatoblastoma and gastric adenocarcinoma.

Answer: A, D, E

6. Match the following statements concerning steroid hormones:

A. Increased in obesity and hyperthyroidism	a. Estrogens
B. Precursors of estrogen	b. Progesterone
C. Stimulate epithelial changes in the uterus, fallopian tube, vagina, and breast	c. Androgens
D. Mostly secreted after ovulation	

Sabiston: 1607
Schwartz: 1739

Comments: All of the steroid hormones (glucocorticoids, mineralocorticoids, and sex steroids) have cholesterol as their parent molecule. Estrogens, progesterones, and androgens are found in varying amounts in both males and females; indeed, progesterones and androgens are direct precursors of estrogens. In the female, most sex hormone production and secretion occurs in the ovary, with the adrenal providing only a small additional amount. Conversion of androgens to estrogens by adipose tissue, muscle, and liver also occurs, which may explain, in part, the increased circulating estrogen levels that can be seen in obesity and liver disease. Hyperthyroidism also may produce a hyperestrogenemic state. In the normal menstrual cycle, estrogen reaches its peak production just prior to ovulation. Among its many effects are the epithelial changes that occur in the mucosa of the vagina, uterus, and fallopian tubes, as well as the parenchymal changes that occur within the breast. Progesterone is secreted primarily following ovulation and plays a significant role in preparing the endometrium for implantation and supporting the endometrium during pregnancy.

Answer: A–a; B–b, c; C–a; D–b

7. Place the following events of female puberty in their proper chronologic order:

A. Increased height
B. Breast budding
C. Menstruation
D. Development of pubic hair

Schwartz: 1740

Comments: The physiologic events that initiate puberty are incompletely understood. There is a moderate degree of variability in the actual age at which the entire process occurs, with 95% of females having their menarche between the ages of 9½ and 16 years. Despite this variability, the actual order of physiologic changes in puberty is fairly constant, beginning with thelarche (breast budding) and followed shortly thereafter by adrenarche (the development of pubic and axillary hair). Subsequent to this is the beginning of a rapid increase in height, which usually precedes the start of menstruation by 6 to 12 months.

Answer: B, D, A, C

8. Match each of the following hormones or events with the appropriate letter on the chart of a typical menstrual cycle.

A. Estrogen
B. Progesterone
C. FSH
D. LH
E. Menses

Sabiston: 1606
Schwartz: 1739

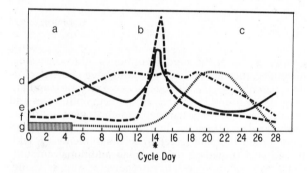

Cycle Day

Comments: See Question 9.

9. Which of the following statements is/are true regarding the events of a typical menstrual cycle?

A. Follicular development occurs during the secretory phase
B. Oocyte degeneration occurs late in the luteal phase
C. Cervical mucus production increases at ovulation
D. Menstruation involves the shedding of the mucosa down to the submucosal plane
E. The LH surge and ovulation bear a fairly constant relationship to each other

Sabiston: 1606
Schwartz: 1741

Comments: The typical menstrual cycle occurs as a result of fluctuating levels of gonadotropic and steroid hormones, as indicated in the diagram. The physiologic events stimulated by these hormonal fluctuations can be considered in two phases: the **proliferative phase**, which is that period of time from the first day of menses to the day of ovulation, and the **secretory** or **luteal phase**, which lasts from ovulation to the onset of subsequent menses. During the proliferative phase, the follicle develops and the endometrium proliferates to ready itself for possible implantation. Ovulation occurs as a direct result of the LH surge late in the proliferative phase, and these two events bear a very constant relationship to each other. At the time of ovulation, cervical mucus production increases to provide a more hospitable environment for sperm cells. If fertilization does not occur, the oocyte begins to degenerate within 24 hours. Finally, in the absence of an implanted fertilized ovum, the superficial layers of the endometrium are shed, leaving the stratum basale and a significant portion of the stratum spongiosum behind, which begin to regenerate in preparation for the next cycle.

Answer: Question 8: A–e; B–g; C–d; D–f; E–a
Question 9: C, E

10. Which of the following statements is/are true regarding menopause?

A. The primary physiologic event is a depletion of the number of ovarian follicles
B. Menopausal symptoms tend to be of gradual onset, with marked variability in age of onset
C. Osteoporosis may result
D. Progesterones should not be used to treat the symptoms of menopause because of the risk of inducing vaginal bleeding

Sabiston: 1607
Schwartz: 1741

Comments: Menopause refers to the gradual cessation of ovarian function, which occurs at an average age of 50 years, varying within a wide range. The initial event is thought to be a decrease in the number of ovarian follicles. As a result, there is a loss of estrogen-producing capacity, with subsequent manifestations of estrogen depletion, which include hot flashes, drying of the vaginal mucosa, and osteoporosis. Estrogen administration during menopause is highly effective in ameliorating these side effects; however, the use of unopposed estrogens over long periods of time has been implicated in a slightly higher incidence of breast and endometrial cancer. Some evidence supports the use of cycled estrogens and progesterones to treat menopausal symptoms to reduce this possible cancer risk. One must be aware that progesterones can cause vaginal bleeding, which may be difficult to distinguish from abnormal bleeding caused by endometrial pathology; however, this alone is not enough reason to preclude their use. Further, a thorough history and an endometrial biopsy should clearly differentiate hormonally induced bleeding from that due to malignancy.

Answer: A, B, C

11. Which of the following statements is/are true regarding pain associated with the menstrual cycle?

A. The term primary dysmenorrhea refers to painful menses associated with identifiable predisposing gynecologic causes
B. Dysmenorrhea is often effectively treated by ibuprofen and/or oral contraceptives
C. Premenstrual tension syndrome may produce symptoms throughout the entire menstrual cycle
D. Mittelschmerz is pain occurring between the 10th and 14th days of the cycle from rupture of a graafian follicle and may be confused with ectopic pregnancy

Schwartz: 1742

Comments: A careful history of the time course of pain presumed to be of menstrual cycle origin is useful in determining the cause of it. Dysmenorrhea refers to pain occurring during menses and is considered to be either primary (idiopathic) or secondary. Although no exact cause of primary dysmenorrhea has been identified, prostaglandins have been implicated in the cause. As a result, treatment involving prostaglandin synthetase inhibitors, such as ibuprofen, have been used successfully in many instances. In secondary dysmenorrhea, specific abnormalities such as endometriosis, congenital malformations, and uterine myomas have been identified as causes of pain. The use of oral contraceptives has also been effective in reducing the severity of dysmenorrhea, possibly through the inhibition of endometrial development and prostaglandin synthesis. The premenstrual tension syndrome refers to a constellation of systemic and psychologic abnormalities (e.g., anxiety, depression, irritability, edema, acneform eruptions) that occur within the 10-day period preceding menses. The diagnosis can be excluded if the symptoms occur earlier in the cycle. Mittelschmerz (midcycle pain) occurs between the 10th and 14th days of the cycle and is thought to be related to local pelvic peritoneal irritation from a ruptured ovarian follicle. Its characteristic timing and fairly abrupt onset may also mimic the presence of an ectopic pregnancy or gastrointestinal pathology such as appendicitis.

Answer: B, D

12. Match the following:

A. A 76-year-old diabetic woman with frequent involuntary loss of urine, even at rest	a. Stress incontinence
	b. Overflow incontinence
	c. Urgency incontinence
B. A 50-year-old woman with urinary leakage when coughing	
C. A 25-year-old woman with complaints of frequent urination, occasionally uncontrolled, associated with burning	

Sabiston: 1617
Schwartz: 1743

Comments: Urinary incontinence refers to the involuntary loss of urine and may be considered in terms of the three categories listed. **Stress incontinence** refers to the loss of urine during maneuvers that increase abdominal pressure, and its most significant predisposing factor is inadequate pelvic support due to stretching or relaxation of the perivesical and periuterine fascial structures. **Overflow incontinence** is seen in patients with large bladders and large volumes of residual urine, usually due to primary neurologic causes such as diabetes, in whom either impaired sensation or motor weakness of the bladder may exist. **Urgency incontinence** refers to involuntary urine loss associated with the frequent urge to urinate and is commonly seen in inflammation of the bladder or with urinary tract infection.

Answer: A–b; B–a; C–c

13. Which of the following therapeutic approaches to the problem of urinary stress incontinence in the female is/are considered acceptable?

A. Voiding exercises
B. Vaginal pessary
C. Transvaginal surgical repair
D. Transabdominal surgical repair

Schwartz: 1744

Comments: The principles of management are to control the incontinence by providing proper pelvic support to the bladder, uterus, and vagina. Voiding exercises (Kegel exercises), in which the patient practices starting and stopping the urinary stream, may occasionally be effective. A vaginal pessary may be successful in providing pelvic support, but generally this therapy is reserved for the elderly or debilitated patient in whom the risk of operation is prohibitive. An operation is indicated in cases of persistent and/or socially limiting stress incontinence. Numerous operations, performed both transvaginally and transabdominally, have been described. The basic goals are to support the uterus and bladder and to restore the proper urethrovesical angle. Almost all procedures will necessitate a hysterectomy. The Marshall-Marchetti suspension procedure is currently the most favored. This operation involves retropubic dissection in the space of Retzius and the placement of paraurethral sutures sewn to the undersurface of the symphysis pubis to provide anterior support to the bladder neck and urethra.

Answer: A, B, C, D

14. Match the following clinical situations with their likelihood of representing significant pathology:

A. Brief midcycle bleeding in a 25-year-old	a. Probably functional; initial observation warranted
B. Vaginal bleeding in a 65-year-old	b. Probably pathologic; investigation warranted
C. Brisk but brief bleeding within a week of fertilization	
D. Intermittent bleeding occurring in the second month of pregnancy	

Schwartz: 1745

Comments: Vaginal bleeding may be completely normal and expected, as with normal menstrual flow; it may be abnormal in timing but easily explained based on functional aberrations; or it may be the hallmark of underlying significant pathology. A careful history of the timing and nature of the bleeding in light of the patient's age, menstrual history, and pregnancy history will often determine whether the vaginal bleeding is of clinical significance. Any bleeding occurring in a postmenopausal woman is of clinical concern and warrants investigation. It may be due to such benign conditions as cervicitis, vaginitis, or benign cervical and/or uterine polyps; one must be alert, however, to postmenopausal bleeding as a sign of cervical or endometrial carcinoma. In premenopausal women, brief midcycle bleeding, probably related to hormonal changes at the time of ovulation, is not uncommon. Menstrual periods may be missed entirely or, in contrast, may be extremely heavy. If these are not persistent changes, however, they usually can be explained by normal hormonal variation or by the occasional anovulatory cycle. The implantation of the blastocyst shortly after fertilization may be accompanied by bleeding; if this does not persist, it is of no concern. Bleeding that occurs in early pregnancy subsequent to implantation, however, may be a sign of threatened abortion, missed abortion, or the presence of trophoblastic disease and warrants immediate investigation, usually with ultrasonography and/or vaginal examination.

Answer: A–a; B–b; C–a; D–b

15. Which of the following may cause hypomenorrhea or amenorrhea?

A. Hyperthyroidism
B. Cushing's syndrome
C. Excessive aspirin use
D. Recent death in the family
E. Sheehan's syndrome
F. Low body weight
G. Recent weight gain
H. Training for the marathon

Sabiston: 1630
Schwartz: 1746

Comments: Amenorrhea or hypomenorrhea may be due to a number of abnormalities of the CNS-hypothalamic-pituitary-ovarian axis. **Hyperthyroidism** is characteristically associated with hypomenorrhea. Although hypothyroidism classically causes menorrhagia, progressive or persistent hypothyroidism may eventually result in amenorrhea. **Cushing's syndrome** can cause amenorrhea, possibly through the inhibitory effect of excessive adrenal androgen production. Primary pituitary problems, such as **Sheehan's syndrome** (postpartum pituitary necrosis) or pituitary tumors, may also cause amenorrhea. **Severe stress**, either psychologic or metabolic, commonly causes aberrations in the menstrual cycle and may result in temporary amenorrhea. These entities have in common altered pituitary function causing abnormal hormonal interplay. For example, it is not uncommon for women having a major operation to miss a menstrual period. **Significant weight loss** or persistence of marked low body weight has also been commonly associated with amenorrhea. **Female athletes**, especially those involved in endurance sports, also have a significant likelihood of being amenorrheic. Investigation of the amenor-

rheic patient involves a careful medical and social history, as well as an appropriate endocrinologic assessment.

Answer: A, B, D, E, F, H

16. Match the following:

A. True hermaphrodite	a. Primary adrenal defect
B. Female pseudohermaph-rodite	b. Abnormal testosterone responsiveness
C. Male pseudohermaphrodite	c. Inadequate testosterone production
D. Testicular feminization	d. Normal karyotype; both ovarian and testicular tissue present

Sabiston: 1613, 1692
Schwartz: 1748

Comments: Abnormal sexual development may result from the fusion of germ cells with abnormal karyotypes, causing karyotypic abnormalities (e.g., Turner's syndrome—XO, Klinefelter's syndrome—XXXY) or may result from abnormal sexual morphologic development in instances in which the karyotypic pattern is normal. In **true hermaphroditism**, the peripheral karyotype may be either 46,XX or 46,XY, but both ovarian and testicular tissue can be found in the same or opposite gonads. The clinical manifestations vary, with the majority of affected patients having ambiguous genitalia. **Female pseudohermaphrodites** have ovaries and a 46,XX karyotype, but because of androgen excess, appear clinically with masculine traits. This may be the result of exogenous drug ingestion during pregnancy or may result from virilizing adrenal dysfunction in which there is excess androgen production. **Male pseudohermaphrodites** have a 46,XY karyotype but a deficiency in testosterone production, leading to clinical feminization. In **testicular feminization**, a 46,XY karyotype is present and the testes, which are usually undescended, secrete normal amounts of testosterone. However, there appears to be a lack of responsiveness to testosterone in the areas that would normally be receptive to its effects. The result is a phenotypic female who may undergo normal secondary sexual changes at puberty but who is sterile. Other considerations of sexual ambiguity are pure gonadal dysgenesis and mosaicism of sexual chromosomes.

Answer: A–d; B–a; C–c; D–b

17. Which of the following statements is/are true regarding various causes of uterovaginal outflow obstruction?

A. A pelvic mass associated with imperforate hymen does not appear until menarche
B. Treatment of imperforate hymen is appropriately performed when diagnosed, even in infancy
C. Surgical treatment of complete absence of vagina should be undertaken just before puberty
D. Intrauterine synechiae are usually post-traumatic
E. Cervical stenosis may be both caused and treated by cervical dilatation

Sabiston: 1611
Schwartz: 1749

Comments: The two most common causes of vaginal outflow obstruction are imperforate hymen and complete absence of the vagina. **Imperforate hymen** in an infant may present with a pelvic or an abdominal mass, which may be confused with bladder distension or neoplasm. Normal secretions from the uterus and vagina may be trapped above the imperforate hymen, even in the premenstrual patient. One must be careful not to explore an infant for an abdominal mass without first excluding the diagnosis of imperforate hymen; when diagnosed, relief is obtained easily with hymenotomy and release of the trapped fluid. **Congenital absence** of the vagina can be treated with surgical reconstruction; this should be delayed, however, until the late teens or early twenties, when the patient is sufficiently mature psychosexually. **Intrauterine synechiae** (Asherman's syndrome) may cause uterine outflow obstruction and are most commonly the result of postpartum or postabortion trauma or endometritis. Hysteroscopic lysis of adhesions is probably the treatment of choice, with placement of an IUD to maintain patency. **Cervical stenosis** may also be posttraumatic and is most often seen following dilatation and curettage or cervical conization. Stenosis is usually asymptomatic but may cause abnormal genital bleeding, dysmenorrhea, and infertility.

Answer: B, D, E

18. Match the following:

A. Severe first trimester bleeding; no tissue passed; HCG positive	a. Incomplete abortion
B. First trimester bleeding; some tissue passed	b. Complete abortion
C. Intact sac passed	c. Septic abortion
D. Abdominal pain, fever, uterine tenderness	d. Missed abortion
E. Uterus shrinks; no discharge; HCG negative	e. Threatened abortion

Schwartz: 1752

Comments: Several types of spontaneous abortion can occur during the first trimester of pregnancy, and they are characterized by the nature of the material passed through the cervix, the clinical status of the uterus, and the result of the HCG assay. Although a small amount of bleeding or spotting in the first trimester of pregnancy is fairly common, persistent or more copious bleeding may be an early sign of an impending abortion. If this occurs without the passage of fragments of tissue and the HCG is positive, this should be considered a **threatened abortion**. If some fragments of tissue are passed in association with the bleeding, an **incomplete abortion** has occurred, and curettage is indicated to prevent further hemorrhage and infection. If all of the products of conception within an intact sac are passed, a **complete abortion** has occurred, and further treatment is usually not necessary. The above notwithstanding, it is very unusual to have a complete spontaneous abortion. More often than not, decidua and placental fragments are still present; therefore dilatation and curettage should be performed on all abortions. A **septic abortion** refers to the clinical signs of abdominal pain, fever, uterine tenderness, and leukocytosis, which almost invariably occur as a result of instrumentation used to induce abortion. Treatment involves aggressive supportive therapy, including antibiotics, followed by gentle curettage once the patient is stabilized. Hysterectomy is sometimes required to control the infection. A **missed abortion** refers to loss of viability of the fetus, unaccompanied by any bleeding or external signs of loss of pregnancy. The uterus shrinks back to normal size, and the HCG returns to negative. Once diagnosed, this is usually treated by uterine curettage.

Answer: A–e; B–a; C–b; D–c; E–d

19. A 25-year-old woman goes to the emergency room complaining of breast tenderness, nausea, mild pelvic pain, and having had no menses for 6 weeks. She has a palpable, tender right adnexal mass. Her serum beta HCG test result is positive, but her urine pregnancy test result is negative. The most likely diagnosis is:

A. Endometriosis
B. Early tubo-ovarian abscess
C. Ectopic pregnancy
D. Duplication of the right fallopian tube, with obstruction

Sabiston: 1630
Schwartz: 1753

Comments: See Question 20.

20. Which of the following statements is/are true concerning ectopic pregnancies?

A. They occur in less than 1% of all pregnancies
B. Results of urine and serum assays to confirm pregnancy are nearly always positive
C. They may be complicated by hemorrhagic shock
D. Unilateral salpingectomy is the only reasonable surgical therapy
E. There is a 10% likelihood of recurrent ectopic pregnancy

Sabiston: 807, 1630
Schwartz: 1753

Comments: Improper transport of a fertilized ovum results in its abnormal implantation in the tube, in the abdomen, or on the ovary. This occurs in less than 1% of pregnancies. The usual signs and symptoms of early pregnancy are often present, including breast tenderness, uterine enlargement, morning nausea, and absent menses. When compared with a normally progressing pregnancy, however, the uterus is usually smaller, and the serum beta HCG level is usually lower for the expected date of gestation; this, however, is not very helpful. In addition, although urine assays for pregnancy have a false negative rate of approximately 50%, the more recent ICON and/or monoclonal antibody tests are considerably more reliable. The most significant complication of ectopic pregnancy is rupture at the ectopic implantation site (usually the fallopian tube). This may result in hemorrhagic shock and is a surgical emergency. In the nonemergency situation, the diagnosis is usually made with ultrasonography and/or laparoscopy. The nonruptured ectopic pregnancy is most often treated by unilateral salpingectomy; however, if the tube is distended to less than 3 cm in size, a conservative salpingostomy, with evacuation of the products of conception and preservation of the involved tube, may be done. Regardless of the surgical approach, recurrent ectopic pregnancies occur in approximately 10% of cases, and subsequent successful pregnancies occur in approximately 50%.

Answer: Question 19: C
Question 20: A, C, E

21. A 25-year-old woman has persistent vaginal bleeding, mild pelvic discomfort, a uterus that is markedly enlarged, high serum level of HCG, and multiple parenchymal nodules on chest x-ray. The most likely diagnosis is:

A. Leiomyosarcoma of the uterus, with pulmonary metastases
B. Malignant trophoblastic disease
C. Meigs' syndrome
D. Adenocarcinoma of the ovary, with metastases
E. Germ cell tumor of the ovary, with metastases

Sabiston: 1629
Schwartz: 1753

Comments: See Question 22.

22. Which of the following statements is/are true regarding trophoblastic disease?

A. Chorioadenoma destruens is associated with a 25% incidence of distant metastatic disease
B. The clinical behavior of trophoblastic disease correlates fairly well with its histologic appearance
C. The use of actinomycin D and methotrexate has resulted in very high response rates in cases of malignant trophoblastic disease
D. The prognosis for metastatic trophoblastic disease is generally favorable

Sabiston: 1629
Schwartz: 1753

Comments: Trophoblastic disease occurs in approximately 0.05% of pregnancies in the United States. It generally takes one of three forms: a **benign hydatidiform mole**, which can be successfully treated with curettage or hysterotomy; **chorioadenoma destruens**, which is a locally invasive process; and the truly malignant and distantly metastasizing form, **choriocarcinoma**. Patients with trophoblastic disease usually present with persistent vaginal bleeding and a uterus that is much larger than expected for gestational age, as well as HCG levels that are inappropriately high. Although many of these patients present with distant disease (most often in the lung), the high response rates attained with appropriate chemotherapy (most often actinomycin D, methotrexate, and/or vinblastine sulfate [Velban]) have resulted in a high likelihood of cure, even in the presence of disseminated disease.

Answer: Question 21: B
Question 22: C, D

23. Match the following:

A. *Trichomonas* vaginitis
B. Monilial vaginitis
C. *Haemophilus* vaginitis
D. Atrophic vaginitis
E. Bartholinitis

a. Acid environment; marked itching; often seen in diabetics; thick, white discharge
b. Discrete tender area; benefits from surgical drainage
c. Green discharge; alkaline environment; metronidazole medication
d. Grayish discharge; clinically nonspecific vaginitis; gram negative organisms; metronidazole treatment
e. Reduced ovarian function; vinegar douches and estrogens helpful

Sabiston: 1616
Schwartz: 1755

Comments: There are numerous inflammatory and infectious conditions of the vagina and vulva; most can be recognized by their clinical history and the gross and microscopic appearance of the discharge. **Monilial** vaginitis can occur at any time but is particularly common after courses of antibiotic therapy and in diabetic patients. It flourishes in an acid environment and is characterized by a thick, white discharge. Examination of the discharge reveals the characteristic mycelial budding. Local antifungal agents provide effective treatment. *Trichomonas* vaginitis is caused by the trichomonad parasite, which is easily identified microscopically by its active flagella. This infection flourishes in an alkaline pH and produces a green, malodorous discharge. It can be effectively treated with vinegar douches or metronidazole. *Haemophilus* is being recognized with increasing frequency as the cause of what was formerly considered to be a nonspecific vaginitis. It produces a gray, malodorous discharge, examination of which reveals gram negative organisms. Metronidazole is effective in treating this infection also. **Atrophic** vaginitis is seen commonly in the postmenopausal patient or in younger patients who have undergone oophorectomy. The associated estrogen depletion results in atrophy of the vaginal mucosa, which permits secondary bacterial invasion to occur. It can be treated effectively with small doses of estrogens or vinegar douches. **Bartholinitis** represents infection of Bartholin's glands and associated ducts in the vulva. Simple dilatation of the duct may be asymptomatic, but superimposed infection usually results in a discrete area of marked tenderness, which may require surgical drainage or excision.

Answer: A–c; B–a; C–d; D–e; E–b

24. Match the following venereal infections with their appropriate characteristics:

A. Syphilis
B. Gonorrhea
C. Chancroid
D. Granuloma inguinale
E. Lymphogranuloma venereum
F. Condyloma acuminatum
G. Genital herpes

a. Painful ulcer; *Haemophilus*
b. Purulent discharge; intracellular diplococci
c. Virus; podophyllin
d. Adenitis; *Chlamydia*
e. Painless ulcer; darkfield examination
f. Painful vesicle; acyclovir
g. Nontender ulcer; Donovan bodies

Sabiston: 1614
Schwartz: 1756

Comments: Changing sexual practices in recent years have resulted in an increase in the frequency of venereal infections. Many of the infections listed above are easily treated if diagnosed early, but they have potentially serious and long-term sequelae if neglected. **Primary syphilis** usually presents as a painless ulcer (chancre) and may be diagnosed by identifying spirochetes on darkfield examination. Serologic tests (VDRL, FTA-ABS) will also suggest the diagnosis. The treatment of choice is penicillin. • **Gonorrhea** appears as a purulent discharge caused by infection with *Neisseria gonorrhoeae*. The diagnosis can be made by identifying intracellular gram negative diplococci within a smear of the vaginal discharge. Culturing the *Neisseria* organism requires careful anaerobic techniques. The treatment of choice is penicillin; however, resistant strains of the bacteria are being recognized with increased frequency. Careful follow-up of the patient with gonorrhea is important, as failure to eradicate the process totally may result in subsequent serious pelvic inflammatory disease. • **Chancroids** are painful ulcers of the vulva that are caused by *Hameophilus ducreyi* and are treated with sulfonamides or streptomycin. • **Granuloma inguinale** is a chronic infection presenting as nontender ulcers, from which can be identified intracellular inclusion bodies (Donovan bodies). Tetracycline is effective treatment. • **Lymphogranuloma venereum** is caused by *Chlamydia trachomatis*. This is an infiltrative process involving the lymphatics and regional lymph nodes, and it presents as inguinal and perineal adenitis. The diagnosis is confirmed by a positive skin test (Frei) result or serology. Tetracycline is effective therapy. • **Condyloma acuminatum** (venereal wart) is caused by papilloma viruses. It can be effectively treated chemically with podophyllin or by electrocoagulation, laser, or surgical excision; unfortunately, recurrence of venereal warts is fairly common. • **Genital herpes** caused by herpes simplex virus Type II is increasing in prevalence. This infection begins as multiple painful vesicles, which may subsequently ulcerate and become associated with systemic symptoms of fever and malaise. Treatment with topical creams and ointments has yielded poor results. More recently, an antiviral agent (acyclovir) has been used with some success.

Answer: A–e; B–b; C–a; D–g; E–d; F–c; G–f

25. Which of the following statements is/are true regarding endometriosis?

A. Reflux of endometrial tissue through the patent fallopian tubes is the only recognized explanation for the occurrence of endometriosis
B. The severity of pain bears a fairly direct relationship to the size of the endometrial nodules present
C. Gastrointestinal bleeding and/or obstruction may be caused by endometriosis
D. Inducing a "pseudopregnant" state with hormone manipulation may relieve the symptoms of endometriosis

Sabiston: 1001
Schwartz: 1757

Comments: Endometriosis refers to the presence of functioning endometrial tissue in locations other than the lining of the uterine cavity, most often in the pelvis and lower abdomen. Reflux of endometrial tissue through the patent fallopian tubes is one explanation for this phenomenon; however, the presence of endometriosis in the lung and other areas distant from the uterus suggests that endometriosis may also result from the activation of embryologic rests of tissues present at birth. The most common symptom of endometriosis is severe dysmenorrhea thought to be related to the cyclic bleeding within the ectopic tissue. Many patients with documented endometriosis, however, are without symptoms. There does not appear to be any correlation between the size of the endometrioma and the severity of pain. Endometrial implants on the serosa of the small and large bowel (most often rectosigmoid areas) can result in bowel obstruction and bleeding. If possible, treatment should be directed at the underlying endometriosis. Medical treatment of this entity usually involves hormone manipulation, including the establishment of a "pseudopregnancy" state with appropriate doses of estrogen and progesterone so that long periods of amenorrhea may be experienced. A "pseudomenopause" may also be induced with such drugs as danazol through inhibition of ovarian function. Symptomatic endometriosis in older patients who desire no further children may also be treated by total abdominal hysterectomy and bilateral salpingo-oophorectomy.

Answer: C, D

26. Complete the following phrase to make one or more true statements: Leiomyomas of the uterus:

A. Being mesenchymal rather than epithelial in origin, are not under hormonal influence
B. Being found within the wall of the uterus rather than within the endometrial cavity itself, are not associated with bleeding
C. May be the cause of habitual abortion or infertility
D. If over 2 cm in size, have a significant likelihood of malignant degeneration

Sabiston: 1623
Schwartz: 1759

Comments: Uterine leiomyomas (fibroids) are fairly common, occurring in approximately 50% of women. They present as whorls of interlacing smooth muscle and are characterized according to their location within the uterus: submucosal, intramural, or subserosal. Although mesenchymal in origin, they are under definite hormonal influence and have been seen to grow in response to estrogen administration. The simple presence of leiomyomas is not an indication for treatment, as the majority are probably asymptomatic. Complications may develop, however, as a result of the size and specific location of the tumor. In the submucosal location, fibroids may bleed significantly, resulting in iron deficiency anemia. They may be pedunculated and undergo a twist of their stalk, with subsequent infarction. They may also be the source of infertility and habitual abortion because of their interference with normal uterine function during pregnancy. Only 1 to 2% of uterine leiomyomas are thought to undergo malignant transformation, but this must be considered whenever there is a rapid increase in size of a previously stable tumor. Leiomyomas causing significant problems may be managed by either local excision or hysterectomy, depending on other clinical circumstances.

Answer: C

27. Regarding carcinoma of the cervix, which of the following statements is/are true?

A. It is by far the most common malignancy of the female genital tract
B. The vast majority are squamous carcinomas
C. Early childbearing and multiple sexual partners appear to be risk factors
D. There is a possible viral etiology
E. The death rate from this disease has declined in recent years

Sabiston: 1619
Schwartz: 1760

Comments: Although the cervix formerly was the leading anatomic site of female genital cancer, it now shares that position with the endometrium. Carcinoma of the cervix and endometrial carcinoma each account for approximately 40% of gynecologic malignancies. Approximately 95% of cervical cancers are squamous carcinomas, and usually they begin at the squamocolumnar junction of the cervix. Early pregnancy and multiparity appear to be risk factors for the development of cervix carcinoma. Further, there is an increased incidence in women with a history of multiple sexual partners, suggesting a possible venereal etiology. This has been supported by the association of cervix carcinoma with several viruses (herpes simplex Type II, papilloma virus, and cytomegalic virus). Early detection has led to increased cure rates and better survival rates in recent years.

Answer: B, C, D, E

28. Regarding the Papanicolaou (Pap) smear, which of the following statements is/are true?

A. It is approximately 95% accurate in screening for cervical carcinoma
B. A negative smear effectively rules out the presence of carcinoma
C. Abnormal appearing epithelial cells that are not frankly malignant suggest an underlying inflammatory process
D. A definitive histologic diagnosis cannot be made on the basis of the smear alone

Sabiston: 1610
Schwartz: 1760

Comments: Wide use of the Papanicolaou smear has afforded the opportunity to screen large populations of women for cervical carcinoma and is a major factor in the recent trend toward earlier detection of cervix carcinoma. The Pap smear is approximately 95% accurate; however, one must be alert to the possibility of sampling error, resulting in false negative or false positive readings. Since this is a cytologic technique, it may indicate the presence of malignant cells but does not give information about the degree of invasiveness. Definitive diagnosis, there-

fore, requires histologic examination of a cervical biopsy specimen. Additionally, an important application of the Pap smear is in the detection of varying degrees of cellular dysplasia, as it alerts the clinician about patients who may require either a more invasive biopsy technique or a closer follow-up because of their higher risk for developing cancer of the cervix in the future.

Answer: A, D

29. Which of the following statements is/are true regarding carcinoma-in-situ of the uterine cervix?

A. It may be diagnosed by Papanicolaou smear
B. It has a predisposition for developing into invasive carcinoma
C. Its proper treatment requires hysterectomy
D. Local radiation therapy is the treatment of choice

Sabiston: 1620
Schwartz: 1761

Comments: Carcinoma-in-situ of the cervix is usually asymptomatic and, therefore, most often suspected because of abnormal results of a pelvic examination and/or a Pap smear. The definitive diagnosis necessitates cervical biopsy with results showing malignant cells confined to the superficial layers of the cervical epithelium without invasion through the basement membrane. As with in situ carcinomas in other sites, carcinoma-in-situ in the cervix is associated with a high incidence of concurrent or future development of invasive carcinoma. For this reason, aggressive therapy is indicated and usually involves either hysterectomy or (in those women who wish to retain the capability to bear children) conization of the cervix. Other cytodestructive techniques, such as laser therapy, cryosurgery, and electrocoagulation, have been used but generally are reserved for treatment of cellular dysplasia. Radiotherapy has also been employed but offers no benefit over conization and has considerably more significant side effects.

Answer: B

30. Match the clinical finding for carcinoma of the cervix with the appropriate clinical stage.

Findings	Clinical Stage
A. Bladder mucosal involvement	a. I
B. Involvement of the lower one third of the vagina	b. II
C. Hydronephrosis	c. III
D. Parametrial involvement	d. IV
E. Attachment to the pelvic sidewall	

Sabiston: 1621
Schwartz: 1762

Comments: As with other malignancies, clinical staging of carcinoma of the cervix influences treatment and bears a strong relationship to prognosis. For cervical malignancies, clinical staging of the primary tumor is accomplished with physical examination, intravenous pyelography, cystoscopy, and proctoscopy. **Stage I** tumors are confined to the cervix. **Stage II** tumors may involve the upper two thirds of the vagina (IIA) or the parametrial tissues (IIB). **Stage III** tumors extend through the parametrial tissues to the pelvic sidewall or extend to the lower one third of the vagina or result in ureteral obstruction. **Stage IV** tumors may invade the bladder or rectal mucosa or have spread outside the pelvis.

Answer: A–d; B–c; C–c; D–b; E–c

31. Match each of the following clinical presentations of cervix cancer with its appropriate treatment:

Presentation	Treatment
A. 2 cm carcinoma confined to the cervix	a. Total abdominal hysterectomy
B. Carcinoma confined to the cervix and upper vagina	b. Radical hysterectomy with pelvic node dissection
C. Parametrial involvement	c. Anterior pelvic exenteration
D. Pelvic sidewall involvement	d. Total pelvic exenteration
E. Extension to the bladder mucosa	e. Radiation therapy

Sabiston: 1621
Schwartz: 1763

Comments: There is a general trend away from surgery and toward radiation therapy for the more advanced carcinomas of the cervix. Stage I and IIA lesions are most often treated by radical (Wertheim) hysterectomy, which includes pelvic lymph node dissection. Radiation therapy has also been employed for these early stage tumors, but generally operation is preferred. Some have treated IA tumors (microinvasive carcinomas less than 3 mm in size) with "nonradical" abdominal hysterectomy. Stage IIB, Stage III, and Stage IV tumors are usually treated with radiation therapy, and most often a combination of external beam and intracavitary or interstitial techniques is used. The exception is the patient with Stage IV cancer who has involvement of the bladder or rectal mucosa; in such cases the appropriate pelvic exenteration should be performed.

Answer: A–b; B–b; C–e; D–e; E–c

32. Match the following characteristics with the tumor(s) with which an association has been suggested:

Characteristics	Tumor
A. Nulliparity	a. Carcinoma of cervix
B. Late first pregnancy	b. Carcinoma of endometrium
C. Obesity	c. Carcinoma of breast
D. Prolonged use of estrogens	
E. Primarily adenocarcinoma	
F. Positive family history	

Sabiston: 1624
Schwartz: 1764

Comments: Endometrial and breast cancers share a number of epidemiologic characteristics in that nulliparity and late first pregnancy increase the risk of developing these cancers. This is in contrast to cancer of the cervix, which occurs with greater frequency in patients with early pregnancies or with multiparity. There is an association between obesity and carcinoma of the endometrium and breast, although the association is much stronger for endometrial cancer. Prolonged, unopposed use of estrogen in the management of menopausal symptoms is thought to increase the risk of breast carcinoma slightly (birth control pills have not been shown to increase this risk); however, once again, this association is much more pronounced in endometrial carcinoma. Cancers of the cervix, endometrium, and breast can certainly affect more than one member of a given family; however, only with breast cancer is a positive family history considered a significant risk factor.

Answer: A–b, c; B–b, c; C–b, c; D–b, c; E–b, c; F–c

33. Match the following clinical findings with the appropriate stage for endometrial carcinoma:

Clinical Findings	Stage
A. Confined to corpus; uterus greater than 8 cm	a. IA
B. Confined to corpus; uterus less than 8 cm	b. IB
C. Rectal mucosal involvement	c. II
D. Cervix involvement	d. III
E. Ovary involvement	e. IV

Sabiston: 1625
Schwartz: 1765

Comments: As implied by the clinical findings listed above, staging for endometrial carcinoma confined to the corpus (Stage I) depends upon the size of the uterus (determined by uterine sounding). Involvement of the cervix alone (Stage II), involvement of other structures in the true pelvis (Stage III), and cancer involving the bladder or the rectal mucosa or its spread outside the true pelvis (Stage IV) complete the staging assessment. Biologic behavior and prognosis for endometrial carcinoma also depend in part on the degree of differentiation of the tumor and whether the tumor lies near the cervix or near the fundus. If the tumor lies near the cervix, regional spread is similar to that for cervix carcinoma; if the tumor lies near the fundus, spread is to the periaortic or inguinal lymph nodes.

Answer: A–b; B–a; C–e; D–c; E–d

34. Which of the following treatment modalities has/have demonstrated effectiveness in the management of endometrial carcinoma?

A. Surgery
B. Radiation therapy
C. Estrogen administration
D. Progesterone administration
E. Cytoxic chemotherapy

Sabiston: 1625
Schwartz: 1765

Comments: Surgery and radiation therapy, alone or in combination, are the principal treatment modalities for endometrial carcinoma. As with carcinoma of the cervix, surgery alone is reserved for the early stages of the disease. Extension of the tumor beyond the corpus (Stage II, Stage III, or Stage IV) is most often treated by surgery and radiation in combination. Extremely advanced disease or recurrent endometrial carcinoma has benefited from the use of progestational agents. Estrogens are generally contraindicated because of their suspected role in the promotion of endometrial carcinoma. Cytotoxic chemotherapeutic agents have had little success. The overall 5-year survival rate for endometrial carcinoma is in the range of 50%, but it is as high as 80% for Stage I disease.

Answer: A, B, D

35. Which of the following is the most common form of uterine sarcoma?

A. Mixed müllerian tumor
B. Endolymphatic stromal myosis
C. Stromal sarcoma
D. Leiomyosarcoma

Sabiston: 1626
Schwartz: 1766

Comments: Uterine sarcomas are not common, accounting for less than 5% of all uterine malignancies. They tend to occur in the postmenopausal patient and generally carry a poor prognosis. Mixed müllerian tumors contain both adenocarcinomatous and sarcomatous elements. Endolymphatic stromal myosis and its more aggressive counterpart, stromal sarcoma, represent invasion of the myometrium by stromal cells of the endometrium. Leiomyosarcoma is the most common uterine sarcoma. It rarely arises from a previous leiomyoma, but when it does, the prognosis appears to be more favorable. All of these tumors, when confined to the uterus, are treated by hysterectomy.

Answer: D

36. Which of the following vulvar abnormalities is/are considered to be risk factor(s) for invasive malignancy?

A. Leukoplakia
B. Lichen sclerosus et atrophicus
C. Bowen's disease
D. Paget's disease

Sabiston: 1615
Schwartz: 1766

Comments: Of the entities listed above, lichen sclerosus et atrophicus stands alone as having no significant relationship to vulvar malignancy. It is a pruritic, patchy, white lesion that is thought to relate to chronic irritation. **Leukoplakia** may present in a similar manner but is differentiated histologically by varying degrees of dysplasia. There is a significant incidence of leukoplakia in patients who also have vulvar malignancies (up to 50%). As with oral cavity leukoplakia, a direct degeneration to malignancy is not always identifiable; however, the association between the two is sufficiently strong that patients with vulvar leukoplakia should be monitored carefully for the development of invasive carcinoma. **Bowen's disease** is considered to be a preinvasive or in situ squamous carcinoma that requires surgical excision. It is also characterized by a high association (up to 35%) with a second ma-

lignant lesion of the female genital tract, usually involving the vagina or cervix. **Paget's disease** appears as an ulcerative, eczematoid vulvar lesion, with the histologic finding of large, foamy pagetoid cells. As in Paget's disease of the breast, this finding is highly suggestive of an underlying adenocarcinoma. With vulvar lesions, this is thought to arise from the apocrine sweat glands. Paget's disease usually requires wide surgical excision and careful follow-up.

Answer: A, C, D

37. True statements regarding invasive squamous cell carcinoma of the vulva include:

A. The "typical" patient is elderly, nulliparous, and obese
B. The primary tumor is usually unilateral
C. The regional lymph nodes most likely involved are those along the ipsilateral common iliac vein
D. Bilateral regional lymph node metastases rarely occur
E. The proper treatment for most cases is radical vulvectomy, with bilateral superficial inguinal lymph node dissections

Sabiston: 1615
Schwartz: 1767

Comments: Invasive vulvar malignancies account for approximately 5% of all cancers of the female genital tract and, among these, squamous carcinomas account for the vast majority. Epidemiologically, these tumors occur with greater frequency in elderly, nulliparous, and obese individuals. They may present anywhere on the vulva but are usually unilateral. Despite this, however, the rich lymphatic networks that interdigitate across the midline result in a high incidence of bilateral lymph node metastases, which appear most often in the inguinal region (inferior to the inguinal ligament). For this reason, proper curative treatment for this tumor involves a total radical vulvectomy, with bilateral inguinal lymph node dissection. The role of prophylactic iliac lymph node dissection is controversial, but most reserve this for cases in which the superficial inguinal nodes are grossly involved. Overall cure rate for invasive squamous carcinoma of the vulva is approximately 50%, but it may be as high as 80 to 90% in individuals with negative nodes.

Answer: A, B, E

38. Match the following vaginal cancers with their appropriate characteristics:

Vaginal Cancer	Characteristics
A. Clear cell carcinoma	a. Most common primary vaginal malignancy
B. Sarcoma botryoides	b. Most common vaginal malignancy
C. Squamous cell carcinoma	c. Diethylstilbestrol (DES) exposure in utero
D. Involvement from malignancies of adjacent organs	d. Seen in young children

Sabiston: 1617
Schwartz: 1768

Comments: Primary cancer of the vagina is rare; most commonly, cancerous involvement is the result of extension from primary tumors of the adjoining vulva, cervix, or endometrium. The most common primary vaginal malignancy is squamous carcinoma. This is not unexpected, since the vagina is lined by squamous epithelium. These tumors most often occur in postmenopausal women. There are notable exceptions: sarcoma botryoides, which is a bulky, polypoid sarcoma occurring in infants and young children; and clear cell carcinoma (mesonephroma), which is an adenocarcinoma frequently occurring in the adolescent and young adult offspring of women who took diethylstilbestrol (DES) during pregnancy. Treatment for these tumors may be by operation (frequently necessitating partial or total pelvic exenteration) or radiation therapy or a combination of the two.

Answer: A–c; B–d; C–a; D–b

39. Which one or more of the following accurately characterize(s) Meigs' syndrome?

A. Hydrothorax
B. Ascites
C. Chylothorax
D. Benign ovarian tumor
E. Malignant ovarian tumor
F. Curable by excising the ovarian tumor

Sabiston: 1628
Schwartz: 1771

Comments: Meigs' syndrome refers to the coexistence of hydrothorax, ascites, and an underlying benign ovarian tumor, usually a fibroma. The pathophysiology of the ascites and pleural fluid is unclear but may result from lymphatic obstruction of the ovary. Excision of the ovarian fibroma is usually accompanied by resolution of the findings. Many ovarian malignancies are also associated with ascites and pleural effusion, which some refer to as "pseudo-Meigs'" or "malignant Meigs'" syndrome.

Answer: A, B, D, F

40. Regarding the evaluation of ovarian masses, which of the following statements is/are true?

A. In infants and young children these are most often malignant germ cell tumors
B. During the reproductive years, masses less than 5 cm in size may be observed through one or two menstrual cycles
C. Clinical characteristics usually suffice to differentiate malignancy from benignity
D. Laparoscopy provides little practical information, since patients with ovarian masses all require laparotomy for management

Sabiston: 1627
Schwartz: 1768

Comments: Pelvic masses in females may arise from the genital tract, the lower urinary tract, the gastrointestinal tract, or the mesenchymal structures of the pelvis; they may be developmental, inflammatory, or neoplastic. The evaluation of a pelvic mass that is thought to represent ovarian pathology is best accomplished initially with careful bimanual pelvic examination (when appropriate according to age) and with ultrasonography. In the absence of extensive disease in the pelvis or fixation of the mass, the clinical diagnosis of ovarian malignancy may be difficult. **Ultrasonography** may demonstrate features suggestive of malignancy, but obviously a firm diagnosis depends upon tissue examination. **Laparoscopy** is a safe method of evaluating pelvic masses and may provide sufficient diagnostic information to preclude the need for laparotomy (e.g., cases of simple ovarian cyst or endometriosis). In **infants and young children**, one must be alert to nonovarian causes of pelvic masses, including Wilms' tumor, imperforate hymen, and bladder abnormalities. Ovarian tumors in this age group are rarely malignant and are most likely to be a benign teratoma. In **women of reproductive age**, masses under 5 cm in size usually represent benign follicle cysts and may be followed through one or two menstrual cycles. Larger masses, those with hard consistency, or those that persist should be further investigated with laparoscopy or laparotomy. Ovarian masses in the **postmenopausal** age group should be investigated when they are discovered. A number of factors enter into the decision-making process as to when and how this should be done. In summary, a plan of observation and follow-up is not applicable to the infant or young girl. In these patients, any enlargement mandates surgical exploration; the same is true for the postmenopausal woman. The probability of malignancy increases sharply after the age of 50 years, and all ovarian enlargements in postmenopausal women should be investigated surgically. In the young woman, however, a careful repeat examination may make operation unnecessary.

Answer: B

41. Which of the following are non-neoplastic benign cysts?

A. Follicular cyst
B. Corpus luteum cyst
C. Endometrioma
D. Wolffian duct remnant
E. Müllerian duct remnant

Sabiston: 1627
Schwartz: 1769

Comments: Except for endometrioma, all of the above represent non-neoplastic cystic enlargements of the ovary or periovarian tissues. When small, they are usually asymptomatic. Sometimes, however, the cysts can become quite large; they may undergo twisting with subsequent infarction, or they may rupture, spilling material into the pelvis, which may result in clinical peritonitis. This normally happens with the diminutive wolffian and müllerian duct remnants.

Answer: A, B, D, E

42. Match the extent of involvement with the stage of ovarian adenocarcinoma.

Extent of Involvement	Stage
A. One ovary involved	a. Stage I
B. Both ovaries involved	b. Stage II
C. Studding of outer surface of bladder	c. Stage III
D. Malignant ascites	d. Stage IV
E. Involvement of undersurface of diaphragm	
F. Liver metastases	

Sabiston: 1628
Schwartz: 1769

Comments: See Question 43.

43. Which of the following statements is/are true regarding ovarian adenocarcinoma?

A. At laparotomy, peritoneal fluid or washings should be routinely sent for cytologic assessment
B. Total abdominal hysterectomy and bilateral salpingo-oophorectomy should be reserved for patients with bilateral ovarian involvement
C. "Debulking" (removing as much gross tumor as possible) ovarian tumors and their abdominal metastases may contribute to improved survival
D. Chemotherapy has done little to improve survival
E. Primary carcinoma of the breast, stomach, and colon are the most common sources of metastases to the ovary

Sabiston: 1628
Schwartz: 1770

Comments: Primary adenocarcinomas of the ovary may be serous, mucinous, or endometrioid. They are staged as follows: Stage I = one or both ovaries; Stage II = extraovarian involvement but contained within the true pelvis; Stage III = involvement of the abdomen outside the true pelvis but not including the liver; Stage IV = spread beyond the abdominal cavity or within the liver. One of the fairly common manifestations in Stage III is that of malignant ascites; malignant cells, however, may be present free within the peritoneal cavity, even without significant ascites. Ascites, therefore, may be present in Stage IC and Stage IIC ovarian cancer. As a matter of fact, ascites differentiates Stage IA and IB from Stage IC, and Stage IIA and IIB from Stage IIC. Peritoneal washings, therefore, should be obtained for cytologic assessment when the abdomen is opened for suspected ovarian carcinoma. With rare exception (e.g., a small, unilateral ovarian tumor in a patient who insists on retaining childbearing capabilities), the operative therapy of ovarian carcinoma is total abdominal hysterectomy and bilateral salpingo-oophorectomy with debulking of as much gross intra-abdominal disease as possible. This usually involves an omentectomy, which often is performed prophylactically because of the omentum being a favored site for ovarian metastasis not apparent at the time of laparotomy (later such involvement becoming clinically manifest can produce disabling symptoms of ascites and obstruction). Some evidence suggests that cytoreductive "debulking" surgery improves the response to chemotherapy and hence improves survival. Ovarian carcinoma is frequently quite responsive to chemothera-

peutic agents, and it is not uncommon for patients with Stage III disease to be rendered free of disease following debulking and chemotherapy. One must always remember that the ovary may also be the site of metastasis from other epithelial tumors; about 6% of ovarian cancers encountered during exploration for a pelvic or abdominal mass are metastatic, usually from primary cancers of the gastrointestinal tract, breast, thyroid, or lymphatic tissue.

Answer: Question 42: A–a; B–a; C–b; D–a, b, c; E–c; F–d
Question 43: A, C, E

44. Match the following ovarian tumors with their appropriate characteristics:

Tumor	Characteristics
A. Teratoma	a. Masculinizing
B. Granulosa-theca cell tumor	b. Totipotential cell
C. Sertoli-Leydig cell tumor	c. Thyroid tissue
D. Struma ovarii	d. HCG
E. Choriocarcinoma	e. Elaborate estrogen

Sabiston: 1627
Schwartz: 1770

Comments: Many of the more unusual ovarian tumors are characterized by their capacity to elaborate humoral substances or to manifest pleuripotentiality in their growth patterns and have varying malignant potential. **Teratoma** is a germ cell tumor that arises from the totipotential ovarian germ cell and may contain differentiated tissues that are grossly or histologically recognizable (e.g., brain, teeth, hair, muscle, bone). In its benign form (cystic teratoma or dermoid), simple excision suffices. Careful inspection or bivalving of the opposite ovary must be performed because of the high incidence (12%) of bilaterality. **Granulosa-theca cell** tumors usually elaborate estrogen and have been associated with precocious puberty in young patients and endometrial carcinoma in the older age groups. Sertoli-Leydig cell tumors (arrhenoblastomas) are associated with androgen output and masculinization and have a malignant potential of 25%. **Struma ovarii** refers to the presence of thyroid tissue and is considered a component element in some dermoid cysts. Occasionally hyperthyroidism may result. **Choriocarcinoma** is a rare primary tumor of the ovary that elaborates chorionic gonadotropin, as also occurs in this variation of trophoblastic disease. Treatment for all of these tumors depends upon the extent of disease when diagnosed, but in their early stages, many are appropriately managed by a unilateral oophorectomy.

Answer: A–b; B–e; C–a; D–c; E–d

CHAPTER 53

Neurosurgery

1. Regarding diagnostic procedures used to evaluate the central nervous system, which of the following is/are true?

A. X-rays of the skull should be taken only when fracture is suspected
B. Tomography has been completely replaced by CT scan
C. Digital subtraction angiography decreases the risk associated with cerebral angiography
D. Pneumoencephalography has been replaced by CT scan
E. Water-soluble contrast material has decreased the incidence of arachnoiditis following myelography
F. MRI produces less bony artefact than does a CT scan

Sabiston: 1366
Schwartz: 1783

Comments: Routine x-rays of the skull can be useful in detecting tumor opacification, shifts of the calcified pineal gland, altered shape of the pituitary fossa, and abnormal appearance of sutures in infants, as well as fractures. **Tomography,** although largely replaced by CT scans, still is useful in the evaluation of CSF rhinorrhea, spinal trauma, and bony infection. **Angiography** is the main method of demonstrating vascular lesions and is useful in the preoperative evaluation of neoplasms and certain cases of trauma. Its major danger, a cerebrovascular accident secondary to vessel manipulation, may be decreased by the use of computer-assisted digital subtraction angiography (DSA), but the images obtained with DSA are usually of inferior quality. **Pneumoencephalography,** once used to enhance definition of the subarachnoid spaces, has been almost completely replaced by the CT scan; this definition can be enhanced even further, if necessary, by the injection of soluble contrast material prior to performance of the CT scanning. **Myelography** is the x-ray study of the spinal cord after the subarachnoid injection of contrast material; the use of water-soluble contrast media has decreased the incidence of post-procedure arachnoiditis. In some institutions, myelography has been replaced by the CT scan, including its use in the evaluation of intervertebral disc disease.

The **CT scan** is at present the most useful diagnostic tool for evaluation of the CNS; modern units provide resolution in the range of 1 mm. The major disadvantage of CT scans is the artefact created by the bony coverings of the central nervous system. **Magnetic resonance imaging** (MRI) may supplant CT scan because it does not expose the patient to radiation, is associated with minimal bony artefacts, yields high-grade differentiation of gray-white matter, and can directly scan in multiple planes.

Answer: C, D, E, F

2. True statements regarding scalp injuries include:

A. The blood supply to the scalp lies between the periosteum and the galea
B. Most scalp laceration hemorrhages can be controlled by applying direct pressure
C. Subgaleal hematomas must be drained to avoid abscess formation and extensive scalp elevation
D. Major scalp lacerations should be drained to avoid subgaleal hematoma formation
E. Galeal lacerations should be closed when possible.

Sabiston: 1386
Schwartz: 1785

Comments: The scalp consists of five layers (Skin, subCutaneous, galea Aponeurotica, Loose areolar tissue, Periosteum). The skin and galea are the layers of surgical importance, with the blood supply lying between the skin above and the galea below. The blood supply to the scalp is rich, so its lacerations can be accompanied by significant blood loss. When the underlying skull is intact, this blood loss can be controlled by simple pressure. If the skull is fractured, direct pressure may be hazardous to the underlying brain; pulling the retracted galea back over the wound edge with forceps often will control such hemorrhage. Contusions causing subgaleal hemorrhage can lead to the formation of large subgaleal hematomas that can elevate extensive portions of the scalp off the skull. In this setting, compression dressings can reduce the extent of hematoma formation. If the overlying scalp is viable and there is no evidence of infection, subgaleal hematomas should be left alone to resolve naturally, a process that may require several weeks. If the hematoma is infected, it is necessary to evacuate it. The occipitalis and frontalis muscles insert on the galea, and their contraction tends to separate any areas of galeal disruptions; therefore, even small lacerations of the galea should be closed. As in the nonoperative treatment of subgaleal hematomas, large lacerations with significant loss of galeal or subgaleal tissue should be treated with compression dressings after appropriate débridement and closure so as to minimize the chances of postoperative galeal hematoma and infection.

Answer: B, E

3. Which of the following statements is/are true regarding intracranial pressure?

A. Monitoring can be accomplished by the insertion of a catheter into the ventricular system
B. Monitoring can be accomplished by insertion of a transducer into the subarachnoid or epidural space
C. Normal pressure usually is below 10 mm Hg
D. Prolonged pressures greater than 20 mm Hg are pathologic

Sabiston: 1370

Comments: Intracranial pressure monitoring is a continuous record of the pressure within the cranial cavity. The degree and pattern of pressure elevation can provide important diagnostic, therapeutic, and prognostic information. Pressures elevated above 20 mm Hg for a prolonged period of time are pathologic, and pressures greater than 60 mm Hg are generally incompatible with survival owing to restriction of parenchymal blood flow. The monitoring devices are placed in the ventricular system or in the subarachnoid or epidural space, using strict sterile technique, and are useful in monitoring patients with increased intracranial pressure secondary to head trauma, tumor, or hemorrhage. In cases of severe brain swelling, ventricular monitoring catheters can allow removal of cerebrospinal fluid to decrease pressure.

Answer: A, B, C, D

4. Regarding skull fractures, which of the following statements is/are true?

A. Linear, nondisplaced skull fractures, in and of themselves, require no special therapy
B. The raccoon sign (periorbital ecchymosis) is associated with basilar skull fractures of the anterior fossa
C. Battle's sign (ecchymosis of the mastoid process) is associated with fractures of the temporal bone
D. The term skull fracture refers to fractures of the cranial or facial bones

Sabiston: 1386
Schwartz: 1786

Comments: The term skull fractures refers to fractures of the bones of the cranium, including the frontal, occipital, temporal, and parietal bones. Most linear, nondisplaced skull fractures do not, in themselves, require treatment. They may, however, extend to the base of the skull,

crossing the middle meningeal artery and causing epidural hemorrhage, or they may occur in association with an underlying dural tear, both situations requiring treatment. Basilar skull fractures are difficult to see on x-ray and often are associated with leakage of cerebrospinal fluid. They should be suspected in patients with the raccoon sign; Battle's sign; air-fluid levels in the frontal, sphenoid, or mastoid sinuses; blood or CSF visible behind the tympanic membrane; or CSF otorrhea or rhinorrhea. Generally, depressed skull fractures should be elevated, particularly those overlying the motor strip, or those that are small with sharp edges that may tear the dura. When present, if there is an associated brain laceration, it should be débrided and the dural tear closed. Fractures with minimal depression (<1 cm) or those located over the major dural sinuses and without evidence of tear may be observed. Compound fractures should be cleansed thoroughly and débrided and the soft tissue closed. Replacement of skull fragments is a matter of surgical judgment; when there is doubt, it is better to remove rather than to replace them.

Answer: A, B, C

5. True statements regarding traumatic cerebrospinal fluid (CSF) leaks include which one or more of the following?

A. Most are due to basilar skull fracture
B. Most close spontaneously
C. The risk of infection is greater with rhinorrhea than with otorrhea
D. They require immediate surgical repair to avoid infection
E. They may be observed for up to 14 days if there is no evidence of infection

Sabiston: 1386
Schwartz: 1786

Comments: Most traumatic CSF fistulas close spontaneously. They should be managed under close medical supervision with the head maintained at a 30-degree elevation. The risk of persistent drainage and of infection is greater with rhinorrhea than with otorrhea. Otorrhea or rhinorrhea that persists for longer than 10 to 14 days is an indication for repair of the torn dura.

Answer: A, B, C, E

6. Regarding brain injury, which of the following statements is/are true?

A. The extent of brain injury is a function of the mechanism of injury
B. Contusions may occur on the side of the brain opposite the side of initial impact
C. Contusions tend to involve the anterior portions of the frontal and temporal lobes
D. Contusions may be clinically silent
E. The effects of secondary edema may be delayed for several days

Sabiston: 1383
Schwartz: 1787

Comments: Localized force can cause damage to the scalp, skull, and underlying brain in the immediate area of injury. The resulting neurologic deficit relates to the area of the brain directly involved and usually produces brief or no loss of consciousness. Applications of generalized force to the skull, such as that caused by the impact of a head against an immovable object, allows diffuse transmission of energy, causing injury to the whole brain. In such a case, the brain insult is more generalized, often producing altered consciousness, and its severity relates to the mechanism of injury. For example, the injury may be due to linear or rotational acceleration/deceleration of the brain against the confining cranium, as when the head hits an immovable object. When the brain strikes the rigid skull, contusions occur in the area where the force is applied as well as against the opposite inner surface of the skull (contrecoup injury). Rotation of the brain within the skull may cause tearing of axons, resulting in diffuse axonal injury within the white matter—a so-called shearing injury. The undersurface of the frontal lobes, the anterior portions of the temporal lobes, the posterior portions of the occipital lobes, and the upper portion of the midbrain are more likely to suffer contusions because they are relatively more confined by bone or dural shelves. The contusion may be clinically silent initially, if the involved area of the brain has no demonstrable clinical function. These injuries often become apparent days after the injury, as edema accumulates, creating the effects of an intracranial mass. Occasionally, a hematoma may accumulate in the area of contusion 24 to 72 hours after injury, a situation seen more commonly in elderly persons.

Answer: A, B, C, D, E

7. True statements in regard to the evaluation and care of head-injured patients include:

A. Hypotension is often the direct result of intracranial trauma
B. Decerebrate posturing is a common response to diffuse cortical injury
C. A score of 5 on the Glasgow coma scale is associated with a poor prognosis
D. Inappropriate secretion of ADH should be suspected when the serum sodium level exceeds 150 mEq/l
E. Inappropriate secretion of ADH should be treated with administration of exogenous solute

Sabiston: 1384
Schwartz: 1788

Comments: The initial care of the head-injured patient must focus on the maintenance of ventilation, the control of hemorrhage, and the maintenance of peripheral circulation. Continued hypotension and tachycardia is rarely the direct result of head trauma and should alert the examiner to the existence of extracranial hemorrhage. In fact, intracranial hemorrhage with elevated intracranial pressure is often manifested by hypertension and bradycardia. As soon as possible, there should be a careful neurologic examination and documentation of the level of consciousness; it is a baseline against which the patient's progress is measured. Decerebrate posturing (extension and internal rotation of the extremities, neck extension, and arching of the back) implies compression of

or damage to the brain stem and often requires immediate therapy. In a patient unconscious for more than 6 hours, the Glasgow coma scale is useful in predicting eventual outcome. It measures motor (M), verbal (V), and eye (E) response on a scale of 1:6, 1:5, and 1:4 respectively. It is recorded as a sum of the highest score in each category. Patients with a score less than 5 have a mortality rate greater than 50%. Patients who have lost the reflex capability to protect their airway should be intubated and their stomachs decompressed by a nasogastric tube. A Foley catheter should be placed, and serum and urine electrolytes and osmolality values should be monitored. Inappropriate secretion of ADH should be suspected when serum osmolality and sodium levels fall in association with an increase in urinary osmolality. Restriction of water intake or the use of solute diuretics may be necessary to control this problem. The body temperature must be closely monitored, as head injuries may be accompanied by the loss of superficial cutaneous vasodilation and sweating, leading to hyperthermia.

Answer: C

8. Which one or more of the following is/are true regarding the treatment of cerebral edema?

A. CT scans should be obtained to rule out the diagnosis of intracranial hemorrhage or a mass lesion before starting therapy
B. Barbiturates are used to capture free radicals
C. The inflammatory response can be decreased by steroids
D. Hypercapnia induces cerebral vasoconstriction and is useful in decreasing intracerebral blood volume
E. Lumbar puncture to drain cerebrospinal fluid is contraindicated

Sabiston: 1383
Schwartz: 1790

Comments: The brain responds to injury by the formation of edema. The bony confines of the skull impose a narrow tolerance for swelling before the intracranial pressure equals arterial pressure. When this occurs, perfusion stops and neuronal death follows in 4 to 5 minutes. The onset of edema usually is slow and reaches a maximum in 36 to 48 hours. The progress of cerebral edema is best followed by the use of intracranial pressure monitoring devices. These are commonly used in monitoring patients with altered consciousness following head injury or in patients with Glasgow coma scale scores of less than 6. After a baseline CT scan is obtained to rule out intracranial hemorrhage or a mass lesion, treatment should be started as soon as possible to minimize the progression of edema. Systemic arterial pressure must be at least 50 mm Hg greater than intracranial pressure in order to preserve cerebral perfusion. The goal of treatment is to maintain this differential by reducing intracranial pressure rather than by elevating systematic arterial pressure. This can be accomplished by: (1) elevating the head of the bed 15 to 20 degrees, (2) intermittent drainage of cerebrospinal fluid via a pressure monitoring catheter placed in the frontal horn of the lateral ventricle, (3) hyperventilation to pCO_2 levels of 25 to 30 mm of mercury to induce vasoconstriction, and (4) the use of fluid restriction and solute diuretics to minimize intracellular edema. Barbiturates are thought to provide protection for the injured brain by decreasing metabolic demands and by capturing free radicals that have been released through cell destruction. Steroids are thought to decrease inflammation and swelling, but their effectiveness in the treatment of cerebral edema secondary to head trauma has not been established. Lumbar puncture is contraindicated becaues the nonuniform distribution of elevated pressure between supratentorial space, infratentorial space, and spinal canal may lead to herniation of the cerebellum through the foramen magnum or temporal lobe herniation with consequent compression of the brain stem.

Answer: A, B, C, E

9. Which one or more of the following is/are true regarding subdural hematomas?

A. Acute subdural hematomas are usually unilateral
B. Adequate treatment of an acute subdural hematoma generally consists of drainage through burr holes
C. Subacute, subdural hematomas occur between 2 and 14 days after injury
D. The diagnosis of subacute subdural hematomas can reliably be made by CT scan
E. Chronic subdural hematomas should be suspected in elderly patients with progressive changes in mental status even without a definite history of trauma

Sabiston: 1387
Schwartz: 1791

Comments: Subdural hematomas are caused by the rupture of veins traversing the subdural space or by arterial bleeding from parenchymal laceration. Their presentation and treatment depends on the rapidity of hematoma formation. All types of subdural hematoma (acute, subacute, and chronic) have in common the presence of a decreased level of consciousness out of proportion to the focal neurologic deficit observed. **Acute subdural hematomas** are those that cause progressive neurologic deficit within 48 hours of injury. They usually follow severe head trauma, have both arterial and venous sources of bleeding, and can progress very rapidly. The diagnosis should be considered in any patient with a severe head injury who shows deterioration in neurologic status or who is unresponsive and with a focal neurologic deficit. The hematomas are solid and easily visualized by CT scan. They may also produce a pineal gland shift visible on skull films. They can be bilateral, and adjacent intracerebral hematomas are often present. Treatment requires formal craniotomy with removal of solid clot and control of bleeding points. **Subacute subdural hematomas** are defined as being more than 48 hours but less than 2 weeks old. The patients usually are less severely injured than those with acute subdural hematomas and marked fluctuation of level of consciousness or headache should alert one to the diagnosis. With large hematomas third nerve paresis with pupil dilatation is a warning that midbrain compression due to temporal lobe herniation is occurring. CT scans may not identify the mass, since the hematoma becomes isodense 10 to 12 days after its formation and there may be bilateral hematomas. If the diagnosis is suspected strongly in a patient with a normal CT scan, the use of multiple burr holes may be indicated

as a method of diagnosis, although MR imaging will clearly delineate the hematoma. If the clot is completely liquefied, burr holes are therapeutic as well. If solid clot is found, craniotomy is indicated. **Chronic subdural hematomas** most often occur in infants and the elderly, frequently without a clear history of antecedent trauma. They can occur months to years after the initial injury and should be suspected in patients with a decreasing or fluctuating mental status out of proportion to the focal neurologic deficit. The hematoma is liquid, and drainage via burr holes is usually all that is necessary.

Answer: A, C, E

10. Concerning epidural hematomas, which of the following is/are true?

A. Epidural hematomas are caused by venous or arterial bleeding
B. Most patients present with brief loss of consciousness followed by a lucid period, then lapse again into unconsciousness and further deterioration
C. Most surgically significant epidural hematomas are arterial, originating from the middle meningeal artery or its branches
D. The middle meningeal artery enters the skull at the foramen ovale
E. Diagnostic burr holes are placed over the temporal region on the side opposite the dilating pupil

Sabiston: 1386
Schwartz: 1793

Comments: Epidural hematomas may be caused by venous or arterial bleeding. Surgically important epidural hematomas usually arise from arterial bleeding due to disruption of the middle meningeal artery or its branches. This may be caused by direct arterial injury due to temporal bone fracture over the course of the middle meningeal artery or due to the shearing effect of angular acceleration causing disruption of the artery along its epidural course. The hematoma, therefore, can occur without a concomitant skull fracture. The classic clinical picture is that of a brief loss of consciousness followed by a lucid interval lasting from a few minutes to a few hours, followed by rapid progressive loss of consciousness as the rapidly expanding hematoma causes tentorial herniation, midbrain compression, and pupillary dilatation on the side of the lesion. The intervening lucid period is seen in less than 30% of patients. A CT scan will demonstrate the presence of hematoma, but often the rapid progression of symptoms precludes its use. In rapidly deteriorating patients suspected of having an epidural hematoma, a diagnostic burr hole may be necessary; this should be placed one fingerbreadth above the zygoma and one fingerbreadth in front of the ear on the side of the dilating pupil. If a clot is found, the burr hole is converted to a craniotomy to allow evacuation of the solid clot and control of the bleeding artery. This may require identification of the foramen spinosum where the middle meningeal artery enters the skull.

Answer: A, C

11. Which one or more of the following choices are correct regarding post-traumatic intracerebral hematomas?

A. They often mimic the symptoms of an acute or sub-acute subdural hematoma
B. They are most commonly found in the anterior third of the temporal lobe
C. They may not be readily apparent clinically and can resolve without the need for surgical intervention
D. A CT scan is the most useful diagnostic test
E. When diagnosed, they may be adequately treated by needle aspiration

Schwartz: 1793

Comments: Post-traumatic intracerebral hematomas occur most frequently in patients suffering from severe head trauma; they may mimic the symptoms of acute or subacute subdural hematoma and frequently are found in conjunction with them. They are most commonly found in the anterior third of the temporal lobe and less frequently in the tips of the frontal or occipital lobes. Some may not be clinically apparent and remain undiagnosed; thus they resolve by liquefaction, phagocytosis, and gliosis. Those that produce focal deficits such as third nerve palsy and hemiparesis associated with progressive alteration in consciousness require surgical attention. As with acute subdural hematomas, the clots are solid and are best detected by CT scanning. The treatment for clinically significant intracerebral hematoma is craniotomy or even craniectomy. Aspiration is not possible since the hematoma is usually a solid clot.

Answer: A, B, C, D

12. Which of the following statements is/are true regarding subarachnoid hemorrhage?

A. It is the most common intracranial hemorrhage following head trauma
B. It usually produces meningismus (stiff neck and headache)
C. Rapid dilution of the blood by the CSF prevents accumulation of a mass-producing clot
D. It may produce communicating hydrocephalus as a late complication

Sabiston: 1375
Schwartz: 1791

Comments: One of the most common intracranial hemorrhages following head injury is subarachnoid hemorrhage. It usually causes signs of meningismus (stiff neck, headache) and occasionally maniacal behavior in young males. Because the bleed is small and rapidly diluted by the cerebrospinal fluid, no localized mass effect occurs; therefore, this type of hemorrhage has little surgical significance. Rarely, it can lead to progressive communicating hydrocephalus requiring shunting.

Answer: A, B, C, D

13. Which statement(s) is/are true regarding convalescence after head injury?

A. Changes in personality and mood are rarely organic and require intensive psychologic counseling
B. Thirty to 45% of patients with an injury involving a brain laceration will have seizures if not placed on anticonvulsive medication

C. The incidence of convulsions after closed head injury is approximately 30%
D. Prolonged elevation of CSF pressure requiring shunting is unusual after closed head injury

Schwartz: 1794

Comments: Problems of the convalescing head-injured patient include psychologic disorders, convulsions, and abnormalities in cerebrospinal fluid dynamics. Patients commonly encounter changes in personality and mood during recovery from head injury and commonly have complaints of headache, fatigue, loss of memory, and depression. Possible organic causes are persistent temporal and frontal lobe malfunction. Anxiety over persistent physical and mental fatigue may have debilitating psychologic effects. Convulsions occur in 30 to 45% of patients who suffer compound injuries that produce lacerations of the brain. These are usually well controlled with dilantin and phenobarbital. Of patients sustaining closed head injuries, 1 to 10% will experience difficulty with postoperative convulsions; they can develop over many years following the injury and at times may be difficult to diagnose. Abnormalities in CSF circulation producing headache, postural vertigo, and feelings of lightheadedness may be common in the early recovery period following head injury, but prolonged elevation of cerebrospinal fluid pressure is rare. When it does occur, however, it can present weeks or months after injury with gradual dementia, motor apraxia, or loss of coordination of motor movements. In such cases, the use of ventriculoperitoneal or ventriculocaval shunts is indicated.

Answer: B, D

14. Which one or more of the following is/are true regarding spinal cord injuries?

A. Fracture dislocations most commonly occur in the lower cervical and upper lumbar regions
B. Cervical stabilization is best accompanied by open fusion
C. A bony fragment in the spinal canal is considered a contraindication to reduction by manipulative maneuvers
D. Spinal cord injuries routinely require decompressive laminectomy

Sabiston: 1431
Schwartz: 1795

Comments: Most spinal cord damage occurs at the time of the bone injury, and is most likely to occur where the relatively fixed thoracic spine joins the relatively mobile lower cervical or upper lumbar spine. Progressive damage to the white matter may occur during the first 4 to 6 hours after injury, but most secondary damage is due to movement of the unstable vertebral column, or the effects of bony fragments displaced into the spinal canal, or the effects of continued compression of the spinal cord. Therapy, therefore, is directed at vertebral stabilization, removal of bone fragments from the canal, and decompression of the spinal cord when indicated. Cervical stabilization is achieved best by skeletal traction and placement of the patient on a firm surface. Six weeks of strict immobilization followed by 6 to 8 weeks of continued support are needed for firm union of unstable cervical fractures. Fixation in a halo vest may be used to obtain earlier mobilization of the patient with an unstable cervical spine fracture. Fracture dislocations of the thoracic or lumbar spine should not be reduced unless the cord is first exposed by laminectomy because of the risk of cord injury during a closed reduction. Compression fractures of these areas may respond to gentle extension, but this maneuver is contraindicated if there is evidence of bony fragments within the canal. Unstable fractures may require open fusion; when indicated, this is best delayed for 2 to 3 weeks so that the reaction within the canal from the primary injury can subside. If any function remains across an area of spinal cord adjacent to or in contact with a bony fragment, decompression, removal of fragments, and spinal stabilization are indicated. Decisions regarding the role of spinal cord decompression in the early care of the spinal cord injury are controversial. Some advocate routine decompressive laminectomy to relieve the pressure caused by edema and swelling that accompanies all spinal cord injuries. Others argue that neuronal loss is complete within a short period of time and that the routine use of laminectomy offers little hope of improving spinal cord function. Most agree, however, that when there is evidence of compression causing progression in the neurologic deficit or obstruction of CSF circulation, decompression is indicated. This decision is based on repeat neurologic assessment and contrast myelography.

Answer: A, C

15. True statements regarding peripheral nerve injuries include:

A. Neurapraxia requires surgical resection of the nerve root involved if one is to eliminate pain
B. Denervation atrophy of muscles becomes irreversible after 12 to 15 months
C. Restoration of sensory loss is not possible after muscle atrophy due to denervation is complete
D. Axonal regeneration progresses at a rate of 1 mm per day after a 10- to 20-day lag period
E. Reduction of the area of sensory loss is considered absolute evidence of re-establishment of anatomic continuity of an injured nerve

Sabiston: 1404
Schwartz: 1797

Comments: There are several classifications of nerve injuries. The Seddon classification uses three terms to classify nerve injuries: neurapraxia, axonotmesis, and neurotmesis. With **neurapraxia,** anatomic continuity of the nerve is preserved and typically there is complete motor paralysis with very little muscle atrophy and considerable sparing of sensory and autonomic function. Operative repair is not indicated and the quality of recovery is excellent. **Axonotmesis** is the loss of axonal continuity without interruption of the investing axonal tissue. There is complete motor, sensory, and autonomic paralysis and progressive muscle atrophy. Operative repair is not indicated and recovery occurs at the rate of about 1 mm per day. **Neurotmesis** is a more severe injury with significant disorganization within the nerve or actual disruption of continuity of the nerve and its investing tissues. Recov-

ery is impossible without operative repair. After disruption, axonal sprouting begins in 10 to 20 days. If not repaired, scar tissue blocks entrance of axonal sprouts into the distal nerve; instead, they coil into a disorganized neuroma that can be quite painful. After operative repair, distal growth occurs at the rate of 1 mm per day after the initial 10- to 20-day lag described above. The degree of recovery is a function of patient age (younger is better), the type of nerve involved (pure motor or sensory nerves recover better than do mixed nerves), the level of nerve injury (distal is better) and the duration of denervation (shorter is better). If more than 12 to 15 months is required for regenerating axons to reach a denervated muscle, a significant degree of denervation atrophy will have occurred, which is irreversible. In contrast, sensory loss may be recovered after prolonged periods of denervation, so a nerve repair can provide protective sensory function in the atrophied distal extremity.

Answer: B, D

16. True statements regarding the assessment of recovered peripheral nerve function include:

A. Shrinkage of the area of sensory loss is not in itself considered evidence of re-establishment of anatomic continuity of an injured sensory nerve
B. Muscle contraction after electrical stimulation of the nerve distal to the point of injury can occur without the occurrence of nerve regeneration
C. Tinel's sign is accurate in predicting the degree of ultimate functional recovery
D. The distal phalanx of the little finger has no area of sensory overlap and can be used to measure the recovery of a sensory deficit in that area

Sabiston: 1404
Schwartz: 1798

Comments: Recovery of voluntary motor function of a muscle innervated by an injured nerve or recovery of sensation in an autonomous area of sensory innervation provides evidence of functional recovery after nerve repair. Similarly, muscle contraction after electrical stimulation of the nerve bundle distal to the point of injury can provide evidence of regeneration, since the distal segment will conduct impulses for only 5 to 6 days after injury unless regeneration has occurred. Tinel's sign (paresthesias felt in the cutaneous distribution of the injured nerve when the nerve is lightly percussed) can be used to follow distal progression of a regenerating nerve; however, this sign requires activation of only a small percentage of fibers and is not accurate in predicting the degree of ultimate functional recovery. Shrinkage of the area of sensory loss is not prognostic for functional recovery since marked sensory overlap in all but a few areas of the body allows re-establishment of sensation in the denervated area without reinnervation by the injured nerve.

Answer: A, B, D

17. Which one or more of the following statements is/are true regarding brain tumors?

A. There is no uniformly accepted system of classification for brain tumors

B. Brain tumors may be classified according to tissue of origin, location, and malignant potential
C. Gliomas are the most common type of brain tumor
D. Glioblastoma multiforme is the most common type of glioma in adults

Sabiston: 1371
Schwartz: 1800

Comments: No uniformly accepted system of classification for brain tumors has been developed. One developed by Kernohan and Sayre is based on naming the tumor for the cells present in the adult nervous system, vascular tissue, and developmental defects (e.g., astrocytoma, medulloblastoma, oligodendrocytoma) combined with a grading of malignancy (where appropriate) from Grade I (least malignant) to Grade IV (most malignant). Another method classifies tumors according to location: intra-axial neuroectodermal (gliomas), intra-axial non-neuroectodermal (e.g., metastases, blood vessel tumors), and extra-axial (meningiomas). The majority of brain tumors are gliomas, the most common of which, in adults, is the highly malignant glioblastoma multiforme (astrocytoma Grades III and IV). Other gliomas include astrocytomas Grades I and II, medulloblastomas, oligodendrogliomas, and ependymomas Grades I to IV. Nonglial tumors include meningiomas, pituitary tumors, neurilemmomas, blood vessel tumors, and metastatic tumors (comprising up to 15% of all brain tumors) most notably arising from lung, breast, melanoma, and kidney.

Answer: A, B, C, D

18. Which one or more of the following statements is/are true regarding brain tumors?

A. Most adult brain tumors are located in the posterior fossa
B. Most childhood tumors are located in the middle or anterior fossa
C. The most common adult brain tumor is the glioblastoma multiforme (astrocytoma Grades III and IV)
D. The most common childhood brain tumor is the Grade I or II astrocytoma
E. All astrocytomas tend to recur after excision with the exception of the cystic astrocytoma of the cerebellum in children

Sabiston: 1372
Schwartz: 1800

Comments: The majority of adult tumors (70%) are supratentorial (middle or anterior fossa) while the majority of childhood tumors (75%) are infratentorial (posterior fossa). The most common primary brain tumor of adults is the Grade III or IV astrocytoma (glioblastoma multiforme), followed by meningiomas, pituitary tumors, and neurilemmomas. In children, the most frequent lesion is the astrocytoma Grade I or II of the posterior fossa followed (in decreasing frequency) by malignant medulloblastoma, ependymomas, and craniopharyngiomas. Adult gliomas occur most commonly in the cerebral hemisphere, while meningiomas have a predilection to occur near the sagittal sinus, the sella, the olfactory groove, and the tentorium and along the petrous ridges. Tumors of childhood characteristically occur near the

midline of the brain. Intracranial tumors very rarely metastasize to other organs, but medulloblastomas and ependymomas may spread through the subarachnoid space. Low-grade gliomas tend to recur even after complete excision, and recurrent low-grade gliomas can degenerate into malignant variants. The median survival of patients with high-grade astrocytomas (glioblastoma multiforme) is less than 12 months.

Answer: C, D, E

19. Which one or more of the following statements is/are true regarding the presentation of brain tumors?

A. The basic pattern of presentation is one of progressive neurologic deficit
B. Unlike metabolic processes, brain tumors produce only focal neurologic deficits
C. Brain tumors produce symptoms by pushing rather than invading adjacent brain tissue
D. The neurologic deficits produced by brain tumors tend to be partial rather than complete

Sabiston: 1372
Schwartz: 1801

Comments: While brain tumors may produce a wide variety of presenting symptoms, the basic pattern is one of progressive neurologic deficit. Compression of neural tissue, infiltration and destruction of neural tissue, alterations in neural blood supply or irritability, alterations in CSF circulation, and mass effect are the mechanisms by which brain tumors produce their symptoms. Often, the neurologic deficit is partial rather than complete (e.g., hemiparesis rather than hemiplegia). The onset of convulsive seizures (35% of adults with brain tumors develop seizures) or progression in the frequency or severity of seizures or in the postictal neurologic deficit is suggestive of brain tumor. Increased intracranial pressure can result in generalized manifestations such as cloudy mentation and headache accompanied by papilledema, vomiting, bradycardia, and hypertension. This increased pressure may be caused by the tumor mass itself, cerebral edema, impaired CSF circulation, or a combination of all. Examples of focal manifestations secondary to brain tumors include focal jacksonian seizures, anosmia caused by olfactory groove meningioma, monocular visual loss caused by optic nerve glioma, bitemporal visual field defects caused by tumor compression of the optic chiasma (pituitary adenoma, craniopharyngioma), unusual facial pain caused by tumors in the vicinity of the trigeminal nerve, and tinnitus and hearing loss caused by acoustic neuromas.

Answer: A, D

20. Which one or more of the following statements is/are true regarding evaluation and treatment of brain tumors?

A. CT scan and angiography are the primary diagnostic methods used in evaluating brain tumors
B. MRI may yield important metabolic as well as anatomic information
C. Nonmalignant intracranial tumors are observed rather than resected to avoid the risk of surgically related neurologic deficits

D. Most tumors of the central nervous system are radio-sensitive

Sabiston: 1373
Schwartz: 1801

Comments: CT and angiography are the diagnostic main-stays for evaluating brain tumors, although MRI is becoming more useful, not only for its anatomic accuracy, but also because it has the potential to provide information about various regional metabolic events. When possible, brain tumors should be removed, regardless of the degree of malignancy, since the tolerance for expanding intracranial masses is very low. When tumors are unresectable or recurrent, secondary alterations in CSF circulation may be treated by placement of a CSF shunt. With the exception of pituitary adenomas, craniopharyngiomas, and certain pineal region tumors, intracranial tumors are relatively insensitive to radiation therapy. However, the modality is useful for unresectable or incompletely resected tumors since some do respond transiently. Brain necrosis may occur 12 to 24 months after total brain radiation; therefore, in patients expected to survive beyond 2 years, this risk must be weighed against the possible benefits of radiation therapy. To date, no combination of radiation therapy, chemotherapy, and immunotherapy has been developed that effectively treats glioblastoma multiforme.

Answer: A, B

21. Which one or more of the following statements is/are true regarding pituitary tumors?

A. The classification of pituitary tumors depends solely on their aniline dye affinity
B. The most common pituitary tumor is endocrine-inactive
C. Common parasellar symptoms include cerebrospinal fluid obstruction
D. Prolactin excess in males causes decreased potency and infertility
E. Surgery and radiation therapy are the mainstays of treatment

Sabiston: 650
Schwartz: 1802

Comments: Pituitary tumors formerly were classified according to their affinity for aniline dyes (chromophobe, eosinophilic, or basophilic adenomas). The more recent classification divides them into endocrine-active and endocrine-inactive tumors. The most common pituitary adenoma is the prolactin-producing adenoma, followed (in decreasing order of frequency) by endocrine-inactive tumors, growth hormone–producing tumors, ACTH-producing tumors, TSH-producing tumors, and, finally, LSH-FSH–producing tumors. Tumors less than 1 cm in diameter are termed microadenomas, while those greater than 1 cm in diameter are called macroadenomas. Symptomatology depends on the type of hormone produced, the degree of compromise of the surrounding anterior pituitary (symptoms of hormone insufficiency), and the mass effect of the tumor itself producing parasellar neurologic deficits. In the female, prolactin excess causes menstrual irregularities, infertility, and galactorrhea. In

the male, they lead to decreased potency and infertility. Growth hormone excess causes gigantism in young patients and acromegaly in patients whose epiphyses are closed. ACTH-producing adenomas cause Cushing's disease. TSH-producing adenomas are associated with thyroid insufficiency, while LSH-FSH–producing adenomas lead to gonadal insufficiency. Parasellar deficits include optic nerve dysfunction, extraocular motor loss, hypothalamic dysfunction, or frontal and medial temporal lobe signs and symptoms. The most effective therapies for symptomatic pituitary adenomas remain surgery and radiation therapy, although TSH-producing and FSH-LSH–producing adenomas may decrease in size in response to exogenous hormone therapy. Similarly, prolactin-producing adenomas may decrease in size in response to bromocriptine therapy.

Answer: D, E

22. True statements regarding spinal cord tumors include:

A. Spinal cord tumors occur as frequently as intracranial tumors
B. Like intracranial tumors, most spinal cord tumors are malignant
C. Spinal cord tumors are divided according to location into extradural and intradural tumors
D. Intradural tumors are divided by location into extramedullary and intramedullary tumors

Sabiston: 1392
Schwartz: 1804

Comments: Spinal cord tumors are one sixth as common as intracranial tumors. While most intracranial adult tumors are malignant, 60% of spinal cord tumors are benign. Many of the malignant spinal cord tumors seem to have a better prognosis than their intracranial counterparts. Metastatic tumors occur as frequently as primary tumors. Spinal metastases and primary spinal neoplasms (malignant and benign) are classified according to their relationship to the dura and spinal cord. They are divided into extradural and intradural groups, the intradural group being divided into the extramedullary and intramedullary locations.

Answer: C, D

23. True statements regarding spinal cord tumors include which one or more of the following?

A. Most intradural tumors are benign
B. Most extradural tumors are malignant
C. Most extradural neoplasms are metastatic tumors
D. Extradural tumors tend to progress rapidly
E. Intradural tumors tend to progress slowly

Sabiston: 1393
Schwartz: 1804

Comments: The majority of extradural tumors are malignant (90%), while most intradural tumors are benign (60%). Most extradural tumors are metastatic (75%), while most intradural tumors are primary (98%). Extradural tumors (usually metastatic) present with pain and rapid spinal cord compression (due to either tumor effect or vertebral collapse), leading to progressive flaccid paralysis and sensory loss. Surgical decompression can provide significant palliation only when performed prior to the occurrence of advanced neurologic loss. Intradural tumors usually present more slowly over months or years. Their motor deficit is often a spastic paralysis accompanied by sensory loss. Despite these differences, spinal cord lesions should be considered when any progressive neurologic loss occurs distal to any transverse level in the spinal cord.

Answer: A, B, C, D, E

24. True statements regarding the signs and symptoms of spinal cord tumors include:

A. Local signs can result from involvement of the anterior motor horn cells
B. Local signs occur in a segmental distribution, allowing localization of the tumor in a rostral caudal orientation
C. Flaccid paralysis is the result of slow onset of tumor compression
D. Spastic paralysis is the result of slow onset of tumor compression
E. Tract signs allow localization of the tumor to a point at or cephalad to the highest level of involvement

Sabiston: 1393
Schwartz: 1804

Comments: Local signs are segmental changes that allow rostral caudal localization. Local motor signs result from involvement of the anterior motor horn cells or anterior spinal roots and leads to weakness and loss of reflexes, fasciculation, and atrophy in a dermatome pattern. Local sensory signs are due to involvement of the dorsal root or dorsal root entry zone, producing localized pain, radicular or radiating pain, and loss of sensation over a dermatome distribution. Local sensory signs may result from involvement of fibers crossing in the anterior commissure secondary to a central lesion of the spinal cord. In this setting the sensory deficit is loss of pain and temperature sensation with persistence of touch, a situation called sensory dissociation. Tract signs indicate the lesion is at or cephalad to the highest point of involvement. Motor changes depend on the rapidity of onset, with rapid loss of function leading to flaccid areflexic paralysis and slow progressive loss leading to spastic paralysis. Other tract signs can include loss of pain and temperature sensation (anterolateral fasciculus involvement), loss of position and vibratory sense (dorsal column involvement), weakness, spasticity, hyperreflexia, and Babinski sign (resulting from posterolateral fasciculus involvement).

Answer: A, B, D, E

25. Match spinal location in the left-hand column with the most common tumor type in the right-hand column.

Spinal Location	Type
A. Extradural	a. Usually metastatic
B. Intradural, extramedullary	b. Usually neurofibroma or meningioma
C. Intradural, intramedullary	c. Usually gliomas

Sabiston: 1393
Schwartz: 1805

Comments: As previously stated, with the exception of a rare benign meningioma, neurofibroma, hemangioma, giant cell tumor, or osteoma of the vertebrae, extradural tumors are malignant, usually metastatic. More than half of all intradural tumors are extramedullary, and of these the majority are neurofibromas or meningiomas. Neurofibromas show no sex predilection, are often multiple, and are more common in the thoracic and cervical area. Meningiomas are more common in females and in the thoracic region. Like extradural tumors, intradural extramedullary tumors cause local and radicular pain associated with progressive spinal cord malfunction. One pattern of dysfunction is the Brown-Séquard syndrome with loss of sensitivity to temperature and pinprick on one side below the lesion with weakness and spasticity more marked on the opposite side. Nearly all intradural intramedullary tumors are gliomas, which tend to be more benign histologically than their intracerebral counterparts. In contrast to intradural extramedullary tumors, intramedullary tumors rarely cause local or radicular pain and can lead to damage of the crossing fibers of the anterior column, creating loss of pain and temperature sensation with preservation of touch (sensory dissociation).

Answer: A–a; B–b; C–c

26. True statements regarding the anatomy of the blood supply to the brain include:

A. The cervical portion of the internal carotid artery gives off the internal and external maxillary arteries
B. The petrous portion of the internal carotid artery gives off branches to the orbit
C. The circle of Willis is fully developed in only 18% of the population
D. The vertebral artery has communications with the thyrocervical trunk and posterior branches of the external carotid artery

Sabiston: 1847
Schwartz: 1806

Comments: The major blood supply to the brain is via the paired internal carotid and vertebral arteries. The internal carotid artery is divided into the cervical portion (which has no branches) and the petrous, cavernous, and intradural portions. The petrous portion has branches that anastomose with the internal maxillary artery, a branch of the external carotid artery. Branches of the cavernous portion include arteries to the cavernous sinus, semilunar and meningeal arteries (which anastomose with meningeal branches of the internal maxillary artery), and the ophthalmic artery (which has anastomoses with terminal branches of the external maxillary artery). These communications create important extracranial-intracranial anastomoses that become significant with certain types of occlusive lesions. The intradural branches of the internal carotid artery include the anterior cerebral, middle cerebral, posterior communicating, and anterior choroidal arteries. The vertebral arteries have anastomotic branches to the thyrocervical trunk of the subclavian artery and to the posterior branches of the external carotid artery. After crossing the dura, the vertebral arteries join to form the basilar artery that supplies the brain stem. This ultimately divides into the posterior cerebral arteries. The circle of Willis, fully developed in 18% of the population, is therefore formed by branches of the internal carotid and vertebral arteries: the anterior cerebrals (joined by the anterior communicating artery) and the posterior communicating arteries of the internal carotid join the posterior cerebral arteries of the vertebral artery to create the circle of Willis.

Answer: C, D

27. True statements regarding cerebral ischemia and infarction include:

A. To fill the criteria as a transient ischemic attack (TIA), symptoms must resolve in 12 hours or less
B. TIA's produced by emboli originating in the carotid arteries can produce hemiparesis, hemisensory disturbances, and amaurosis fugax
C. Vertebral basilar TIA's may produce vertigo, dysarthria, facial paresthesias, diplopia, and occasionally paresis and "drop attacks"
D. One third of patients with carotid TIA's progress to full stroke in 5 years
E. The immediate mortality for intracerebral thrombosis is greater than that for intracerebral embolism

Sabiston: 1848
Schwartz: 1808

Comments: A transient ischemic attack (TIA) produces focal neurologic signs and symptoms that resolve within 24 hours. TIA's tend to recur and produce symptoms according to the region of perfusion involved (as above). One third of patients with carotid TIA's progress to complete stroke within 5 years. The incidence of stroke is less frequent in patients with vertebral basilar TIA's. The immediate mortality for intracerebral hemorrhage, embolism, and thrombosis is 93, 60, and 37%, respectively. Survivors have an annual death rate of 16 to 18%. Some patients with carotid ischemia and infarction are helped with surgery. The ideal candidate is the patient with carotid TIA's, an isolated extracranial lesion, and no neurologic deficit. Some patients with intracranial lesions may be treated by one of a number of extracranial-intracranial bypass procedures (such as the superficial temporal artery–middle cerebral artery bypass), but long-term follow-up suggests that there is no significant impact on the natural history of the underlying disease. Another group of patients who may be helped by surgery are those with completed infarcts or intracerebral hemorrhage in whom progressive focal deficits and brain stem involvement occur usually 12 to 36 hours post-stroke. In these cases the deterioration is caused by the mass effect of brain swelling or clot and occasionally can be reversed by craniotomy.

Answer: B, C, D

28. Which of the following statements is/are true regarding intracerebral aneurysms?

A. The most common site is the middle meningeal artery
B. Most are multiple
C. Rupture occurs with equal frequency in patients with and without hypertension
D. Silent aneurysms occur with equal frequency in patients with and without hypertension
E. Focal neurologic deficit with headache is the usual clinical presentation of ruptured intracerebral aneurysms

Sabiston: 1376
Schwartz: 1810

Comments: Most intracranial aneurysms arise from the large intracerebral arteries of the circle of Willis and at the origin of the vertebrobasilar arteries. The most common sites in decreasing order include the internal carotid artery, the anterior cerebral artery, the middle cerebral artery, and the vertebrobasilar system. Multiple aneurysms are present 20% of the time. When multiple, they tend to be symmetrical in distribution or arise from the same parent artery. Most aneurysms are congenital and are probably due to defects in the muscular and elastic layers of the intracerebral arteries. They have a saccular or berry-like shape, hence the name berry aneurysm. The incidence of silent aneurysms is the same in patients with and without hypertension. However, rupture is more common in patients with hypertension. The majority of ruptures occur between the ages of 40 and 60. Sudden headache followed by altered consciousness is the usual clinical pattern following subarachnoid hemorrhage. Focal neurologic deficits may occur, but are less common than those occurring after occlusion of major intracranial arteries. The sequelae vary depending on the size of the bleed and range from headache to death. The goal of treatment is to isolate the aneurysm from the force of systolic blood flow. This should be attempted as early as possible, since the likelihood of secondary rupture increases with time. A contraindication to early surgical intervention is the presence of neurologic deficit due to spasm of the circle of Willis caused by the irritating effect of blood in the cerebrospinal fluid.

Answer: D

29. Which of the following statements is/are true regarding intracranial arteriovenous malformations?

A. The majority of AV malformations result from closed head trauma
B. Most are silent unless they bleed
C. Rupture due to AV malformations tends to occur at a younger age than that due to intracranial aneurysms
D. Surgical excision is contraindicated unless there is a history of hemorrhage

Sabiston: 1379
Schwartz: 1811

Comments: AV malformations are the second most common congenital vascular abnormality of the central nervous system following intracranial aneurysm. They are frequently associated with neurologic deficits and seizures of varying severity due to shunting of blood from the surrounding brain tissue. In addition, they may cause subarachnoid or intracerebral hemorrhage. Hemorrhage due to AV malformations occurs at a younger age (20 to 49 years of age) than that due to intracranial aneurysm. Hematomas secondary to AV malformations tend to occur in the white matter of the cerebral hemisphere as well as in the cerebellum, spinal cord, and brain stem. When possible, exploration and resection of AV malformations is indicated. Feasibility of resection is determined by the size of the malformation, its position within the brain, and the source of its arterial supply.

Answer: C

30. Which of the following statements is/are true regarding surgical treatment of seizure disorders?

A. Two thirds of patients have their first seizure before the age of 20
B. The incidence of tumor as an etiologic cause increases with age
C. Frontal lobe foci respond best to surgical intervention
D. Gliosis is the most common pathologic finding in resected seizure foci

Sabiston: 1419
Schwartz: 1812

Comments: Two thirds of patients have their first seizure before the age of 20 years. The older the patient at presentation, the more likely it is that a focal etiologic cause such as tumor or an AV malformation can be found. The efficacy of medical control is variable in several series, with 50% of patients achieving total control and 25% achieving partial control. This leaves a large number of patients with seizure disorders that cannot be controlled by medicine. Surgery is reserved for patients in whom medical treatment fails and who have findings suggestive of a focal source of their seizures. Before surgery is indicated, therefore, medical management is developed optimally, the presence of multifocal disease is excluded, and structural CNS abnormalities are searched for. Of patients with intractable seizure disorders, 15 to 25% are eventually found to have an intracranial mass. In patients without radiographic findings, gliosis is the most common pathologic finding in the resected seizure focus. After surgery, anticonvulsants are continued for 5 years; then, if the patient remains seizure-free, they are gradually discontinued. Patients with well localized temporal lobe foci enjoy the most success following operation, while patients with foci of the frontal, parietal, or occipital lobes do less well. In patients with unresectable mass lesions, the severity of the seizure disorder can be reduced by partial excision and, if the lesion is malignant, radiation therapy. For patients with multifocal seizure disorders, several experimental procedures hold promise, including subcortical radiofrequency ablation, and limited or complete section of the corpus callosum.

Answer: A, B, D

31. Which of the following statements is/are true regarding infections of the skull and epidural space?

A. They commonly result from extension of infection from the paranasal sinuses, mastoid air cells, or middle ear
B. Skull infection can be adequately treated with antibiotics because of the rich blood supply
C. Epidural abscesses can cause meningitis and brain abscesses

D. Focal neurologic deficits are rarely seen with epidural abscesses

Sabiston: 1389
Schwartz: 1813

Comments: Central nervous system infections become surgically significant when they produce a mass effect (due to pus, edema, or effusion), osteomyelitis, or hydrocephalus. Osteomyelitis develops (1) as a direct extension of infection in the paranasal sinuses, middle ear, or mastoid air cells, (2) secondary to infected scalp wounds that extend below the galea, or (3) by hematogenous spread. The most common organisms involved are *Staphylococcus aureus* and the gram-negative bacteria of ear infection. Spread usually occurs along the diploic and epidural spaces, and can result in inflammation of the brain. The treatment is excision of involved bone and drainage of the area, combined with appropriate antibiotics. Epidural abscesses usually occur adjacent to skull infections in the vicinity of the middle ear, mastoid air cell, and nasal sinuses. When they break through the dura, meningitis and brain abscesses can occur. Unlike simple skull infections, focal neurologic deficits and seizures are more common. Treatment consists of drainage, excision of involved bone, and the appropriate antibiotics.

Answer: A, C

32. Which of the following statements is/are true regarding subdural empyema?

A. Subdural empyema most commonly occurs as the result of hematogenous spread
B. The most common organisms involved are staphylococci and streptococci
C. Dural attachments prevent rapid spread
D. Drainage of the pus and systemic antibiotics are the treatment of choice

Sabiston: 1389
Schwartz: 1814

Comments: Subdural empyema most commonly arises from infections of the paranasal sinuses. It is most commonly caused by acute staphylococcal or streptococcal infection superimposed on a chronic sinusitis. When this occurs, it can lead to serious neurologic deficit within a matter of hours since there is no structural barrier to spread of infection in the subdural space. The infection can cause thrombosis of the veins traversing the subdural space from cortex to the dural sinuses as well as irritation of the underlying brain, leading to acute meningitis and encephalitis. A mass effect is often produced secondary to inflammation, venous thrombosis, and pus accumulation. The typical symptom pattern is rapid development of seizures, meningitis, and neurologic deficits in a patient with a previous history of chronic sinusitis or middle ear infection. Because the entire subdural space over one side of the cortex can be involved, and because of the reactive inflammation and swelling below the dura, treatment includes drainage of the subdural space by craniotomy and prolonged antibiotic therapy.

Answer: B, D

33. Which of the following statements is/are true regarding brain abscesses?

A. The brain is highly susceptible to infection owing to its high glucose content
B. The brain is extremely effective in walling off infections
C. Brain abscesses are classified as acute, chronic, and subacute
D. Prompt drainage is indicated for all types of brain abscesses

Sabiston: 1389
Schwartz: 1815

Comments: The brain is generally resistant to infection unless previously damaged by trauma, hemorrhage, or anoxia. Once infected, the brain is very effective in walling off infection and is capable of isolating the abscess from the uninvolved brain and systemic circulation, making sterilization by systemic antiobiotics nearly impossible. The three major sources of brain abscesses include: (1) direct extension from middle ear, mastoid, and nasal sinus infections (commonly affecting the temporal lobe and cerebellar hemispheres), (2) hematogenous spread (as occurs in cyanotic heart defects with right-to-left shunts), and (3) direct trauma. The most common organisms are streptococci, pneumococci, and staphylococci. Brain abscesses are classified as **acute**—which follows a course similar to and difficult to differentiate from subdural empyema; **chronic**—often presenting with progressive neurologic deficit and an expanding mass with a short (2- to 3-week) history; and **subacute**—presenting with a picture somewhere between acute and chronic. CT scanning is the most accurate means of making the diagnosis and is mandatory before surgical drainage. Treatment of a "walled off" abscess is surgical drainage by needle aspiration, open drainage, or excision of the abscess cavity. Treatment of acute abscesses is supportive (antibiotics and anti-inflammatory agents such as steroids) until a capsule forms (usually in 10 to 12 days) followed by drainage, although newer antibiotics may prevent the need for surgery in many cases.

Answer: B, C

34. Which of the following statements is/are true regarding neurologic problems in premature infants?

A. The major risk in this group of patients is intraventricular hemorrhage
B. The risk of intraventricular hemorrhage varies from 40 to 50% depending on birth weight
C. Hydrocephalus due to bacterial infection is a common problem in this age group
D. Hydrocephalus present at the time of birth in a premature infant may improve with time and not require chronic drainage

Sabiston: 1408
Schwartz: 1824

Comments: Preterm infants weighing less than 1500 gm face a 40 to 50% risk of intraventricular hemorrhage at birth. This risk depends on the weight of the infant. Hydrocephalus is also a common problem and is caused by

either blockage of cerebrospinal fluid flow by clot, or decreased cerebrospinal fluid absorption due to immaturity of the arachnoid granulation tissue. In some infants, this cause of decreased absorption gradually improves, sometimes resulting in return to normal ventricular pressures.

Answer: A, B, D

35. Which of the following statements is/are true regarding hydrocephalus?

A. It represents a primary process in up to two thirds of patients
B. It is classified as communicating or noncommunicating
C. In communicating hydrocephalus, obstruction to cerebrospinal fluid flow is outside the ventricular system
D. With proper shunting, patients with hydrocephalus usually have intelligence equal to that of matched control groups without hydrocephalus

Sabiston: 1408
Schwartz: 1826

Comments: Hydrocephalus is a secondary, not a primary, problem. Causes of hydrocephalus include aqueductal stenosis, dysfunction of arachnoidal granulations, subarachnoidal scarring, and cerebrospinal fluid blockage by clot or tumor. Hydrocephalus is classified as communicating or noncommunicating. In communicating hydrocephalus, obstruction to flow is outside the ventricular system. In noncommunicating hydrocephalus, there is obstruction of flow of the cerebrospinal fluid from inside the ventricular system. Most cases of hydrocephalus are treated by pressure-activated shunts, the most common being the ventriculoperitoneal (VP) shunt. Although treated patients usually attain acceptable intelligence (and some in fact are very bright), overall, shunted patients do not do as well intellectually as nonhydrocephalic matched control groups.

Answer: B, C

36. Which of the following statements is/are true regarding neurosurgery in children between the ages of 2 and 10?

A. Trauma is the most common neurosurgical problem in this age group
B. Closed head trauma in young children can produce hypovolemic shock
C. Headaches more frequently indicate surgical pathology in adults than in young children
D. Vascular abnormalities found in children should be left untreated until the patient reaches middle age

Schwartz: 1825

Comments: Trauma is the most common neurologic problem in young children. Prior to closure of cranial suture lines, head injury is more likely to cause shock than in adults because an open fontanelle and expansile sutures allow intracranial sequestration of enough blood to cause hypovolemia. Because of the flexibility of the immature skull, dural vessels may be torn and significant cerebral damage occur without evidence of fracture. For this reason, in-hospital observation following loss of consciousness is indicated in this age group. Also in this age group, closed head injury without clear etiology should suggest the possibility of child abuse. In adolescents and adults, headache may often occur without significant pathology, whereas in children headaches are more likely to be due to significant underlying pathology. Tumors in this age group tend to occur in the midline and include medulloblastomas and ependymomas, pineal gland tumors, craniopharyngiomas, and neural ectodermal tumors. Laterally placed tumors in this age group include the choroid plexus papilloma. Vascular malformations and aneurysms do occur in this age group, and the approach to their treatment is essentially the same as in adults.

Answer: A, B

37. Which of the following statements is/are true regarding neurosurgical treatment in the newborn?

A. Neurosurgery in newborns is primarily treatment of congenital abnormalities
B. The most common congenital midline abnormality is the myelomeningocele
C. The most common congenital abnormalities are the craniosynostoses
D. For maximum effectiveness, procedures to correct craniosyntosis should be performed as soon as possible

Sabiston: 1407
Schwartz: 1824

Comments: Pediatric neurosurgery is mainly the treatment of congenital abnormalities. However, in this age group, there are several acquired problems including hemorrhagic hydrocephalus, subdural hematoma, and fractures of the skull. The most common of the dysraph- isms (failure of the structures of the CNS to join properly in the midline) is the myelomeningocele. This disorder occurs in utero between 21 and 25 days after conception. Its diagnosis is suggested by elevated alpha-fetoprotein levels found in maternal serum or in amniotic fluid. The area most commonly affected is the lumbosacral area, where surgical closure protects the underlying nervous system from mechanical trauma and infection, but does not generally improve lower extremity function. Craniosynostosis is another common congenital problem noted in the postnatal period. It results from premature closure of skull sutures that do not allow expansion as the underlying brain grows. Total craniosynostoses are rare; metopic, coronal, and lambdoidal synostoses are more common. Sagittal is the most common of all and fortunately is not associated with the concern of possible diminished intelligence. The most important diagnostic procedure is a good clinical examination that raises suspicion based on premature closure of fontanelles (an altered shape of the head is a later sign). Since only 50% of abnormal sutures will appear on x-ray or bone scan, the importance of physical examination cannot be overemphasized. Uncorrected synostoses will give rise to one of the following abnormalities: **sagittal**—a long, narrow head with a ridge along the sagittal suture; **coronal**—a narrow anterior cranial vault with angled orbits such that their lateral margins are well posterior of the medial margins; **metopic**—resembles coronal synostosis with an additional midline forehead ridge; **lambdoidal**—a flattening of the ipsilateral occiput and protrusion and anterior displacement of ipsilateral ear. One treatment of synostoses is linear craniectomy to create an artificial suture line that is then lined with Silastic film. This procedure allows the brain to grow normally, or to reshape the head if it is deformed. For maximum effectiveness, these procedures are performed as soon as circulating blood volume is adequate (to allow for blood loss at surgery).

Answer: A, B, D

CHAPTER 54

Amputations

1. Match the amputations with their characteristics.

Characteristics	Amputations
A. Tissues are cut circularly and allowed to retract	a. Conventional
B. The periosteal flap is developed and is closed to seal the marrow, and antagonist muscles are sutured across the bone end	b. Osteomyoplastic
C. Transected muscles are attached to bone by suturing through drill holes placed at the distal bone	c. Myodesis
D. Skin (curved), fascia, and muscle transection based at level of amputation, then closed over the bone	d. Open "guillotine"

Schwartz: 2045

Comments: The **conventional** amputation utilizes curved skin and fascial flaps based at the level of amputation. Fitting for a prosthesis is delayed until healing has occurred. The **osteomyoplastic** amputation and the **myodesis** amputation provide for improved function and allow the application of immediate postsurgical prosthetic devices. The **open** or "**guillotine**" amputation should be regarded as an emergency or drainage procedure. The results are usually poor, and reamputation is often necessary. If infection is likely, it is preferable to perform a conventional amputation with slightly longer than usual flaps, which are left open initially but then revised and closed 3 to 5 days postoperatively.

Answer: A–d; B–b; C–c; D–a

2. Principles of postoperative management after amputation include:

A. Splinting of the stump dressing to avoid shifting in position
B. Compression dressing over the stump to avoid postoperative edema and hematoma
C. Exercise and positioning to avoid contracture

D. Early evaluation and care by a qualified physical therapist and prosthetist

Sabiston: 1491
Schwartz: 2045

Comments: Conventional postoperative care begins with the application of a light compression dressing in the operating room followed by repeated application of elastic dressings to avoid stump edema. Stump exercises and stretching prevent contracture after primary wound healing has taken place. Progressive training after suture removal allows the eventual application of a permanent prosthesis. Alternately, application of a rigid dressing in the operating room allows the immediate use of a prosthetic device; immediate prosthetic fitting, however, need not be employed in order to utilize the rigid dressing. Rigid dressings offer the advantage of immediate use of the extremity, and wound healing may be enhanced by maximum control of edema and hematoma as well as by better tissue immobilization. When treatment is successful, resumption of full activity can be expected to occur within 4 to 6 weeks.

Answer: A, B, C, D

3. Regarding the proper selection of the level of amputation, which of the following is/are true?

A. The extent of resection for malignant tumors must not be compromised for functional considerations
B. The use of skin grafts and flaps to conserve bony length is appropriate in healthy, stable trauma patients
C. Unless 4 inches or more of tibia can be preserved, the knee joint should be sacrificed
D. The presence of contracture should not influence the level of amputation

Sabiston: 1490
Schwartz: 2043

Comments: As a general principle, the longer the amputation stump, the more functional the limb. However, when performing amputations for malignancy, adequate tumor excision, not preservation of stump length, is the primary concern. The irregular damage to skin caused by trauma can be treated by skin grafts and flaps to preserve bony length. Amputations in patients with peripheral vascular disease succeed when performed at levels having adequate nutritional blood flow to the skin. Below-knee stumps as short as 2 inches can be successfully fitted with prostheses. Preservation of the knee joint allows a bent-knee, end-weight–bearing prosthesis to be used and is sometimes preferable to a long above-knee stump. Amputations above the knee should remove at least 4 inches of femur to facilitate fitting of a prosthetic knee joint. It is preferable to amputate above the level of contracture to enhance rehabilitation.

Answer: A, B

4. Useful preoperative tests to evaluate adequacy of blood flow in patients with peripheral vascular disease undergoing amputation include:

A. Clinical assessment of cutaneous blood flow
B. Cutaneous radioxenon clearance
C. Status of peripheral pulses
D. Doppler systolic blood pressure

Sabiston: 1490
Schwartz: 2044

Comments: The healing ability of an amputation stump is determined by the adequacy of the nutritional blood flow to the skin. This can be assessed clinically (skin temperature, capillary refill, status of cutaneous appendages) as well as empirically by measurement of radioxenon clearance at the level of the anticipated line of incision (a flow of greater than 0.6 mg per gram of tissue is desired). Palpable popliteal pulses are associated with a higher success rate for below-knee amputations, but their absence is not considered a contraindication. A Doppler systolic blood pressure in the calf of greater than 74 mm Hg is associated with a high success rate for below-knee amputations, but has a high false negative rate and should not be used as the single criterion for evaluation. Ankle to brachial pressures may be useful in predicting the outcome of forefoot amputations.

Answer: A, B, C, D

5. True statements regarding amputations of the toes or feet include:

A. Transphalangeal amputations may be used as long as the necrosis is distal to the metatarsophalangeal joint
B. When the entire toe must be removed, disarticulation is preferred over transmetatarsal amputation
C. Toe amputations should never be attempted in patients who do not have pedal pulses
D. Rehabilitation after a transmetatarsal amputation requires no special prosthesis

Sabiston: 1492
Schwartz: 2046

Comment: Transphalangeal amputations may be used if the necrosis is distal to the proximal interphalangeal joint

and if the proximal skin is free of cellulitis and edema. When the entire toe must be amputated, a transmetatarsal level is preferred over disarticulation to avoid problems with the bulky metatarsal head and with the poor vascular supply to the articular cartilage. Patients with palpable popliteal and pedal pulses who have transmetatarsal amputations do better than those without, but their absence is not considered an absolute contraindication. Ambulation may be started after the incision is healed; no special shoe is required, but a shoe filler improves gait.

Answer: D

6. Syme's amputation is best suited for:

A. Males
B. Most peripheral vascular disorders involving the feet
C. A foot destroyed by trauma
D. Anticipation of lower extremity weight-bearing

Sabiston: 1493
Schwartz: 2047

Comments: Syme's amputation is created at a bone level just proximal to the tibial flare with preservation of the heel pad. It maintains the length of the lower extremity and allows creation of an end-weight–bearing stump. It is usually performed when the majority of the foot is destroyed by trauma. Rarely, it is successful in the dysvascular or diabetic patient. In the majority of cases it requires a complex prosthesis that some patients may find cosmetically unacceptable.

Answer: A, C, D

7. Advantages of a below-knee (BK) amputation over an above-knee (AK) amputation include:

A. Enhanced patient mobility
B. A prosthesis more compatible with complete rehabilitation
C. Less phantom limb pain
D. A higher percentage of patients ultimately able to ambulate on their prosthesis

Sabiston: 1493
Schwartz: 2048

Comments: The BK amputation offers many advantages, including those listed above. Even if a BK stump is too short for a conventional BK prosthesis, when fitted with a bent-knee prosthesis, it is preferred over a long AK stump. Ischemic lesions of the foot extending above the malleoli and ischemic rigor of calf muscles are considered contraindications to the BK amputation. Relative contraindications include knee or hip contracture, since these negate the functional advantages of the BK amputation. The patient's general health and potential for rehabilitation and the vascular supply at the level of amputation should determine the choice between BK and AK amputations.

Answer: A, B, C, D

8. Knee disarticulation has which of the following advantages?

A. In children it is useful for maintaining the epiphysis for bony growth
B. In adults it is used to preserve bony length when severe ischemia contraindicates a BK amputation
C. It provides maximal length with good end-weight–bearing characteristics
D. It is easily fitted with a simple prosthesis

Sabiston: 1495
Schwartz: 2050

Comments: Knee disarticulation is most often used in children because it allows maintenance of the epiphysis for bony growth. It is rarely used in situations in which there is impaired circulation. The procedure preserves maximum length, provides a good end-weight–bearing stump, and lends itself to a good fit between stump and socket. However, since the femoral condyles are preserved, the stump is bulky, and this can make prosthesis fitting difficult. The anterior flap is left longer than the posterior flap and the patella is preserved, if not involved by disease.

Answer: A, C

9. Indications for an above-knee amputation include:

A. Absent popliteal pulses
B. Diabetes mellitus
C. Gangrene proximal to the malleoli
D. Calf muscle rigor
E. Knee or hip contractures

Sabiston: 1495
Schwartz: 2051

Comments: Assessment of the vascular status at the level of amputation is important, but the absence of popliteal pulses or the presence of diabetes are not in themselves absolute indications for an AK amputation. Rigor of the calf muscles and the presence of gangrene of the skin at the level the flaps would be constructed for the below-knee amputation are sufficient indications for an AK amputation. Because knee and hip contractures make rehabilitation after BK amputation unlikely and since the AK amputation has the highest healing rate and the lowest reamputation rate in patients with peripheral vascular disease, patients so afflicted do best with an AK amputation.

Answer: C, D, E

10. Which of the following statements is/are true regarding hip disarticulation and hemipelvectomy?

A. Prostheses are unavailable for ambulation
B. The usual indications are bone tumors, soft tissue tumors, and, occasionally, extensive trauma
C. Flaps are brought together posteriorly after hip disarticulation
D. The entire ilium must be removed during hemipelvectomy

Sabiston: 1496
Schwartz: 2052

Comments: The indications for hip disarticulation are tumors of bone or soft tissue and, in some cases, extensive trauma. Hemipelvectomy is indicated when an upper thigh tumor cannot be excised by disarticulation alone. The posterior flap after hip disarticulation is closed anteriorly so that the patient can sit comfortably in the socket of the prosthesis. Whenever possible, a leaf of ilium and the pelvic rami are preserved during the hemipelvectomy so as to act as support points for the prosthesis. Both amputations can be fitted with a special (Canadian) prosthesis that allows ambulation.

Answer: B

11. Of the following statements, which is/are true regarding lower limb prostheses?

A. They require less energy to use than does crutch walking
B. The shorter the stump, the greater the stump tip pressure
C. The main pressure point in the BK prosthesis is the stump end
D. A suspension belt is mandatory for all above-knee prostheses

Sabiston: 1489
Schwartz: 2053

Comments: Prostheses are designed to restore function, mobility, and appearance. Except in cases involving diabetics with above-knee amputations, properly fitted prostheses have lower energy requirements when compared with crutch walking. Socket design has as its goals patient comfort and an even distribution of forces upon the stump. The longer the stump, the greater the surface area over which these forces can be distributed. Above-knee sockets are usually of the quadrilateral total contact design and are suspended either by stump suction or by pelvic belts. Below-knee prostheses most commonly used are the patellar tendon–bearing (PTB) type or the patellar tendon supracondylar (PTS) type.

Answer: A, B

12. In the order of decreasing frequency, amputations of the arm are performed for:

A. Tumor
B. Trauma
C. Peripheral vascular disease

Sabiston: 1496
Schwartz: 2055

Comments: Trauma and malignant tumors are the two most common indications for arm amputations. Only rarely are peripheral vascular diseases indications for arm amputation, the most common of these being thromboangiitis obliterans. The goal of amputation of the proximal arm is preservation of as much viable tissue as possible; for distal arm amputations it is preservation of the grasping function of the hand.

Answer: B, A, C

13. Regarding amputations about the hand, which of the following statements is/are true?

A. Digital tourniquets should be avoided when possible
B. Scar placement is of little concern
C. After suprametacarpal amputation, opposing tendons should be fixed to preserve muscle tone and strength
D. The precise nature of the operation requires a general anesthetic

Sabiston: 1496
Schwartz: 2056

Comments: Most patients undergoing lower extremity amputations have peripheral vascular disease, and the use of tourniquets is contraindicated. In the upper extremity, however, tourniquets (cuff pressure best tolerated at 280 mm Hg) are frequently used to provide a blood-free field, so that critical nerve and tendon structures can be identified. Because of the risk of thrombosis, digital tourniquets such as rubber bands should be avoided. Scars should be minimized and placed as far as possible from bone, tendon, nerve, and points of pressure. To best preserve muscle strength, tone, and hence function, opposing tendons should be fixed anatomically. In general, arm amputations are more precise operations than are leg amputations. Adequate anesthesia can often be accomplished by regional block; this is preferred in trauma patients, who may present with a full stomach, as it avoids the risk of vomiting and aspiration.

Answer: A, C

14. Which of the following statements is/are true regarding amputations of digits?

A. A shorter volar flap and a longer dorsal flap are desired
B. The root of the nail should always be preserved
C. In removal of the distal phalanx, the middle phalangeal cartilage should be preserved
D. Amputation at the metacarpophalangeal joint is preferable to amputation through the proximal phalanx
E. Even the smallest stump of the thumb is preferable to complete amputation with prosthesis

Sabiston: 1497
Schwartz: 2056

Comments: A longer volar flap is desired so that the scar can be positioned away from pressure-bearing surfaces. However, bone and viable tissue should never be sacrificed to obtain ideal scar placement. Unless more than half the nail bed can be preserved, the nail root should be removed. If the distal phalanx must be removed, the exposed middle phalangeal cartilage should be resected. Given a choice, resection through the proximal phalanx is preferred over a metacarpophalangeal amputation; as is the case with the thumb, any stump, no matter how short, has function. When a digit must be removed in its entirety, preservation of function of the hand as a unit is the goal and may require a variety of secondary procedures.

Answer: E

15. Which of the following statements is/are true regarding wrist disarticulation?

A. It provides better prosthesis control than does a long forearm amputation
B. The stump is stronger than that left when the amputation is through the carpal bones
C. The severed tendons and ligaments of the hand must be fixed to prevent their retraction and atrophy
D. Preservation of the styloid processes is necessary for prosthetic fitting

Sabiston: 1498
Schwartz: 2057

Comments: Wrist disarticulation has several advantages over more proximal amputations. It preserves length and provides better control of prosthesis. While it is less strong than when the carpal bones remain, it accommodates a less conspicuous prosthesis. The styloid processes are removed to permit a smoother fit. The tendons of the hand are transected with the muscles at rest and fixed to periosteum to prevent retraction and atrophy.

Answer: A, C

16. Which of the following statements is/are true regarding forearm amputations?

A. Unless adequate muscle mass and length can be preserved, an above-elbow amputation is preferred so as to enhance prosthetic function
B. Skin mobility is preserved by avoiding excessive dissection between skin and fascia
C. A short stump of the ulna or radius can be lengthened secondarily by a bone graft or flap
D. Cineplastic operations using biceps or pectoralis muscles can provide function to artificial limbs when the amputation stump is very short

Sabiston: 1498
Schwartz: 2057

Comments: Dissection should be kept to a minimum to avoid immobilization of skin by subsequent scar formation. Pronation and supination should be preserved by striving for a longer stump. Also, the procedure should be conducted as atraumatically as possible to avoid fibrosis. Even a very short below-elbow stump is preferable to an above-elbow amputation. Functional control of a prosthesis fitted over a short stump can be provided by a cineplastic operation using the ipsilateral biceps or pectoralis muscle after the initial stump has healed. Other secondary procedures include the use of bone flaps or grafts to lengthen short stumps of the ulna or radius.

Answer: B, C, D

CHAPTER 55

Orthopedics—General Principles

1. Herniation of a cervical intervertebral disc can produce:

A. Nerve root compression
B. Spinal cord compression
C. Both nerve root and spinal cord compression
D. Local and referred pain without nerve root compression

Sabiston: 1398
Schwartz: 1834

Comments: Most patients with cervical disc degeneration have only symptoms of local and referred pain. **Lateral herniation** of a cervical disc may produce nerve root compression with radicular symptoms. **Posterior herniation** occurs less commonly and may result in spinal cord compression. There are eight cervical nerve roots: the first exits from the spinal canal between the occiput and the atlas. Therefore, nerve root compression produced by herniation of a cervical disc affects the nerve root immediately below it.

Answer: A, B, C, D

2. Which of the following diagnostic studies may be useful in the evaluation of hand/arm pain?

A. Adson test for thoracic outlet syndrome
B. Chest x-ray for Pancoast's tumor
C. Nerve conduction studies for carpal tunnel syndrome
D. Cervical spine x-rays for radicular compression
E. Finkelstein test

Sabiston: 1398, 1548
Schwartz: 937, 1834, 2087

Comments: Pain in the hand and/or forearm may result from various musculoskeletal or neurologic disorders. Neurogenic pain may reflect involvement at any level from the spinal cord to peripheral nerves. The cause can be determined from the history, physical examination,

382

and appropriate laboratory tests. Radiologic studies are important for the evaluation of cervical vertebral abnormalities and lung tumors. Nerve conduction studies confirm the clinical diagnosis of median nerve compression. The Adson test and other studies may be positive with thoracic outlet syndrome but are not diagnostic. The Finkelstein test produces pain in patients with entrapment of the abductor pollicis longus and extensor pollicis brevis (de Quervain's disease).

Answer: B, C, D, E

3. Acute cervical nerve root compression due to disc herniation may be treated by which of the following?

A. Bed rest and cervical traction
B. Prompt institution of active resistance exercises
C. Radiotherapy for progression of any neurologic deficit
D. Surgical decompression to prevent progression of deficit

Sabiston: 1399
Schwartz: 1836

Comments: In most acute cases, recumbency, sedation, and traction immobilization of the neck are indicated. When pain has subsided, or the attacks are less severe, exercises may be initiated to improve flexibility. Progression of the neurologic deficit and evidence of spinal cord compression are indications for an operative procedure, usually laminectomy and sometimes spinal fusion or disc removal. Radiotherapy is given for relief of symptoms caused by malignant disease and if there is bony stability; if not, bony stability may be obtained by a surgical procedure.

Answer: A, D

4. Match each spinal condition in left column with the appropriate phrase from the right column.

A. Spondylolisthesis
B. Spondylolysis
C. Both spondylolisthesis and spondylolysis
D. Neither spondylolisthesis nor spondylolysis

a. Defined as subluxation of a vertebral body
b. Defined as a bony defect of the neural arch
c. Commonly involves L5
d. Usually results from trauma

Sabiston: 1395
Schwartz: 1838

Comments: Spondylolisthesis is an anterior subluxation of one vertebral body, most commonly involving the fifth lumbar vertebra. It usually results from a structural defect in the vertebra that often is the result of spondylolysis, which is a defect of the bony neural arch and is believed to be inherited. Degenerative joint disease or stress fractures are other causes of spondylolisthesis. Neither of these terms should be confused with spondylosis, which is a general term for degenerative vertebral disease.

Answer: A–a; B–b; C–c; D–d

5. The tumor most commonly metastatic to the vertebral spine is:

A. Prostatic
B. Renal
C. Breast
D. Skin

Sabiston: 1393
Schwartz: 1845

Comments: The most common tumors of the vertebral column are metastatic. Multiple myelomas are among the most common primary tumors that involve the vertebral column. Most primary bone tumors occur less frequently in the vertebral column than in other parts of the skeleton; the exceptions are aneurysmal bone cyst, benign osteoblastoma, and chordoma.

Answer: C

6. The most common cause of sciatica is:

A. Intervertebral disc herniation
B. Alcoholism
C. Diabetic neuritis
D. Rheumatoid arthritis
E. Intraspinal tumor

Sabiston: 1396
Schwartz: 1840

Comments: Sciatica refers to a radicular type of pain involving the legs as a result of compression followed by simple inflammation of lumbosacral nerve roots. The most common cause, **compression,** can occur intraspinally, within the intervertebral foramen or within the pelvis or buttock. Herniation of a lumbar intervertebral disc is the most common cause of compression. Many **inflammatory** conditions may cause similar symptoms, but nonetheless, are less often responsible.

Answer: A

7. Coccydynia:

A. May be of traumatic origin
B. Is often associated with radicular symptoms
C. Is best treated by excision of the coccyx
D. Is often associated with anal sphincter incompetence

Schwartz: 1833

Comments: Pain in the coccyx or lower sacrum can be caused by trauma, arthritis, or disc protrusion. The pain must be clinically differentiated from other forms of perineal pain including proctalgia fugax, intergluteal fold inflammation, low pilonidal cyst infection, or dorsal perirectal abscess. The symptoms of coccydynia may be aggravating and progressive, but there is no radicular component or impairment of sphincter function. Treatment is usually nonoperative, consisting of heat, cushioned seating, and anti-inflammatory medications. Only rarely is operative intervention required.

Answer: A

8. Common initial symptoms of lumbar intervertebral disc herniation include:

A. Low backache
B. Radicular sciatic pain
C. Simultaneous backache and sciatic pain
D. Incontinence

Sabiston: 1397
Schwartz: 1841

Comments: Herniation of an intervertebral disc may proceed either vertically or horizontally. Vertical herniation into the body of the vertebra (Schmorl's node) has no clinical significance. Horizontal involvement can be a bulge in the annulus, herniation of the nucleus, or actual extrusion of the nucleus. Usually herniation is posterolateral and therefore accompanied by unilateral nerve root compression. About one half of patients initially have presenting symptoms of low back pain and later may develop sciatic pain. Approximately one third of patients first develop sciatica, however, and in the remainder, sciatica and back pain occur simultaneously. Anterolateral nuclear herniation is often associated with spondylosis.

Answer: A, B, C

9. In the physical examination of a patient with a prolapsed intervertebral disc:

A. The straight leg–raising test is usually positive on the side of prolapse
B. Dorsiflexion of the foot during straight leg–raising may aggravate pain
C. Sensory deficit is often present
D. Knee jerk is often absent

Sabiston: 1397
Schwartz: 1842

Comments: Examination of a patient with low back pain includes careful observation of movement, spinal curvature, and range of motion. Straight leg–raising with the patient in the supine position will produce ipsilateral pain when there is nerve root compression. Aggravation by subsequent dorsiflexion of the foot is known as Lasègue's sign. Neurologic examination may reveal hypesthesia and weakness according to the nerve root involved. Herniation at the L5–S1 level may be accompanied by a diminished ankle jerk. If the knee jerk is absent, compression is occurring at a higher level than usual.

Answer: A, B, C

10. Which of the following statements is/are true regarding the treatment of a herniated intervertebral disc?

A. Heat, rest, and analgesics provide relief in most cases
B. Laminectomy should be performed when the diagnosis is confirmed because of the risk of paraplegia
C. Epidural steroids are contraindicated
D. Injection of chymopapain may reduce the size of a protruding disc

Sabiston: 1397
Schwartz: 1844

Comments: An initial trial of conservative therapy is first recommended for most patients. Operative treatment involving laminectomy with removal of the herniated nucleus pulposus and possible concomitant spinal fusion is indicated for patients who fail to respond to an appropriate conservative regimen or who have frequent or severe attacks. Both epidural steroids and proteolytic enzyme injections have been beneficial in patients whose herniation has not progressed to frank extrusion.

Answer: A, D

11. Pyogenic osteomyelitis of the vertebral column is

A. Most commonly caused by tuberculosis
B. Usually associated with paravertebral abscess
C. Most common in the thoracic region
D. Most common in the elderly
E. Most common in men

Sabiston: 1500
Schwartz: 1845

Comments: Pyogenic osteomyelitis of the vertebral column is most commonly caused by hematogenous spread of *Staphylococcus aureus* from other sites. These infections most commonly occur in adolescents and young male adults, and most commonly involve the lumbar region. Paravertebral abscess formation as occurs with tuberculous osteomyelitis is uncommon. Treatment includes immobilization, antibiotics, and surgical débridement or drainage. An anterior operative approach is usually advised. Bone grafting may be required.

Answer: E

12. Principles of tendon transfer include:

A. The muscle used should retain its full strength after transfer
B. Joint contractures should be corrected prior to operation

C. Synergistic muscles provide better results
D. The selected muscle must have adequate excursion

Sabiston: 1538
Schwartz: 1853

Comments: Tendon transfer is used to restore function, muscle balance, and strength to joint motions in patients with various paralytic conditions. There are four main requirements for tendon transfer: (1) A muscle with adequate strength must be available, since one grade of strength is lost following transfer owing to loss of the direct line of action between the muscle origin and insertion. (2) The muscle must have adequate excursion to allow sufficient range of motion of the joint. (3) The joint must have passive range of motion prior to transfer. (4) Synergistic muscles generally provide better results, although tendon transfers of nonsynergistic muscles can be successful with proper rehabilitation.

Answer: B, C, D

13. Which of the following statements is/are true regarding orthopedic surgical treatment for patients with cerebral palsy?

A. It is usually indicated for the athetoid type of cerebral palsy
B. It is most often performed for treatment of spasticity
C. Stabilization procedures are more likely to be successful than tendon transfer
D. None of the above

Schwartz: 1855

Comments: In cerebral palsy, there is a nonprogressive, permanent upper motor neuron lesion of variable etiology. About one half of the patients have a spastic condition, and it is this group that is most likely to benefit from some form of operation. One fourth of patients have athetosis characterized by repetitive involuntary movements; operative correction is rarely useful, since correction of the deformity at one level may result in expression at a more proximal level. Orthopedic approaches to patients with cerebral palsy include weakening of spastic muscles by tendon lengthening, improving joint motion by tendon transfer, stabilization of deformed or contracted joints by arthrodesis, correction of deformities by osteotomy, and correction of leg-length inequality. Stabilization procedures are usually more successful, since tendon transfer requires muscle re-education which these patients may not be capable of achieving.

Answer: B, C

14. Which of the following statements is/are true regarding the role of orthopedic surgery in the patient with a stroke?

A. Peripheral nerve block may control spasticity
B. Muscle release procedures for the relief of spasticity are contraindicated owing to the consequent loss of muscle strength
C. Elongation of the Achilles tendon or transfer of the

tibialis anterior tendon is useful for treating foot deformities
D. Prophylactic shoulder release procedures are indicated to prevent "frozen" shoulder

Schwartz: 1859

Comments: Proper positioning, nursing care, and early physical therapy are vital to prevent many of the deformities that may occur in the arms and legs following stroke. Operative correction may be required for disabling spasticity or fixed deformities such as flexion contractures; the most useful for spasticity involves peripheral muscle release. As this is irreversible and produces muscle weakness, one must be certain that the resulting weakness will not produce a worse disability than the spasticity already present. The foot and ankle are the most common sites of deformity in stroke patients. A painful "frozen" shoulder is a major impediment to successful rehabilitation. Correct positioning and a program of active assisted exercise can help maintain a proper range of shoulder motion, preventing this complication and the need for release procedures.

Answer: A, C

15. Which of the following statements is/are true regarding spinal deformities?

A. Adolescent kyphosis may result from abnormalities of muscle, bone, or intervertebral disc
B. Senile kyphosis results from disc degeneration of the intervertebral disc or from osteoporosis
C. Postural scoliosis is seen most commonly in adolescent females
D. Structural scoliosis may be congenital, paralytic, or idiopathic in origin

Schwartz: 1862

Comments: Both kyphosis and scoliosis have numerous causes. The etiology, type, and degree of deformity and age of the patient are all important considerations that determine the most appropriate form of treatment. These may include postural training, general spinal exercises, and various braces or operations.

Answer: A, B, C, D

16. Which of the following statements is/are true regarding Dupuytren's contracture?

A. It results from severe tenosynovitis
B. It is most common among manual laborers
C. It may be treated with steroid injection and physical therapy
D. Successful surgical treatment requires complete excision of the palmar fascia

Schwartz: 1871

Comments: Contraction of the palmar aponeurosis is believed to be inherited, although other factors are involved in determining its expression. There is an association with epilepsy, tuberculosis, and alcoholism.

Contrary to common notion, its incidence is not higher in manual laborers. There are several clinical types of involvement that vary in severity. Nonoperative treatment consisting of exercise, local injections, and even radiotherapy has been successful. Fasciotomy is useful for limited contractures; more severe cases will require radical excision of the palmar fascia.

Answer: C

17. Which of the following statements is/are true regarding Volkmann's ischemic contracture?

A. Ischemic injury is greatest along the axis of the posterior interosseous artery
B. The ulnar nerve is the most commonly involved nerve
C. The deformity may result as a complication of supracondylar humeral fracture
D. Prompt surgical decompression and exploration of the brachial artery may be preventive

Sabiston: 1520
Schwartz: 1872, 2083

Comments: Volkmann's contracture is the result of ischemic damage to the muscles of the deep flexor compartment of the forearm (flexor digitorum profundus and flexor pollicis longus) secondary to compromised flow in the anterior interosseous artery. This can be a complication of supracondylar fracture, forearm fracture, brachial artery puncture, hemophilia, and various forms of trauma. The median nerve, which lies close to the anterior interosseous artery, may be involved in this process, and in severe cases the ulnar nerve can be involved as well. Since the damage occurs within a few hours of the insult, initial treatment must be prompt and definitive.

Answer: C, D

18. Match the items in the two columns.

Disease	Area Involved
A. Legg-Calvé-Perthes	a. Tibial tuberosity
B. Osgood-Schlatter	b. Upper femoral epiphysis
C. Köhler's	c. Navicular bone

Schwartz: 1873

Comments: All of the above conditions are forms of epiphysitis, also known as osteochondritis, and involve a derangement of growth at an ossification center. Numerous etiologic factors have been implicated, particularly trauma with a subsequent vascular disturbance. These conditions are seen clinically, usually soon after the appearance of the particular ossification center or during the adolescent growth spurt. They are more common in men and most often involve weight-bearing bones. There are potential long-term complications, particularly arthritis with Legg-Calvé-Perthes disease. Treatment may include immobilization with plaster cast and bracing or osteotomy for problems at the upper femoral epiphysis.

Answer: A–b; B–a; C–c

19. Which of the following statements is/are true regarding scoliosis:

A. Congenital scoliosis is the form most likely associated with paraplegia
B. The prognosis for both paralytic and idiopathic scoliosis is related to age of onset
C. Idiopathic scoliosis is progressive
D. The site of curvature affects the prognosis of idiopathic scoliosis

Schwartz: 1863

Comments: The specific treatment of scoliosis depends on several clinical considerations. Since untreated congenital scoliosis is the form that most often results in paraplegia, these patients must be closely observed throughout their growth period. The two most important prognostic factors in **idiopathic scoliosis** are age of onset and site of the curve; this form progresses during growth, and with an onset before the age of 10 years, the prognosis is poor and the deformity often severe. In **paralytic scoliosis,** the prognosis depends more on age of onset than on location of the primary curve.

Answer: A, B, C, D

CHAPTER 56

Orthopedics—Trauma

1. Proper care of an open fracture generally includes:

A. Culture of the wound
B. Antibiotic prophylaxis
C. Tetanus prophylaxis
D. Complete surgical débridement
E. Immobilization of bony fragments

Sabiston: 1430
Schwartz: 1952

Comments: In an open fracture, the skin or mucosal barrier is broken, introducing the possibility of infection from contamination of the fracture site. Management is aimed at preventing infection and providing bony union. The aforementioned goals can best be attained through identification of the potential contamination, antibiotic prophylaxis, débridement of devitalized tissues, and immobilization of fractures. Soft tissue management is based on the same principles as in other types of injury, depending upon wound size, degree of contamination, and time interval between injury and treatment. All wounds associated with open fractures should be cultured when the patient presents; some wounds can be closed primarily or in delayed fashion.

Answer: A, B, C, D, E

2. Which of the following injuries involve(s) a significant risk of vascular injury?

A. Supracondylar fracture of the humerus
B. Distal femoral shaft fractures
C. Knee dislocation
D. Gunshot wound
E. Open fractures

Schwartz: 1952

Comments: Although arterial injury may accompany any fracture or dislocation, certain injuries have a higher incidence. Vascular trauma should, therefore, be suspected on the basis of the type of injury or the findings of vascular compromise known as the five P's: Pain, Pallor, Pulselessness, Paralysis, and Paresthesia. Even if there is no initial suggestion of vascular trauma, the injured limb must be re-evaluated frequently, since delayed thrombosis may occur. In many patients with pain that is out of proportion to that anticipated, or is not relieved by standard analgesic techniques, vascular injury should also be suspected and looked for. Arteriography should be performed if there is any question of vascular injury. Definitive therapy must be instituted promptly, since irreversible muscle ischemia may occur in 6 to 8 hours.

Answer: A, B, C, D, E

3. In which of the following fractures is there at least partial continuity of the cortex?

A. Stress fracture
B. Torus fracture
C. Greenstick fracture
D. Compound fracture

Sabiston: 1428
Schwartz: 1950

Comments: A **stress** fracture is the result of cumulative stress resulting in bony failure. The diagnosis frequently cannot be made by x-ray and requires a bone scan. By definition, therefore, there is at least partial continuity of the cortex. A **torus** fracture is a wrinkle or buckle of the cortex, usually found in the metaphyseal region of children, specifically in the distal radial area. There is maintenance of alignment and no displacement. **Greenstick** fractures almost always occur in children and by definition involve disruption of only one cortex with the opposite cortex remaining intact. A **compound** fracture may be any or all of the above or may be completely displaced. The term compound refers to direct communication between the fracture site and skin surface.

Answer: A, B, C

4. Which of the following is/are true regarding peripheral nerve injury associated with extremity trauma?

387

A. Neurapraxia or axonotmesis may be seen with closed trauma
B. Nerve injury associated with closed fractures usually requires primary repair
C. Digital nerves are best repaired secondarily
D. Nerve suture may be technically easier 10 days after injury

Schwartz: 1953

Comments: In peripheral nerve injuries associated with closed bone or soft tissue trauma, continuity of the nerve is generally preserved; complete nerve division (neurotmesis) may accompany open injuries. Usually, in-continuity nerve injuries will heal spontaneously and repair is not required. However, expectant observation with electrodiagnostic studies is mandatory. Recent advances in cases of nonhealing include reconstructive procedures by microsurgical cable graft technique. In the case of peripheral nerve transection, precise approximation is required for proper axonal regeneration. In clean transections, primary repair may be successful. In other cases, it may be better to delay repair until soft tissue has healed.

Answer: A, D

5. Nonunion of fractures is more common with:

A. Children
B. Adults
C. Extensive soft tissue injury
D. Closed reduction

Sabiston: 1431
Schwartz: 1955

Comments: Nonunion occurs when a fracture does not heal based upon time and radiologic and pathologic criteria. There may be avascularity, soft tissue interposition, or excessive motion accounting for failure of a bone to heal. There may be osteosclerosis or osteoporosis at the bony fragments where nonunion has taken place. Excessive soft tissue disruption, infection, or pre-existing orthopedic conditions (such as neurofibromatosis, diabetes, syphilis) can account for nonunion. At the time of operative reduction of fractures, it is important to minimize periosteal stripping or devitalization of the fracture region.

Answer: B, C

6. True or False: Pathologic fractures are rarely the result of benign conditions.

Sabiston: 1428
Schwartz: 1955

Comments: Pathologic fractures occur spontaneously or as a result of minor trauma in bones with a pre-existing pathologic condition. Although any primary or metastatic malignant process may be responsible for this, benign conditions frequently are the cause. In adults, osteoporosis may result in pathologic fractures; in children, developmental diseases such as osteogenesis imperfecta, osteopetrosis, or nutritional deficiencies may be respon-

sible. Benign bone cysts or tumors also may be associated with fractures.

Answer: False

7. Stress fractures:

A. Are associated with an underlying congenital disorder of bone formation
B. Commonly affect the metatarsal shafts and femoral neck
C. Are best detected by strong clinical suspicion and a positive bone scan
D. Usually require internal fixation for adequate union

Sabiston: 1429
Schwartz: 1956

Comments: Repeated trauma results in accelerated osteoclastic resorption with loss of normal structural bone mass and subsequent weakening and fracture if the trauma continues. The usual locations for such injuries include the distal second and third metatarsal shafts, proximal tibia, distal fibula, and calcaneus. Appropriate treatment is immobilization and cessation of the offending activity.

Answer: C

8. Match the Salter and Harris classification with the corresponding epiphyseal injury.

A. Salter I
B. Salter II
C. Salter III
D. Salter IV
E. Salter V

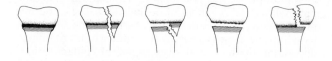

Schwartz: 1956

Comments: The classification of Salter and Harris is as follows: Salter I: Complete separation of the epiphyseal plate from the metaphysis without recognized fracture on x-ray. Salter II: Partial separation of epiphyseal plate with metaphyseal fracture. Salter III: Partial separation of epiphyseal plate with associated fracture of the epiphysis into the joint. Salter IV: Fracture of epiphyseal plate with metaphyseal and epiphyseal bony involvement. Salter V: Crush injury to epiphyseal plate. It is important to recognize the presence and type of epiphyseal plate injury, since the epiphyseal plate is the center of longitudinal bone growth and injuries may result in abnormalities of length or in deformities. Type I and type II fractures are treated by closed reduction and usually have an excellent prognosis. Accurate reduction is necessary for type III injuries, but the prognosis is good if the blood supply to the fractured portion is not impaired. Type IV and type V injuries are more likely to cause growth disturbances.

Whenever an epiphyseal fracture exists, the patient and/or the parents should be cautioned that growth abnormalities may result.

Answer: A–d; B–c; C–e; D–b; E–a

9. Which of the following is/are true regarding fractures in children?

A. Nonunion is rare
B. Healing is more rapid than in adults
C. Long-bone shaft fractures generally require open reduction
D. Compound fractures occur more often than in adults

Schwartz: 1958

Comments: Fractures in children are approached differently than in adults. Certain degrees of angulation, displacement, and shortening can be accepted, depending upon the fracture site and the age of the child, because some correction will occur with the patient's remaining growth. Epiphyseal injuries must be recognized, however, because of the possibility of growth disturbance. Compound fractures and nonunion are much less common in children. In general, shaft fractures in long bones should not be opened because of the risk of infection or epiphyseal disturbance.

Answer: A, B

10. Persistent pain after closed reduction and casting may result from:

A. Neural injury
B. Muscle spasm
C. Pressure point necrosis
D. Ischemia
E. Inadequate immobilization

Schwartz: 1958

Comments: Although there are several factors that may be responsible for limb pain after casting, vascular insufficiency is the most serious. Following plaster casting, the extremity should be elevated and the digits exposed. Adequate immobilization should significantly relieve pain. Unrelenting pain should always suggest ischemia and is an indication for splitting the cast with parallel cuts through the padding on both sides of the extremities. Localized burning pain may occur as a result of pressure point necrosis from the cast and is treated by cutting the cast window.

Answer: A, B, C, D, E

11. Sternoclavicular dislocations:

A. Are usually anterior
B. Require reduction when retrosternal
C. May require partial excision of the clavicle
D. None of the above

Sabiston: 1441
Schwartz: 1963

Comments: The most common type of sternoclavicular dislocation is anterior; the reduction is not as critical as it is for posterior dislocations, which may produce neurovascular compression. Old, unreduced symptomatic subluxations may require resection of the proximal clavicle.

Answer: A, B, C

12. Match the following regarding clavicular fractures.

A. Figure-of-8 splint
B. Nonunion common
C. Junction of middle and distal thirds
D. Open reduction for cosmetic defect

a. Children
b. Adults
c. Both
d. Neither

Sabiston: 1441
Schwartz: 1963

Comments: Clavicular fractures most commonly occur at the junction of the middle and distal thirds of the clavicle, although in older patients, fractures of the distal tip are more common. Both children and adults may be treated with a figure-of-8 apparatus, although accurate reduction is difficult to maintain. Reduction is not important in children because of remodeling with age; in adults, a cosmetic deformity may result but it is most often well tolerated and masked by overlying soft tissue. Open reduction of clavicular fractures is associated with a 50% incidence of nonunion and is generally not indicated for a cosmetic deformity.

Answer: A–c; B–d; C–c; D–d

13. Subluxation of the acromioclavicular joint:

A. Results from injury to the superior and inferior acromioclavicular ligaments
B. Is best detected with the patient examined in the supine position
C. Is usually the result of a direct blow to the shoulder from a sports injury
D. Is usually treated symptomatically

Schwartz: 1964

Comments: In young patients, downward force on the shoulder produces acromioclavicular separation as a result of disruption of the acromioclavicular and coracoclavicular ligaments. In elderly patients, a similar mechanism of injury results in fracture of the distal clavicle. The patient is best examined in the upright position, and radiologic confirmation may require stress views. Treatment is largely symptomatic; operative treatment may be necessary for severe dislocations, cosmetic deformity, or persistent pain.

Answer: C, D

14. Match the following concerning dislocations of the shoulder.

A. Immediate reduction
B. Axillary nerve injury
C. Seizures
D. Most common

a. Anterior
b. Posterior
c. Both
d. Neither

Sabiston: 1439
Schwartz: 1965

Comments: Dislocations of the humeral head from the glenoid fossa may occur in any direction. The most common mechanism involves an extension force applied to the abducted arm with subsequent anterior dislocation so that the humeral head lies in the subglenoid or subcoracoid position. Axillary nerve injury may occur and is assessed by examining for an area of sensory loss over the deltoid muscle. Posterior dislocations may be seen with seizures, during electroconvulsive therapy, or sometimes as a result of motor vehicle accidents. An axillary x-ray is the best view for identifying either an anterior or a posterior dislocation. However, the patient with a posterior dislocation is usually unable to mobilize the arm for this view, so that a proper x-ray is best obtained with a transthoracic lateral view. Acute dislocations should immediately be reduced with subsequent shoulder immobilization. Recurrent dislocations may require operative correction.

Answer: A–c; B–a; C–b; D–a

15. Fractures of the proximal humerus:

A. Most commonly involve the surgical neck
B. Are associated with minimal deformity
C. Usually require open reduction and internal fixation
D. Require prolonged immobilization to achieve healing in elderly patients

Sabiston: 1440
Schwartz: 1967

Comments: The surgical neck (below the tuberosities) is the most common site of a proximal humeral fracture. Fractures of the anatomic neck (above the tuberosities) may occur in children, and these involve the epiphysis. There may be considerable displacement with a proximal humeral fracture owing to opposing actions of the pectoralis major, the deltoid, and the subscapularis musculature in addition to the latissimus dorsi and the teres major. Closed reduction and immobilization is the usual method of treatment. In elderly patients, shoulder motion should begin as early as 7 to 10 days after reduction to prevent shoulder stiffness.

Answer: A

16. Which of the following are indications for immediate open operative treatment of humeral shaft fractures?

A. Radial nerve injury
B. Brachial artery injury
C. Median nerve injury
D. Unsuccessful closed reduction
E. Fractures in adults

Sabiston: 1440
Schwartz: 1968

Comments: Neurovascular injuries are not uncommon with humeral shaft fractures, the most common being traction injury to the radial nerve, which usually recovers spontaneously but constitutes a surgical indication if nerve function is not recovered in 4 to 6 months. If brachial arterial injury is suspected, primary exploration is indicated; internal fixation of the humeral shaft may be necessary, but not all orthopedic surgeons perform internal fixation when there has been a vascular repair. Primary open reduction of closed shaft fractures is also necessary if bony apposition cannot be obtained. Most of these fractures can be treated by closed reduction using some form of casting or traction.

Answer: B, D

17. Fractures of the proximal radius:

A. Most often involve the radial head in adults
B. Most often involve the radial neck in children
C. May require excision of the radial head in adults
D. May require excision of the radial head in children

Sabiston: 1446
Schwartz: 1969

Comments: A fall on an outstretched hand may produce a fracture of the radial head in adults or a fracture of the radial neck in children. Early joint motion should be established for the successful treatment of radial head fractures. Radial neck fractures are treated by closed reduction, but may require open reduction if the resulting angulation is severe. In adults, limitations of pronation and supination may require excision of the radial head; in children, however, the radial head should never be excised because of the deformity due to lack of growth from loss of the epiphysis.

Answer: A, B, C

18. Which of the following is/are true regarding supracondylar fractures of the humerus?

A. Volkmann's contracture usually results when the brachial artery is injured by the distal fragment
B. Gunstock deformity may result when angulation or rotation of the distal fragment is not corrected
C. Treatment always requires hospitalization
D. The affected limb is usually immobilized in extension

Sabiston: 1444
Schwartz: 1969

Comments: Supracondylar fractures of the humerus are often considered a most serious fracture of the upper extremity because of the potential for brachial artery injury. The result is an ischemic injury to the entire forearm. Usually, these fractures are caused by a fall on the extended elbow and therefore should be immobilized in flexion. However, the causal mechanism may be a fall with the elbow in flexion, in which instance immobilization in extension is required. The latter is relatively infrequent. Reversal of the carrying angle (so-called gunstock deformity) is another potential complication.

Answer: B

19. Which one or more of the following humeral fractures in children usually requires an operation for correction?

A. Anatomic neck
B. Surgical neck

C. Shaft
D. Supracondylar
E. Lateral epicondyle

Sabiston: 1445
Schwartz: 1971

Comments: Supracondylar fractures are common fractures about the elbow in children. Fractures of the lateral epicondyle in children are Salter type IV epiphyseal injuries and require anatomic reduction by either closed or open means. If they are undisplaced, they still may require internal fixation because of the high incidence of nonunion. All of the other types of fractures listed above are best treated by closed reduction.

Answer: E

20. Monteggia's fracture is best described as which of the following?

A. Ulnar styloid fracture, radial head subluxation
B. Proximal ulnar fracture, radial head subluxation
C. Radial head fracture, ulnar styloid subluxation
D. Radial neck fracture, ulnar styloid subluxation

Sabiston: 1446
Schwartz: 1972

Comments: This deformity results from forced pronation or from a direct blow on the ulna. The radial head usually dislocates anteriorly. Treatment is by closed reduction with the forearm placed in supination to maintain reduction of the radial head. When the radial head is anterior, the elbow is placed in flexion; when posterior, the elbow is placed in extension. In adults with ulnar displacement, intramedullary fixation is required.

Answer: B

21. Which of the following statements is/are true in regard to fractures of the forearm?

A. They are most common in children
B. They require anatomic reduction
C. Supination usually provides greatest stability for proximal fractures
D. Pronation usually provides greatest stability for distal fractures

Sabiston: 1446
Schwartz: 1973

Comments: As a general rule, whenever a fracture or dislocation of one bone of the forearm is present, one should check for associated subluxation or fracture of the other bone. Because of the interrelationship necessary for normal function, anatomic reduction is necessary. If this cannot be accomplished by closed technique in adults, open reduction is indicated. Open reduction is not indicated in children. Fractures that most often require open reduction are displaced fractures of the proximal third of the forearm and oblique fractures of the radius. Following reduction, the arm is immobilized with the elbow at 90 degrees and the hand at the position of greatest stability, which varies according to the site of the fracture. Some degree of angulation at the fracture site may be ac-

cepted in children, depending upon their age and the proximity to the epiphysis.

Answer: A, B, C, D

22. Which three of the following best describe the position of immobilization for a Colles fracture?

A. Radial deviation
B. Ulnar deviation
C. Pronation
D. Supination
E. 30-degree palmar flexion
F. Full palmar flexion

Sabiston: 1447
Schwartz: 1975

Comments: Fractures of the distal radius 1 inch proximal to the articular surface with associated fracture of the ulnar styloid or rupture of the ulnar collateral ligament are common. They are best treated by closed reduction and plaster immobilization with the wrist in 30-degree palmar flexion to maintain the correction from the dorsal angulation and maximal ulnar deviation to maintain proper length of the compressed, shortened radius and with the forearm pronated (although a school of thought has accepted supination as a proper position of immobilization). An appropriate cast is applied.

Answer: B, C, E

23. Complications of Colles' fractures include:

A. Shoulder stiffness
B. Wrist stiffness
C. Carpal tunnel syndrome
D. Avascular necrosis of the ulnar styloid

Sabiston: 1449
Schwartz: 1976

Comments: Colles' fracture is common in older patients, and residual shoulder or wrist stiffness following plaster immobilization may cause significant disability. Patients should therefore engage daily in exercise of the interphalangeal and metaphalangeal joints as well as range of motion of the shoulder. If immobilization is carried out with excessive palmar flexion, median nerve compression may occur.

Answer: A, B, C

24. A 25-year-old skater complains of wrist pain after slipping on the ice and falling on an outstretched hand. There is no deformity. A likely diagnosis is:

A. Colles' fracture
B. Navicular fracture
C. Lunate subluxation
D. Scaphoid-lunate subluxation

Sabiston: 1449
Schwartz: 1976

Comments: The same mechanism that produces Colles' fracture in older patients results in navicular fracture in young adults. It is not uncommon for this fracture to go undetected on initial radiographs. Less commonly, hyperextension injuries of the wrist may cause lunate dislocation or disruption of the normal scaphoid-lunate relationship.

Answer: B

25. Which of the following x-rays should be obtained on the patient described in Question 24?

A. AP view of the wrist
B. Lateral view of the wrist
C. Oblique view of the wrist
D. 17-degree angle AP view of the wrist

Sabiston: 1449
Schwartz: 1976

Comments: In addition to standard views of the carpal bones, a special angled x-ray may help in the assessment of navicular injuries. AP and lateral views will demonstrate displacement of the lunate.

Answer: A, B, C, D

26. X-rays of the patient described in Question 24 reveal no fracture or dislocation. Appropriate treatment at this time should be:

A. Ice packs, elastic wrap, and rest
B. Dorsal wrist splint
C. Plaster cast, including the thumb, up to the elbow
D. Plaster cast, including the thumb and elbow

Sabiston: 1450
Schwartz: 1976

Comments: If the patient has tenderness over the navicular bone, a fracture should be suspected despite negative x-rays. The patient should be treated by plaster cast immobilization, including the thumb and elbow. After 3 weeks, x-rays out of plaster should be repeated. If they are still negative and the tenderness is gone, the cast can be removed. Adequate treatment is important because of the risk of avascular necrosis of the proximal fragment, which is inherent in the nature of the fracture itself, or of nonunion, whether the fracture be displaced or nondisplaced. Both complications inherent in this fracture can produce post-traumatic arthritis at the wrist.

Answer: D

27. Which of the following statements is/are true regarding fractures of the hand?

A. In the reduction of metacarpal neck fractures, correction of rotational deformity is most important
B. Bennett's fracture involves an intra-articular fracture of the carpometacarpal joint of the thumb
C. An avulsion fracture associated with mallet finger requires reduction of one third of the articular surfaces involved
D. Metacarpal fractures with overlying skin disruption on the dorsal hand are open fractures

Sabiston: 1455, 1467
Schwartz: 1977

Comments: Fractures of the hand are among the most common problems encountered in the emergency room; they must be treated properly in order to avoid or minimize any subsequent disability. Correction of rotational deformities with metacarpal fractures is important and is determined clinically; each finger when flexed should point toward the navicular. Correction of angulation in the ulnar and radial planes may also be very important. Intra-articular fractures generally require anatomic reduction. Open fractures, such as metacarpal neck fractures with an overlying tooth bite, must be recognized because of the potential for serious infection.

Answer: A, B, C, D

28. The preferred primary treatment of a nondisplaced femoral neck fracture is:

A. Skeletal traction
B. Internal fixation
C. Femoral head prosthesis
D. All of the above are equally effective

Sabiston: 1473
Schwartz: 1980

Comments: Preferred primary treatment of a femoral neck fracture is internal fixation if the fracture is nondisplaced. If the femoral neck fracture is displaced, then femoral head prosthetic treatment is appropriate. Early internal fixation of nondisplaced fractures relieves pain, permits mobilization, and facilitates union. While there may be some influence on the prevention of avascular necrosis, one must be aware that avascular necrosis is inherent in the nature of the fracture itself and for the most part is determined at the time the injury occurs. There is a very high incidence of avascular necrosis and nonunion in femoral neck fractures in children whether they are treated by traction or internal fixation. Reduction and internal fixation of displaced fractures carries a high risk of avascular necrosis, so that primary arthroplasty is indicated in this situation. Prosthetic arthroplasty is also indicated for cases of avascular necrosis or nonunion.

Answer: B

29. Appropriate initial treatment of a femoral shaft fracture commonly includes which one or more of the following?

A. Open reduction in children
B. Intramedullary nailing in adults
C. Skeletal traction
D. Application of a cast brace

Sabiston: 1473
Schwartz: 1983

Comments: Skeletal traction and closed intramedullary nailing are felt to be superior to methods of internal fixation that involve operation at the fracture site because they carry a lower risk of infection. Femoral shaft fractures in children are treated by closed methods because of the risk of damage to the epiphyseal plate and subsequent growth abnormalities. A cast brace may allow earlier mobilization of patients with midshaft or distal femoral fractures who have been initially treated with skeletal traction. Primary cast brace treatment, however, is receiving increased emphasis in certain areas.

Answer: B, C

30. Which of the following statements is/are true regarding the technique of insertion of a Steinmann pin for skeletal traction and femoral shaft fractures?

A. The pin is placed in the proximal tibia when there is associated knee injury
B. The pin is inserted lateral to medial at the tibial tubercle
C. The pin is inserted medial to lateral in the supracondylar femur
D. The pin should be placed as anterior as possible in the supracondylar position

Schwartz: 1984

Comments: Steinmann pins for skeletal traction are easily inserted after administration of a local anesthetic and may be placed proximal to the femoral condyles or across the proximal tibia. In the supracondylar position, the pin is placed as far posterior as possible to avoid the suprapatellar pouch. Insertion at the tibial tubercle must avoid injury to the lateral popliteal nerve. When there is associated knee injury, the pin is inserted above the knee so that traction is not applied across the injured joint.

Answer: B, C

31. A direct lateral blow (valgus force) to the knee may produce injury to the:

A. Medial collateral ligament
B. Lateral collateral ligament
C. Anterior cruciate ligament
D. Posterior cruciate ligament

Schwartz: 1985

Comments: Injuries to the supporting ligamentous structures of the knee commonly occur in young athletes. Accurate diagnosis depends upon knowledge of the mechanism and the position of injury, and careful clinical examination to assess abnormal mobility. Diagnostic arthroscopy is useful for the assessment of intra-articular injuries, such as torn cruciate ligaments or menisci. With a direct valgus force applied to the knee, the medial collateral ligament is disrupted first and, with continuing force, the anterior cruciate may rupture.

Answer: A, C

32. Match the statements on the left with the location of the tibial fracture on the right.

A. Associated ligamentous injury
B. Usually requires open reduction
C. Compound fracture

a. Shaft
b. Plateau
c. Both
d. Neither

Sabiston: 1481
Schwartz: 1989

Comments: Tibial fractures are usually the result of direct trauma. They occur at any age, although plateau fractures are more common in the middle-aged or elderly. With certain exceptions, treatment is by closed methods. Tibial plateau fractures may require surgical repair if the medial collateral ligament is disrupted or if there is severe displacement of the lateral tibial plateau. About 30% of tibial shaft fractures are open and therefore require operative intervention.

Answer: A–b; B–d; C–a

33. Which of the following statements is/are true regarding the assessment of ankle injury?

A. AP and lateral x-rays are adequate for radiologic evaluation
B. Medial tenderness following inversion injury suggests injury to the deltoid ligament
C. Stress x-ray views may require anesthesia
D. Ability to walk immediately following injury excludes ligamentous disruption

Sabiston: 1485
Schwartz: 1991

Comments: Ligamentous and bony injuries of the ankle frequently result from rotational or inversion/eversion forces. An important goal of treatment is to maintain ankle stability. Initial evaluation should include a history of the mechanism of injury and examination for the location of tenderness, swelling, or deformity. If the patient was able to walk following the injury, the ankle may be stable, but an undisplaced fracture or ligamentous disruption may still be present. Adequate radiologic evaluation requires standard AP and lateral views as well as a mortise view obtained in a 30-degree medial oblique position. The most common ankle injury involves a portion of the lateral collateral ligament injured as the result of an inversion force. Associated medial tenderness suggests a force sufficient to produce damage to the deltoid ligament as well. Integrity of the lateral collateral ligament can be assessed with stress films, which may require the help of local or general anesthesia.

Answer: B, C

34. Which of the following statements is/are true regarding the treatment of ankle injuries?

A. Anatomic reduction of fractures is mandatory
B. Operation is contraindicated if closed anatomic reduction is achieved
C. Disruption of the tibiofibular ligaments usually requires open reduction
D. Plaster cast should be applied with the ankle in 90-degree dorsiflexion

Sabiston: 1485
Schwartz: 1992

Comments: The principles of treatment of ankle fractures include anatomic reduction of all fractures, rigid fixation, and early motion. The concept of closed reduction and maintenance by casting has been the standard. However, there is an inherent instability to all bi- and trimalleolar fractures, which has led to more aggressive treatment practices including operative intervention to achieve greater security, even if anatomic reduction has already been achieved. The most common isolated malleolar fracture involves the lateral malleolus and is treated with closed reduction and casting for 6 to 8 weeks. Bimalleolar fractures involving the medial and lateral malleoli usually result from a combination of pronation/supination and external rotation. The posterior malleolus is important in maintaining the anterior/posterior stability of the ankle joint. In trimalleolar fractures with small posterior fragments, surgical intervention is determined primarily by the status of the medial and lateral malleoli. When the posterior fragment involves 30% or more of the articular surface, however, or when there is AP instability, anatomic reduction usually requires internal fixation. The distal tibial fibular joint is important to ankle stability, and disruption generally requires operative correction.

Answer: A, C, D

35. Match the following types of hip injury with the characteristic position of the limb.

A. Anterior hip dislocation
B. Posterior hip dislocation
C. Femoral neck fracture
D. Intertrochanteric femoral fracture

a. External rotation, shortened
b. Internal rotation, shortened
c. Abduction, flexion, external rotation
d. Adduction, flexion, internal rotation

Schwartz: 1980, 1996

Comments: Proximal femoral fractures and hip dislocations present with the injured limb in characteristic positions. When combined with a history of mechanisms of injury, this should suggest the diagnosis even before radiologic confirmation. Note the difference between anterior and posterior dislocations; posterior dislocations are less common and result from an axial force applied to a flexed hip, as may occur with dashboard injuries.

Answer: A–c; B–d; C–a; D–a

36. Complications of hip dislocation include:

A. Sciatic nerve injury
B. Avascular necrosis
C. Degenerative arthritis
D. Fat embolism
E. Compartment syndromes

Schwartz: 1996

Comments: Avascular necrosis of the femoral head and the later development of degenerative traumatic arthritis are the most common complications of hip dislocations. Avascular necrosis occurs in about 20% of patients; the incidence is directly related to delay in reduction. Approximately one half of patients can develop later traumatic arthritis. Sciatic nerve injury is a potential complication when the hip dislocates posteriorly.

Answer: A, B, C

37. Appropriate initial management of a patient with a pelvic fracture may include:

A. Fluid resuscitation
B. Peritoneal lavage
C. Retrograde urethrogram/cystogram
D. Open reduction of pelvic fracture

Sabiston: 1469
Schwartz: 1998

Comments: Pelvic fractures most often are the result of automobile accidents and frequently are associated with injury to abdominal or pelvic viscera and significant retroperitoneal or pelvic hemorrhage. Initial management is directed at the resuscitation and assessment of a patient with multiple injuries. Associated urethral and bladder injuries are not uncommon and must be assessed. Most pelvic fractures are treated by bed rest and pelvic sling; open reduction is rarely indicated.

Answer: A, B, C

38. Indications for operation in patients with acute fracture-dislocations of the cervical spine include:

A. Unstable fractures or dislocations
B. Progressive neurologic deficits
C. Persistent bony fragments in spinal canal
D. There is no indication for operative intervention in patients who present with associated neurologic deficit

Sabiston: 1434
Schwartz: 2001

Comments: Patients with unstable fractures or dislocations may be treated by stabilization procedures. Reduction and stabilization is indicated in patients who present with minimal neurologic findings that subsequently progress. In patients with fragments in the spinal canal, operative intervention is mandatory in the face of a neurologic deficit. The role of surgery for patients with acute fracture-dislocations and established neurologic deficits is controversial.

Answer: A, B, C

CHAPTER 57

Orthopedics—Congenital Disease

1. Which of the following are appropriately considered in the differential diagnosis of congenital hip dislocation?

A. Coxa vara
B. Pathologic dislocation
C. Septic arthritis
D. Paralytic dislocation from poliomyelitis

Schwartz: 1883

Comments: All of the above should be considered in the differential diagnosis of congenital hip abnormalities, but an accurate history and careful physical examination will usually differentiate among them. In **paralytic dislocation** there is a waddling gait, but also muscular weakness and a shortness of limb; the acetabular development is relatively normal. In **pathologic dislocation** there is a history of hip joint trouble developing at birth, hip movement generally is limited, and the x-rays show an acetabulum usually adequately developed but with a head that is absorbed or deformed. **Septic arthritis** has accompanying signs and symptoms of infection. In **coxa vara** the limp is less pronounced, the head is not palpable, and the appearance on x-ray is characteristic.

Answer: A, B, C, D

2. Which of the following clinical signs are indicative of congenital hip dislocation or dysplasia?

A. Ortolani's sign
B. Limitation of hip adduction
C. A waddling gait
D. Trendelenburg's sign

Schwartz: 1884

Comments: Although x-ray examination is essential to establishing the diagnosis, certain clinical signs are characteristically present. Among these are: Ortolani's sign—a click heard during abduction of the flexed hip; limitation of hip *ab*duction; asymmetry in the skin crease of the gluteal and perineal areas (more pronounced on the affected side), producing a waddling gait; and Trendelenburg's

sign—when standing on the dislocated leg the opposite buttock drops (instead of rising) and the trunk leans toward the dislocation (instead of remaining straight).

Answer: A, C, D

3. Regarding the management of congenital hip dysplasia and dislocation, which of the following is/are true?

A. Abduction splinting is usually adequate in infants with dislocatable hips
B. Open reduction is best performed after the age of 6 years
C. Osteotomy is most useful between the ages of 6 and 10 years
D. Hip fusion may be indicated for control of arthritic pain in older patients
E. Total hip replacement carries too great a morbidity to be considered in managing this abnormality

Schwartz: 1885

Comments: In patients with a dislocatable hip, pillow or harness splints are usually adequate to correct congenital hip dysplasia. Operative reduction of congenital dislocations is rarely indicated before 1 year of age and is contraindicated as the sole form of surgical therapy after the age of 6. Used alone, osteotomy of the innominate bone or of the femur does not correct the hip dislocation, but it is useful in altering the angulation of the femur or acetabulum to maintain the reduced hip joint. In older patients with significant associated arthritic pain, fusion of the involved hip may provide excellent palliation. Total hip replacement may be indicated in middle-aged patients who present primarily with pain. While the methods of hip fusion described above are sound and have stood the test of time, their use is quickly fading in the face of rapid advancements, particularly arthroplasty.

Answer: A, D

4. Which of the following statements is/are true regarding the management of congenital club foot?

A. The approach to management does not vary with the patient's age
B. Attention should be focused solely on the correction of the anatomic deformity
C. Physical manipulation is contraindicated because of the risk of associated fracture
D. Treatment may require tendon transfers and bone resection

Schwartz: 1888

Comments: The likelihood of success in correcting club foot deformities decreases as the patient becomes older, and the method of management varies with age as well. In infants and young children, manipulation with casting or shaping is successful (at least 50%) and carries little risk; in recalcitrant club foot, aggressive soft tissue release is carried out. At age 3 to 8 years, tendon transfers and other manipulations of the associated soft tissue may be required for correction and to balance muscle power. At age 8 to 12 years, a wedge osteotomy often is a better choice for a club foot resistant to lesser measures. In adults, manipulation and surgery of the soft tissues is unlikely to help, and triple arthrodesis is the most common procedure to correct the symptomatic residual deformity. Management in all these settings should be focused not only on the correction of the anatomic deformity, but also on the development of sufficient muscular strength to maintain the anatomic correction.

Answer: D

5. True statements regarding torticollis include:

A. It is felt to be a result of trauma
B. The pathophysiology is thought to involve ischemic contracture
C. Its clinical manifestations do not appear until approximately 2 years of age
D. Manipulation of the neck is the preferred treatment in the earliest stages of the process

Schwartz: 1892

Comments: Congenital wry neck (torticollis) is thought to represent an ischemic event within the midportion of the sternocleidomastoid muscle, the initiation of which is thought to be traumatic. Initially it presents as a "tumor" of the muscle as a consequence of localized swelling. This then goes on to ischemic contracture of the muscle, often with contractures of the associated musculofascial elements on the involved side. Clinical manifestations usually appear within the early months of life. In the early stage, massage and physical therapy are recommended and are usually successful in preventing permanent deformity. In the later stages, however, manipulation may not correct the deformity, and operative division of the fibrosed musculofascial structures may be required.

Answer: A, B, D

6. Match the items in the two columns:

Clinical Characteristics	Congenital Anomaly
A. May be bilateral	a. Congenital radioulnar synostosis
B. Abnormal bony fusion	b. Madelung's deformity
C. Disproportionate bony growth	c. Both
D. Osteotomy helpful	d. Neither

Schwartz: 1893

Comments: Both of these entities are congenital anomalies of the distal forearm and wrist, and both are often bilateral. **Congenital radioulnar synostosis** involves an abnormal fusion of the proximal radius and ulna, resulting in fixation of the forearm in a position midway between pronation and supination. **Madelung's deformity** is a congenital subluxation of the wrist due to defective growth of the inner third of the distal radius. This results in a bowing of the radius, increasing the interosseous space. Appropriately directed osteotomy may be beneficial in both deformities.

Answer: A–c; B–a; C–b; D–c

7. Characteristics of cleidocranial dysostosis syndrome include:

A. Associated severe mental retardation
B. Delayed closure of the fontanelles
C. Increased transverse diameter of the cranium
D. Marked limitation of shoulder motion

Schwartz: 1892

Comments: This entity is usually inherited and is characterized by aplasia of the clavicles, increased transverse cranial diameter, and delayed closure of the fontanelles. There are usually no other associated anomalies and no associated disability. Patients with this syndrome are frequently able to approximate the tips of the shoulders to each other below the chin.

Answer: B, C

8. Which of the following represent deformities resulting from the in-utero position of the fetus?

A. Metatarsus adductus
B. Valgus foot
C. Tibial pseudoarthrosis
D. Unilateral externally rotated leg
E. Bilaterally internally rotated tibias

Schwartz: 1881

Comments: All of the above except tibial pseudoarthrosis are examples of deformity of an extremity that may result from fetal position within the uterus. These are usually evident at birth. Initial treatment involves passive stretching exercises and, occasionally, soft splints. Soft tissue contractures may develop if the correct anatomic position cannot be achieved within 6 weeks.

Answer: A, B, D, E

CHAPTER 58

Orthopedics—Acquired Diseases

1. Match the type of joint with its appropriate example:

Type of Joint	Example
A. Fibrous joint	a. Knee
B. Fibrocartilaginous joint	b. Skull sutures
C. Synovial joint	c. Pubic symphysis

Schwartz: 2007

Comments: Joints may be categorized according to the type of tissue by which they are joined. A **fibrous** joint (synarthrosis) represents two bones joined by fibrous tissue, as exemplified by the suture lines in the skull. **Fibrocartilaginous** joints (symphyses) are those in which the bones are joined by hyalin cartilage or fibrocartilage, examples being the pubic symphysis and the intervertebral discs. **Synovial** (diarthrodial) joints are movable joints in which cartilage-covered bone ends are united by a synovial-lined capsule, permitting motion to occur. Most joints of the extremities are synovial joints. The type of motion that a synovial joint permits is determined by the contour of the articular surfaces, the anatomy of the supporting connective tissues (capsule and ligaments) and the supporting musculature.

Answer: A–b; B–c; C–a

2. The two organisms most commonly found in pyogenic arthritis are:

A. *Escherichia coli*
B. *Staphylococcus aureus*
C. *Haemophilus influenzae*
D. Hemolytic streptococci

Sabiston: 1504
Schwartz: 2011

Comments: Pyogenic or septic arthritis is a severe joint condition which if not diagnosed and managed very early in the clinical course will likely result in permanent joint disability. It is most often caused by hematogenous spread from other infected sites, direct infection by way of traumatic wounds, or extension of adjacent osteomyelitis. The most common offending organisms are *Staphylococcus aureus* and hemolytic streptococci, although in children *Haemophilus influenzae* is also commonly seen. The clinical presentation is that of local tenderness, swelling, and extreme pain on motion. The specific diagnosis is made by joint aspiration with immediate Gram stain and culture. Systemic antibiotics should be started promptly and drainage of the joint carried out on an urgent basis.

Answer: B, D

3. The most common site of skeletal tuberculosis is the:

A. Knee
B. Hip
C. Spine
D. Humerus

Schwartz: 2012

Comments: Skeletal tuberculosis remains a significant problem in the Asian and African populations but, fortunately, it is rare in the United States, although it has increased in recent years. The most common site of involvement is the spine. Peripheral joint tuberculosis may also occur and usually involves synovium, bone, and cartilage. Untreated, joint tuberculosis usually results in complete joint destruction, deformity, and pain. In contrast to septic arthritis, the clinical course in skeletal tuberculosis is insidious, with symptoms lasting weeks to months before the patient seeks medical advice. A worsening of the pain at night is a characteristic feature. The diagnosis requires recovery of organisms from the involved joint or bone. Treatment involves antituberculous drug therapy, general supportive and nutritional measures, joint or back immobilization, drainage of tuberculous abscesses, and occasionally surgical débridement.

Answer: C

4. Regarding Pott's disease (tuberculous spondylitis):

A. This is the most common form of skeletal tuberculosis

B. Paraplegia may result
C. The anterior vertebral structures are most often involved
D. Posterior laminectomy is the preferred route of surgical management

Schwartz: 2014

Comments: Tuberculous spondylitis is the most common form of skeletal tuberculosis and usually occurs in the thoracic region. The infection is most often located in the vertebral bodies and may result in destruction of the anterior elements of the spinal column with subsequent abscess formation and/or angular deformity. Paraplegia may develop with progressive vertebral destruction and deformity, from pressure from an epidural abscess, or from direct involvement of the neural elements. Since the early x-ray findings are similar to those seen in staphylococcal disc space infection, diagnosis depends upon recovery of organisms from the involved site. Treatment includes appropriate antituberculous chemotherapy and bed rest with spinal immobilization. Surgery is performed for the purposes of draining abscesses, excising associated necrotic tissue, and stabilizing the anterior elements of the spinal column. Laminectomy is contraindicated since it decreases posterior spinal column stability.

Answer: A, B, C

5. Which of the following statements is/are true regarding the clinical features of gonococcal arthritis?

A. It occurs predominantly in females
B. It usually begins as a migratory polyarthralgia
C. The hip, knee, and shoulder are the most common sites of infection
D. Even with proper treatment, mild residual loss of joint motion usually results

Schwartz: 2015

Comments: In contrast to gonococcal urethritis in males, which is usually symptomatic and results in the early seeking of medical treatment, gonococcal cervicitis or vaginitis in females is frequently asymptomatic, and the sequelae of septicemia and arthritis are therefore more common. Initial symptoms usually include a migratory polyarthralgia with a variable febrile course. The infection usually localizes in the knee, elbow, or wrist. Diagnosis requires recovery of gonococcal organisms from the septic joint; treatment includes a 2-week course of penicillin as well as appropriate joint immobilization. With proper treatment, full recovery of joint function usually occurs.

Answer: A, B

6. Radiographic findings of rheumatoid arthritis include:

A. Subluxation
B. Osteoporosis
C. Bony erosions
D. Joint deformity

Schwartz: 2016

Comments: There are many radiographic abnormalities in patients with rheumatoid arthritis, depending on the stage of the disease process and the specific joints involved. The earliest findings are those relating to the destructive effects of the hyperplastic synovia and are best seen in x-rays of the hands. Fusiform swelling, particularly in the area of the proximal interphalangeal or metacarpophalangeal joints, is common. As the disease progresses, bony erosions produced by osteoclastic resorption occur. This cortical irregularity is made more apparent by the development of periosteal new bone formation in response to the synovial inflammation. Osteoporosis occurs as a result of the adjacent inflammation as well as by disuse atrophy. Further progression results in subluxation of the involved joints and joint deformity (particularly ulnar deviation at the metacarpophalangeal joints).

Answer: A, B, C, D

7. Joint pain:

A. Is always well localized
B. Often has a component of sensation from the articular cartilage
C. Is often referred distally within the extremity
D. Is due primarily to afferents from the subarticular bone, the most pain-sensitive structure in a joint

Schwartz: 2009

Comments: The innervation of a synovial joint is by way of articular branches from the nerves that supply the muscles controlling that joint. There is marked variability in the distribution and location of these branches and, as a result, joint pain is frequently difficult to localize. Furthermore, it is often referred to distal locations within the extremity (e.g., knee pain is frequently seen in primary pathologic processes involving the ipsilateral hip). Articular cartilage is without sensation, but the underlying subarticular bone does contain pain fibers which account for the bone pain experienced in certain inflammatory joint conditions. The most pain-sensitive joint structures, however, are the joint capsule and associated ligaments.

Answer: C

8. Regarding joint fluid assessment:

A. Joints should be aspirated with a No. 22 or smaller needle to prevent hemarthrosis
B. The mucin clot test helps differentiate inflammatory from degenerative joint abnormalities
C. The normal gradient of glucose concentration between plasma and joint fluid is approximately 50 mg/100 ml
D. Most joint fluid crystals of clinical significance can be adequately assessed with standard microscopic illumination techniques

Schwartz: 2010

Comments: Aspiration of a joint to obtain fluid for testing is commonly required in the evaluation of joint abnormalities. This should be done using scrupulously sterile technique, and it is generally recommended that a No.

18 or larger needle be used in order to be able to aspirate the more viscous fluid associated with certain forms of pathology. The fluid obtained should be routinely examined for color, appearance, and viscosity, and sent for a Gram stain examination, bacterial culture, mucin clot test, white blood cell count, crystal examination, and measurement of glucose concentration. The mucin clot test is a good qualitative assessment of the character of the protein-polysaccharide complex of synovial fluid. A firm, ropy clot that does not easily fragment suggests normal polymerization and is seen in normal joints and those with degenerative arthritis. Poor mucin clots suggest the presence of one of the inflammatory arthritides. Similarly, the gradient between joint fluid and plasma glucose concentration may suggest the presence of infection or rheumatoid arthritis. In such conditions, this gradient may be 50 mg/100 ml or greater; in the normal situation the gradient is less than 10 mg/100 ml. Assessment of joint fluid crystals is also important, particularly if gouty arthritis and/or crystal synovitis (pseudogout) is considered a possible cause of the joint disorder. This requires examination of the joint fluid utilizing polarized light in order to see the rod-shaped urate crystals, which manifest a strong negative birefringence.

Answer: B

9. Which of the following statements is/are true regarding rheumatoid arthritis?

A. It has a peak incidence in the sixth and seventh decades
B. It occurs more commonly in women
C. It is easily distinguished from other autoimmune disorders
D. A negative rheumatoid factor assay rules out the disease
E. The clinical manifestations of rheumatoid arthritis are limited to joint disorders

Schwartz: 2015

Comments: Rheumatoid arthritis is a systemic disease that may involve the musculoskeletal, cardiovascular, respiratory, and nervous systems. Its peak incidence is in the fourth and fifth decades, and it has a marked female predominance. Because it can involve multiple systems, at times it is difficult to differentiate rheumatoid arthritis from other systemic autoimmune disorders. A positive rheumatoid factor may be seen in 90% of adult patients and only 20% of juvenile patients with rheumatoid arthritis; thus, a negative assay does not exclude the presence of the disease. From a surgical standpoint, the most significant changes in rheumatoid arthritis are those affecting the synovial joints, as well as the adjacent tendons, tendon sheaths, and bursae. The surgeon treating these disorders must be aware of the cardiopulmonary and other systemic effects of rheumatoid arthritis as well as the side effects of drugs (e.g., steroids, aspirin) used to treat this disease.

Answer: B

10. Which of the following statements is/are true regarding the management of rheumatoid arthritis?

A. Medical management is the mainstay of treatment of early rheumatoid arthritis
B. Appropriate physical therapy will reduce the pain of rheumatoid arthritis but will not affect the progress of the underlying disease
C. Synovectomy of involved joints should be performed along with initial medical therapy in newly diagnosed cases in order to prevent progress of the disease
D. Synovectomy is most effective at the knee joint

Schwartz: 2017

Comments: The rheumatoid arthritic is best managed in a multidisciplinary way with input from the rheumatologist, orthopedist, and physical and occupational therapists. While management of early or less severe cases revolves around appropriate medical intervention (analgesics and anti-inflammatory medications), physical therapy and counseling regarding physical activities may be of great benefit early in the course of the disease process. Such therapy not only relieves the associated pain, but also plays a major role in maintaining strength, maintaining joint mobility, preventing flexion contractures, and delaying joint deformity. Synovectomy has been beneficial in relieving pain and preventing or delaying joint destruction in selected patients. Synovectomy, however, should be performed only when there is evidence of progression of disease in spite of adequate anti-inflammatory treatment and activity modification. Synovectomy appears to have the greatest benefit in the management of knee involvement and does not appear to modify the disease process when it involves the metacarpophalangeal or metatarsophalangeal joints.

Answer: A, D

11. Which of the following joints (when severely damaged by rheumatoid arthritis) may benefit from resection arthroplasty or total joint replacement?

A. Hip
B. Knee
C. Ankle
D. Shoulder
E. Metatarsophalangeal (MTP) joints
F. Metacarpophalangeal (MCP) joints

Schwartz: 2019

Comments: When medical management has failed to control the disease process and joint pain, immobility, deformity, and contracture are disabling to the patient, surgical intervention may be warranted. Benefit has been achieved in the surgical management of arthritis involving all of the joints listed above, but with varying success. Total replacements of the hip, knee, ankle, shoulder, and MCP joints have been reported with success. Surgical intervention for arthritis of the MTP joints has been successfully achieved with resection of the metatarsal heads and proximal portions of the phalanges. The success of these procedures depends on many factors, including the general health of the patient, severity of the arthritic process, ability to undergo appropriate postoperative physical therapy, and degree of soft tissue involvement associated with the joint in question.

Answer: A, B, C, D, E, F

12. Which of the following procedures may be indicated in the surgical management of the rheumatoid hand?

A. Tenosynovectomy
B. Interphalangeal joint fusion
C. Joint arthroplasty
D. Distal ulnar shaft resection

Schwartz: 2020

Comments: As with other joints involved with rheumatoid arthritis, those of the hand and wrist may require surgical intervention when the disease progresses in spite of appropriate medical management. The type of intervention elected depends on the joint affected and the nature and severity of involvement.

Answer: A, B, C, D

13. In osteoarthritis:

A. The earliest recognizable changes occur in the subchondral bone
B. The articular cartilage is involved late in the disease process
C. There is a strong correlation between clinical symptoms and radiographic changes
D. Chondroitin sulfate is increased in the articular cartilage
E. None of the above

Schwartz: 2023

Comments: Osteoarthritis is a term that refers to degenerative changes in synovial joints. The earliest changes seen are those in the articular cartilage. Grossly, the cartilage may appear softer and more yellow than usual, and biochemically it is found to have a decrease in the normal amount of chondroitin sulfate. Since cartilage is not normally seen on x-ray, these early changes, which may be quite symptomatic, are not seen radiographically. Thus, at times there is poor correlation between the clinical and radiographic findings. Since this process is more one of degeneration than of inflammation, some have felt that the terms "degenerative joint disease" and "osteoarthrosis" are more appropriate names for the process.

Answer: E

14. The classical clinical presentation of osteoarthritis includes:

A. Joint pain occurring on motion and relieved by rest
B. Frequent involvement of the MCP joints
C. Normal synovial fluid/blood glucose gradient
D. Fairly abrupt onset of symptoms

Schwartz: 2024

Comments: Osteoarthritis may be considered to occur as a primary disease in which there are no antecedent forms of joint pathology or as a secondary entity, usually related to previous joint trauma, rheumatoid disease, gout, or other forms of inflammatory arthritis. The onset is usually insidious, and the symptoms primarily relate to joint pain that is brought on by motion and weight-bearing and relieved by rest. Primary osteoarthritis is a disease of the elderly, usually presenting in persons 60 years and older. Secondary osteoarthritis may be found in any joint that has been previously injured by trauma, rheumatoid arthritis, or other inflammatory conditions, whereas primary osteoarthritis tends to involve the large weight-bearing joints (most notably the hips and knees). The elbows, wrists, and MCP joints are rarely involved. Laboratory examinations are usually unrevealing, and in the absence of underlying inflammatory processes, the synovial fluid reveals few abnormalities.

Answer: A, C

15. True statements regarding the nonoperative management of osteoarthritis include:

A. Rest of the clinically involved joint is the key to successful nonoperative management
B. Weight loss in the obese patient may significantly improve symptoms
C. Anti-inflammatory medications present risks (gastric ulceration and antiplatelet effects) greater than the benefit they confer, and should be avoided in this form of arthritis
D. Range of motion and muscle strengthening exercises aggravate the osteoarthritic joint and should be avoided

Schwartz: 2025

Comments: The majority of patients with osteoarthritis are successfully treated with conservative management, the basic principle of which is rest and/or immobilization of the involved joint(s). A careful search should be made for possible aggravating factors (e.g., occupational trauma, obesity), and modification of such lifestyle-related factors should be made if possible. There is some controversy over the risk vs. benefit of intra-articular steroid injections, but most agree that oral nonsteroidal anti-inflammatory medications are helpful and frequently indicated in treatment. When the acute symptoms have resolved, range of motion and muscle strengthening exercises should be employed to maintain as full function of the joint as possible and to promote joint stability.

Answer: A, B

16. Match the following surgical procedures used for osteoarthritis of the hip with their appropriate descriptive statement

Procedure	Description
A. Arthrodesis	a. Has the best short- and medium-term results
B. Displacement osteotomy	b. Joint sepsis is the most frequent indication
C. Femoral head replacement arthroplasty	c. Best procedure for young patients with early osteoarthritis
D. Total hip arthroplasty	d. Contraindicated when the acetabulum is severely diseased

Schwartz: 2026

Comments: A number of operative procedures are available to treat osteoarthritis of the hip. **Arthrodesis**, which involves a fusion of the hip joint, is most frequently indicated when the presence of pyogenic or tuberculous sepsis makes prosthetic arthroplasty contraindicated. It also presents an alternative in the young patient with severe joint changes. **Displacement osteotomy** of the femur involves transection of the proximal femoral shaft and medical displacement of the shaft on the femoral head. This usually results in excellent pain relief and improvement in joint motion, but generally is reserved for the treatment of young patients with fairly early osteoarthritis who are still capable of producing at least 70 degrees of hip flexion. **Arthroplasty** by femoral head replacement is utilized mainly in subcapital fractures of the femur and requires a normal acetabulum. **Total hip replacement** is indicated when both the femoral head and acetabulum are involved. It has the best short- and medium-term results of all of the procedures available. However, complications due to infection or loosening of the prostheses may be severe and quite debilitating. The tendency to avoid its use in the younger population has been based on unanswered questions regarding the long-term performance of the prostheses, particularly the risk of loosening. Research in the fields of bioengineering and bioprosthetics is extremely active in this regard.

Answer: A–b; B–c; C–d; D–a

17. Absorption of methyl methacrylate (bone cement) constituents during a cemented total hip replacement is associated with:

A. Rare late carcinogenic effects
B. Hepatotoxicity
C. Hypotension
D. Inhibition of platelet function
E. None of the above

Schwartz: 2029

Comments: The cementing substance most often used in the fixation of orthopedic prosthetic devices is methyl methacrylate, which is an acrylic polymer. During mixing of the components of the cement, a marked exothermic reaction develops which can produce temperatures as high as 90° C. This results in some local tissue damage, which may be a factor associated with prosthetic loosening. Hypotension has been reported to occur as a result of absorption of the methacrylate constituents at the time of surgery. There has been no evidence, however, of other toxic or carcinogenic sequelae to the use of methyl methacrylate.

Answer: C

18. The loss of mobility in a hip joint involved with osteoarthritis results from:

A. Articular cartilage destruction
B. Loss of joint space
C. Capsular contracture
D. Muscle spasm and fibrosis of musculotendinous structures
E. Mechanical blocking from osteophytes or loose bodies

Schwartz: 2026

Comments: Osteoarthritis of the hip may produce a wide spectrum of functional disability ranging from mild discomfort with no functional loss to a completely immobile joint. All of the factors listed above may contribute to the functional disability associated with osteoarthritis.

Answer: A, B, C, D, E

19. Which of the following statements is/are true regarding chondromalacia of the patella?

A. The initial changes usually occur on the lateral aspect of the patella
B. The pain is aggravated by knee flexion, kneeling, and descending stairs
C. Radiographs show characteristic changes early in the course of the disease process
D. The progressive nature of the disease warrants early surgical intervention
E. Patellectomy is the only proven successful form of surgical therapy

Schwartz: 2030

Comments: Chondromalacia of the patella, as its name implies, is a disease process of the cartilage of the patella, which has several similarities to osteoarthritis. The initial changes are usually seen on the medial aspect of the patella, and the characteristic clinical presentation is that of an insidious onset of medial knee or peripatellar pain aggravated by knee flexion, direct pressure (as in kneeling), and descending stairs. As with other forms of osteoarthritis and cartilage injury, radiographs are frequently negative and not diagnostic, especially early in the disease process. The majority of patients with this problem are adequately managed by conservative treatment, which involves avoiding knee flexion and performing quadriceps strengthening exercises. When the disease process progresses, surgical intervention may be warranted. Patellectomy may be required in severe chondromalacia with osteoarthritis of the patellofemoral joint; however, excision of the cartilage itself or realignment of the quadriceps patellar mechanism has been successful in less severe forms of the disease.

Answer: B

20. Regarding hallux valgus:

A. Exostosis removal is usually effective
B. Most patients are asymptomatic
C. It is much more common in populations in which shoes are not worn
D. Silastic arthroplasty is the surgical procedure of choice in most instances

Schwartz: 2031

Comments: Hallux valgus refers to the lateral deviation of the great toe and is popularly considered synonymous with bunion, which actually refers more specifically to the large exostosis and overlying soft tissue bursa that frequently occurs in association with hallux valgus. This is primarily a disease of the shoe-wearing population (improper shoe fitting). Whereas the anatomic abnormality is fairly common, the associated symptoms of intermittent pain over the involved MTP joint occur relatively infrequently. Conservative treatment with the use of molded insoles and metatarsal arches to redistribute the weight is usually successful. When symptoms persist despite conservative measures, surgical intervention may be warranted. The most common surgical procedure employed is the Keller arthroplasty, which involves excision of the proximal half of the proximal phalanx with excision of the osteophyte associated with the dorsomedial metatarsal head. Prosthetic arthroplasty is not generally used for this condition, and procedures involving only excision of the bursa and metatarsal exostosis usually fail to relieve symptoms.

Answer: B

21. Which of the following statements regarding gout is/are true?

A. It commonly presents as a monoarticular arthritis of the MTP joint of the great toe
B. Diagnosis requires demonstration of urate crystals in synovial fluid
C. There is a direct correlation between clinical evidence of gout and serum uric acid level
D. Because of the inability of medical management to control chronic disease, surgical intervention is usually required at some point in the clinical course

Schwartz: 2032

Comments: Gout is a metabolic disease which may present in a primary form (inborn error of metabolism) or a secondary form (e.g., myeloproliferative disorders, leukemia, hemolytic anemia). The clinical manifestations of gouty arthritis are presumed to be secondary to the inflammatory sequelae of urate crystal deposition in cartilage, subchondral bone, and periarticular soft tissues. Although the likelihood of clinical symptoms increases with increasing serum uric acid levels, it is not uncommon to have significant hyperuricemia without clinical symptoms and to have clinical symptoms without hyperuricemia. The classic clinical presentation is that of an acute attack of monoarticular arthritis, most often involving the MTP joint of the great toe, most often occurring in males over the age of 30. Management of the acute attack involves rest and anti-inflammatory medication (e.g., colchicine, nonsteroidal anti-inflammatory drugs). Upon resolution of the acute symptoms, long-term management with allopurinol to reduce serum uric acid levels may be indicated. Surgery is rarely indicated in the management of acute or chronic gouty arthritis; however, excision of large tophaceous deposits may provide symptomatic relief, and joints that are severely involved may require arthrodesis or arthroplasty.

Answer: A, B

22. A 5-year-old boy presents with symptoms of an upper respiratory infection, fever, and a painful hip. X-rays are negative, and a CBC shows a slightly elevated white count. The next step in management is:

A. Repeat the CBC in 4 hours
B. Obtain a bone scan

C. Obtain tomograms of the involved hip
D. Aspiration of the hip
E. None of the above

Sabiston: 1504
Schwartz: 2036

Comments: The causes of painful hip in children and adolescents are numerous. Since a septic joint must always be considered among these causes, and since delay in treatment of a septic joint can result in significant permanent disability, aspiration of acutely symptomatic joints in children should be performed early in the diagnostic management. Once the diagnosis of infection has been excluded, a clinical and radiographic search for other causes (e.g., Legg-Calvé-Perthes disease, acute synovitis) should be undertaken.

Answer: D

23. Slipped capital femoral epiphysis:

A. Is more prevalent in males
B. Is rarely bilateral
C. Commonly presents with knee pain
D. Is often associated with loss of normal internal rotation
E. Is rarely managed surgically because of the risk of permanent epiphyseal damage

Schwartz: 2036

Comments: Slipped capital femoral epiphysis is a relatively rare entity which most often occurs in adolescent males. It represents a separation of the proximal capital femoral epiphysis in the region above the zone of calcified cartilage. The actual cause of the epiphyseal disruption is unknown, but the associated muscular forces across the hip result in the characteristic medial and posterior displacement of the capital epiphysis. The clinical sequelae include pain in the area of the hip aggravated by motion, pain referred to the knee, and loss of normal internal rotation. The process is bilateral in 25% of cases. Treatment is based on the principles of preventing further slippage and minimizing existing deformity. This is achieved most often by surgical pinning of the femoral head and neck to engage the epiphysis.

Answer: A, C, D

24. Which of the following statements accurately characterize(s) Charcot joint?

A. It occurs as a consequence of various forms of neurologic disorders
B. It is usually of acute onset
C. Characteristic x-ray findings are those of dense sclerosis of the subchondral bone
D. Treatment may necessitate arthrodesis

Schwartz: 2037

Comments: A Charcot or neuropathic joint is one in which there has been significant articular and periarticular destruction thought to be secondary to repeated trauma on structures rendered insensitive by underlying neurologic disorders (e.g., tabes dorsalis, diabetes). The clinical course is usually of insidious onset and the patient is often unaware of the joint disability until it becomes quite severe with gross instability and significant effusion. Radiographically, there is usually marked bone destruction and widening of the joint space, which may contain loose bony fragments. The knee and hip are frequently involved; and when conservative management with a properly fitted weight-bearing brace fails, arthrodesis is frequently indicated.

Answer: A, D

25. Shoulder pain may be caused by which of the following entities?

A. Spinal arthritis
B. Lung cancer
C. Umbilical hernia
D. Diaphragmatic irritation
E. Angina

Schwartz: 2038

Comments: See Question 26.

26. Match the following primary shoulder disorders with their appropriate clinical characteristics

Disorder	Characteristic
A. Subacromial bursitis	a. Pain extending along the proximal humeral groove
B. Bicipital tendinitis	b. Unrelenting pain unimproved by position
C. Supraspinatus tendinitis	c. Limitation of internal rotation and full abduction
D. Rotator cuff tear	d. Surgical repair may be required

Schwartz: 2038

Comments: In evaluating shoulder pain, one must be alert to the numerous clinical entities that, although anatomically unrelated, may cause referred pain to the shoulder. These include cervical arthritis with brachial plexus irritation, Pancoast's tumor, cardiac angina, and abdominal conditions associated with diaphragmatic irritation. Of the primary shoulder disorders that characteristically produce pain, lesions of the rotator cuff, bicipital tendinitis, and subacromial bursitis are the most common. The **rotator cuff** consists of the common tendinous insertion of the supraspinatus, infraspinatus, teres minor, and subscapularis tendons. In positions of full elevation or abduction, the rotator cuff may contact the coracoacromial ligament and cause irritation of the intervening bursa. Repeated injury may cause degeneration and lead to **subacromial bursitis**. This entity is usually characterized by fairly severe and unrelenting pain that is unimproved by position and may even require narcotics for relief. A **rotator cuff tear** represents a physical disruption of the tendinous structure with varying degrees of associated inflammation. Most rotator cuff tears are partial, and initial conservative management with shoulder immobilization is usually successful. With total rupture, open surgical repair of the tear is often preferred, but conservative management can be successful. With **supraspinatus tendinitis**, the pain is more insidious in onset and of lesser degree. It frequently limits the motions of internal rotation and full abduction, which are painful. **Bicipital tendinitis** produces symptoms that are quite similar to those of supraspinatus tendinitis. However, the distribution of pain and tenderness is more distal over the bicipital groove. In these four inflammatory entities, treatment with rest, analgesics, nonsteroidal anti-inflammatory drugs, and occasionally steroid injections are usually successful.

Answer: Question 25: A, B, D, E
Question 26: A–b; B–a; C–c; D–d

CHAPTER 59

Orthopedics—Neoplasms

1. Which of the following statements is/are true regarding the biologic properties of bone tumors?

A. They have a bimodal age peak
B. Paget's disease is the only known example of premalignant change in bone
C. The age incidence of primary bone tumors in men and women is the same
D. Only cells contributing to primary skeletal bone formation are capable of malignant degeneration
E. All of the above
F. None of the above

Sabiston: 1505
Schwartz: 1934

Comments: The incidence of bone tumors peaks in two age groups. The first peak (10 to 25 years) is due mainly to primary tumors, while the second peak (40 to 70 years) is due to secondary tumors arising from pre-existing conditions (such as Paget's disease, previously irradiated bone, fibrous dysplasia, and diaphyseal aclasis) or metastatic cancer. True bone tumors arise from cells of mesenchymal origin whose function is primarily formation of skeletal bone. These cells include the osteoblast, the osteoclast, and the fibroblast. Tissues found in bone but not participating in bone formation can also give rise to malignant bone tumors. These include tumors arising from supportive fibrous tissue, bone marrow, blood vessels, and nervous and adipose tissue. The highest incidence of bone tumors in females is between the ages of 5 and 14 years, whereas in males it is between ages 15 and 24 years. This difference in incidence is felt to relate to differences in growth patterns and hormonal influences between the sexes.

Answer: A

2. Which of the following statements is/are true regarding osteoma and osteoid osteoma?

A. Both represent benign tumors arising from the osteoblast
B. Osteoma is a relatively common benign tumor in ad-

olescents, occurring with equal distribution throughout the skeletal system
C. Osteoid osteoma occurs in young males between the ages of 10 and 30 years, particularly in the bones of the lower extremities
D. Both lesions are considered premalignant

Sabiston: 1509
Schwartz: 1934

Comments: Both tumors arise from the osteoblast and are not considered premalignant. Osteoma is rare; it is found in the orbit, nasal sinuses, external auditory meatus, and the oral side of the mandible and is believed to result from abnormal growth or from imperfect remodeling after trauma. An example of traumatic osteoma is the so-called rider's bone found on the femur in relationship to the adductor magnus. Patients with osteoid osteoma frequently present with local nocturnal pain relieved by salicylates. When possible, complete resection of this lesion will provide cure.

Answer: A, C

3. Features of osteogenic sarcoma include:

A. The most common site of involvement is the diaphesis of the femur
B. It may occur in 10% of patients with Paget's disease
C. Metastases occur mainly via the lymphatic system
D. The first symptom usually is pain resulting from a pathologic fracture
E. "Sun-ray" appearance on x-ray is a frequent finding

Sabiston: 1509
Schwartz: 1935

Comments: Osteogenic sarcoma is rare, occurring about 1 in 775,000 of the population. As a primary tumor, it is seen most commonly in the second decade of life. The most common site of involvement is the metaphysis of the femur, followed by the upper end of the tibia and the humerus; the radius, ulna, ilium, and scapula are less frequently affected. Osteogenic sarcoma in older patients frequently arises from pre-existing Paget's disease. Such sarcomatous degeneration occurs in 10% of male patients with Paget's disease; it carries a poorer prognosis than primary osteogenic sarcoma, and often arises simultaneously at multiple sites. When the tumor extends to or originates beneath the periosteum, the periosteum is raised off the bone, producing a soft tissue swelling. Spicules of bone within the tumor produce a "sun-ray" appearance on x-ray. When the tumor extends towards the medulla, it rarely transgresses the cartilage of the epiphysis. Usually, the first symptom is night pain secondary to periosteal irritation. This pain often precludes ambulation, making pathologic fractures an uncommon occurrence. Metastatic spread is primarily hematogenous and most commonly is to the lung, often producing a clinical picture of bronchitis or pneumonia. In the past, standard treatment was local radiation therapy with delayed amputation, giving a 5-year survival rate of 20%. Current treatment combines surgery with high-dose methotrexate with citrovorum "rescue." The 5-year survival now is over 50%. Considerable success is being reported with limb salvage surgery in combination with chemotherapy.

Answer: B, E

4. Match the clinical statement with the disease.

Clinical Statement	Disease
A. History of painful swelling with loss of joint function; occurs most commonly in patients 10 to 30 years old	a. Chondroma b. Benign chondroblastoma c. Chrondrosarcoma d. Osteoclastoma (giant cell tumor) e. Juvenile bone cyst
B. Slow-growing tumor arising from cartilaginous elements, frequently undergoing calcification	
C. Occurs as a primary tumor in the later age groups and as a secondary tumor in osteochondroma, Paget's disease, and diaphyseal aclasia	
D. Occurs during the years of active bone growth and often presents as a pathologic fracture without previous symptoms	
E. Occasionally behaves malignantly despite having a benign histologic appearance	

Sabiston: 1506
Schwartz: 1936

Comments: **Chondroma** is a benign neoplasm arising from cartilaginous elements of developing bone and frequently undergoes calcification. In the small bones of the hand or foot, it is known as an enchondroma or Ollier's disease. On x-ray it appears as a dense shadow with a feathery outline of calcified spicules. Malignant degeneration occurs only in multiple enchondromas. **Benign chondroblastoma** occurs in the first and second decades of life, before closure of the epiphyseal line. There is often a history of painful swelling with loss of joint function. On x-ray, it appears as an osteolytic lesion contain-

ing calcium deposits. Treatment consists of curettage and grafting with cancellous bone. **Chondrosarcoma** arises from chondroblasts and may be either primary (in older patients) or a secondary malignant change in such pre-existing conditions as osteochondroma, Paget's disease or diaphyseal aclasia. The pelvis, ribs, sternum, and femur are the bones most commonly involved. X-rays show destruction of trabecular bone or cortex associated with an expanding soft tissue mass containing irregular areas of calcified tissue. A grading system based on the degree of cellularity, the amount of matrix formed, and the severity of nuclear irregularities seems to correlate with survival, which ranges from good to poor. **Osteoclastoma,** or giant cell tumor, contains a highly vascular cellular stroma with many giant cells. They are seen commonly in the ends of long bones in the vicinity of the knee and the lower end of the radius and on x-ray appear as a clear cystic tumor in the metaphyseoepiphyseal area. They may penetrate the articular cartilage but only rarely extend into the joint. Occasionally these tumors behave with malignant characteristics despite a benign histologic appearance. Local recurrence is as high as 50% with curettage, and therefore complete excision is recommended. Radiotherapy does not decrease the recurrence rate. **Juvenile bone cyst** occurs in the metaphyseal area of long bones, such as the upper end of the humerus and femur. It often presents as a pathologic fracture without previous symptoms. In contrast to the giant cell tumor, the juvenile bone cyst is relatively avascular. Treatment consists of curettage of the cystic cavity and of bone grafting to restore continuity.

Answer: A–b; B–a; C–c; D–e; E–d

5. Which of the following statements is/are true regarding Ewing's tumor and reticulum cell sarcoma?

A. Both tumors mostly affect patients under 20 years of age
B. Ewing's tumor is frequently associated with febrile attacks
C. Ewing's tumor begins in the diaphyseal marrow, and, as it extends to the periosteum, new bone formation occurs, creating so-called onion layers.
D. Reticulum cell sarcoma responds well to radiation but tends to recur; therefore, this treatment should be followed by amputation or radical resection.

Sabiston: 1512
Schwartz: 1942

Comments: Ewing's tumor is a small, round-cell malignancy arising from the diaphyseal marrow of long bones in patients under 20 years of age. The tumor extends from the medulla to the periosteum and as new bone is deposited "onion-layering" parallel to the shaft is visible on x-ray. A history of trauma is not uncommon and there are frequently associated febrile attacks and leukocytosis. The tumor is capable of lymphatic as well as hematogenous spread, and death usually results from pulmonary metastases. The tumors are radiosensitive but tend to recur. Newer treatments using various chemotherapeutic agents have improved survival; in carefully selected patients, the limb can be salvaged. **Reticulum cell sarcoma** occurs in patients between ages 20 and 40 and affects most commonly the femur, tibia, and humerus. Pain, preceding formation of a visible tumor, is often the first complaint. On x-ray, the lesions appear osteolytic at the end of the diaphysis, later extending throughout the length of the bone. Sometimes there is a pathologic fracture. Radiation therapy combined with surgery and chemotherapy has given the best survival rates.

Answer: B, C, D

6. Match the clinical statement with the corresponding lesion.

Clinical Statement	Lesion
A. Most often located in the jaw	a. Aneurysmal bone cyst
B. Located in the metaphysis, this lesion histologically consists of cavernous spaces interspersed with osteoid tissue	b. Adamantinoma
	c. Neurilemmoma
	d. Chordoma
C. Presents as a single cystic swelling associated with destruction of bone	e. Hemangioma
D. Most commonly found in the sacrococcygeal region	
E. A benign vascular tumor more commonly found in the skull and vertebral column than in other bones	

Sabiston: 523, 1356
Schwartz: 1944

Comments: **Aneurysmal bone cyst** is an osteolytic lesion found in the metaphyses of long bones in young people. Histologically, the characteristic findings are cavernous spaces within fibrous tissue, without endothelial lining. Local curettage with or without bone graft usually is adequate treatment. **Adamantinoma** occurs most frequently as an enamel-containing tumor in the jaw. This tumor is treated with wide excision, which often requires bone grafting. A rare histologically similar tumor that occurs in the tibia or other long bones is also designated adamantinoma, although this type does not contain enamel. The treatment of choice for adamantinoma of a long bone is amputation through a bone higher on the affected limb. **Neurilemmoma** is a nerve sheath tumor that may grow in bone. In that setting, it presents on x-ray as cystic swelling with associated destruction of bone. Usually it occurs singly and the clinical course is benign, and local removal, when possible, provides adequate treatment. Deformity of bone and fracture may occur. **Chordoma** is a rare malignant neoplasm arising from embryonic remnants of the notochord and is found in the spheno-occipital or sacrococcygeal region. The tumor is radioresistant, the only hope for cure being complete surgical excision. **Hemangioma** is a vascular tumor that rarely affects bone, most commonly doing so in the skull and vertebral column; in the latter location, this can lead to collapse of the vertebral body. The majority of these tumors are benign, but excision is advised whenever possible.

Answer: A–b; B–a; C–c; D–d; E–e

7. Correctly match the statement with the corresponding soft tissue tumor.

Statement	Soft Tissue Tumor
A. Occurs in the deep muscle masses as a painful swelling, is locally invasive, but does not metastasize	a. Fibrosarcoma of muscle
B. Is a malignant small-cell tumor with a high incidence of blood-borne metastases	b. Liposarcoma
	c. Rhabdomyosarcoma
	d. Synovial sarcoma
C. Arises from embryologically sequestered synovioblastic cells	e. Desmoid tumor
D. Usually presents as a large painful tumor mass, most commonly in the musculature of the thigh	
E. Is one of the more common malignant soft tissue tumors and occurs primarily in the soft tissues of the extremities	

Sabiston: 522
Schwartz: 1945

Comments: **Fibrosarcoma** of muscle can occur either as a well-differentiated or as an anaplastic tumor. Usually it presents as a large painful tumor mass in the thigh. **Liposarcoma** also occurs either as a differentiated or as an anaplastic tumor arising from the soft tissues of the extremities. Liposarcomas most commonly occur in middle-aged patients and equally in men and women. The thigh-popliteal area and the inguinal and gluteal regions are the most commonly involved. These tumors arise de novo and do not represent malignant transformation of a lipoma. Their radiosensitivity is variable; curative treatment is best achieved by wide surgical excision. **Rhabdomyosarcoma** is a small-cell malignancy originating from striated muscle cells. It is a tumor of infants and young adults and has very high incidence of hematogenous spread. It is rarely radiosensitive; treatment is multimodal, combining systemic chemotherapy with local surgical resection. **Synovial sarcoma** arises from sequestered synovial blastic cells present in subcutaneous tissue as well as in muscle. There is no obvious continuity with joint tissue. It is capable of local infiltration and should be excised radically to include the main muscle mass surrounding the tumor. **Desmoid tumor** is a very low grade fibrosarcoma capable of local invasion but not hematogenous metastases. Usually it presents as a painful tumor in the deep muscles, tends to occur in younger people, and can recur following inadequate resection; treatment therefore is radical surgical excision.

Answer: A–e; B–c; C–d; D–a; E–b

8. Which of the following statements is/are true regarding the treatment of malignant tumors of soft tissue?

A. Because they are generally well encapsulated, excisional biopsy around the capsule is the procedure of choice to establish diagnosis

B. Biopsy is generally unnecessary, since the diagnosis can be made on the basis of physical examination and radiographic findings

C. Incisional biopsy, when required, should be performed through an incision that can easily be encompassed at the time of definitive surgical treatment

D. When soft tissue sarcomas are diagnosed in the extremity, they are best treated by forequarter or hindquarter amputation

Sabiston: 522
Schwartz: 1946

Comments: Rapidly growing soft tissue tumors compress surrounding normal tissue to form a pseudocapsule. Microscopic nests of cells are often found beyond this pseudocapsule, making simple enucleation unacceptable. Although characteristics consistent with malignancy are often detectable on physical examination and on x-ray, a tissue diagnosis is essential prior to definitive surgical therapy, as the natural history of the various soft tissue tumors varies widely. Low-grade tumors such as desmoid tumor or low-grade fibrosarcomas or liposarcomas are locally invasive, but rarely metastasize. Thus, aggressive primary surgical excision is the treatment of choice. In contrast, osteosarcoma, Ewing's tumor, and rhabdomyosarcoma are examples of tumors with high propensity for distant metastases. For these, treatment by operation alone does little to prolong life; multimodal treatment utilizing antineoplastic drugs and radiation is indicated. An incisional biopsy for diagnosis should be performed in a manner that does not preclude wide excision of the tumor through undissected tissue planes. Because many of these tumors are capable of distant metastases, radical amputation does little to prevent death from distant disease. Amputation is indicated when the anatomic location requires it, examples being tumors arising high in the buttock, high in the thigh, or near the shoulder.

Answer: C

9. Which of the following statements is/are true regarding metastatic tumors of bone?

A. Skeletal metastases can originate from virtually all types of malignant tumors, but most frequently are from tumors of the breast, prostate, thyroid, kidney, and lung
B. Metastatic bone tumors are the result of hematogenous spread ending in bony capillary beds
C. The vast majority of patients with bone metastases complain of pain
D. Bone metastases are a grave prognostic sign and once they appear, survival is rarely longer than three months

Schwartz: 1946

Comments: While the most common cancers metastasizing to bone are those of the breast, prostate, thyroid, kidney, and lung, nearly all types of malignant tumors can do this. The usual route is via the blood stream, originating in veins leaving the primary tumor, then passing through the pulmonary circulation and on to the systemic capillary beds. The high incidence of metastasis to the axial skeleton probably is due to hematogenous dissemination through the vertebral venous plexus (of Battson). Only 65% of patients with x-ray evidence of bone metastases complain of pain; tenderness to palpation is present in fewer than 20%. Many patients with bone metastases may live for many months or years, particularly those with breast cancer responsive to hormonal manipulation.

Answer: A, B

10. Tumors of which organ(s) listed below give rise to bony metastases that may respond to hormonal manipulation?

A. Breast
B. Prostate
C. Kidney
D. Thyroid
E. All of the above
F. None of the above

Schwartz: 1946

Comments: Bone metastases from breast or from prostate are often hormonally dependent, so that progression of disease can frequently be retarded or symptoms relieved by hormonal manipulation. Treatment with diethylstilbestrol diphosphate, orchiectomy, or both frequently relieves the pain caused by prostatic metastases. Approximately 30% of patients with bone metastases from breast respond to hormonal manipulation therapy. Treatment in this setting is variable; it may include pharmacologic agents such as diethylstilbestrol, androgens, antiestrogen (tamoxifen), progesterones, or corticosteroids, as well as endocrine ablative surgery such as oophorectomy, adrenalectomy, or pituitary ablation.

Answer: A, B

11. Which method of diagnosis is the most sensitive for the detection of bony metastases?

A. History and physical examination
B. X-ray
C. Technetium bone scan
D. Measurement of serum alkaline phosphatase
E. Measurement of serum calcium

Schwartz: 1946

Comments: About 65% of patients with bony metastases complain of pain and about 15% have palpable tenderness. The alkaline phosphatase may be normal in up to 40% of patients. X-rays are unreliable since at least 50% of the medulla must be destroyed before a lesion will be seen on a bone x-ray; tomograms of the bone are more sensitive. Far and away the most sensitive screening test for bony metastases in the technetium bone scan. Hypercalcemia may be the result of bone destruction by metastases, but when the kidneys are functioning, one usually finds hypercalciuria associated with normal serum calcium levels. Hypercalcemia due to bronchogenic carcinoma may be due to a parathormone-like hormone secreted by the tumor. Mammary carcinomas frequently produce hypercalcemia, which may be due to the excretion of specific osteolytic steroids derived from the mammary carcinoma.

Answer: C

12. Which of the following is/are true concerning treatment of skeletal metastases?

A. The pain that arises from skeletal metastases may be diminished if the hypercalcemia is treated

B. There is an 80% chance of pain relief following hormonal therapy
C. Radiotherapy to the localized area of pain is indicated when hormonal therapy is ineffective
D. Large lytic lesions, particularly of the femur, should be treated initially with radiation followed by internal fixation to avoid a pathologic fracture

Schwartz: 1946

Comments: In most instances, treatment of skeletal metastases is palliative. Pain may occur only in association with hypercalcemia, and once this is treated, the pain may be relieved. Patients with hormonally dependent tumors often have significant relief of pain following hormonal manipulation. If hormonal therapy fails or for tumors that are not hormonally dependent, radiotherapy to a localized area of pain often produces relief. Large lytic lesions with impending fracture should have internal fixation followed by radiation. Radiotherapy given preoperatively may predispose to pathologic fracture, lessening the effectiveness of the fixation. Vertebral metastases with subsequent compression fracture involving the spinal cord may be treated by decompression laminectomy. Radiotherapy only in this setting can control pain, but does not improve an established paraplegia.

Answer: A, C

CHAPTER 60

Hand Surgery

1. Match each of the following nerves with the correct labeled structure on the diagram.

A. Median nerve
B. Radial nerve
C. Ulnar nerve

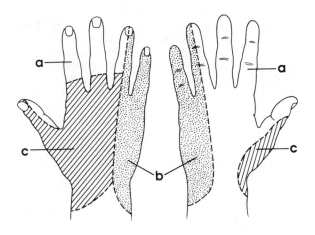
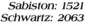

Sabiston: 1521
Schwartz: 2063

Comments: There is considerable overlap in the sensory innervation of the hand. The usual innervation is as depicted in the illustration. Despite the overlap, there are certain autonomous zones useful in evaluating nerve function: the **median** nerve on the flexor aspect of the index finger beyond the distal interphalangeal joint; the **ulnar** nerve on the flexor aspect of the little finger beyond the distal interphalangeal joint; the **radial** nerve on the dorsal web space of the thumb. Light touch with a piece of cotton and point discrimination are the most valuable sensory tests. Light touch is preferred in assessing sensation after acute injury or when examining children.

Answer: A–a; B–c; C–b

2. True statements regarding the intrinsic muscles of the hand include:

A. The intrinsic muscles originate in the forearm and insert on the metacarpals
B. The palmar interossei pull the fingers to the midline and flex the metacarpophalangeal joints of the index, ring, and little fingers
C. Their innervation is derived from the radial, median, and ulnar nerves
D. The dorsal interosseous muscles spread the fingers and flex the proximal phalanges
E. The intrinsic muscles of the index, long, and ring fingers consist of the palmar and dorsal interossei and the lumbrical muscles

Sabiston: 1518, 1522
Schwartz: 2065

Comments: The intrinsic muscles have their entire course confined to the hand and include the thenar and hypothenar muscles, the lumbricals, and the interosseous muscles. Together, they flex the metacarpophalangeal joints, extend the interphalangeal joints (lumbricals), provide elevation, rotation, and apposition of the thumb (thenar muscles), and spread the fingers. When functioning normally, they provide the hand with a transverse and longitudinal arch. Their innervation is derived from the median and ulnar nerves, the distribution of which is variable. The classic pattern is median innervation of the first two lumbricals and the muscles of the thenar eminence excluding the ulnar head of the flexor pollicis brevis. The ulnar nerve innervates the hypothenar muscles, the interosseous muscles, and the ulnar head of the flexor pollicis brevis. The median nerve is tested by palmar abduction of the thumb and opposition. The ulnar innervated intrinsics are responsible for finger abduction and adduction.

Answer: B, D

3. True statements regarding the techniques of hand surgery include:

A. Epinephrine should never be used with local anesthesia

B. Digital blocks are best placed using the ring technique

C. When providing pain relief to allow assessment of digital movement, a radial, ulnar, or median wrist block is employed

D. A rubber-band tourniquet at the base of the digit is a safe, effective means to provide a bloodless field

E. Tourniquet ischemia is tolerated for 30 minutes in the unanesthetized arm and for 2 hours in the anesthetized arm

Sabiston: 1457
Schwartz: 2065

Comments: Because of possible irreversible vascular complications, epinephrine should never be used in local anesthetics employed during hand surgery. The ring block raises venous pressure and may compromise digital vascularity. Digital blocks therefore are established by injecting the web space on both sides of the involved finger. The nerves to the radial side of the index and the ulnar side of the little finger are located in the subcutaneous tissue on the volar surface of the corresponding metacarpal head. Wrist blocks anesthetize intrinsic muscles, and therefore digital blocks should be used to provide pain relief during assessment of digital motion. Tourniquets are applied as high on the arm as possible over adequate padding. Arm exsanguination is accomplished by distal-to-proximal wrapping with an elastic bandage before tourniquet pressure is applied. Rubber-band tourniquets at the level of the finger should never be used; they apply high pressure over a narrow area and can cause irreversible neurovascular damage.

Answer: A, E

4. True statements regarding the dressing of hand wounds include:

A. Hand dressings must begin with an occlusive layer to avoid infection

B. Hand dressings must be conforming and absorptive, not occlusive

C. The "safe position" of immobilization places the wrist in 20 to 30 degrees of extension, the metacarpophalangeal joints in 60 to 90 degrees of flexion, and the interphalangeal joints in extension

D. The arm must be immobilized in a sling after hand surgery to avoid increased arterial blood flow

Schwartz: 2068

Comments: Hand dressings must be applied smoothly and without pressure. The layer next to the skin must be conforming and absorptive, not occlusive, to encourage drainage of blood into the dressing. The next layer should be longitudinally applied, soft gauze dressings. Conforming gauze dressings then help mold the gauze in place. Plastic splints and rolls are then applied without pressure, with the hand in the "safe position." The thumb (if not involved in injury or operation) and uninvolved digits should protrude from the dressing. It may be necessary to include the adjacent digit in the dressing to provide adequate immobilization. The hand must be kept elevated at all times after surgery or injury, even during ambulation. Slings should be avoided, except in very young children.

Answer: B, C

5. True statements regarding the placement of hand incisions include:

A. Palm incisions should parallel the skin creases or cross them obliquely

B. It is better to err on the volar rather than the dorsal aspect in placement of incisions on the side of the digit

C. Incisions on the volar side of the digit must cross the interphalangeal flexion creases transversely

D. Dorsal skin incisions should cross skin creases transversely or obliquely

Schwartz: 2067

Comments: There are several principles one must follow in planning hand incisions. Those on the palm should run parallel to the skin creases or cross them obliquely. Digital incisions should be placed dorsal to the midlateral line on the side of the digit (through the midaxial line at the finger joints). Given a choice, it is far better to err in placing an incision dorsally rather than on the volar aspect of the side of the digit. Volar incisions may form a bridging scar. The line marking the change in character between the dorsal and volar skin on the side of the digit is a useful landmark. Incisions crossing the flexor creases of the digit must avoid the diamond-shaped area where the skin surfaces on each side of the interphalangeal and metacarpal joints touch during maximal digital flexion (see diagram). Skin incisions on the dorsum of the hand and digits should cross skin creases transversely or obliquely. In the rheumatoid hand, incisions that cross the skin of the dorsal wrist should be longitudinal or minimally curved to avoid slough of a distal-based flap.

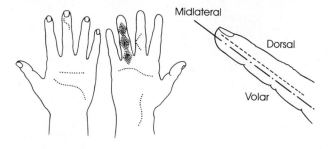

Answer: A, D

6. True statements regarding evaluation of the extrinsic flexors and extenders of the hand include:

A. The flexor digitorum profundus flexes the proximal interphalangeal joint

B. The flexor digitorum profundus flexes the distal interphalangeal joint

C. The flexor digitorum superficialis inserts on the proximal end of the distal phalanx

D. The flexor pollicis longus flexes the first metacarpophalangeal joint

E. There are two extensor tendons to the little finger

Sabiston: 1531
Schwartz: 2064

Comments: The extrinsic muscles of the hand originate in the forearm and their tendons insert on the phalanges (flexor digitorum profundus, flexor digitorum superficialis, extensor digitorum communis) and thumb (flexor pollicis longus, abductor pollicis longus, extensor pollicis brevis). The flexor digitorum profundus inserts on the base of the distal phalanx and flexes the distal interphalangeal joint. The function of the flexor digitorum profundus to the index finger is isolated in 85% of patients. The tendons to the ulnar three digits often act as a single unit and should be tested both simultaneously and individually. Profundus function is evaluated by holding the proximal interphalangeal and metacarpophalangeal joints of the finger being examined in extension. The flexor digitorum superficialis inserts on the entire volar surface of the middle phalanx and flexes the proximal interphalangeal joint. It is evaluated by holding the adjacent fingers in extension. Injuries to the little finger should be examined by simultaneous flexion of the ring and little fingers, since their superficialis tendons may share a common muscle belly. The flexor pollicis longus is responsible for flexion of the distal phalanx of the thumb. The main extensors of the metacarpophalangeal joints are the extensor digitorum communis passing to each of the four fingers, the extensor digiti minimi to the little finger, and the extensor indicis proprius to the index finger. Transection of an extensor tendon results in extensor lag of that digit at the metacarpophalangeal joint. The frequent presence of double tendons to the index and little fingers may confuse the diagnosis. The extensor pollicis brevis extends the proximal phalanx of the thumb, while the abductor pollicis longus extends the first metacarpophalangeal joint. Damage to either of these tendons results in loss of their corresponding function.

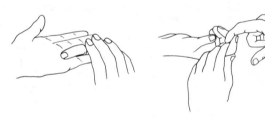

Superficialis testing   Profundus testing

Answer: B, D, E

7. Match the muscle tendon unit with its innervation.

Muscle Tendon Unit	Innervation
A. Flexor digitorum superficialis	a. Median nerve
B. Extensor digitorum communis, extensor indicis proprius, extensor digiti minimi, extensor pollicis brevis, abductor pollicis longus	b. Radial nerve
C. Flexor digitorum profundus to index and middle fingers	c. Ulnar nerve
D. Flexor digitorum profundus to ring and little fingers	

Sabiston: 1521

Comments: The innervation of the extrinsic muscles is derived from the radial, median, and ulnar nerves. The usual pattern of innervation to the extrinsic muscles of the hand is as given above. The innervation of the flexor digitorum superficialis is entirely median, while that of the extensor group is entirely radial. The ulnar nerve innervates the flexor digitorum profundus tendons to the fingers on the ulnar half of the hand, while the median nerve innervates the profundus tendons to the index and middle fingers. Injury to the forearm can potentially lead to abnormalities of digit and thumb flexion and extension due to nerve damage. Flexion and extension of the digits and thumb should always be evaluated in patients presenting with forearm injuries.

Answer: A–a; B–b; C–a; D–c

8. You are called to examine a 30-year-old painter who cut the palm of his right hand with a fresh razor blade. On examination you note a 2-cm clean laceration at the base of the long finger. Metacarpophalangeal joint flexion is intact, but he cannot flex either interphalangeal joint in that finger. The injury is 1 hour old. Your diagnosis is:

A. Lacerated flexor digitorum superficialis tendon
B. Lacerated flexor digitorum profundus tendon
C. Combined flexor digitorum superficialis and profundus laceration
D. Laceration of the intrinsic muscles to the long finger
E. Radial nerve transection

Sabiston: 1529
Schwartz: 2072

Comments: See Question 9.

9. Your immediate treatment plan for the patient described in Question 8 should include:

A. Plans for immediate tendon repair to avoid the hazards of delayed tendon anastomosis
B. Establishment of a wrist block, extension of the skin wound, and exploration to confirm your diagnosis
C. Careful cleansing of the wound, placement of an appropriate dressing, and hand immobilization prior to definitive primary surgical repair
D. Cleansing of the wound, primary skin closure, hand immobilization, and discharge; wounds in this area require free tendon graft reconstruction 6 weeks after injury

Sabiston: 1529
Schwartz: 2072

Comments: Flexion of the metacarpophalangeal joint is a function of the intrinsic muscles and can persist in the face of extrinsic flexor tendon injury. The goal of flexor tendon repair is restoration of interphalangeal joint flexion. Flexor tendon repair demands meticulous attention to detail and, whenever possible, should be performed by a hand surgeon. The character of the wound, the nature of the injury, the degree of contamination, and the time between injury and definitive treatment determine whether primary or delayed repair is performed.

Proper wound cleansing, dressing, immobilization, and prophylactic antibiotics allow delay of primary repair for up to 24 hours if a hand surgeon is not immediately available. If there is a question about the degree of contamination or if the initial wound treatment has been delayed beyond several hours, making primary closure hazardous, delayed repair after 2 to 6 days may be performed. This allows the presence or absence of infection to be clearly established. Many experts feel this type of delay does not significantly alter the ultimate outcome of the repair. Grossly contaminated wounds, those with significant tendon disruption, or wounds with significant associated injuries to soft tissue, bone, nerve, or blood vessels are treated by secondary repair in 3 to 6 weeks, after the wound has healed and edema and callus formation subside.

Answer: Question 8: C
Question 9: C

10. True statements regarding the repair of flexor tendon injuries include:

A. The level of skin laceration determines the level of underlying tendon laceration
B. The flexor tendons run through a fibro-osseous tunnel extending from the distal palm crease to the distal end of the middle phalanx
C. Injuries in Verdan's Zone I carry a good prognosis
D. Free tendon grafts should be considered a procedure of last resort
E. Active range of motion exercises immediately after surgery have significantly improved results
F. The fibro-osseous tunnel is lined by synovium and reinforced by a series of annular and cruciate pulleys that prevent bow-stringing during flexion

Sabiston: 1529
Schwartz: 2072

Comments: Several rules hold for flexor tendon repair: Maximal postoperative function requires full thickness skin coverage. Injuries adjacent to fixed fibrous structures (the flexor tendon pulleys, the palmar fascia, or the wrist retinaculum) or tendons with injuries repaired next to each other can become adherent as healing occurs. The annular pulley at the base of the proximal phalanx (A-2) and at the midportion of the middle phalanx (A-4) must be preserved to prevent bow-stringing during flexion. Precise apposition of tendon ends and avoidance of trauma to the tendon and its underlying bed are extremely important. The level of the flexor tendon injury is very important, and Verdan has described six zones relating the level of injury to prognosis. In Zone I, distal to the digital fibro-osseous tunnel, the prognosis for primary profundus repair is good. In Zone II, the region of the digital fibro-osseous tunnel or "no man's land" (running from the distal palm crease to the proximal end of the middle phalanx), results are not as good. It is an area of controversy regarding appropriate repair of tendon lacerations. For children all surgeons primarily repair the profundus tendon, while some will repair the superficialis tendon as well. In adults, if the wound is clean and the tendon laceration sharp, most surgeons will repair the profundus tendon and, now, usually the flexor superficialis as well. In Zone V on the palm, the superfi-

cial and profundus tendons are both repaired. In Zone VI at the wrist, only the profundus is usually repaired. ● Tendon injuries requiring delayed secondary repair are often treated with free flexor tendon grafts. Tendons heal slowly, and aggressive early mobilization after **free tendon graft** repair may lead to anastomotic disruption or increased scar. After **primary** repair, some surgeons begin immediate active extension and passive flexion with the joint dynamically protected by a rubber band from the wrist to the nails. Active assisted muscle exercise is usually tolerated at 3 weeks, but splinting and elastic extension traction should be delayed for at least 7 weeks.

Answer: B, D, C, F

11. True statements regarding metacarpal fractures include:

A. They are commonly known as Bennett's fracture
B. They are commonly known as the "boxer's fracture"
C. They most often involve the distal metacarpal of the little and ring fingers
D. Physical examination is the most effective means of assessing the degree of angulation
E. The fractures most commonly require open reduction and internal fixation to avoid severe rotation and angulation

Sabiston: 1464
Schwartz: 2069

Comments: Metacarpal fractures commonly result from hitting an object with a clenched fist. They normally involve the distal metacarpal of the fourth and fifth fingers and are known as the boxer's fracture. The metacarpal head is displaced palmward, and pain, swelling, and some loss of knuckle prominence are the usual physical findings. Associated lacerations should be treated as human bites until proven otherwise. Swelling usually masks the degree of angulation, and a lateral x-ray is needed for accurate evaluation. Each finger should be individually flexed to the palm to assess the degree of rotational deformity. During flexion, the fingers normally point to the scaphoid in the anatomic snuff box. Deviation from this alignment allows estimation of the rotational deformity. The usual treament is closed reduction followed by immobilization of the involved and adjacent digits, placing the metacarpophalangeal joint in 60 to 90 degrees of flexion and the interphalangeal joints in full extension. Unstable or multiple metacarpal fractures often need intramedullary fixation. Metacarpal shaft fractures require reduction and immobilization: sometimes percutaneous internal fixation, or even open reduction and internal fixation (especially if a wound already makes the fracture "open") is needed if the fracture is unstable.

Answer: B, C

12. True statements regarding injuries of the thumb include:

A. Bennett's fracture is an avulsion fracture of the base of the first metacarpal
B. Abduction force applied to the thumb most often injures the interphalangeal joint

C. The valgus stress test is used to diagnose disruption of the ulnar collateral ligament system at the first metacarpophalangeal joint

D. The term "gamekeeper's thumb" refers to injuries of the distal phalanx of the thumb

E. The valgus stress test should not be performed when a fracture is suspected or in children suspected of having epiphyseal injury

Sabiston: 1465
Schwartz: 2070 .

Comments: Bennett's fracture is an intra-articular avulsion fracture at the base of the thumb metacarpal. The ligaments remain attached to the bone fragment, the abductor pollicis longus subluxes the metacarpal laterally, and the fracture is unstable. The usual treatment is traction reduction with percutaneous wire fixation of the metacarpal to the trapezium and adjacent carpus. Abduction force applied to the thumb may result in disruption of the ulnar collateral ligament system at the first metacarpophalangeal joint. It commonly occurs in skiing and football injuries. It also may result from repetitive low-grade abduction force as is encountered when using the thumb to dislocate rabbit's necks; hence the name "gamekeeper's thumb." The diagnosis is based on the finding of valgus instability of the metacarpophalangeal joint. When this diagnosis is made, open repair of the ligament is indicated.

Answer: A, C, D, E

13. True statements regarding phalangeal fractures include:

A. Volar angulation of proximal phalangeal fractures causes a flexion deformity of the proximal interphalangeal joint

B. Collateral ligament tears of the interphalangeal joints require open repair

C. Fractures of the base of the middle phalanx tend to have apical dorsal angulation

D. Fractures of the neck of the middle phalanx tend to have apical volar angulation

E. In the presence of distal phalangeal fracture, an associated subungual hematoma must not be opened to avoid osteomyelitis

Sabiston: 1458
Schwartz: 2070

Comments: Closed distal phalangeal fractures are often the result of crush injury and involve nail bed damage as well. If the nail bed and plate are intact, subungual hematomas are drained after careful antiseptic preparation of the digit. Displaced fractures involving injury to the nail matrix may require exploration to ensure that no matrix is interposed in the fracture. Failure to do so predisposes to chronic osteomyelitis. The most important aspect of open fractures of the distal phalanx is not the bone, but rather the repair of skin and soft tissue damage. Fractures of the middle phalanx may or may not involve damage to the collateral ligaments at the interphalangeal joints. Tears of these ligaments with or without small chip fractures usually respond to closed realignment and splinting. Dorsal and volar dislocations at

these joints require precise reduction, and open procedures with internal fixation are frequently necessary. Distal fractures of the middle phalanx usually have apex volar angulation because the proximal segment is flexed by the flexor digitorum superficialis. Fractures at the base of the middle phalanx usually have apical dorsal angulation because of distal segment flexion by the flexor digitorum superficialis and proximal segment extension by the central slip of the extensor mechanism. Most middle phalangeal fractures respond to closed reduction and external immobilization.

Answer: A, C, D

14. True statements regarding extensor tendon injuries include:

A. Extensor tendon lacerations have a good prognosis because of their subcutaneous location

B. The extensor retinaculum must be closed over extensor tendon repairs to prevent bow-stringing

C. Avulsion of the extensor tendon at the base of the distal phalanx results in the boutonnière deformity

D. Disruption of the central extensor tendon at the base of the middle phalanx results in the mallet deformity

Schwartz: 2076

Comments: The extensor tendons occupy a subcutaneous position except at the wrist. The overlying skin is nearly as mobile as the excursion of the extensor tendons and, after repair, rarely restricts their function. An exception to this is at the wrist, where the extensor retinaculum overlies the tendons. Injuries at this level are repaired by transposition of the tendons into the subcutaneous tissue with closure of the retinaculum deep to the repair. The boutonnière deformity results from disruption of the central extensor tendon near its insertion into the dorsum of the base of the middle phalanx. This is accompanied by tears allowing lateral separation of the two lateral bands. The lateral bands are displaced toward the palm, lose their extensor function, and become proximal interphalangeal joint flexors. The patient is unable to initiate full extension from the flexed position but sometimes can maintain extension if the digit is passively placed in that position. Without treatment, the PIP joint becomes fixed in flexion and the DIP joint assumes a position of hyperextension. Immobilization of the proximal interphalangeal joint at 0 degrees of extension for 6 to 8 weeks achieves good results. An alternative treatment is immobilization for 4 weeks, followed by dynamic extension splinting for another 4 weeks; this, obviously, does not shorten the time needed for post-injury splinting or exercise. Injuries to the extensor insertion into the dorsum of the distal phalanx result in the mallet deformity. If the fracture fragment is small, dorsal splinting with the joint in 0 degrees to minus 10 degrees of extension for 6 to 8 weeks provides good results. If more than one third of the articular surface is displaced with the avulsed tendon, and volar subluxation of the distal phalanx occurs, open reduction and internal fixation may be advised.

Answer: A

15. True statements regarding hand infections include:

A. The relatively avascular environment of the synovial sheaths makes them resistant to infection
B. One third of hand infections have a mixed flora
C. Treatment of human bite wounds includes aggressive cleansing and antibiotic therapy before suturing
D. Cellulitis of the hand must be drained before loculation occurs
E. The organisms most commonly isolated from hand infections are penicillinase-producing staphylococci

Sabiston: 1522
Schwartz: 2078

Comments: Hand infections are potentially serious because of the superficial location of the hand's bones and joints, the high density of relatively avascular tendons, and the ease of spread through the synovial sheaths due to constant flexion and extension. Staphylococci are present in nearly 80% of hand infections and are frequently penicillin-resistant. One third of hand infections contain mixed flora and frequently include beta-hemolytic streptococci, *Escherichia coli*, *Proteus*, and *Pseudomonas*. Drainage procedures are reserved to decompress loculations of pus, while cellulitis without fluctuance is treated with immobilization, elevation, antibiotics, and frequent re-examination. The empiric use of antibiotics is indicated in severe infections, with appropriate changes in therapy being made when culture and sensitivity results are available. All complex infections should be drained in the operating room with proximal tourniquet control. Distal-to-proximal wrapping to obtain a bloodless field, as used in elective hand surgery, is contraindicated. Human bites should be vigorously cleansed, treated with antibiotics, and allowed to close secondarily.

Answer: B, E

16. Which of the following statements is/are true?

A. Paronychia occurs in the digital pulp of the finger
B. A felon is an infection around the margin of the nailbed
C. Finger felon or paronychia has the potential to cause tenosynovitis
D. The deep structures of the hand are protected from subcutaneous abscesses of the palm by the superficial palmar fascia

Sabiston: 1522
Schwartz: 2080

Comments: Subcutaneous abscesses of the volar surface of the hand often follow small puncture wounds or infection of superficial blisters. Pain and swelling are confined to the area of inflammation and are not increased with minor tendon motion. Loculations should be drained since they have the potential of tracking to the dorsum of the hand. A felon is an infection of the pulp of the fingertip that can lead to deep ischemic necrosis because of the presence of compartmentalizing septa that prevent expansion as pressure increases. Sharp pain and tenderness out of proportion to the amount of swelling are characteristic. The pulp space must be drained by dividing the septa before tissue necrosis occurs. Paronychia are infections around the margins of the nail plate, often

caused by hangnails, manicure trauma, or small foreign bodies. *Staphylococcus* is the usual offending organism. Early cases can be treated with warm soaks and antibiotics, but abscesses must be drained, often requiring resection of the overlying proximal nail plate.

Answer: C

17. True statements regarding tenosynovitis include:

A. Infections of the flexor sheath of the little finger more often extend to the thumb than to the adjacent ring finger
B. A flexor tendon sheath infection causes the involved finger to assume a position of mild extension at all joints
C. The involved digit becomes uniformly swollen, and active or passive extension elicits pain
D. By definition, deep palmar space infections involve the flexor tendons

Sabiston: 1524
Schwartz: 2081, 2084

Comments: Infection of the synovial sheaths of the flexor tendons is a serious problem. The tendons are relatively avascular and are characterized by poor natural resistance to infection. The potential to spread to other fingers within the ulnar bursa places fingers remote from the initial injury at risk. Although anatomy varies, the sheath of the little finger is often continuous with the ulnar bursa, which in turn is directly adjacent to the radial bursa, which extends to the flexor sheath of the thumb. The infected digit becomes uniformly swollen and assumes a position of mild flexion at all joints. Active or passive extension elicits local pain. Surgical drainage is mandatory and is accomplished by a longitudinal incision on the side of the digit along the axis of joint motion. The incision is placed on the radial side of the digit if palmar spread is suspected. Placement of irrigating catheters within the sheath and systemic antibiotics are important adjuncts to surgical therapy. The deep palmar space is located between the flexor tendons and the metacarpals in the palm. It is divided into the thenar space and midpalmar space at the level of the third metacarpal. Infections here present as localized, tender swellings and must be drained, using an appropriate incision.

Answer: A, C

18. True statements regarding the forearm compartment syndrome include:

A. The classic four P's—pain, pallor, paralysis, and pulselessness—accurately describe the syndrome
B. The underlying cause is increased tissue pressure in the deep flexor compartment of the forearm
C. The deep flexor compartment is fed only by the anterior interosseous artery that becomes occluded as tissue pressure rises
D. The median, radial, and ulnar nerves become strangulated by deep flexor compartment fibrosis
E. The hand loses intrinsic muscle function and becomes numb in the median and ulnar distributions

Schwartz: 2083

Comments: The elevation of tissue pressure in the deep flexor compartment of the forearm leads ultimately to occlusion of flow through the anterior interosseous artery. The result of this occlusion is a dense, fibrotic degeneration of the muscular contents of the deep flexor compartment. Originally described by Volkmann as a result of tight bandaging at the elbow, it can be caused by a number of insults that have elevation of tissue pressure as their common denominator. The fibrosis that results causes a fixed flexion contracture of the wrist and fingers and a "strangulation neuropathy" of the median and ulnar nerves. The nerve involvement causes loss of intrinsic muscle function and numbness in the respective sensory distributions of the ulnar and median nerves. The radial artery does not pass through the deep flexor compartment and maintains its patency. The early clinical signs of increasing tissue pressure are tenderness over the forearm muscles, pain with passive finger extension, and paresthesias in the distribution of the median and ulnar nerves. Once the diagnosis is made, complete fasciotomy from elbow to wrist is indicated. Treatment of late cases involves major reconstructive surgery.

Answer: B, C, E

19. True statements regarding replantation of the hand include:

A. Single digits (other than the thumb) are rarely replanted except in children
B. The amputated part may tolerate cool ischemia for up to 24 hours if there is no significant avascular muscle mass
C. Bleeding from the proximal part is ideally treated with pressure, rather than clamping
D. A history of heavy smoking, diabetes mellitus, hypertension, and Raynaud's phenomenon are relative contraindications to replantation
E. Replantation above the elbow is contraindicated

Sabiston: 1564
Schwartz: 2085

Comments: Replantation is a highly specialized procedure best performed by a team of replantation surgeons. The procedure is long and requires that the patient be carefully evaluated for associated injuries before committing to a replantation attempt. Distal amputations properly cooled immediately after injury may be viable for up to 24 hours. The part should be wrapped in sterile dressings and placed in a plastic container, which is then submerged in ice water. This part should never be frozen or come in contact with the surrounding liquid. Only rarely are single digits replanted except in children. The hand and thumb are always considered for replantation unless definite contraindications exist or the extremity was not properly preserved. Amputations above the elbow are considered for replantation (particularly in children) since even partial success can convert an above-elbow to a below-elbow stump for future rehabilitation. Guillotine amputations are the injuries that present most favorably for replantation.

Answer: A, B, C, D

20. False statements regarding digit amputations include:

A. Any length of thumb that can be saved should be preserved
B. The middle finger can assume the role of primary pinch if the index finger is lost
C. Any length of index finger that can be saved should be preserved to maintain its pinching function
D. Metacarpophalangeal joint amputations of the middle and ring fingers leave a space open in the clenched fist through which objects held in the palm may fall
E. Traumatic loss of the thumb can be treated by digital transposition or by toe transfer

Schwartz: 2086

Comments: Planned or traumatic amputations within the hand must take into consideration a number of factors including the patient's handedness, age, occupation, and concern for esthetics. The thumb is the most important digit, and as much as possible of its length should be preserved. The index finger amputated proximal to the proximal interphalangeal joint loses its ability to pinch. All attempts to preserve length distal to the proximal interphalangeal joint should be made, but the need for shorter amputations may be best served by transection through the middle metacarpal (ray amputation) since the long finger can assume the role of primary pinch. Loss of little finger length proximal to the proximal interphalangeal joint may also be best treated by ray amputation. Central finger amputations (long and ring fingers) near the metacarpophalangeal joint can cause bothersome spaces in the clenched fist that can be treated by the transfer of the adjacent peripheral finger with its metacarpal to fill the space.

Answer: C

21. True statements regarding carpal tunnel syndrome include:

A. The carpal tunnel syndrome is entrapment of the ulnar nerve in the carpal canal
B. It is most commonly traumatic in origin
C. The associated pain and numbness is often nocturnal, with reference of the pain to the shoulder and neck
D. Injection of steroids into the carpal canal is contraindicated
E. Electromyography helps confirm the diagnosis and exclude more proximal nerve entrapment

Sabiston: 1548
Schwartz: 2087

Comments: Carpal tunnel syndrome is entrapment of the median nerve in the carpal canal with resultant neurapraxia. Most commonly it is idiopathic in origin, but it can be seen following Colles' and Smith's fractures or lunate and perilunate dislocations. It can be part of the presenting symptoms of rheumatoid arthritis, gout, diabetes mellitus, hypothyroidism, or amyloidosis. Proximal entrapment due to Pancoast tumors, cervical spine disease, or pronator teres abnormalities must be excluded as a diagnosis. Presenting symptoms include pain and numbness of the median nerve distribution, often nocturnal, with reference of pain to the shoulder and neck. Physical findings include thenar atrophy, increased symptoms with forced wrist flexion, and a positive Tinel's sign over the nerve at the wrist. Initial treatment consists of splinting, nonsteroidal anti-inflammatory agents, and possibly a steroid injection into the carpal canal. Thenar atrophy, weakness, and failure to respond to conservative therapy are indications for surgery, which involves release of the portion of the flexor retinaculum that is entrapping the nerve.

Answer: C, E

22. True statements regarding de Quervain's disorder include:

A. It is an entrapment syndrome within the first extensor compartment at the wrist
B. It involves the abductor pollicis longus and extensor pollicis brevis
C. It causes pain over the radial styloid at the wrist
D. Finkelstein's test is usually negative
E. Medical treatment includes splinting, anti-inflammatory agents, and change in pattern of hand use

Schwartz: 2088

Comments: The de Quervain syndrome is an idiopathic tenosynovitis involving the abductor pollicis longus and extensor pollicis brevis, causing a painful entrapment in the first extensor compartment at the wrist. It causes pain over the radial styloid with local tenderness and swelling. Having the patient grasp the thumb with the fingers of the same hand and then perform ulnar deviation of the wrist causes increased pain (positive Finkelstein's sign). Treatment is splinting, nonsteroidal anti-inflammatory agents, and change in the pattern of hand use. Failure to respond to medical therapy is an indication for surgical decompression. Great care must be taken to avoid injury to the radial sensory branches during decompression.

Answer: A, B, C, E

23. True statements regarding stenosing tenosynovitis include:

A. It is also known as trigger finger
B. It is also known as the swan-neck deformity
C. It can cause locking of the digit in flexion or extension
D. Surgical correction should be performed with wrist-block anesthesia

Schwartz: 2089

Comments: Trigger finger is caused by the passage of swollen flexor tendons beneath the pulley system of the fibro-osseous tunnel. It is associated with a snapping sensation that, in the extreme situation, can occur with locking of the digit in extension or flexion. Treatment is with nonsteroidal anti-inflammatory agents and steroid injections. Failure to respond to medical treatment is an indication for surgical decompression. Wrist-block anesthesia is used for operation so that free active excursion

of the tendon can be demonstrated following release of the constricting area.

Answer: A, C, D

24. True statements regarding Dupuytren's contracture include:

A. Dupuytren's contracture is contracture of the palmar aponeurosis
B. Males are affected more often than females, and the contracture is primarily caused by excessive alcohol consumption
C. It begins as nodule formation ultimately leading to contracture at the metacarpophalangeal and proximal interphalangeal joints
D. Four clinical types have been described
E. Aggressive nonsurgical treatment can influence the course of the disease

Sabiston: 1520
Schwartz: 2091

Comments: Dupuytren's contracture occurs two times more frequently in males and primarily affects people of northern European origin. It appears to be transmitted as an autosomal gene influenced by multiple exogenous factors, such as injury, liver disease, alcoholism, pulmonary disease, and chronic bowel disease. It begins as nodule formation within the palmar fascia in line with the pretendinous bands. Gradually, the skin becomes dimpled and contractures form at the level of the metacarpophalangeal and proximal interphalangeal joints. Four clinical types—the senile, middle-aged, young fulminant, and feminine types—have been identified. There is no known effective medical therapy. Surgical options include open fasciotomy, radical excision of the palmar fascia, and partial palmar fasciectomy. Postoperative splinting and hand therapy are extremely important to the success of such therapy.

Answer: A, C, D

25. Which of the following statements is/are true concerning peripheral nerve injury?

A. Nerve repair is progressively less effective if performed 2 months following surgery
B. Nerve repair is best performed using 4 to 15× magnification
C. Nerve repair is best performed in a fashion that minimizes tension across the repair
D. Regeneration may be followed clinically by observation of the distal progression of Tinel's sign

Sabiston: 1554
Schwartz: 2077

Comments: Nerve injuries result from stretching or compression (neurapraxia) or transection. Neurapractic injuries carry a better prognosis than do transection injuries. Nerve injuries do not need to be repaired at the time of injury, but the results are progressively worse if repair is delayed beyond 6 months. Occasionally, repair delayed for up to 2 years may be successful, especially in children. Although it is a matter of choice, most surgeons perform a careful epineural repair rather than repair the individual fascicular bundles. Recovery after repair begins with return of sensitivity starting proximally. Regenerating axons grow down the distal nerve sheath at an approximate rate of 1 mm per day. Distal progression of Tinel's sign (tingling felt after percussion over the growing nerve) usually follows the start of regeneration.

Answer: B, C, D

26. Regarding burns of the hands, which of the following statements is/are true?

A. Full thickness dorsal burns cause scarring, which prevents flexion contractures
B. Loss of the extensor tendons is often treated by joint fusion to prevent contractures due to unopposed flexion forces
C. An important part of treatment includes splinting in the "safe" position
D. Partial thickness burns are best treated with whirlpool débridement and splinting

Sabiston: 1538
Schwartz: 2082

Comments: Treatment of hand burns must begin as soon as possible. Although the injury to the hand may be complex, certain principles bear comment: Proper dressing should be applied and the hand splinted in a "safe" position whenever possible. Destruction of extensor tendons will result in flexion contractures unless the joints are fused in the appropriate position. Partial thickness burns should be débrided of superficial necrotic tissue, using whirlpool baths. Full thickness burns are best treated by early excision and skin grafting.

Answer: B, C, D

27. Neuroma is appropriately treated by:

A. Alcohol injection
B. Primary nerve root repair
C. Ligation of proximal nerve end
D. Burial of the nerve end in soft tissue

Schwartz: 2093

Comments: The proximal ends of unrepaired peripheral nerves have the potential to form a tumor mass consisting of sprouting axons and fibroblasts (neuroma). They are tender to palpation and can be the source of electric-like sensations interpreted as coming from the previously innervated area. The best treatment is resection and primary nerve repair. If repair is impossible, the nerve ends should be placed deep in the soft tissue away from points of pressure or trauma.

Answer: B, D

28. Match the following:

A. Median nerve palsy
B. Ulnar nerve palsy
C. Radial nerve palsy

a. Claw deformity of ring and little fingers
b. Loss of wrist extension
c. Loss of thumb abduction and apposition

Sabiston: 1538
Schwartz: 2093

Comments: **Median nerve** palsy at the wrist results in inability to perform proper pulp-to-pulp pinch. Transfer of the flexor digitorum superficialis of the ring finger (median nerve innervation proximal to the wrist) to the insertion of the abductor pollicis brevis is frequently the treatment of choice. Median nerve injuries at the elbow result in denervation of the flexor digitorum superficialis, and in this case transfer of the abductor digiti minimi (ulnar innervation) is utilized. **Ulnar nerve** palsy at the wrist results in a claw deformity in the third and fourth fingers. This results from metacarpophalangeal joint hyperextension with secondary flexion of the interphalangeal and distal phalangeal joints. The flexor digitorum superficialis to the little finger can be moved to the base of the proximal phalanx of the ring and little fingers to restore metacarpophalangeal joint flexion. **Radial nerve** disruption over the mid or distal humerus causes loss of wrist extension, metacarpophalangeal joint finger extension, and thumb abduction and extension. The common transfer used to repair this deformity is the pronator teres to the extensor carpi radialis brevis, the flexor carpi ulnaris to the extensor digitorum communis, and the palmaris longus to the extensor pollicis longus.

Answer: A–c; B–a; C–b

29. Which of the following statements regarding syndactyly is/are true?

A. Syndactyly is often associated with polydactyly
B. Release should be accomplished by the age of 1 year if digits of differing growth rates are involved
C. It may be related to an autosomal dominant genetic pattern
D. Males are more frequently affected than females

Sabiston: 1544
Schwartz: 2094

Comments: Syndactyly is a common congenital deformity that varies in severity from a thin skin web between normal digits to complete fusion of bony elements with a common nail. It may be inherited in an autosomal dominant pattern and is associated with several different syndromes, including Poland's and Apert's syndromes. Often, both hands and feet are involved, and males are affected more frequently than females. The timing of operation is debatable. Syndactyly involving distal bony structures in digits of differing growth rates is often treated by surgical division of the distal syndactyly before 1 year of age. When there is no concern for differential growth rate, surgery is delayed 2 to 3 years. Complete release of syndactyly before age 1 frequently results in an unacceptable degree of scarring. When more than two digits are involved, the releases are staged with 6 months between operations to avoid compromise of the fingers' blood supply. When both sides of a digit must be released, full thickness skin grafts are needed to close a portion of the surgical defect.

Answer: B, C, D

30. Match the hand lesions with their descriptive common features.

Lesion	Common Features
A. Ganglion cyst	a. Arises from the short vinculum near the interphalangeal joints
B. Giant cell tumor of tendon	b. When arising from the distal interphalangeal joint it is called a mucous cyst
C. Inclusion cyst	c. A fibrous capsule lined with squamous epithelium found on the flexor aspect of the palm and fingers
D. Lipoma	d. Most commonly found around the thenar eminence
E. Sebaceous cyst	e. Most commonly found in the dorsum of the hand

Sabiston: 1545
Schwartz: 2095

Comments: **Ganglion cysts** are often seen in any of four different locations: the dorsum of the hand, the flexor side of the wrist adjacent to the radial artery, arising from the flexor sheaths (often at the base of the digit), or arising from the distal interphalangeal joints (where they are known as mucous cysts). **Giant cell tumors** of the tendons are benign and arise from the short vinculum near the interphalangeal joints. Both tendons in the flexor sheath are usually involved by the tumor, which lies deep to the neurovascular bundle. **Inclusion cysts** result from implantation of the epithelium with or without a foreign body and present as a cyst on the flexor aspect of the palm or finger. **Lipomas** often present over the thenar eminence. **Sebaceous cysts** most often occur on the dorsum of the hand.

Answer: A–b; B–a; C–c; D–d; E–e

31. Match the common anatomic defect with the associated type of arthritis.

Common Anatomic Defect	Type of Arthritis
A. Metacarpophalangeal joint anterior subluxation-dislocation with extensor lag and ulnar drift	a. Rheumatoid arthritis
B. Interphalangeal joint, boutonnière, or swan-neck deformity	b. Osteoarthritis
C. Radial deviation of the wrist	
D. Interphalangeal joints of fingers and thumb and the metacarpophalangeal joint of the thumb often affected	
E. Heberden's nodes	
F. Bouchard's nodes	

Sabiston: 1541
Schwartz: 2097

Comments: **Rheumatoid arthritis** is a systemic disease that can involve any or all of the tendon systems and joints of the hand. Often there is significant involvement at the wrist as well as in the metacarpophalangeal and interphalangeal areas. The management of rheumatoid arthritis is complex and involves the hand surgeon, rheumatologist, hand therapist, and social worker. **Osteoarthritis** commonly involves multiple hand joints and most frequently occurs in postmenopausal women. The joints most commonly involved are the interphalangeal joints of the fingers and thumb as well as the metacarpophalangeal joint of the thumb. Heberden's nodes are osteophytes at the distal interphalangeal joint, while Bouchard's nodes are of the proximal interphalangeal joint. Disabling involvement of the distal interphalangeal joint is often treated with arthrodesis. Severe involvement of the proximal interphalangeal joints of the fingers and the metacarpophalangeal joint of the thumb is often treated with implant arthroplasty.

Answer: A–a; B–a; C–a; D–b; E–b; F–b

CHAPTER 61

Plastic and Reconstructive Surgery

1. Which of the following statements regarding the orientation of skin incisions is/are correct?

A. Skin incisions should usually be oriented parallel to the long axis of the underlying muscle
B. Lines of minimal tension parallel skin lines
C. The long axis of underlying muscles is usually perpendicular to skin lines
D. In some anatomic locations the best incision is chosen independent of the orientation of the underlying muscle

Sabiston: 1575
Schwartz: 2101

Comments: In most anatomic areas, skin lines represent lines of minimal tension, and incisions in these areas should be made parallel to these lines in order to result in the narrowest possible scar. These lines of minimal tension generally run perpendicular to the long axis of underlying muscles. In some circumstances, however, the choice of an incision is made independent of the underlying orientation. Examples would be vertical incisions in the preauricular area and circumareolar incisions of the breast.

Answer: B, C, D

2. Which of the following statements regarding the techniques of wound closure is/are correct?

A. Forceps with fine teeth are less traumatic to skin than are forceps without teeth
B. Questionably viable tissue at the wound margin should be preserved, as this will frequently regain vascularity within 2 days of the injury
C. In general, sutures should be kept in approximately 10 to 14 days in order to reduce the tension on the wound during that time
D. Even modest undermining of skin edges should be avoided, as this devascularizes the overlying skin and impedes wound healing

Schwartz: 2102

Comments: Successful closure of a surgically created or traumatic wound involves the proper coaptation of well-vascularized tissues without tension. Gentle handling of tissues is always recommended and is facilitated by the use of small "piercing" forceps rather than "crushing" forceps (i.e., those without teeth). Devitalized or questionably viable tissue should always be removed prior to closure. Tension on a wound impedes healing and leads to widening of the scar. This can be avoided in most circumstances by undermining the wound edges. A rich network of subdermal vessels will provide quite adequate vascular supply to the skin edges, so long as the undermining has not been too excessive. Sutures are removed at variable times, depending on the vascularity and tension of the tissues coapted as well as the cosmetic results desired. On the face, sutures are usually removed after 3 to 5 days. On the back and distal extremities it may be prudent to leave sutures in longer, up to 10 to 14 days. On the abdomen sutures are usually removed at 5 to 7 days. Early removal of sutures and support of the wound with adhesive strips is becoming popular and allows for support of the wound without leading to the cross-hatch marks created by the sutures themselves.

Answer: A

3. Which one or more of the following recipient beds will be unlikely to support a split-thickness skin graft?

A. Muscle with its overlying fascia intact
B. Muscle without overlying fascia
C. Tendon with its paratenon intact
D. Tendon without its paratenon
E. Bone with its periosteum intact
F. Bone without its periosteum

Sabiston: 485, 1575
Schwartz: 2105

Comments: Proper "take" of a split-thickness skin graft applied to a recipient bed depends upon adequate vascularization of the bed, avoidance of dead space or tenting of the graft over the bed, and absence of infection within the wound (defined as greater than 10^5 bacteria/gram of tissue). Muscle, with or without its fascia intact, is an excellent recipient site for split-thickness skin grafts. Although apparently less well vascularized, tendon with its paratenon intact and bone with its periosteum intact will also support a split-thickness skin graft in most circumstances. Tendon without paratenon and bone without periosteum, however, will usually not support a skin graft. Closure over these structures must be achieved by providing a vascularized tissue over the exposed bone or tendon (e.g., omentum, muscle) prior to skin grafting.

Answer: D, F

4. Which of the following statements is/are correct regarding the use of split-thickness and full-thickness skin grafts?

A. A split-thickness skin graft undergoes approximately 10% shrinkage of its surface area immediately after harvesting
B. A full-thickness skin graft undergoes approximately 40% shrinkage of its surface area immediately after harvesting
C. Secondary contracture is more likely to occur after adequate healing of a full-thickness skin graft than a split-thickness skin graft
D. Sensation does not recur to areas that have undergone skin grafting
E. Skin grafts may be exposed to moderate amounts of sunlight without changing pigmentation

Sabiston: 1575
Schwartz: 2107

Comments: Skin grafts are considered to be full thickness when they are harvested at the dermal/subcutaneous junction. Split-thickness skin grafts are those which contain epidermis and variable thicknesses of underlying dermis. These may be considered as thin, medium, or thick split-thickness skin grafts and usually are in the range of 0.012 to 0.018 inch in thickness. When a skin graft is harvested, there is immediate shrinkage of the surface area of the graft because of the presence of elastic fibers within the skin. The thicker the skin graft, the greater this immediate shrinkage, with full-thickness skin grafts shrinking approximately 40% of their initial surface area and split-thickness skin grafts shrinking approximately 10% of their initial surface area. This must be considered when planning the amount of skin to harvest for coverage of a given size defect. After adequate healing of the skin graft on the recipient site, secondary contracture occurs. In contrast to the initial shrinkage, the secondary contracture occurs to a greater degree in split-thickness skin grafts than in full-thickness skin grafts. Quite adequate, although perhaps not completely normal, sensation may return to areas that have been grafted. This process begins at about 10 weeks and is maximal at 2 years. Skin grafts appear to be more sensitive to the effects of sunlight than is the normal surrounding skin. Early exposure to sunlight after grafting will lead to a permanent increased pigmentation of the graft and should be avoided.

Answer: A, B

5. Match the type of flap in the left-hand column with the appropriate nature of its blood supply in the right-hand column.

A. Z-plasty
B. Forehead flap
C. Deltopectoral flap
D. Omental flap
E. Limberg flap

a. Random pattern
b. Axial pattern

Sabiston: 1577
Schwartz: 2107

Comments: See Question 6.

6. Match the type of flap in the left-hand column with the appropriate description or example from the right-hand column:

A. Transposition flap
B. Interpolation flap
C. Advancement flap
D. Island flap
E. Free flap

a. V-Y flap
b. Microvascular anastomosis required
c. Rotation to an adjacent defect
d. Rotation to nearby but not adjacent defect
e. Attached pedicle of vessels

Sabiston: 484
Schwartz: 2107

Comments: Flaps are defined according to the nature of their blood supply: A **random flap** derives its blood supply from the dermal-subdermal plexus; an **axial flap** derives its blood supply by a direct, usually named, cutaneous artery. **Random flaps** usually are those used to reorient a wound in a different direction or to close small defects. Examples are a Z-plasty, a simple rotation flap, an advancement flap, and a transposition flap. A Limberg flap is a particular type of transposition flap involving the transposition of a rhomboid flap to cover an adjacent defect with primary closure of the donor site. A random flap may be defined by the manner in which it is moved to its recipient site. A simple rotation flap is usually semicircular and is "slid" over the recipient site for closure. An advancement flap is moved directly forward to cover a defect without rotation around a pivot point. A V-Y flap, frequently used to close small defects in the finger or eyelid areas, is a commonly employed advancement flap. Transposition flaps are those that involve rotation around a pivot point to a defect that is adjacent to the donor site. An interpolation flap also involves rotation around a pivot point but is used to cover a defect that is nearby but not directly adjacent to the donor site. **Axial flaps** generally are used to cover larger defects more distant from the donor site. Examples are a forehead flap (superficial temporal artery), deltopectoral flap (perforating branches of the internal mammary artery), or omental flap (gastroepiploic arteries). An island flap is an axial-pattern type of flap in which tissue is removed from the donor to recipient site on a pedicle that contains the nutrient vessels. **Free flaps** involve complete severing of the nutrient vessels with reanastomosis to vessels in the vicinity of the recipient site. This nearly always requires microvascular surgical technique.

Answer: Question 5: A–a; B–b; C–b; D–b; E–a
Question 6: A–c; B–d; C–a; D–e; E–b

7. Which one or more of the following statements is/are true regarding myocutaneous flaps?

A. A myocutaneous flap is a free graft of full-thickness skin with a small shaving of underlying muscle
B. Both the supplying artery and draining vein must be intact for survival of a myocutaneous flap
C. In some circumstances, bone may be included with a myocutaneous flap
D. These flaps may be transferred as free flaps with microvascular anastomoses
E. Myocutaneous flaps are of theoretical importance but of little practical use because of the increasing use of synthetic materials in reconstruction

Schwartz: 2109

Comments: The development of myocutaneous flaps for reconstruction of soft tissue defects is based on the fact that skin frequently receives blood supply from vessels perforating the underlying somatic musculature. When the blood supply to the underlying muscle is by way of a discrete vessel, the muscle and its overlying skin paddle may be transferred to a distant site on a pedicle containing the nutrient vessels. It is critical that both the artery and vein within the pedicle remain patent for successful transfer of the flap. In some circumstances, bone that is closely associated with the muscle and skin may be transferred en bloc, providing an osseomyocutaneous flap (e.g., rib and overlying pectoralis muscle and skin used for mandible reconstruction). When the arc of rotation or the length of vessels within the pedicle does not permit the graft to reach the recipient site, division of these vessels with reanastomosis utilizing microvascular techniques may be carried out. These myocutaneous flaps are widely used in head and neck reconstruction, breast reconstruction, and other areas of reconstructive surgery where well-vascularized soft tissue covering over bone or neurovascular structures is required.

Answer: B, C, D

8. For which of the following breast conditions may surgery be an appropriate form of therapy?

A. Macromastia
B. Gynecomastia
C. Hypomastia
D. Ptosis
E. None of the above

Sabiston: 576
Schwartz: 2113

Comments: Surgery may appropriately play a role in any of the breast conditions listed above. **Macromastia** is an abnormal enlargement of the breast which may be a result of hormonal imbalance or obesity. For some women, the breasts become so large that chronic back, shoulder, or neck pain and skin changes of the shoulders and inframammary areas may result. In such circumstances, reduction mammoplasty, involving resection of portions of the breast parenchyma and overlying skin with reposi-

tioning of the nipple and areola, may be carried out. **Ptosis** of the breast exists when the nipple is present at a level below that of the inframammary crease. This may occur in any size breast and may lead to chronic skin changes in the inframammary crease. Reduction mammoplasty similar to that described above can alleviate the ptosis. **Gynecomastia** is enlargement of the male breast due to increase in glandular tissue. In the adolescent, it is frequently a physiologic response to the hormonal changes of puberty and usually reverses itself. In the adult, gynecomastia may result from underlying liver disease; pituitary, testicular, or adrenal tumors; or certain drugs (e.g., digitalis). It must be differentiated from male breast carcinoma, especially when it is unilateral in presentation. Resection of the breast tissue will confirm the diagnosis and correct the cosmetic abnormality. **Hypomastia** refers to insufficient volume of breast tissue and may be corrected, for cosmetic reasons, by the placement of a prosthesis.

Answer: A, B, C, D

9. Which one or more of the following techniques may be employed for breast reconstruction following mastectomy?

A. Placement of a silicone gel prosthesis
B. Placement of an expanding (saline-filled) prosthesis
C. Latissimus dorsi myocutaneous flap
D. Trapezius myocutaneous flap
E. Rectus abdominis myocutaneous flap

Sabiston: 573
Schwartz: 2115

Comments: See Question 10.

10. Which of the following statements is/are true regarding post-mastectomy breast reconstruction?

A. The presence of positive axillary nodes is a contraindication to reconstruction
B. Delayed reconstruction (i.e., 3 months or more post-mastectomy) is generally preferred over immediate reconstruction
C. The status of the skin flaps (vascular supply and degree of tension) is the key consideration in proceeding with immediate reconstruction
D. Nipple reconstruction is usually delayed for several months following reconstruction of the breast mound
E. In most cases excellent symmetry can be achieved without the need for surgery on the uninvolved breast

Sabiston: 573
Schwartz: 2115

Comments: Breast reconstruction following mastectomy is an important aspect in breast cancer therapy for obvious cosmetic and psychological reasons. The basic principle involved in breast reconstruction centers on the placement of a prosthesis (usually silicone gel) in a subpectoral/subserratus pocket with closure of the skin and subcutaneous tissue over the muscle. If an appropriately sized prosthesis cannot be placed without undue tension on the closure of the skin, an expanding prosthesis may be placed which is gradually filled with saline over a several-month period. This leads to stretching of the muscle and overlying skin and allows for placement of a larger permanent prosthesis at a later date. As an alternative to the expanding prosthesis or in cases in which the pectoralis major muscle has been taken (Halsted mastectomy), a myocutaneous flap may be utilized to provide bulk, muscular cover over the prosthesis, and additional skin for closure. The latissimus dorsi myocutaneous flap pedicled on the thoracodorsal vessels and the rectus abdominis myocutaneous flap pedicled on the superior epigastric vessels have been popularly used for this purpose. In the latter case, a prosthesis is frequently not required because of the bulk of muscle brought up into the mastectomy defect. The limited length and arc of rotation of the trapezius myocutaneous flap make it inappropriate for use in breast reconstruction. The presence of positive axillary lymph nodes and the anticipated need for adjuvant chemotherapy or postoperative chest wall radiation are not in and of themselves absolute contraindications to reconstruction. However, one must weigh the possible increased risk of infection (related to chemotherapy-induced leukopenia) and the possibility of a suboptimal cosmetic result from post-reconstruction radiation against the psychological advantage to the patient of the reconstruction itself. Post-mastectomy reconstruction may be carried out immediately or in a delayed fashion (at least 3 months after mastectomy), depending on the desires of the patient, the anticipated need for adjuvant treatment, and, most importantly, the status of the skin flaps in terms of vascular supply and degree of tension on closure. There does not appear to be any significant difference in the final cosmetic outcome comparing immediate with delayed reconstruction. The nipple may also be reconstructed, usually by grafting skin from the upper medial thigh and labia, but this is deferred for several months following completion of the breast mound reconstruction. The ultimate goal in breast reconstruction is to achieve symmetry of both breasts. In many patients, this necessitates a reduction mammoplasty on the uninvolved side.

Answer: Question 9: A, B, C, E
Question 10: C, D

11. Which of the following statements is/are true regarding reconstruction of major chest wall and abdominal wall defects?

A. The morbidity of surgery for major chest wall defects is greater than that for abdominal defects because of the prolonged period of postoperative intubation required for stabilization of the bony chest wall
B. The omentum is an excellent flap for abdominal wall reconstruction, but will not adequately reach most areas of the chest wall
C. Single-stage reconstruction is usually possible for chest and abdominal wall defects
D. Synthetic materials should be avoided in the reconstruction of large defects because of the inherent risk of infection

Schwartz: 2122

Comments: The two goals of reconstruction of major chest and abdominal wall defects involve (1) the closure

of the bony or musculofascial defect to prevent exposure and/or herniation of the chest or abdominal wall contents, and (2) the provision of soft tissue and skin coverage over the bony or fascial repair. In large defects, the former goal usually necessitates the use of synthetic materials sutured to the perimeter of the defect. Autologous tissues (e.g., fascia lata) may also be used; however, in the absence of established infection at the time of surgery, the use of synthetic materials has been associated with a low and very acceptable rate of subsequent infection. In cases of very large chest wall defects, the use of "bone cement" in association with prosthetic mesh provides for a rigid chest wall reconstruction that usually results in excellent pulmonary mechanical dynamics and the ability to extubate the patient within 24 hours of operation. Following the musculofascial reconstruction, soft tissue coverage may be provided by simple advancement or rotation flaps for small defects or myocutaneous flaps (e.g., latissimus dorsi, rectus abdominis) for larger defects. The omentum may be used for coverage of bone or prosthetic material, and with proper dissection of the gastroepiploic pedicle, the omentum can be made to reach most areas of the chest and abdomen. Split-thickness skin grafting over the omentum is frequently employed. The increased use of these synthetic materials, as well as myocutaneous flaps, has allowed most major chest and abdominal wall reconstructions to be performed in a single stage.

Answer: C

12. Which of the following statements is/are true regarding decubitus ulcers (pressure sores)?

A. Pressure of 40 to 80 mm Hg applied to tissue continuously for 4 hours will result in permanent microvascular changes and an ischemic ulcer
B. After débridement of devitalized tissues, closure of decubitus ulcers is usually satisfactorily achieved with local skin flaps
C. Superficial ulcers often heal spontaneously after débridement if subsequent pressure can be avoided
D. Long-standing decubitus ulcers are usually partially epithelialized, which promotes spontaneous healing

Schwartz: 2123

Comments: Continuous pressure on tissues, if severe enough for a long enough period of time, will result in venous, capillary, and arterial compression with subsequent ischemic necrosis of the tissue leading to a decubitus ulcer. A pressure of 40 to 80 mm Hg applied continuously to tissue over 4 hours will result in temporary microvascular changes and edema. If this continues for an 8-hour period, it may lead to permanent microvascular changes, subsequently resulting in a decubitus ulcer. Superficial ulcers will usually heal spontaneously if devitalized tissue is débrided and subsequent pressure is avoided. Deeper ulcers, especially those involving exposed bone in the base of the ulcer, require débridement and the grafting of well-vascularized tissues into the defect. Local skin flaps often fail owing to tension and poor vascularity. The most successful closure of deep decubitus ulcers involves the placement of myocutaneous skin flaps into the defect. Partial epithelialization of a long-standing ulcer impedes subsequent healing, and débridement of the ulcer must be carried back to nonepithelialized tissue in order for a graft to be successfully placed.

Answer: C

13. Which of the following statements is/are true regarding extremity lymphedema?

A. Lymphedema represents an abnormal accumulation of lymph within the intercellular spaces
B. Postoperative lymphedema is usually temporary and with proper management will resolve completely with no permanent sequelae
C. Lymphangiosarcoma can occur in cases of long-standing extremity lymphedema
D. Surgical therapy is the treatment of choice for chronic lymphedema

Sabiston: 1700
Schwartz: 2133

Comments: Lymphedema is an abnormal accumulation of lymph in the intercellular spaces, resulting either from a congenital obstruction or absence of lymphatics or from surgical removal of regional lymph nodes (e.g., axillary dissection, inguinal dissection). Some factors that may increase the likelihood or severity of lymphedema include the application of radiation therapy to the extremity, circumferential or nearly circumferential incisions, and infections within the extremity. Once significant lymphedema occurs in an extremity, it is unusual for the extremity to return entirely to normal size. Some degree of residual permanent swelling usually remains and is related to a chronic fibrosis that occurs within the soft tissues. For reasons that are not fully understood, some extremities with chronic long-standing lymphedema may develop lymphangiosarcoma (Stewart-Treves syndrome). Most lymphedematous extremities are managed medically with compression sleeves or stockings, elevation, diuretics, and the early recognition and treatment of infection. When these measures fail and the edema is quite severe, successful results can be achieved in some instances with omental flaps (to provide lymphatic outflow) or resection of lymphedematous tissue.

Answer: A, C

14. Which of the following statements regarding the reconstruction of genitourinary anomalies is/are correct?

A. A newborn with hypospadias should undergo circumcision as the first stage of the definitive three-stage repair
B. Single-stage repair for hypospadias should be avoided
C. Repair of epispadias frequently involves closure or resection of the bladder
D. Reconstruction of the penis and scrotum is not possible without prosthetic materials
E. Reconstruction of the vagina in cases of vaginal agenesis is not possible because it causes injury to the pelvic organs

Sabiston: 1688
Schwartz: 2124

Comments: Reconstructive surgery of the external genitalia may be required because of congenital abnormalities or trauma. **Hypospadias** is one of the more common congenital abnormalities in males and occurs when the urethral meatus opens onto the ventral surface of the penis, frequently in association with chordee (ventral curvature of the penis). Circumcision should be avoided in such cases, as the foreskin may be needed for reconstructive purposes in the future. Correction of hypospadias may be achieved in a multiple-stage or single-stage procedure, the goal of each being to release the fibrous tissue causing the chordee and to position the urethral meatus at the tip of the glans penis. This is accomplished with local skin flaps, and the success rate is approximately 85%. **Epispadias** occurs when the urethral meatus opens abnormally on the dorsum of the penis; frequently it is associated with exstrophy of the bladder and failure of fusion of the pubic symphysis. Treatment as regards the penis and urethra is similar to that for hypospadias. Attention to the exstrophy of the bladder is also required and involves closure of the bladder if possible. If this is not possible, bladder resection with creation of a urinary diversion conduit should be performed. Reconstruction of the penis and scrotum is possible with the use of local abdominal or gracilis myocutaneous flaps. **Vaginal agenesis** may be treated by creation of a perineal pocket lined with a split-thickness skin graft.

Answer: C

15. Which of the following statements is/are true regarding facial cosmetic surgery?

A. After rhytidectomy, a significant hematoma will occur in approximately 4% of patients
B. After rhytidectomy, an injury to the facial nerve or its branches will occur in approximately 8 to 10% of patients
C. After dermabrasion, ultraviolet therapy is useful in helping the return of normal pigmentation
D. Local vasoconstricting agents should not be employed in the course of cosmetic facial surgery
E. A properly performed rhinoplasty involves the resection or repositioning of the nasal soft tissues, not the nasal bones and cartilage

Schwartz: 2127

Comments: For purely cosmetic facial surgery to be justified, the associated morbidity must be extremely low. In the case of rhytidectomy ("face-lift"), the major sources of operative morbidity include significant hematoma under the flap (approximately 4% of cases) and a possible facial nerve injury (less than 1% of cases). These procedures may be performed using general anesthesia or local anesthesia, and in either case, blood loss can be reduced by the appropriate local injection of vasoconstrictive agents. All incisions, but particularly broad areas of surgical "injury," as is seen with dermabrasion, should be protected from sunlight or other sources of ultraviolet light in order to reduce the likelihood of permanent hyperpigmentation in those areas. Perhaps the most technically challenging aspect of cosmetic facial surgery is rhinoplasty, in which portions of the nasal bones and nasal cartilage are resected and/or repositioned to provide a new nasal contour.

Answer: A

16. Match the following craniofacial anomalies with the most appropriate descriptive statement:

A. Craniofacial microsomia
B. Cranial synostosis
C. Crouzon's syndrome
D. Apert's syndrome

a. Involves coronal suture; normal intelligence
b. Premature closure of one or more cranial sutures
c. Macrostomia; facial nerve dysfunction
d. Involves coronal suture; syndactyly; mental retardation

Sabiston: 1408
Schwartz: 2130

Comments: Craniofacial anomalies may be considered in two categories: facial clefts and cranial synostosis. **Facial cleft** has as its most common entity craniofacial microsomia, which is characterized by a groove present from the oral commissure to the involved ear, producing macrostomia. This is associated with a deformed ear and pre-auricular tags. The trigeminal and facial nerves may be involved, producing difficulties with occlusion and weakness of facial expression. **Cranial synostosis** involves premature closure of one or more of the cranial sutures. The sagittal suture is most commonly involved, and generally this is a benign, readily correctable anomaly. Crouzon's syndrome is one of the cranial synostoses and is characterized by early closure of the coronal suture associated with hypoplasia of the mid-face and protrusion of the eyes. Affected children are generally of normal intelligence. Apert's syndrome is a more severe form of cranial synostosis also involving the coronal suture. In this syndrome, syndactyly is frequently seen and most children have some degree of mental retardation. All of the above anomalies can be partially or completely corrected with craniofacial surgery involving both intra- and extracranial approaches, separation of fused sutures, and the application of interposition and onlay bone grafts.

Answer: A–c; B–b; C–a; D–d

17. Which of the following statements regarding maxillo-mandibular disproportion is/are true?

A. Retrognathia is defined as an abnormally small mandible positioned abnormally posteriorly
B. Prognathism is not satisfactorily correctable without the use of synthetic prostheses
C. Most operative corrections of developmental mandibular problems allow normal use of the mandible within 3 weeks of the surgery
D. Hypoplasia is the most common developmental deformity of the maxilla
E. Maxillary osteotomies are used for correction of both hypoplasia and hyperplasia of the maxilla

Sabiston: 1348
Schwartz: 2133

Comments: Developmental mandibular deformities may result from the mandible being malpositioned or abnor-

mally large or small. In retrognathia, the mandible is of normal size but is malpositioned posteriorly. In micrognathia the mandible is properly positioned but is abnormally small. Both of these entities give a similar clinical appearance of a recessed mandible, and both are correctable by the appropriate osteotomies with anterior repositioning of the mandible. In prognathism, the mandible is overdeveloped and prominent. Surgical treatment involves osteotomy with posterior repositioning. In all of these surgical corrections, intermaxillary fixation of the mandible is required for 10 to 12 weeks for proper healing of the osteotomies. ● Of the maxillary anomalies, hypoplasia is the most common and is often seen in association with cleft palate. This may be treated by a maxillary osteotomy with repositioning of the isolated lower maxillary segment. Maxillary hyperplasia is evidenced clinically by a long face with exposure of the gingiva when smiling. This may be corrected with maxillary osteotomy and a resection of a vertical segment of maxilla with an upward repositioning of the lower segment.

Answer: D, E

18. Match the following vascular abnormalities with one or more appropriate descriptive statements:

A. Port wine stain
B. Strawberry hemangioma
C. Cavernous hemangioma
D. Cystic hygroma

a. A form of capillary hemangioma
b. Associated with gigantism of the affected part
c. May enlarge during periods of infection
d. The majority spontaneously involute

Sabiston: 1336
Schwartz: 2134

Comments: The general surgeon and plastic surgeon must be aware of the differential characteristics of the above-listed vascular lesions insofar as their natural history, size, and location may affect the appropriateness and difficulty of surgical intervention. The **port wine stain** is a form of capillary hemangioma and presents as a flat, uniformly dark red cutaneous lesion which is present at birth and does not involute. **Strawberry hemangioma** also is a form of capillary hemangioma, but it is raised and brighter red in color. It is usually not present at birth but may become apparent within several weeks and then grow rapidly during the early months of life. Observation is appropriate, as the majority of these lesions involute spontaneously. The **cavernous hemangioma** is situated in deeper subcutaneous tissues and appears as a swollen blue mass which may be associated with gigantism of the involved part of the body. It is present at birth and seldom involutes. Excision may be quite hazardous because of the risk of hemorrhage and should be reserved for patients with significant associated functional or cosmetic disability. The **cystic hygroma** is a lymphangioma which most often presents in the head and neck region. These lesions may enlarge and become tender during periods of upper respiratory infection. Some cystic hygromas will involute, but not if there is a hemangiomatous component to the lesion. Complete excision of both cavernous hemangiomas and cystic hygromas is frequently impossible because of the diffuse insinuation of these lesions into local tissues without regard to tissue planes.

Answer: A–a; B–a, d; C–b, D–c

19. Which of the following techniques may be appropriately used in the management of major scalp and/or calvarium defects?

A. Rotation flap utilizing adjacent scalp
B. Allowing intact dura to form granulation tissue, then applying split-thickness skin graft
C. Free microvascular transfer of omentum or muscle followed by skin graft
D. Allowing rib grafts into a calvarium defect to granulate, then placing a split-thickness skin graft

Schwartz: 2135

Comments: Providing soft tissue covering over an intact calvarium may be achieved in many ways, including rotation or advancement flaps of adjacent scalp and the placement of split-thickness skin graft over periosteum. If there is an associated calvarium defect but the dura is intact, skin grafting over dura is possible, although rigid protection of the underlying brain is obviously not achieved. In large calvarial defects, reconstruction with transplanted autologous bone or synthetic material to provide rigid protection to the brain may be necessary. This should be delayed, however, until adequate soft tissues are available for coverage. This may necessitate a temporary rotation flap or skin graft prior to the calvarial reconstruction. Free microvascular transfers of omentum or muscle have been utilized quite successfully in the reconstruction of large scalp and calvarial defects.

Answer: A, B, C

20. Which of the following statements is/are true regarding reconstructive surgery in the periorbital area?

A. Loss of up to one fourth of either eyelid may be closed primarily
B. Large upper eyelid defects may be closed utilizing composite tissue from the lower eyelid
C. The eyebrow may be reconstructed utilizing a free flap of hair-bearing scalp
D. Surgical repair of eyelid ptosis should be avoided, as this will result in fixation of the upper lid in an open position, putting the cornea at risk for exposure keratitis

Schwartz: 2136

Comments: Of the two eyelids, the upper is clearly the more important, as it serves as the principal protector of the eye and specifically the cornea. The tissues of the periorbital area are sufficiently lax that defects of up to one fourth of the transverse dimension of the upper or lower lid may be closed primarily. Large defects of the upper lid may be closed utilizing a composite graft from the lower lid, with the lower lid then reconstructed utilizing adjacent tissues from the cheek. Following traumatic loss the eyebrow may be reconstructed utilizing a free graft of hair-bearing scalp. An island pedicle graft of hair-bearing scalp may also be utilized for this purpose.

Ptosis, or drooping of the upper eyelid, may be caused by injury to the third cranial nerve or the cervical sympathetic chain. Correction of this defect may be successfully achieved by resection of a portion of the levator complex or by fascial suspension of the lid to the frontalis muscle. The ability to close the lids, and thereby protect the eye, is preserved as this function is achieved by the orbicularis oculi muscle, which is innervated by the seventh cranial nerve.

Answer: A, B, C

21. Which of the following statements is/are correct regarding reconstruction of nose and lip defects?

A. A composite graft of cartilage and skin from the ear for nasal alar reconstruction should not be employed because of the high risk of graft necrosis
B. Full-thickness skin graft is an appropriate form of reconstruction for soft tissue loss at the tip of the nose
C. A forehead rotation flap is useful for reconstruction of major nasal defects
D. The most important step cosmetically in the primary closure of a lip defect is the proper apposition of the vermilion border

Schwartz: 2136

Comments: Reconstruction of minor soft tissue defects of the nose (e.g., following excision of a superficial basal cell carcinoma) may be achieved by a split-thickness or full-thickness skin graft or rotation of a nasolabial flap. When there is loss of cartilage, as may occur at the nasal ala, a composite graft of skin and cartilage taken from the ear has resulted in an excellent reconstruction. Major nasal losses require a bone graft for framework as well as provision of internal and external soft tissue lining. This can be achieved by a rotation flap from the forehead, nasolabial flaps, or a scalp flap. Defects of the lip can usually be closed primarily unless they involve more than one third of the length of the lip or are in close approximation to the commissure. The most important aspect cosmetically of primary closure of a lip defect is proper apposition of the vermilion border. Even a slight "step-off" of vermilion apposition will be noticeable. Large lip defects or those near the commissure require rotation flaps from the opposite lip and advancement of buccal mucosa.

Answer: B, C, D

22. Which one or more of the following would be an indication for operation in a patient with a blowout fracture of the orbit?

A. Mechanical entrapment of the extraocular muscles
B. Significant enophthalmos
C. A large fracture seen on x-ray
D. Numbness of the cheek on the involved side

Schwartz: 2143

Comments: A direct blow to the anterior face can significantly increase the pressure within the orbit, causing a "blowout" of the orbital floor. Temporary or permanent injury to the infraorbital nerve may occur as a result, but this alone would not serve as an indication for surgery. Displacement of the globe usually results in enophthalmos or mechanical entrapment of the muscles (usually inferior rectus) and produces double vision or restriction of extraocular motion. These problems would all warrant exploration and repair of the fractures, as would a large fracture seen on x-ray. Repair is usually achieved via dissection of the orbital contents deep to the periosteum and return of the herniated tissue into the orbit. The bony fragments are usually stable after anatomic reduction. If not, a thin bone graft or a Silastic sheet may be employed to reinforce the floor of the orbit.

Answer: A, B, C

This book is dedicated to

    A. Kathryn
    B. Ann
    C. Mary
    D. Linda
    E. All of the above

Comment: Our appreciation is beyond measure.

Answer: E

SE, SB, DD, TW